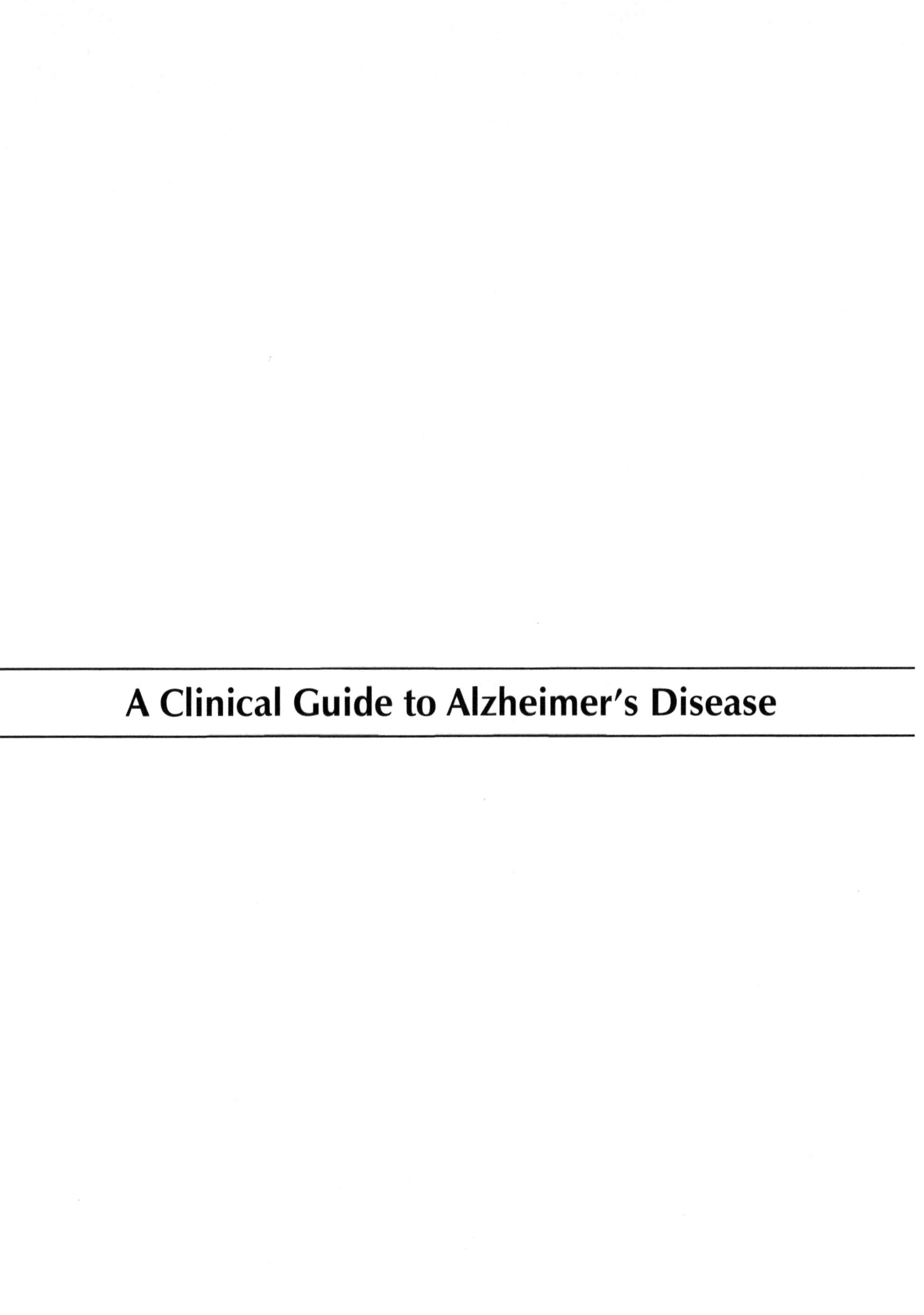

A Clinical Guide to Alzheimer's Disease

A Clinical Guide to Alzheimer's Disease

Editor: Trevor Cornfield

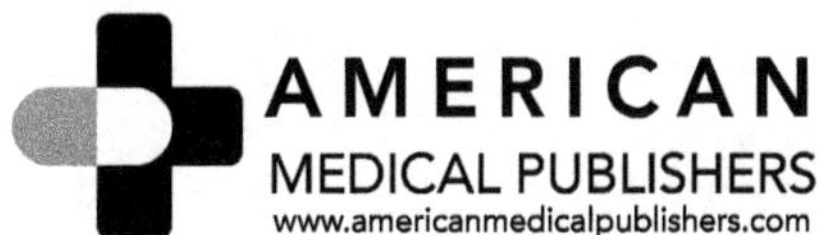

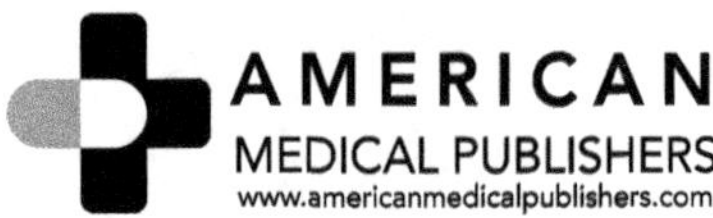

Cataloging-in-Publication Data

A clinical guide to Alzheimer's disease / edited by Trevor Cornfield.
p. cm.
Includes bibliographical references and index.
ISBN 978-1-63927-835-0
1. Alzheimer's disease. 2. Alzheimer's disease--Treatment.
3. Alzheimer's disease--Diagnosis. I. Cornfield, Trevor.
RC523 .C55 2023
616.831--dc23

American Medical Publishers,
41 Flatbush Avenue,
1st Floor, New York,
NY 11217, USA

ISBN 978-1-63927-835-0 (Hardback)

Contents

Preface

Alzheimer's disease (AD) refers to a type of neurodegenerative disease that typically begins slowly and worsens over time. The most usual symptom is trouble remembering recent events. Various other symptoms can also occur with the progression of the disease, such as loss of motivation, behavioral issues, mood swings, problems with language, self-neglect and disorientation. As the health of the patient deteriorates, they frequently withdraw from society and family. There are numerous environmental and genetic risk factors that contribute to the development of this disease. An allele of the apolipoprotein E (APOE) is the most powerful genetic risk factor. There are several other risk factors, such as high blood pressure, a history of head injury and clinical depression. There are no treatments that can reverse or stop the development of the disease, while some can temporarily alleviate symptoms. This book aims to understand the clinical perspectives of Alzheimer's disease. It aims to shed light on some of the unexplored aspects of this disease. Those with an interest in this field would find this book helpful.

All of the data presented henceforth, was collaborated in the wake of recent advancements in the field. The aim of this book is to present the diversified developments from across the globe in a comprehensible manner. The opinions expressed in each chapter belong solely to the contributing authors. Their interpretations of the topics are the integral part of this book, which I have carefully compiled for a better understanding of the readers.

At the end, I would like to thank all those who dedicated their time and efforts for the successful completion of this book. I also wish to convey my gratitude towards my friends and family who supported me at every step.

Editor

1

Auditory Memory Decay as Reflected by a New Mismatch Negativity Score is Associated with Episodic Memory in Older Adults at Risk of Dementia

Daria Laptinskaya[1,2]*, Franka Thurm[2,3], Olivia C. Küster[1,4], Patrick Fissler[1,4], Winfried Schlee[5], Stephan Kolassa[6], Christine A. F. von Arnim[4] and Iris-Tatjana Kolassa[1,2]

[1]Clinical and Biological Psychology, Institute of Psychology and Education, Ulm University, Ulm, Germany, [2]Department of Psychology, University of Konstanz, Konstanz, Germany, [3]Faculty of Psychology, TU Dresden, Dresden, Germany, [4]Department of Neurology, Ulm University, Ulm, Germany, [5]Department for Psychiatry and Psychotherapy, University Hospital Regensburg, Regensburg, Germany, [6]SAP (Switzerland) AG, Tägerwilen, Switzerland

***Correspondence:**
Daria Laptinskaya
daria.laptinskaya@uni-ulm.de

The auditory mismatch negativity (MMN) is an event-related potential (ERP) peaking about 100–250 ms after the onset of a deviant tone in a sequence of identical (standard) tones. Depending on the interstimulus interval (ISI) between standard and deviant tones, the MMN is suitable to investigate the pre-attentive auditory discrimination ability (short ISIs, $\leq$ 2 s) as well as the pre-attentive auditory memory trace (long ISIs, $>$2 s). However, current results regarding the MMN as an index for mild cognitive impairment (MCI) and dementia are mixed, especially after short ISIs: while the majority of studies report positive associations between the MMN and cognition, others fail to find such relationships. To elucidate these so far inconsistent results, we investigated the validity of the MMN as an index for cognitive impairment exploring the associations between different MMN indices and cognitive performance, more specifically with episodic memory performance which is among the most affected cognitive domains in the course of Alzheimer's dementia (AD), at baseline and at a 5-year-follow-up. We assessed the amplitude of the MMN for short ISI (stimulus onset asynchrony, SOA = 0.05 s) and for long ISI (3 s) in a neuropsychologically well-characterized cohort of older adults at risk of dementia (subjective memory impairment, amnestic and non-amnestic MCI; n = 57). Furthermore, we created a novel difference score (ΔMMN), defined as the difference between MMNs to short and to long ISI, as a measure to assess the decay of the auditory memory trace, higher values indicating less decay. ΔMMN and MMN amplitude after long ISI, but not the MMN amplitude after short ISI, was associated with episodic memory at baseline (β = 0.38, p = 0.003; β = −0.27, p = 0.047, respectively). ΔMMN, but not the MMN for long ISIs, was positively associated with episodic memory performance at the

Abbreviations: AD, Alzheimer's dementia; aMCI, amnestic mild cognitive impairment; MCI, mild cognitive impairment; MemTra, Memory Trace; MMN, mismatch negativity; MMN–Dur, mismatch negativity after duration deviants; MMSE, Mini-Mental State Examination; MVGT, Münchner Verbaler Gedächtnistest; naMCI, non-amnestic mild cognitive impairment; NMDA, N-methyl-D-aspartate; Opt1, Optimum–1; SMI, subjective memory impairment; TMT, Trail Making Test; ΔMMN, difference score between MMNs to short and to long ISIs; ΔMMN–Dur, index for auditory memory trace decay, amplitude difference between the MMN after duration deviant in the Optimum–1 paradigm and the Memory Trace paradigm, higher values indicating less auditory memory trace decay.

5-year-follow-up ($\beta = 0.57$, $p = 0.013$). The results suggest that the MMN after long ISI might be suitable as an indicator for the decline in episodic memory and indicate ΔMMN as a potential biomarker for memory impairment in older adults at risk of dementia.

Keywords: mismatch negativity, auditory memory, cognition, episodic memory, mild cognitive impairment, subjective memory impairment, Alzheimer's disease, event-related potentials

INTRODUCTION

The global number of people aged 50 years and older is constantly increasing (e.g., Gerland et al., 2014; United Nations, 2015). Age is the major risk factor of Alzheimer's dementia (AD). Until 2050 about three million older adults will be affected by AD in Germany (Bickel, 2016) and 132 million worldwide (Prince et al., 2015). Alzheimer's pathology is characterized by amyloid-beta and tau deposition in the entorhinal cortex, hippocampus, neocortex and other brain regions (for a review see Ballard et al., 2011). Furthermore, Alzheimer's pathology is associated with deficiencies in neuronal signal transmission and neuronal death and precedes the manifestation of cognitive symptoms by many years or even decades (for a review see Bateman et al., 2012).

Mild cognitive impairment (MCI) can be a prodromal syndrome of AD and is therefore intensively studied in the context of early diagnosis of the disease. Individuals with MCI show cognitive decline in at least one cognitive domain, while overall daily functioning is still intact (Petersen, 2016). MCI is associated with an increased risk of dementia, particularly AD, compared to the general population with a conversion rate to dementia of about 8%–15% per year (Petersen, 2016). Amnestic MCI (aMCI) has a higher progression rate than non-amnestic MCI (naMCI; Petersen, 2016). Furthermore, recent research indicates that subjective memory impairment (SMI) that cannot be confirmed during objective testing is associated with an increased risk for AD up to 6 years later (Jessen et al., 2014).

Event-related potentials (ERPs) can provide further insights into neurophysiological correlates of cognitive decline and neuropathology in old age (e.g., Papaliagkas et al., 2008; Lai et al., 2010; Vecchio and Määttä, 2011; Thurm et al., 2013), with the advantages of being non-invasive and cost-efficient. One of the most widely investigated ERP components in EEG research is the mismatch negativity (MMN; Näätänen et al., 1978). The MMN is elicited when a presentation that has been automatically predicted by the central nervous system is violated (for a review see Näätänen et al., 2011), i.e., when a deviant tone is presented in a sequence of standard tones. It peaks at about 100–250 ms after the onset of the deviant (for a review see e.g., Fishman, 2014). The MMN indicates a generally pre-attentive process, but can be modulated by attention (e.g., Erickson et al., 2016). Previous studies suggest an association between MMN in a passive paradigm and the active deviant tone detection (e.g., Todd et al., 2012). Nevertheless, the MMN elucidation does not depend on the subject's active involvement and can be observed even in the fetus in the womb (e.g., Draganova et al., 2007) or in coma patients (see Morlet and Fischer, 2014 for a recent review). Because of its pre-attentive character the MMN is independent of fluctuations in vigilance and motivation which may be of special importance at long EEG recordings or in older and/or clinical populations (Näätänen et al., 2004).

Depending on the interval length between the standard and deviant tones (interstimulus interval, ISI), the MMN is suitable to determine two different, but strongly interrelated, processes. In case of a short ISI of 2 s or less (see Cheng et al., 2013), the MMN primarily reflects the detection of a mismatch between a stored auditory regularity and the current presentation of the environment and can therefore be considered as an index of the pre-attentive auditory discrimination ability (for a review see Näätänen et al., 2012). With increasing ISI, the MMN provides information on the duration of the pre-attentive auditory memory trace for the standard tone (for a review see Bartha-Doering et al., 2015). In young, healthy adults the auditory memory trace approximates 10 s (Böttcher-Gandor and Ullsperger, 1992; Sams et al., 1993; see Bartha-Doering et al., 2015 for a recent review on MMN in healthy and clinical populations).

A limited number of studies so far investigated the MMN in normal compared to pathological aging, specifically in AD, with equivocal results. While some studies report an attenuated MMN in AD for short (e.g., Schroeder et al., 1995) as well as for long ISIs (e.g., Pekkonen et al., 1994; Papadaniil et al., 2016), others failed to find MMN differences between AD and healthy controls (e.g., Kazmerski et al., 1997; Engeland et al., 2002; Brønnick et al., 2010; Hsiao et al., 2014). Studies investigating MMN in older adults with MCI are even scarcer. The majority of studies report an altered MMN in MCI in comparison to matched controls (e.g., Lindín et al., 2013; Ji et al., 2015; Papadaniil et al., 2016; but see Tsolaki et al., 2017 for contrary results). However, the results vary in MMN parameter (i.e., amplitude, latency), MMN localization (i.e., frontal, temporal), and the applied ISI length (i.e., short, long).

In sum, previous studies suggest that MMN after short as well as after long ISIs has the potential to be a biomarker for cognition, where the results for MMN after long ISIs are more consistent than for short ISIs. On the other hand, the MMN after short ISIs is the most often investigated one in AD research so far. Since the impact of pre-attentive auditory memory processes increases with ISI length, auditory memory processes seem to be an important factor that is responsible for the MMN-cognition relationship. We assumed that the difference score between MMN after short and long ISI (ΔMMN) might be a better and more reliable biomarker for cognitive (especially episodic memory) decline, compared to the simple MMN after long or short ISI, since ΔMMN takes individual differences in auditory discrimination ability as well as auditory memory into account. The difference between MMN after short and after long ISI is strongly determined by the pre-attentive maintenance of the memory trace for the standard tone. On the one hand ΔMMN would be 0 if the MMN amplitude after the short and long ISI is the same and thus the standard tone is well remembered independent of the ISI. On the other hand, the ΔMMN would become higher as the MMN amplitude attenuates as a function of the ISI. Thus, the ΔMMN could constitute a biomarker for automatic auditory memory decay, which in turn seems to be the key index for cognitive decline.

The main aim of the present study was to evaluate the validity of pre-attentive auditory memory decay as well as the MMN after short and long ISI as biomarkers for cognitive decline in an at risk population for AD (i.e., aMCI, naMCI, SMI). MMN after short ISI was assessed using the Optimum-1 (Opt1, stimulus onset asynchrony [SOA] = 0.5 s) paradigm (see Näätänen et al., 2004), whereas the MMN after long ISI (3 s) was investigated using the Memory Trace (MemTra) paradigm (in accordance with Grau et al., 1998). Pre-attentive memory trace decay was assessed by the difference score between the MMN after short and long ISIs (ΔMMN).

We hypothesized that pre-attentive auditory memory decay, reflected by the ΔMMN at baseline, is positively associated with episodic memory performance assessed at baseline as well as episodic memory 5 years later (5-year-follow-up). Further, we expected a smaller MMN in the MemTra paradigm in comparison to the Opt1 paradigm and a more pronounced decay of the pre-attentive auditory memory trace in aMCI compared to naMCI/SMI subjects.

MATERIALS AND METHODS

Participants

The inclusion and exclusion criteria for study participation have previously been described in detail (Küster et al., 2016). In brief, subjects were recruited in the Memory Clinic of the University Hospital Ulm, Germany and the Center for Psychiatry Reichenau, Germany or via public advertisements. Inclusion criteria were: 55 years of age or older, fluency in the German language, subjective memory complaints or MCI, stable antidementive and/or antidepressive medication, normal or adjusted-to-normal hearing, and independent living. Exclusion criteria were: probable moderate or severe dementia (Mini-Mental State Examination, MMSE [Folstein et al., 1975] < 20), a history of other neurological or psychiatric disorders, except mild to moderate depression). Depressive symptoms were assessed with the 15-item short version of the Geriatric Depression Scale (Yesavage et al., 1983). Participants without contraindication were offered structural magnetic resonance imaging (MRI) to exclude other brain abnormalities such as major strokes and brain tumors.

SMI was assessed with the question "Do you feel like your memory is getting worse?" (according to Geerlings et al., 1999; Jessen et al., 2010). The evaluation of objective cognitive impairment was based on encoding (sum of words of the five learning trials) and long-delay free recall scores of the adapted German version of the California Verbal Learning Test (German: Münchner Verbaler Gedächtnistest [MVGT, Munich Vebal Memory Test]; Ilmberger, 1988) for memory functions. For non-memory cognitive functions the following subtests from the Consortium to Establish a Registry for Alzheimer's Disease–plus (Welsh et al., 1994) were used: Trail Making Test (TMT) part A and B, phonematic and semantic word fluency, and Boston Naming Test. Objective cognitive impairment was defined as 1.0 *SD* below the age- and education-adjusted norm; aMCI was assigned if at least one of the memory tests was below average; naMCI was assigned if performance in the memory tests was average while one of the test scores of the other cognitive domains was below average. Subjects with severe objective impairment (≤ 2 *SD* below the norm) in memory and non-memory, indicating probable dementia, were excluded from further analysis ($n = 6$), even if they reached the critical MMSE score ≥ 20.

From altogether 122 subjects who were screened for eligibility, 59 met the inclusion criteria. For 14 participants no MRI scan was available. No participant had to be excluded because of abnormalities in the MRI scan. According to the classification criteria 16 subjects were classified as SMI, 19 as naMCI and 24 as aMCI. Demographic and cognitive characteristics of the groups are listed in **Table 1**. Groups did not differ with regard to distribution of gender or crystallized (premorbid) intelligence as indicated by a Verbal Knowledge Test (German: Wortschatztest; Schmidt and Metzler, 1992; all $ps > 0.05$). However, aMCI subjects showed lower education ($p = 0.041$) and tended to be older than naMCI and SMI which was, however, not significant ($p = 0.098$).

Procedure

The study was approved by the ethics committees of both study centers, University of Konstanz and Ulm University, Germany. The study was part of a controlled clinical trial investigating the effect of physical exercise and cognitive training on cognition as well as on biological and electrophysiological parameters (Küster et al., 2016, 2017; Fissler et al., 2017). All participants provided written informed consent in accordance with the Declaration of Helsinki prior to study participation. The neuropsychological assessment and the EEG examination were carried out by intensively trained assessors (i.e., doctorial and psychology students). Both MMN paradigms were carried out at the same session. Prior to the beginning of the EEG recordings, individual hearing thresholds were assessed using in-house software PyTuneSounds (Hartmann, 2009).

Five years ($M = 5.23$, $SD = 0.19$) after baseline assessment, a telephone interview-based follow-up was obtained for participants of the Konstanz sample. Out of the 32 potential follow-up participants, 28 subjects could be contacted again, five subjects refused participation and another two subjects had to be excluded since they were no longer able to attend the telephone interview due to severe progression of cognitive and functional decline. As a result, 21 complete data sets were available for follow-up analysis with four subjects classified as SMI, 11 as naMCI and six as aMCI at the baseline assessment.

TABLE 1 | Demographic and cognitive data within groups.

Variable	Group values			aMCI vs. naMCI/SMI	
	SMI (n = 14)	naMCI (n = 19)	aMCI (n = 24)	$F_{(1,55)}$	p
Age (y.)	71.9 ± 5.4	68.1 ± 6.1	72.5 ± 6.2	2.83	0.098
Education (y.)	11.1 ± 1.9	10.5 ± 1.8	9.7 ± 1.8	4.37[a]	0.041
WST (z)	1.1 ± 0.8	0.6 ± 0.9	0.6 ± 0.7	0.89	0.349
MMSE (0–30)	28.9 ± 0.9	28.7 ± 1.2	27.5 ± 1.8	10.46	0.002
Episodic memory (cs)	0.6 ± 0.4	0.6 ± 0.7	−0.8 ± 0.5	92.15	<0.001
Attention/EF (cs)	0.6 ± 0.8	−0.1 ± 0.9	−0.3 ± 0.9	4.96	0.030
ADAS free rec. (0–10, error rate)	4.1 ± 1.4	4.8 ± 1.8	5.7 ± 1.4	8.29	0.006
Digit span (0–28)	15.0 ± 3.6	14.4 ± 3.6	13.6 ± 2.5	1.52	0.223
ECB (0–28)	14.7 ± 4.6	16.0 ± 5.0	10.9 ± 5.4	10.20[b]	0.002
MVGT enc. (0–80)	50.5 ± 5.4	52.4 ± 8.1	36.2 ± 5.1	81.57	<0.001
MVGT rec. (0–16)	10.9 ± 2.3	11.0 ± 2.5	4.6 ± 2.8	84.11[a]	<0.001
TMT A (s)	38.0 ± 8.4	53.8 ± 14.7	54.0 ± 19.7	2.32	0.134
TMT B (s)	92.2 ± 22.0	121.3 ± 46.2	129.8 ± 48.5	3.14	0.082
Word fluency (w.)	40.1 ± 7.8	31.3 ± 6.7	32.0 ± 7.8	1.65[a]	0.204

Values are means (M) ± standard deviations (SD). aMCI, amnestic MCI; naMCI, non-amnestic MCI; SMI, subjective memory impairment; WST, Wortschatztest [Verbal Knowledge Test]; MMSE, Mini-Mental State Examination; ADAS free rec., Alzheimer's Diseases Assessment Scale–free recall; Digit span, total value from the forward and backward part; ECB, Everyday Cognition Battery–computation span; MVGT enc., Münchner Verbaler Gedächtnistest [Munich Verbal Memory Test]–encoding (sum of words of the five learning trials); MVGT rec., Münchner Verbaler Gedächtnistest [Munich Verbal Memory Test]–long-delay free recall; TMT, Trail Making Test; Word fluency, total value of the episodic and phonemic word fluency; EF, executive functions; y., years; cs, composite score; w., words. Distribution of gender–aMCI vs. naMCI/SMI: $\chi^2_{(1)} = 3.18$, $p = 0.074$. $^aF_{(1,54)}$; $^bF_{(1,50)}$.

Because of the limited neuropsychological assessment no renewed classification was carried out at the 5-year-follow-up. All participants were asked if they had received an AD diagnosis during the past 5 years, which was not the case for the final $n = 21$.

Neuropsychological Assessment

All participants completed the following assessments: the Alzheimer's Disease Assessment Scale–cognitive subscale (Ihl and Weyer, 1993), phonemic and semantic word fluency as well as TMT part A and B of the Consortium to Establish a Registry for Alzheimer's Disease–plus test battery, the subtests digit span and digit-symbol coding of the Wechsler Adult Intelligence Scale (Tewes, 1991), and the MVGT. Additionally, everyday cognition in an ecologically valid task was assessed using the working-memory subtest of the Everyday Cognition Battery (Allaire and Marsiske, 1999). Crystallized abilities were assessed using the Verbal Knowledge Test (German: Wortschatztest).

In order to assess latent cognitive function scores, a principal component analysis was performed across all participants (n = 59) to reduce multiple testing and thus α-inflation. An oblique rotation technique was chosen for the assumption of correlations between the extracted components. The following test scores were entered: MVGT encoding, MVGT free long-delay recall, free recall of the Alzheimer's Disease Assessment Scale, TMT part A and B (time in sec), Everyday Cognition Battery–computation span, digit span forward and backward (total value), digit-symbol coding, and semantic and phonemic word fluency (total value as indicator for verbal word fluency). Using the Kaiser criterion (eigenvalues $\geq$ 1.0) two components were extracted, the first one showing high loadings of episodic memory scores (MVGT encoding, MVGT long-delay free recall, and free recall of the Alzheimer's Disease Assessment Scale) and the second one showing high loadings of attention and executive functions scores (TMT part A and B, digit span, digit-symbol and verbal word fluency). All variables were z-standardized and two component scores were built, representing the weighted average of those z-standardized variables with loadings of at least a_{ij} = 0.50 on the respective component. Only the Everyday Cognition Battery–computation span did not reach the critical threshold (a_{ij} = 0.48) and was excluded from further component calculation.

For the follow-up investigation we selected tests from the baseline investigation, which were suitable for assessments via telephone (for telephone tools for cognitive assessment see e.g., Castanho et al., 2014; Duff et al., 2015), namely the MVGT, the digit span forward and backward, and the Consortium to Establish a Registry for Alzheimer's Disease–plus subtests phonemic and semantic word fluency. The composite scores were built in the same manner as at baseline using the same weights from the available variables, i.e., MVGT encoding and MVGT long-delay free recall for the memory domain score; and digit span (total value for forward and backward) and verbal word fluency (total value for phonemic and semantic word fluency) for the attention/executive domain score.

MMN Stimuli and Task Procedure

Two passive mismatch-negativity paradigms were applied: the Opt1 paradigm (see, Näätänen et al., 2004) to assess auditory discrimination ability and the newly developed MemTra paradigm (in accordance with Grau et al., 1998) to investigate auditory memory trace. The standard tone, duration and frequency deviant were further used in the MemTra paradigm (see below). The standard tone was a harmonic tone of three sinusoidal partials of 500, 1000 and 1500 Hz with the second partial being 3 dB and the third being 6 dB lower in intensity then the first partial. The standard tone was 75 ms in duration including 5 ms rise and fall times. In comparison to the standard tone, the duration deviant was 50 ms shorter and the gap deviant comprised a 7 ms silent gap (including 1 ms fall and rise times) in the middle of the tone. One half of all frequency deviants were 10% higher (partials: 550, 1100, 1650 Hz) and the other half 10% lower in frequency than the standard tone (partials: 450, 900, 1350 Hz). Intensity deviants were 10 dB louder or lower than the standard tone (50% each). The location deviants had an interaural time difference of 800 μs to the left or to the right ear (50% each).

Optimum–1 Paradigm

In the Opt1 paradigm (Näätänen et al., 2004; **Figure 1**) a total number of 1845 auditory stimuli were presented in three blocks of 5 min each. Every second tone was a standard tone, resulting in a probability of 50% for standard and deviant stimuli and a probability of 10% for each deviant type. A sequence of 15 standard tones was presented at the beginning of each block to allow the formation of the standard tone as such. Stimuli were presented with a constant SOA of 0.5 s. Thus, the Opt1 paradigm is suitable to investigate the MMN after short ISI for five deviant types in a very short administration time.

Memory Trace Paradigm

The MemTra paradigm (Grau et al., 1998; **Figure 1**) was developed to investigate the effect of longer ISIs on the MMN-related memory trace. The paradigm presented 462 auditory stimuli within three blocks of 6 min each. As in the Opt1 paradigm, 15 standard tones were presented consecutively at the beginning of each block. Duration and frequency deviants were presented with one to three standard tones between two deviants. The ISI between standard tone and consecutive deviant was constantly 3 s. The number of standard stimuli between the deviants and the ISI (0.5 s, 1.5 s and 3 s) between standard tones were assigned pseudorandomly. Standard stimuli were presented with 66.2% probability; deviants (duration, frequency) with the probability of 16.9% each. Only MMNs elicited to deviants following a standard tone (ISI = 3 s) were included into MMN analysis.

EEG Recording

EEG was recorded using a high-density 256-channel HydroGel^{TM} Geodesic Sensor Net (HCGSN; Electrical Geodesics, Inc., Eugene, OR, USA) with Cz (vertex) as reference during data acquisition. Continuous data were sampled with 1000 Hz and hardware filters were set to 0.1 Hz high-pass and 100 Hz low-pass. After recording, the data were imported into MATLAB (version 2015b; The MathWorks, 2015) and preprocessed using the FieldTrip toolbox (version 20151012; Oostenveld et al., 2011). During EEG recordings, participants were sitting comfortably in an electrically shielded and sound-attenuated room watching silent Charlie Chaplin videos. All auditory stimuli were presented binaurally through stereo headphones with 50 dB above the individual hearing threshold. All participants were instructed to watch the video carefully and not to pay attention to the delivered tones. The paradigm order was counter-balanced between subjects.

MMN Analysis

For both the Opt1 and the MemTra paradigm, EEG data were band-pass filtered in the range of 1–35 Hz (24 dB/octave) and noisy channels were interpolated using the average method before rereferencing the data to the linked mastoids. Continuous data were further down-sampled to 250 Hz, segmented into epochs starting 100 ms before and ending 350 ms after stimulus onset and baseline-corrected (100-ms pre-stimulus time window). After manually rejecting artifact contaminated epochs, the remaining epochs were averaged for the standard tone and for each deviant type separately. On average, no more than 20% of the trials were excluded. Consequently, the following number of trials was left for averaging in the Opt1 paradigm (values are means ± standard deviations): 753 ± 53 for the standard stimulus, 152 ± 11 for the duration deviant, 151 ± 11 for the frequency deviant, 150 ± 11 for the intensity deviant, 150 ± 11 for the location deviant, and 149 ± 13 for the gap deviant. In the MemTra paradigm the reaction to standard stimulus was averaged over 83 ± 6 trials, for the duration deviant over 65 ± 5 trials, and for the frequency deviant over 65 ± 5 trials. Difference

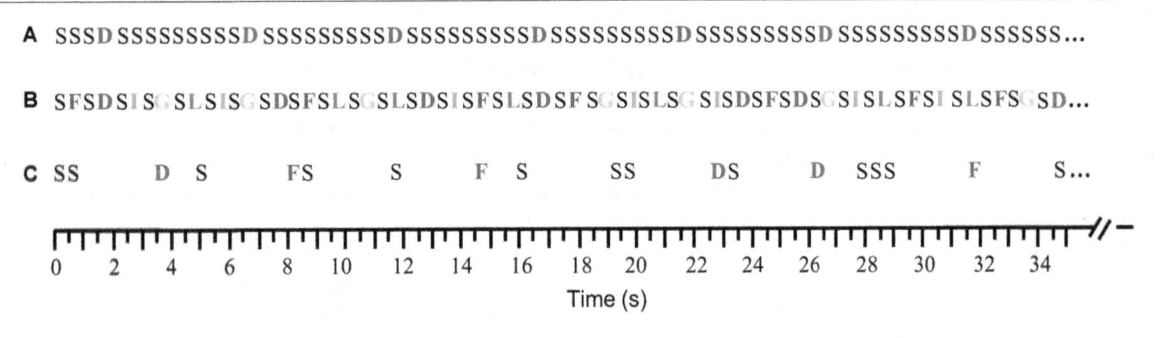

FIGURE 1 | Schematic illustration of the auditory paradigms, compared to the traditional oddball paradigm, which was not used in the study. **(A)** Traditional oddball paradigm (SOA = 0.5 s), **(B)** Optimum–1 (Opt–1) paradigm (SOA = 0.5 s), and **(C)** Memory Trace (MemTra) paradigm (ISI = 0.5, 1.5, and 3 s; $ISI_{standard\text{-}deviant}$ = 3 s).

waveforms between the ERPs to the standard and to the deviant stimuli were carried out for each paradigm and deviant type, respectively. The MMN search window was determined within 100–250 ms, corresponding to previous studies on older adults with MCI (see Mowszowski et al., 2012, 2014; Ji et al., 2015). The MMN amplitude was defined as the mean voltage in a 40 ms time window centered at the peak of the grand-average waveform of each group (SMI, aMCI and naMCI). The MMN latency was defined at the most negative peak within the MMN search window after deviant onset (100–250 ms for frequency, intensity, and location deviants; 125–275 for duration deviant, and 134–284 ms for gap deviant). As the largest MMN is often assessed at fronto-central EEG electrodes and the averaging of electrodes with similar activity has been demonstrated to show more reliable results than the measure of single separate electrodes (Huffmeijer et al., 2014), the average voltage at FCz, Fz, and Cz was computed as mean MMN amplitude for all further analyses. The mean MMN latency was computed accordingly.

In two subjects (both SMI) the MMN amplitude extracted from the difference between standard and deviant tone showed a value above mean (−0.68 for duration and −0.17 frequency deviant) + 1.5 × interquartile range and >2 μV for both deviant types (duration and frequency) in the MemTra paradigm. Because of this abnormally high positive value (the difference score should be negative or around zero), we assumed that the paradigm did not work for them properly. To avoid any inaccuracies we excluded their datasets from all further analyses.

Statistical Analyses

All statistical analyses were performed using R (version 3.2.3; R Core Team, 2016) in RStudio (RStudio Team, 2015). Statistical analyses of the baseline sample were performed with 57 subjects (24 classified as aMCI, 19 as naMCI and 14 as SMI). For one SMI subject only data for the Opt1 paradigm and for one aMCI subject only the MemTra paradigm data were available. All contrasts for group comparisons were set to aMCI vs. naMCI/SMI. Since all model residuals were normally distributed, parametric tests were applied for group comparisons. Comparisons for age, years of education, and cognitive function were conducted with univariate analysis of variance (ANOVA) models. Group differences in gender distribution were assessed by Pearson's Chi-square (χ^2)-test.

As a first step of the statistical ERP analysis, one-tailed *t*-tests for dependent samples for normally distributed data and Wilcoxon signed-rank tests for non-normally distributed data were conducted to determine whether mean MMN amplitudes significantly differed from zero within groups. Second, since both MMN paradigms applied a different number of deviants (five in the Opt1 and two in the MemTra paradigm), we explored differences in mean MMN amplitudes and latencies depending on group and deviant type for each paradigm separately.

The statistical models were carried out as follows: (1) for the MMN after short ISI (i.e., Opt1 paradigm) we conducted Group (aMCI vs. naMCI/SMI) × Deviant Type (duration, frequency, intensity, location, gap) linear mixed effect models with Subject as random intercept (lme4 package in R version 1.1-12; Bates et al., 2015) separately for mean MMN amplitude and mean MMN latency as dependent variable. (2) For the MMN after long ISI, statistical analyses focused only on the duration deviant, since there was no significant MMN component elicited by the frequency deviant in the MemTra paradigm. In order to investigate differences in the mean MMN amplitude for the duration deviant between paradigms (and thus ISIs), we carried out a Paradigm (Opt1/SOA = 0.5 s vs. MemTra/ISI = 3 s) × Group (aMCI vs. naMCI/SMI) linear mixed effects model including Subject as random intercept. (3) Second level (*post hoc*) analyses were conducted using univariate ANOVA models and pairwise *t*-tests with Bonferroni correction for multiple comparisons (multcomp package for R version 1.4-6; Hothorn et al., 2008).

As a final step, hierarchical linear regression models were carried out to investigate associations between MMN after short ISI, MMN after long ISI and pre-attentive auditory memory trace decay (i.e., ΔMMN for the duration deviant; ΔMMN–Dur) and neuropsychological composite scores for episodic memory and attention/executive functions at baseline (n = 57) and follow-up assessment (n = 21) as dependent variables, respectively. Based on previous research indicating higher age as a risk factor and education as a protective factor for cognitive decline (e.g., Ardila et al., 2000; Cansino, 2009; Salthouse, 2009, 2012), we statistically accounted for age and education by entering them into the model first (reduced models), followed by ΔMMN–Dur and MemTra MMN after duration deviants (MemTra MMN–Dur) as predictors in two separate models (full models). To explore the effect of Opt1 MMN we entered an Opt1 MMN × Deviant Type (duration, frequency, intensity, location, gap) term into the model instead of calculating models for each deviant type separately which would increase multiple testing and thus α-inflation. Using ANOVA, the full regression models were then compared to the reduced regression models without MMN indices as additional predictor. Collinearity between predictors was examined by computing the variance inflation factor (VIF) for each predictor's beta score and for the mean beta score as well as the VIF tolerance score (1/VIF). Individual VIF scores > 10, a mean VIF score > 1, and a VIF tolerance score < 0.1 indicated beta score inflation by collinearity in the models (Bowerman and O'Connell, 1990; Myers, 1990; Menard, 1995). For illustration purposes significant associations between auditory memory and cognition are depicted as Pearson's product-moment correlation coefficients (r).

Normal distribution of all models' residuals was confirmed using the Shapiro-Wilk test (W statistic) and visual inspection (Q-Q plots). The statistical significance level (α) was set to 0.05 for all analyses.

The stability of significant associations between MMN indices and cognition was evaluated by the inclusion of the participants who were excluded before because of probable AD (see section "Participants").

RESULTS

ERP Analysis of the MMN

In order to examine whether all deviants elicited a MMN, one-tailed t-tests for dependent samples for normally distributed variables and Wilcoxon signed-rank tests for non-normally distributed data were conducted. **Figure 2** shows the difference waveforms for the Opt1 and MemTra paradigm, respectively. The mean MMN difference waveform in the Opt1 condition significantly differed from zero for all deviant types in all groups (see Supplementary Table S1). In the MemTra paradigm only the difference waveform for the duration deviant significantly differed from zero in all groups (see Supplementary Table S1). Therefore, all further statistical analyses regarding the MemTra paradigm were restricted to the duration deviant (MMN–Dur).

Group Differences between MMN Parameters

MMN after Short ISI

Analysis of the MMN after short ISI focused on the Opt1 paradigm and was conducted with linear mixed-effects models. The mixed-effects models with Group (aMCI vs. naMCI/SMI) as between-subject factor and Deviant Type (duration, frequency, intensity, location, gap) as within-subject factor showed a main effect of Deviant Type for both the mean MMN amplitude, $F_{(4,216)} = 11.65, p < 0.001$, and the mean MMN latency, $F_{(4,216)} = 14.49, p < 0.001$. Mean MMN amplitudes were largest for the duration deviant ($ps \leq 0.029$) and mean MMN latencies were shortest for the duration and gap deviants ($ps \leq 0.131$; $ps \leq 0.002$, respectively).

Neither a main effect of Group nor a Group × Deviant Type interaction was found in both models (amplitude and latency; see **Table 2** for MMN amplitudes and latencies for each group and see Supplementary Table S2 for pairwise comparison of the deviant types).

MMN after Long ISI and ISI Duration Effect

Comparing the MMN amplitudes for the duration deviant between both paradigms, a mixed-effects model of Paradigm (Opt1 vs. MemTra) as within-subject factor × Group (aMCI vs. naMCI/SMI) as between-subject factor revealed a main effect of Paradigm, $F_{(1,55)} = 61.88$, $p < 0.001$, indicating smaller mean MMN–Dur amplitudes in the MemTra compared to the Opt1 paradigm (**Figure 3**), i.e., a stronger pre-attentive auditory memory decay in the long ISI condition. Subjects with aMCI showed a more pronounced pre-attentive auditory memory decay in comparison to naMCI and SMI, even though the Paradigm × Group interaction was only significant at a trend level, $F_{(1,55)} = 3.21$, $p = 0.079$ (see also **Table 2**). No main effect or interaction was found for the mean MMN–Dur latency.

Associations between the MMN Parameters and Baseline Cognition

To investigate the associations between baseline MMN indices and baseline cognitive performance, linear hierarchical regression models were conducted across groups. The models were carried out separately for the episodic memory and the attention/executive functions composite scores as dependent variables, including age and education at baseline (reduced models) and additionally ΔMMN–Dur, MemTra MMN–Dur, or Opt1 MMN × Deviant Type term as predictors (full models; see **Table 3**). In the reduced models, age, but not education was a significant predictor of both episodic memory, $\beta = -0.38$, $t_{(50)} = -2.94$, $p = 0.005$, and attention/executive functions, $\beta = -0.41$, $t_{(50)} = -3.30$, $p = 0.002$, at baseline assessment; indicating worse performance in older participants. According to our hypothesis adding ΔMMN–Dur as predictor to the reduced model explained an additional 14% of the variance in the episodic memory score, $F_{(49,1)} = 10.16$, $p = 0.002$; $\beta_{\Delta MMN\text{–}Dur} = 0.38$, $t_{(49)} = 3.19$, $p = 0.002$ (see also **Figure 4** for correlative association). MemTra MMN–Dur

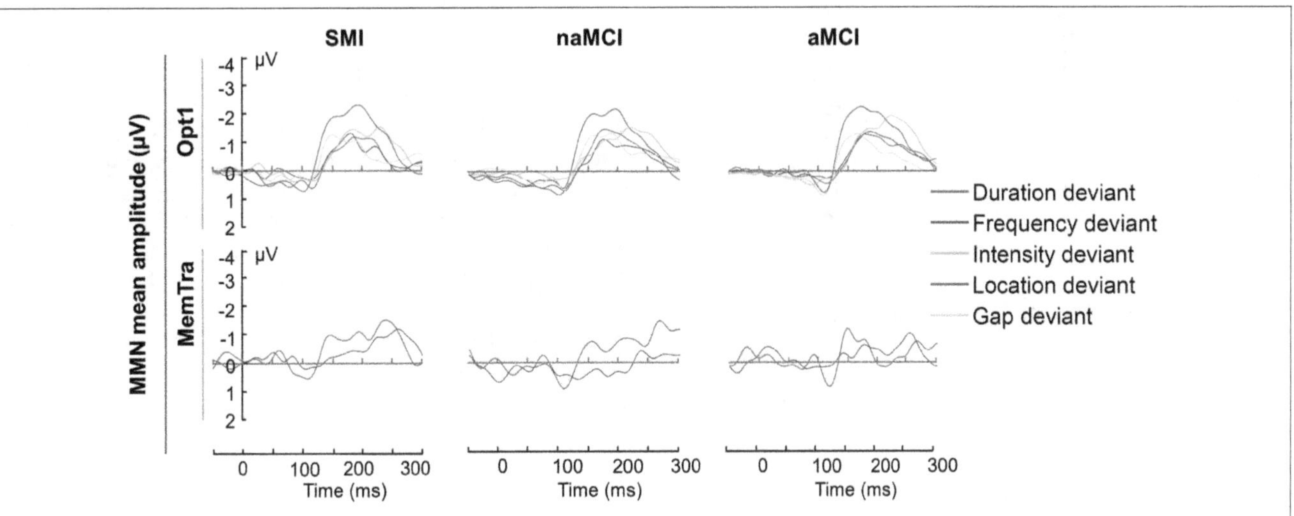

FIGURE 2 | Mean MMN amplitudes for the Opt1 paradigm and MemTra paradigm within groups. Mean values are the averaged signal of the fronto-central electrodes Fz, FCz, and Cz. Opt1, Optimum-1; MemTra, Memory Trace; aMCI, amnestic MCI; naMCI, non-amnestic MCI; SMI, subjective memory impairment.

TABLE 2 | Mean MMN amplitudes and latencies within groups.

MMN parameter	Group values			aMCI vs. naMCI/SMI	
	SMI	naMCI	aMCI	$F_{(1,54)}$	p
		Amplitudes			
Opt–Dur	−2.2 ± 1.1	−2.1 ± 1.2	−2.1 ± 1.1	0.01	0.910
Opt–Freq	−1.1 ± 0.7	−1.1 ± 1.0	−1.3 ± 1.0	1.02	0.317
Opt–Intens	−1.4 ± 1.0	−1.4 ± 1.3	−1.9 ± 1.4	1.76	0.191
Opt–Loc	−1.1 ± 0.8	−1.4 ± 1.6	−1.2 ± 1.1	0.01	0.935
Opt–Gap	−1.1 ± 1.3	−1.2 ± 1.0	−1.2 ± 1.0	0.02	0.880
MemTra–Dur	−1.1 ± 1.2	−1.0 ± 1.4	−0.5 ± 1.2	3.06	0.086
ΔMMN–Dur	−1.0 ± 1.3	−1.1 ± 1.4	−1.7 ± 1.2	3.03[a]	0.087
		Latencies			
Opt–Dur	183.5 ± 23.5	184.5 ± 21.2	190.4 ± 29.8	0.74	0.394
Opt–Freq	191.7 ± 20.5	198.7 ± 21.7	199.0 ± 26.4	0.21	0.651
Opt–Intens	213.0 ± 23.9	208.5 ± 25.4	210.5 ± 29.7	0.50	0.483
Opt–Loc	195.0 ± 28.7	200.4 ± 27.7	199.6 ± 27.4	0.01	0.940
Opt–Gap	174.2 ± 20.6	184.9 ± 24.2	177.2 ± 28.0	0.01	0.913
MemTra–Dur	203.7 ± 34.1	184.4 ± 31.3	187.3 ± 31.9	1.92	0.172

aMCI, amnestic MCI; naMCI, non-amnestic MCI; SMI, subjective memory impairment; Opt–Dur, MMN after duration deviants in the Optimum–1 paradigm; Opt–Freq, MMN after frequency deviants in the Optimum–1 paradigm; Opt–Intens, MMN after intensity deviants in the Optimum–1 paradigm; Opt–Loc, MMN after location deviants in the Optimum–1 paradigm; Opt–Gap, MMN after gap deviants in the Optimum–1 paradigm; MemTra–Dur, MMN after duration deviants in the Memory Trace paradigm; ΔMMN–Dur, difference score between MMN amplitude after duration deviant in the Optimum–1 paradigm and the Memory Trace paradigm, higher values indicating less auditory memory trace decay. [a]$F_{(1,53)}$.

as predictor explained an additional 7% of the variance in the episodic memory score, $F_{(50,1)} = 4.14$, $p = 0.047$; $\beta_{MemTraMMN\text{-}Dur} = -0.27$, $t_{(50)} = -2.04$, $p = 0.047$. There was no additive effect in predicting individual differences in the attention/executive functions score. No additive effect was found for the model including the Opt1 MMN × Deviant Type interaction.

Even when the analysis was repeated with $n = 6$ subjects who were excluded because of probable AD the additive effect of ΔMMN–Dur remained significant, $F_{(54,1)} = 13.93$, $p < 0.001$; $\beta_{\Delta MMN\text{-}Dur} = 0.41$, $t_{(54)} = 3.73$, $p < 0.001$.

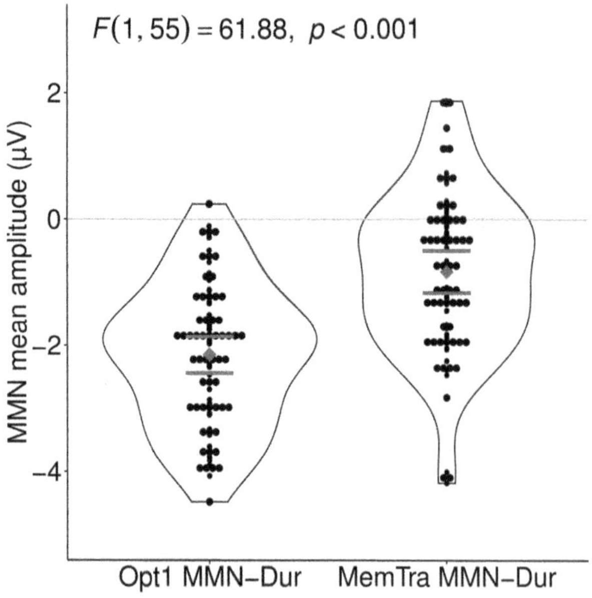

$F(1, 55) = 61.88$, $p < 0.001$

MMN mean amplitude (μV)

2
0
−2
−4

Opt1 MMN–Dur MemTra MMN–Dur

FIGURE 3 | Mean MMN after duration deviants in comparison between the Opt1 and the MemTra paradigm. Mean values build from the averaged signal of the fronto-central electrodes Fz, FCz, and Cz. The depicted F-value is accounted for Group main effect and Group × Paradigm interaction. 95% confidence intervals for the average MMN amplitude are shown as horizontal bars, red dot representing the mean value. Opt1, Optimum–1; MemTra, Memory Trace; MMN Opt–Dur, MMN after duration deviants in the Optimum–1 paradigm; MMN Memtra–Dur, MMN after duration deviants in the Memory Trace paradigm.

Associations between MMN Parameters and Cognition at the 5-Year-Follow-up

To investigate the prognostic effect of baseline auditory memory on cognition, linear hierarchical regression models were carried out across groups, separately for the episodic memory and the attention/executive functions composite score assessed 5 years later (see **Table 4**). In the reduced models including only age and education at baseline as predictors, neither age nor education was a significant predictor for episodic memory or attention/executive functions at the 5-year follow-up. Corroborating our hypothesis, including ΔMMN–Dur as additional predictor explained an additional 36% of the variance in the episodic memory (but not in the attention/executive functions) composite score compared to age and education entered alone, $F_{(16,1)} = 7.91$, $p = 0.013$; $\beta_{\Delta MMN\text{-}Dur} = 0.57$, $t_{(16)} = 2.81$, $p = 0.013$ (see also **Figure 5** for correlative association). No additive effects were found for MemTra MMN–Dur or the model including the Opt1 MMN × Deviant Type interaction. The additive effect of ΔMMN–Dur remained significant after inclusion of one subject ($n = 6$ at baseline) with probable AD, $F_{(17,1)} = 8.63$, $p = 0.009$; $\beta_{\Delta MMN\text{-}Dur} = 0.55$, $t_{(17)} = 2.94$, $p = 0.009$.

DISCUSSION

We investigated the auditory MMN after short and after long ISI as well as a novel pre-attentive auditory memory trace decay index in older adults with SMI, aMCI and naMCI as

TABLE 3 | Baseline associations between auditory memory trace decay and episodic memory as well as executive functions accounting for age and education.

	Episodic memory				Attention/EF			
Predictor	**ΔR^2**	**B**	**β**	**p**	**ΔR^2**	**B**	**β**	**p**
Model 1	0.17			0.010	0.21			0.002
Age		−0.06	−0.38	0.005		−0.07	−0.41	0.002
Education		0.08	0.17	0.187		0.12	0.23	0.073
Model 2	0.14			0.002	0.02			0.214
Age		−0.05	−0.32	0.011		−0.06	−0.39	0.003
Education		0.07	0.16	0.183		0.11	0.22	0.078
ΔMMN-Dur		0.26	0.38	0.002		0.12	0.16	0.214

EF, executive functions. ΔMMN-Dur, difference score between MMN amplitude after duration deviant in the Optimum-1 paradigm and the Memory Trace paradigm, higher values indicating less auditory memory trace decay.

an at risk population of AD. The MMN after short ISI was investigated using the Opt1 paradigm (applying short ISI), with respect to five deviants (duration, frequency, intensity, location, gap). The MMN after long ISI was investigated using the MemTra paradigm (with long ISI) with respect to two different auditory deviant types (duration, frequency). Pre-attentive auditory memory trace decay was assessed by the difference score between the MMN after short and long ISI (ΔMMN). In line with the majority of studies (Verleger et al., 1992; Kazmerski et al., 1997; Gaeta et al., 1999; Brønnick et al., 2010; Cheng et al., 2012; Hsiao et al., 2014), we found no group differences in MMN after short ISI (see Pekkonen et al., 1994; Ruzzoli et al., 2016; but see also Engeland et al., 2002 for contrary results) suggesting preserved pre-attentive auditory encoding in MCI (aMCI and naMCI) in comparison to SMI. As a proof of concept, all groups showed an attenuated MMN in the MemTra (ISI = 3 s) in comparison to the Opt1 paradigm (SOA = 0.5 s) for the duration deviant.

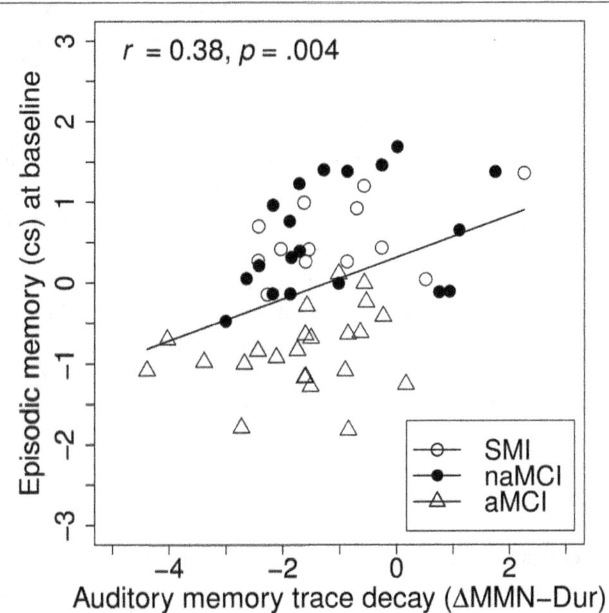

FIGURE 4 | Baseline associations between auditory memory decay and episodic memory. Auditory memory reflected by the difference score between MMN amplitude after duration deviant in the Opt1 paradigm and the MemTra paradigm (ΔMMN-Dur), higher scores indicating less auditory memory trace decay. Opt1, Optimum-1; MemTra, Memory Trace, cs, composite score.

In line with our main hypothesis, the ΔMMN-Dur (indicative of the pre-attentive auditory memory trace decay for the duration deviant) was positively associated with episodic memory performance across groups at baseline and 5 years later even after accounting for age and education. In contrast, no such relation was found for attention/executive functions, which is in line with previous work by Ruzzoli et al. (2012). The authors investigated the MMN for duration deviants in an auditory oddball paradigm with 4 s ISI in a healthy adult sample aged 21–60 years. In this, the frontal MMN for duration deviants was positively correlated with memory performance but not with executive functions. Foster et al. (2013) reported a positive association between MMN employing different ISIs as standard and deviants and verbal memory assessed with the Rey Auditory Verbal Learning Test in older healthy adults.

TABLE 4 | Associations between baseline auditory memory trace decay and follow-up episodic memory as well as executive functions accounting for age and education.

	Episodic memory				Attention/EF			
Predictor	**ΔR^2**	**B**	**β**	**p**	**ΔR^2**	**B**	**β**	**p**
Model 1	0.07			0.556	0.19			0.164
Age		−0.04	−0.25	0.294		−0.05	−0.39	0.090
Education		0.02	0.03	0.885		0.08	0.18	0.431
Model 2	0.31			0.013	0.01			0.592
Age		−0.03	−0.18	0.391		−0.04	−0.38	0.115
Education		0.07	0.11	0.596		0.09	0.19	0.405
ΔMMN-Dur		0.40	0.57	0.013		0.06	0.12	0.592

EF, executive functions. ΔMMN-Dur, difference score between MMN amplitude after duration deviant in the Optimum-1 paradigm and the Memory Trace paradigm, higher values indicating less auditory memory trace decay.

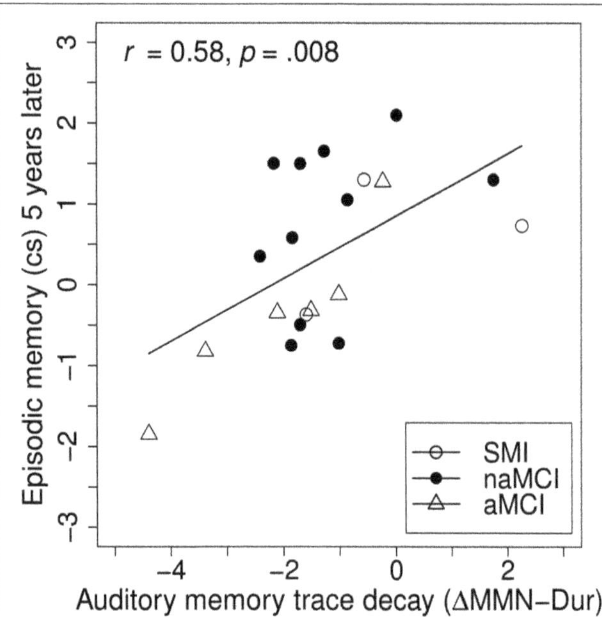

FIGURE 5 | Associations between baseline auditory memory decay and follow-up episodic memory. Auditory memory reflected by the difference score between MMN amplitude after duration deviant in the Opt1 paradigm and the MemTra paradigm (ΔMMN–Dur), higher scores indicating less auditory memory trace decay. Opt1, Optimum-1; MemTra, Memory Trace, cs, composite score.

Shared underlying neurobiological mechanisms might be responsible for the association between pre-attentive auditory memory trace decay and episodic memory. Interestingly, the pre-attentive auditory memory trace, measured with the MMN, especially after long ISIs, and episodic memory are both related to N-methyl-D-aspartate (NMDA) receptor functioning. It is well known that the NMDA receptor is highly involved in neuronal plasticity, long-term-potentiation, as well as learning and episodic memory (for a review see Newcomer et al., 2000). A distorted NMDA receptor-subunit expression and functionality has been reported for healthy older adults and in AD (Mishizen-Eberz et al., 2004; Amada et al., 2005; for a review see Magnusson et al., 2010) and is thought to be involved in age-associated cognitive impairment (for a review see Kumar, 2015). Recently, the decay in the pre-attentive auditory memory trace has also been discussed in the context of NMDA receptor modulation of plasticity, and predictive coding theory (Friston, 2005; Garrido et al., 2009; Näätänen et al., 2014), an integrative model to explain the formation of the MMN within the fronto-temporal network (Friston, 2005; Baldeweg, 2006). Predictive coding considers neuronal activity as a reflection of matches or mismatches between internal predictions based on previous experiences stored in short-term memory and current external events (Heekeren et al., 2008). The theory of predictive coding is well studied in the visual domain (see Stefanics et al., 2014 for a recent review) and has also been increasingly discussed for auditory processing in recent years (e.g., Friston, 2005; Garrido et al., 2009). Regarding the auditory paradigms used in this study, this can be a form of a detection error, indexed by the MMN, whenever the incoming information (deviant tone) does not match the prediction (standard tone). The memory trace formation for the standard tone as well as its changes demand short-term synaptic plasticity which is codetermined by an intact NMDA receptor activity (e.g., Garrido et al., 2009).

The MMN after the duration deviant was significantly larger than the one after the other four deviant types (see also **Figure 2**) in the Opt1 paradigm. Näätänen et al. (2004) report the same finding in healthy young adults. Thus, it seems as if the fronto-temporal network described above is more sensitive to deviations in duration in comparison to deviations in frequency, intensity, location, or a gap in the middle of the tone.

No MMN was detectable in the MemTra paradigm for the frequency deviant, which might indicate that the slope of memory trace decay varies for different tone characteristics (in case of the MemTra paradigm duration and frequency), with the memory trace for frequency deviants fading faster with time compared to duration deviants. Consequently, our results regarding the applicability of ΔMMN are restricted to MMN for duration deviants. To our best knowledge, no study exists to date which investigated MMN after different deviant types and for different ISI lengths within one AD or MCI sample. Contrary to our results, two studies investigating the MMN after duration and frequency deviants for short as well as long ISIs in healthy older adults indicate a faster decay of the pre-attentive auditory memory trace for duration in comparison to frequency deviants (Schroeder et al., 1995; Pekkonen et al., 1996). However, Cooper et al. (2006) failed to find such differences in healthy aging. Interestingly, MMN for duration deviants suggests the best prognostic value in the prediction of psychosis in at risk individuals in comparison to frequency and intensity deviants (see Näätänen et al., 2015 for a recent review and Erickson et al., 2016 for a recent meta-analysis). Notably, the vast majority of studies of MMN in schizophrenia use short ISIs only.

Regarding the fact that subjects with aMCI have the highest risk to develop AD, we expected a more pronounced pre-attentive auditory memory trace decay reflected by the ΔMMN–Dur in aMCI in comparison to naMCI/SMI. This effect was only present at the trend level ($p = 0.079$). Nevertheless, visual inspections indicate a smaller MMN after long ISIs in aMCI compared to the other two groups (**Figure 2**).

It needs to be mentioned that aMCI subjects had a significantly lower education ($p = 0.041$; **Table 1**) in comparison to SMI and naMCI. This finding is in line with the well-studied findings of education as a protective factor against cognitive decline (e.g., Salthouse, 2009).

The following limitations need to be considered for this study: as all participants investigated in this study showed subjective or objective cognitive impairment, our results are restricted to this at risk of developing AD group only. Thus, we cannot draw any conclusion about the prognostic value of ΔMMN–Dur in healthy aging. The sample size of the study, especially in the follow-up investigation, was rather small. Nevertheless, we found hypothesis-confirming significant positive associations between auditory memory trace decay and episodic memory.

As all tests included in the episodic memory composite score were verbal in nature (Alzheimer's Disease Assessment Scale free recall, MVGT), it remains open whether the association between auditory memory and episodic memory is restricted to verbal memory only or if it can be generalized to other memory modalities.

Due to logistic reasons, we had two dropouts from the 5-year-follow-up due to severe cognitive and functional decline, a group of especially great interest. Larger sample sizes in future studies would help to handle dropout analyses. Future studies with larger sample sizes are needed to replicate the effects (including e.g., survival analyses).

CONCLUSION

The strong significant association between ΔMMN–Dur and episodic memory at baseline and at the 5-year-follow-up provides an additional insight into neurobiological processes associated with pathological aging and may help in developing new tools for early diagnosis as well as for treatment monitoring. Since EEG recording is a non-invasive and cost-efficient tool, ΔMMN–Dur might become a useful extension to complement neuropsychological assessment in older populations at risk of developing AD. Further research and longitudinal studies with larger sample sizes and healthy age-matched as well as younger healthy controls are needed to evaluate possible clinical implications.

AUTHOR CONTRIBUTIONS

DL contributed to study conception and design, organized study procedures and acquired data, analyzed and interpreted the data, and wrote the first draft of the manuscript. FT contributed to study conception and design, organized study procedures, acquired data, contributed to data analysis, and critically revised the first draft of the manuscript and the article. PF and OCK contributed to study conception and design, organized study procedures and acquired data, contributed to data interpretation and critically revised the manuscript. SK supervised the statistical analysis of the data and critically revised the manuscript. WS provided support in data analyses and data interpretation and critically revised the manuscript. CAFA and I-TK conceptualized the study, obtained funding, supervised all phases of the study as principal investigators and critically revised the manuscript. All authors read and approved the final manuscript.

FUNDING

This research was funded by the Heidelberg Academy of Sciences and Humanities, Germany. During the data collection, I-TK was a fellow (now alumna) of the Zukunftskolleg of the University of Konstanz, Germany.

ACKNOWLEDGMENTS

DL, FT and I-TK were at University of Konstanz at the time of baseline data acquisition. We thank Thomas Elbert for general advice and support in study conception and implementation as well as Anne Korzowski for her support in data acquisition. We further thank Risto Näätänen and colleagues (University of Helsinki, Finland) who kindly provided all stimuli of the Opt1 paradigm (standard tone and deviants in the types of duration, frequency, intensity, location and gap).

REFERENCES

Allaire, J. C., and Marsiske, M. (1999). Everyday cognition: age and intellectual ability correlates. *Psychol. Aging* 14, 627–644. doi: 10.1037/0882-7974.14.4.627

Amada, N., Aihara, K., Ravid, R., and Horie, M. (2005). Reduction of NR1 and phosphorylated Ca^{2+}/calmodulin-dependent protein kinase II levels in Alzheimer's disease. *Neuroreport* 16, 1809–1813. doi: 10.1097/01.WNR.0000185015.44563.5d

Ardila, A., Ostrosky-Solis, F., Rosselli, M., and Gómez, C. (2000). Age-related cognitive decline during normal aging: the complex effect of education. *Arch. Clin. Neuropsychol.* 15, 495–513. doi: 10.1093/arclin/15.6.495

Baldeweg, T. (2006). Repetition effects to sounds: evidence for predictive coding in the auditory system. *Trends Cogn. Sci.* 10, 93–94. doi: 10.1016/j.tics.2006.01.010

Ballard, C., Gauthier, S., Corbett, A., Brayne, C., Aarsland, D., and Jones, E. (2011). Alzheimer's disease. *Lancet* 377, 1019–1031. doi: 10.1016/S0140-6736(10)61349-9

Bartha-Doering, L., Deuster, D., Giordano, V., am Zehnhoff-Dinnesen, A., and Dobel, C. (2015). A systematic review of the mismatch negativity as an index for auditory sensory memory: from basic research to clinical and developmental perspectives. *Psychophysiology* 52, 1115–1130. doi: 10.1111/psyp.12459

Bateman, R. J., Xiong, C., Benzinger, T. L. S., Fagan, A. M., Goate, A., Fox, N. C., et al. (2012). Clinical and biomarker changes in dominantly inherited Alzheimer's disease. *N. Engl. J. Med.* 367, 795–804. doi: 10.1056/NEJMoa1202753

Bates, D., Mächler, M., Bolker, B., and Walker, S. (2015). Fitting linear mixed-effects models using lme4. *J. Stat. Softw.* 67, 1–48. doi: 10.18637/jss.v067.i01

Bickel, H. (2016). *Die Häufigkeit Von Demenzerkrankungen [The Prevalence of Dementia].* Berlin, Germany: Deutsche Alzheimer Gesellschaft e.V. Available online at: https://www.deutsche-alzheimer.de/

Böttcher-Gandor, C., and Ullsperger, P. (1992). Mismatch negativity in event-related potentials to auditory stimuli as a function of varying interstimulus interval. *Psychophysiology* 29, 546–550. doi: 10.1111/j.1469-8986.1992.tb02028.x

Bowerman, B. L., and O'Connell, R. T. (1990). *Linear Statistical Models: An Applied Approach.* 2nd Edn. Belmont: CA: Duxbury.

Brønnick, K. S., Nordby, H., Larsen, J. P., and Aarsland, D. (2010). Disturbance of automatic auditory change detection in dementia associated with Parkinson's disease: a mismatch negativity study. *Neurobiol. Aging* 31, 104–113. doi: 10.1016/j.neurobiolaging.2008.02.021

Cansino, S. (2009). Episodic memory decay along the adult lifespan: a review of behavioral and neurophysiological evidence. *Int. J. Psychophysiol.* 71, 64–69. doi: 10.1016/j.ijpsycho.2008.07.005

Castanho, T. C., Amorim, L., Zihl, J., Palha, J. A., Sousa, N., and Santos, N. C. (2014). Telephone-based screening tools for mild cognitive impairment and dementia in aging studies: a review of validated instruments. *Front. Aging Neurosci.* 6:16. doi: 10.3389/fnagi.2014.00016

Cheng, C.-H., Hsu, W.-Y., and Lin, Y.-Y. (2013). Effects of physiological aging on mismatch negativity: a meta-analysis. *Int. J. Psychophysiol.* 90, 165–171. doi: 10.1016/j.ijpsycho.2013.06.026

Cheng, C.-H., Wang, P.-N., Hsu, W.-Y., and Lin, Y.-Y. (2012). Inadequate inhibition of redundant auditory inputs in Alzheimer's disease: an MEG study. *Biol. Psychol.* 89, 365–373. doi: 10.1016/j.biopsycho.2011.11.010

Cooper, R. J., Todd, J., McGill, K., and Michie, P. T. (2006). Auditory sensory memory and the aging brain: a mismatch negativity study. *Neurobiol. Aging* 27, 752–762. doi: 10.1016/j.neurobiolaging.2005.03.012

Draganova, R., Eswaran, H., Murphy, P., Lowery, C., and Preissl, H. (2007). Serial magnetoencephalographic study of fetal and newborn auditory discriminative evoked responses. *Early Hum. Dev.* 83, 199–207. doi: 10.1016/j.earlhumdev.2006.05.018

Duff, K., Tometich, D., and Dennett, K. (2015). The modified Telephone Interview for Cognitive Status is more predictive of memory abilities than the Mini-Mental State examination. *J. Geriatr. Psychiatry Neurol.* 28, 193–197. doi: 10.1177/0891988715573532

Engeland, C., Mahoney, C., Mohr, E., Ilivitsky, V., and Knott, V. J. (2002). Acute nicotine effects on auditory sensory memory in tacrine-treated and nontreated patients with Alzheimer's disease: an event-related potential study. *Pharmacol. Biochem. Behav.* 72, 457–464. doi: 10.1016/s0091-3057(02)00711-6

Erickson, M. A., Ruffle, A., and Gold, J. M. (2016). A meta-analysis of mismatch negativity in schizophrenia: from clinical risk to disease specificity and progression. *Biol. Psychiatry* 79, 980–987. doi: 10.1016/j.biopsych.2015.08.025

Fishman, Y. I. (2014). The mechanisms and meaning of the mismatch negativity. *Brain Topogr.* 27, 500–526. doi: 10.1007/s10548-013-0337-3

Fissler, P., Müller, H.-P., Küster, O. C., Laptinskaya, D., Thurm, F., Woll, A., et al. (2017). No evidence that short-term cognitive or physical training programs or lifestyles are related to changes in white matter integrity in older adults at risk of dementia. *Front. Hum. Neurosci.* 11:110. doi: 10.3389/fnhum.2017.00110

Folstein, M. F., Folstein, S. E., and McHugh, P. R. (1975). "Mini-mental state". A practical method for grading the cognitive state of patients for the clinician. *J. Psychiatr. Res.* 12, 189–198. doi: 10.1016/0022-3956(75)90026-6

Foster, S. M., Kisley, M. A., Davis, H. P., Diede, N. T., Campbell, A. M., and Davalos, D. B. (2013). Cognitive function predicts neural activity associated with pre-attentive temporal processing. *Neuropsychologia* 51, 211–219. doi: 10.1016/j.neuropsychologia.2012.09.017

Friston, K. (2005). A theory of cortical responses. *Philos. Trans. R. Soc. Lond. B Biol. Sci.* 360, 815–836. doi: 10.1098/rstb.2005.1622

Gaeta, H., Friedman, D., Ritter, W., and Cheng, J. (1999). Changes in sensitivity to stimulus deviance in Alzheimer's disease: an ERP perspective. *Neuroreport* 10, 281–287. doi: 10.1097/00001756-199902050-00014

Garrido, M. I., Kilner, J. M., Stephan, K. E., and Friston, K. J. (2009). The mismatch negativity: a review of underlying mechanisms. *Clin. Neurophysiol.* 120, 453–463. doi: 10.1016/j.clinph.2008.11.029

Geerlings, M. I., Jonker, C., Bouter, L. M., Adèr, H. J., and Schmand, B. (1999). Association between memory complaints and incident Alzheimer's disease in elderly people with normal baseline cognition. *Am. J. Psychiatry* 156, 531–537.

Gerland, P., Raftery, A. E., Sevčíková, H., Li, N., Gu, D., Spoorenberg, T., et al. (2014). World population stabilization unlikely this century. *Science* 346, 234–237. doi: 10.1126/science.1257469

Grau, C., Escera, C., Yago, E., and Polo, M. D. (1998). Mismatch negativity and auditory sensory memory evaluation: a new faster paradigm. *Neuroreport* 9, 2451–2456. doi: 10.1097/00001756-199808030-00005

Hartmann, T. (2009). *PyTuneSounds.* Konstanz, San Diego, CA: Slashdot Media. Available online at: https://sourceforge.net

Heekeren, H. R., Marrett, S., and Ungerleider, L. G. (2008). The neural systems that mediate human perceptual decision making. *Nat. Rev. Neurosci.* 9, 467–479. doi: 10.1038/nrn2374

Hothorn, T., Bretz, F., and Westfall, P. (2008). Simultaneous inference in general parametric models. *Biom. J.* 50, 346–363. doi: 10.1002/bimj.200810425

Hsiao, F.-J., Chen, W.-T., Wang, P.-N., Cheng, C.-H., and Lin, Y.-Y. (2014). Temporo-frontal functional connectivity during auditory change detection is altered in Alzheimer's disease. *Hum. Brain Mapp.* 35, 5565–5577. doi: 10.1002/hbm.22570

Huffmeijer, R., Bakermans-Kranenburg, M. J., Alink, L. R. A., and van Ijzendoorn, M. H. (2014). Reliability of event-related potentials: the influence of number of trials and electrodes. *Physiol. Behav.* 130, 13–22. doi: 10.1016/j.physbeh.2014.03.008

Ihl, R., and Weyer, G. (1993). *Die Alzheimer Disease Assessment Scale (ADAS).* Weinheim, Germany: Beltz Test.

Ilmberger, J. (1988). *Münchner Verbaler Gedächtnistest (MVGT) [Munich Verbal Memory Test, Unpublished Manuscript].* München: Institut für Medizinische Psychologie, Universität München.

Jessen, F., Wiese, B., Bachmann, C., Eifflaender-Gorfer, S., Haller, F., Kölsch, H., et al. (2010). Prediction of dementia by subjective memory impairment: effects of severity and temporal association with cognitive impairment. *Arch. Gen. Psychiatry* 67, 414–422. doi: 10.1001/archgenpsychiatry.2010.30

Jessen, F., Wolfsgruber, S., Wiese, B., Bickel, H., Mösch, E., Kaduszkiewicz, H., et al. (2014). AD dementia risk in late MCI, in early MCI, and in subjective memory impairment. *Alzheimers Dement.* 10, 76–83. doi: 10.1016/j.jalz.2012.09.017

Ji, L.-L., Zhang, Y.-Y., Zhang, L., He, B., and Lu, G.-H. (2015). Mismatch negativity latency as a biomarker of amnestic mild cognitive impairment in chinese rural elders. *Front. Aging Neurosci.* 7:22. doi: 10.3389/fnagi.2015.00022

Kazmerski, V. A., Friedman, D., and Ritter, W. (1997). Mismatch negativity during attend and ignore conditions in Alzheimer's disease. *Biol. Psychiatry* 42, 382–402. doi: 10.1016/s0006-3223(96)00344-7

Kumar, A. (2015). NMDA receptor function during senescence: implication on cognitive performance. *Front. Neurosci.* 9:473. doi: 10.3389/fnins.2015.00473

Küster, O. C., Fissler, P., Laptinskaya, D., Thurm, F., Scharpf, A., Woll, A., et al. (2016). Cognitive change is more positively associated with an active lifestyle than with training interventions in older adults at risk of dementia: a controlled interventional clinical trial. *BMC Psychiatry* 16:315. doi: 10.1186/s12888-016-1018-z

Küster, O. C., Laptinskaya, D., Fissler, P., Schnack, C., Zügel, M., Nold, V., et al. (2017). Novel blood-based biomarkers of cognition, stress, and physical or cognitive training in older adults at risk of dementia: preliminary evidence for a role of BDNF, irisin and the kynurenine pathway. *J. Alzheimers Dis.* 59, 1097–1111. doi: 10.3233/JAD-170447

Lai, C. L., Lin, R. T., Liou, L. M., and Liu, C. K. (2010). The role of event-related potentials in cognitive decline in Alzheimer's disease. *Clin. Neurophysiol.* 121, 194–199. doi: 10.1016/j.clinph.2009.11.001

Lindín, M., Correa, K., Zurrón, M., and Díaz, F. (2013). Mismatch negativity (MMN) amplitude as a biomarker of sensory memory deficit in amnestic mild cognitive impairment. *Front. Aging Neurosci.* 5:79. doi: 10.3389/fnagi.2013.00079

Magnusson, K. R., Brim, B. L., and Das, S. R. (2010). Selective vulnerabilities of N-methyl-D-aspartate (NMDA) receptors during brain aging. *Front. Aging Neurosci.* 2:11. doi: 10.3389/fnagi.2010.00011

Menard, S. (1995). *Applied Logistic Regression Analysis. Sage University Series on Quantitative Applications in the Social Sciences.* Thousand Oaks, CA: Sage.

Mishizen-Eberz, A. J., Rissman, R. A., Carter, T. L., Ikonomovic, M. D., Wolfe, B. B., and Armstrong, D. M. (2004). Biochemical and molecular studies of NMDA receptor subunits NR1/2A/2B in hippocampal subregions throughout progression of Alzheimer's disease pathology. *Neurobiol. Dis.* 15, 80–92. doi: 10.1016/j.nbd.2003.09.016

Morlet, D., and Fischer, C. (2014). MMN and novelty P3 in coma and other altered states of consciousness: a review. *Brain Topogr.* 27, 467–479. doi: 10.1007/s10548-013-0335-5

Mowszowski, L., Hermens, D. F., Diamond, K., Norrie, L., Cockayne, N., Ward, P. B., et al. (2014). Cognitive training enhances pre-attentive neurophysiological responses in older adults "at risk" of dementia. *J. Alzheimers Dis.* 41, 1095–1108. doi: 10.3233/JAD-131985

Mowszowski, L., Hermens, D. F., Diamond, K., Norrie, L., Hickie, I. B., Lewis, S. J. G., et al. (2012). Reduced mismatch negativity in mild cognitive impairment: associations with neuropsychological performance. *J. Alzheimers Dis.* 30, 209–219. doi: 10.3233/JAD-2012-111868

Myers, R. H. (1990). *Classical and Modern Regression with Applications.* 2nd Edn. Boston: PWS and Kent Publishing Company.

Näätänen, R., Gaillard, A., and Mäntysalo, S. (1978). Early selective-attention effect on evoked potential reinterpreted. *Acta Psychol.* 42, 313–329. doi: 10.1016/0001-6918(78)90006-9

Näätänen, R., Kujala, T., and Winkler, I. (2011). Auditory processing that leads to conscious perception: a unique window to central auditory processing opened by the mismatch negativity and related responses. *Psychophysiology* 48, 4–22. doi: 10.1111/j.1469-8986.2010.01114.x

Näätänen, R., Kujala, T., Escera, C., Baldeweg, T., Kreegipuu, K., Carlson, S., et al. (2012). The mismatch negativity (MMN)—a unique window to disturbed central auditory processing in ageing and different clinical conditions. *Clin. Neurophysiol.* 123, 424–458. doi: 10.1016/j.clinph.2011.09.020

Näätänen, R., Pakarinen, S., Rinne, T., and Takegata, R. (2004). The mismatch negativity (MMN): towards the optimal paradigm. *Clin. Neurophysiol.* 115, 140–144. doi: 10.1016/j.clinph.2003.04.001

Näätänen, R., Shiga, T., Asano, S., and Yabe, H. (2015). Mismatch negativity (MMN) deficiency: a break-through biomarker in predicting psychosis onset. *Int. J. Psychophysiol.* 95, 338–344. doi: 10.1016/j.ijpsycho.2014.12.012

Näätänen, R., Sussman, E. S., Salisbury, D., and Shafer, V. L. (2014). Mismatch negativity (MMN) as an index of cognitive dysfunction. *Brain Topogr.* 27, 451–466. doi: 10.1007/s10548-014-0374-6

Newcomer, J. W., Farber, N. B., and Olney, J. W. (2000). NMDA receptor function, memory, and brain aging. *Dialogues Clin. Neurosci.* 2, 219–232.

Oostenveld, R., Fries, P., Maris, E., and Schoffelen, J.-M. (2011). FieldTrip: open source software for advanced analysis of MEG, EEG, and invasive electrophysiological data. *Comput. Intell. Neurosci.* 2011:156869. doi: 10.1155/2011/156869

Papadaniil, C. D., Kosmidou, V. E., Tsolaki, A., Tsolaki, M., Kompatsiaris, I. Y., and Hadjileontiadis, L. J. (2016). Cognitive MMN and P300 in mild cognitive impairment and Alzheimer's disease: a high density EEG-3D vector field tomography approach. *Brain Res.* 1648, 425–433. doi: 10.1016/j.brainres.2016.07.043

Papaliagkas, V., Kimiskidis, V., Tsolaki, M., and Anogianakis, G. (2008). Usefulness of event-related potentials in the assessment of mild cognitive impairment. *BMC Neurosci.* 9:107. doi: 10.1186/1471-2202-9-107

Pekkonen, E., Jousmäki, V., Könönen, M., Reinikainen, K., and Partanen, J. (1994). Auditory sensory memory impairment in Alzheimer's disease: an event-related potential study. *Neuroreport* 5, 2537–2540. doi: 10.1097/00001756-199412000-00033

Pekkonen, E., Rinne, T., Reinikainen, K., Kujala, T., Alho, K., and Näätänen, R. (1996). Aging effects on auditory processing: an event-related potential study. *Exp. Aging Res.* 22, 171–184. doi: 10.1080/03610739608254005

Petersen, R. C. (2016). Mild cognitive impairment. *Continuum (Minneap Minn)* 22, 404–418. doi: 10.1212/CON.0000000000000313

Prince, M., Wimo, A., Guerchet, M., Ali, G.-C., Wu, Y.-T., and Prina, M. (2015). *World Alzheimer Report 2015.* London: Alzheimer's Disease International. Available online at: https://www.alz.co.uk/research/world-report-2015

R Core Team. (2016). *R: A Language and Environment for Statistical Computing.* Vienna: R Foundation for Statistical Computing. Available online at: http://www.r-project.org

RStudio Team. (2015). *R Studio: Integrated Development for R.* Boston, MA: R Studio, Inc. Available online at: https://www.rstudio.com/

Ruzzoli, M., Pirulli, C., Brignani, D., Maioli, C., and Miniussi, C. (2012). Sensory memory during physiological aging indexed by mismatch negativity (MMN). *Neurobiol. Aging* 33, 625.e21–625.e30. doi: 10.1016/j.neurobiolaging.2011.03.021

Ruzzoli, M., Pirulli, C., Mazza, V., Miniussi, C., and Brignani, D. (2016). The mismatch negativity as an index of cognitive decline for the early detection of Alzheimer's disease. *Sci. Rep.* 6:33167. doi: 10.1038/srep33167

Salthouse, T. A. (2009). When does age-related cognitive decline begin? *Neurobiol. Aging* 30, 507–514. doi: 10.1016/j.neurobiolaging.2008.09.023

Salthouse, T. A. (2012). Consequences of age-related cognitive declines. *Annu. Rev. Psychol.* 63, 201–226. doi: 10.1146/annurev-psych-120710-100328

Sams, M., Hari, R., Rif, J., and Knuutila, J. (1993). The human auditory sensory memory trace persists about 10 sec: neuromagnetic evidence. *J. Cogn. Neurosci.* 5, 363–370. doi: 10.1162/jocn.1993.5.3.363

Schmidt, K.-H., and Metzler, P. (1992). *Wortschatztest [WST, Verbal Knowledge Test].* Weinheim, Germany: Beltz Test.

Schroeder, M. M., Ritter, W., and Vaughan, H. G. Jr. (1995). The mismatch negativity to novel stimuli reflects cognitive decline. *Ann. N Y Acad. Sci.* 769, 399–401. doi: 10.1111/j.1749-6632.1995.tb38155.x

Stefanics, G., Kremláček, J., and Czigler, I. (2014). Visual mismatch negativity: a predictive coding view. *Front. Hum. Neurosci.* 8:666. doi: 10.3389/fnhum.2014.00666

Tewes, U. (1991). *Hamburg-Wechsler-Intelligenztest für Erwachsene [HAWIE-R, Hamburg-Wechsler-Intelligence Test for Adults].* Bern, Stuttgart, Toronto: Huber.

The MathWorks. (2015). *MATLAB and Statistics Toolbox Release 2015b.* Natick, MA: The MathWorks, Inc. Available online at: https://de.mathworks.com

Thurm, F., Antonenko, D., Schlee, W., Kolassa, S., Elbert, T., and Kolassa, I.-T. (2013). Effects of aging and mild cognitive impairment on electrophysiological correlates of performance monitoring. *J. Alzheimers Dis.* 35, 575–587. doi: 10.3233/JAD-121348

Todd, J., Michie, P. T., Schall, U., Ward, P. B., and Catts, S. V. (2012). Mismatch negativity (MMN) reduction in schizophrenia-impaired prediction-error generation, estimation or salience? *Int. J. Psychophysiol.* 83, 222–231. doi: 10.1016/j.ijpsycho.2011.10.003

Tsolaki, A. C., Kosmidou, V., Kompatsiaris, I. Y., Papadaniil, C., Hadjileontiadis, L., Adam, A., et al. (2017). Brain source localization of MMN and P300 ERPs in mild cognitive impairment and Alzheimer's disease: a high-density EEG approach. *Neurobiol. Aging* 55, 190–201. doi: 10.1016/j.neurobiolaging.2017.03.025

United Nations (2015). *World Population Ageing. 1950–2050.* New York, NY: United Nations Publications.

Vecchio, F., and Määttä, S. (2011). The use of auditory event-related potentials in Alzheimer's disease diagnosis. *Int. J. Alzheimers Dis.* 2011:653173. doi: 10.4061/2011/653173

Verleger, R., Kömpf, D., and Neukäter, W. (1992). Event-related EEG potentials in mild dementia of the Alzheimer type. *Electroencephalogr. Clin. Neurophysiol.* 84, 332–343. doi: 10.1016/0168-5597(92)90086-q

Welsh, K. A., Butters, N., Mohs, R. C., Beekly, D., Edland, S., Fillenbaum, G., et al. (1994). The consortium to establish a registry for Alzheimer's disease (CERAD). Part V. A normative study of the neuropsychological battery. *Neurology* 44, 609–614. doi: 10.1212/WNL.44.4.609

Yesavage, J. A., Brink, T. L., Rose, T. L., Lum, O., Huang, V., Adey, M., et al. (1983). Development and validation of a geriatric depression screening scale: a preliminary report. *J. Psychiatr. Res.* 17, 37–49. doi: 10.1016/0022-3956(82)90033-4

2

Alzheimer's Disease and Type 2 Diabetes: A Critical Assessment of the Shared Pathological Traits

Shreyasi Chatterjee and Amritpal Mudher*

Centre of Biological Sciences, University of Southampton, Southampton, United Kingdom

***Correspondence:**
Shreyasi Chatterjee
s.chatterjee@soton.ac.uk

Alzheimer's disease (AD) and Type 2 Diabetes Mellitus (T2DM) are two of the most prevalent diseases in the elderly population worldwide. A growing body of epidemiological studies suggest that people with T2DM are at a higher risk of developing AD. Likewise, AD brains are less capable of glucose uptake from the surroundings resembling a condition of brain insulin resistance. Pathologically AD is characterized by extracellular plaques of Aβ and intracellular neurofibrillary tangles of hyperphosphorylated tau. T2DM, on the other hand is a metabolic disorder characterized by hyperglycemia and insulin resistance. In this review we have discussed how Insulin resistance in T2DM directly exacerbates Aβ and tau pathologies and elucidated the pathophysiological traits of synaptic dysfunction, inflammation, and autophagic impairments that are common to both diseases and indirectly impact Aβ and tau functions in the neurons. Elucidation of the underlying pathways that connect these two diseases will be immensely valuable for designing novel drug targets for Alzheimer's disease.

Keywords: insulin resistance, tau proteins, abeta oligomers, synaptic dysfunction, autophagy, inflammation

INTRODUCTION

Alzheimer's Disease: Neuropathological Alterations and Metabolic Risk Factors

Diagnosed by the German psychiatrist and neuropathologist, Prof. Alois Alzheimer in 1906, Alzheimer's disease is the most prevalent form of dementia in the aging population (van der Flier and Scheltens, 2005). Recently declared as the sixth major cause of death in the world, patients affected with AD suffer a gradual decline of cognitive abilities and memory functions till the disease renders them incapable of performing daily functions (James et al., 2014). Statistical data reveals that over 30 million people are suffering from AD worldwide and this number is estimated to double every 20 years to reach 66 million in 2030 and about 115 million by 2050[1].

Clinically AD can be classified into two subtypes. About 95% 0f AD patients are aged 65 years or older and are diagnosed with "late-onset" or "sporadic AD" (sAD) while 5% of AD patients carry rare genetic mutations associated with "early-onset" or "familial AD" (fAD) that causes the onset of disease symptoms in a person's thirties, forties, or fifties (De Strooper, 2007). In early onset fAD, the disease pathology is caused by mutation in three known genes namely: amyloid precursor protein (APP), presenilin-1 (PS-1), and presenilin-2(PS-2). Although PS-1 mutations account for most of the fAD, there are mutations outside these three genes that are yet unknown. Unlike the fAD, the genetics of sAD is more complex (Dorszewska et al., 2016).

[1] Available online at: https://www.alz.co.uk/research/WorldAlzheimerReport2015.pdf.

Other than aging, which is the strongest risk factor for sAD, GWAS studies reveal that the epsilon four allele of the apolipoprotein E (ApoE4) gene is a significant risk factor for the development of this disease. Two copies of ApoE4 gene increases risk of AD by 12-fold, while one copy of this allele enhances the risk by 4-fold (Bertram and Tanzi, 2009). However, only 50–60% individuals are carriers of this gene suggesting that other factors also confer risk. Studies suggest that these include factors such as cerebrovascular infarction, family history of diabetes, hypertension, and obesity (Li et al., 2015a).

At a cellular level, AD is characterized by a progressive loss of pyramidal cells in the entorhinal cortex and CA1 region of the hippocampus that are responsible for maintenance of higher cognitive functions (Serrano-Pozo et al., 2011). Early symptoms of AD are also marked by synaptic dysfunction that disrupts connectivity between neural circuits, thereby initiating the gradual loss of memory.

Neuropathologically, AD is characterized by extracellular plaques of insoluble amyloid-β protein, and intracellular neurofibrillary tangles (NFTs) of hyperphosphorylated tau protein (Iqbal et al., 2010; Serrano-Pozo et al., 2011). In AD, abnormal cleavage of APP results in the formation of insoluble amyloid-β protein, densely packed with beta sheets, which form the core of the senile plaques (Serpell et al., 2000). Tau protein, in a physiological state serves as a microtubule binding protein and plays an important role in axonal and vesicular transport (Mandelkow and Mandelkow, 1995). Conversely, in the disease state tau protein is hyperphosphorylated and detached from the microtubules. In animal models this phospho-tau-mediated disruption of cytoskeletal integrity manifests in synaptic and behavioral impairments (Mudher et al., 2004; Quraishe et al., 2013; Gilley et al., 2016; Lathuilière et al., 2017). Although a large body of *in vitro* studies have investigated tau-microtubule binding interactions, most of these studies have been conducted *in silico* or in non-neural cellular models (Kadavath et al., 2015; Huda et al., 2017). In a series of elegant experiments involving single-molecule tracking of tau in axonal processes, Niewidok et al. and Janning et al. have shown that the interaction of tau with the microtubules follows a "kiss-and-hop" mechanism. Their studies show that a single tau molecule resides only 40 ms on a particular microtubule and then hops longitudinally and transversely on adjacent microtubules. This novel mechanism has been particularly effective in resolving the paradoxical observation that despite regulating microtubule dynamics, alterations in tau levels may not interfere with axonal transport (Janning et al., 2014; Niewidok et al., 2016). Using pseudo-hyperphosphorylated tau constructs they observed a considerable weakening of the tau-microtubule interactions that corroborated with previous *in vitro* studies.

A large body of evidence supports the idea that the formation of Aβ plaques occurs 15–20 years earlier before the cognitive functions decline, whereas the spatial and temporal spread of tau pathology correlates more strongly with the severity with disease progression (Serrano-Pozo et al., 2011; Vlassenko et al., 2012). Although Aβ and tau are the pathological hallmarks that characterize sAD, it is not yet clear whether these two factors trigger AD or if they are manifested as the effect of the disease.

The drug therapy of AD is still at a nascent stage providing symptomatic relief but not slowing down disease progression. Such treatments include FDA-approved choline esterase inhibitors and NMDA (glutamate) receptor agonists. Thus, from a public health perspective AD exerts a significant healthcare burden that is expected to escalate 5-fold in the coming decades. Hence, the need for early detection and effective treatment is an urgent priority (Yiannopoulou and Papageorgiou, 2013).

In recent times, it has been hypothesized that various risk factors promote Aβ and tau-related pathological changes before the onset of clinical symptoms in AD. One of the formidable challenges of the twenty-first century is to identify these risk factors and enable early detection of pathophysiological alterations at the cellular and biochemical level so that effective treatments can be designed against this devastating disease. A significant risk factor associated with sAD that has received a considerable attention in recent times is Type 2 Diabetes (T2D) (Li et al., 2015a).

Type 2 Diabetes

Diabetes mellitus is a chronic metabolic disorder that is increasing worldwide at an alarming rate. It is estimated that 387 million people are affected by Typel and T2DM and this number is expected to reach 552 million by 2030 (American Diabetes, 2009). The financial costs for the treatment of diabetes and support for the patients presents a significant healthcare challenge for any country across the world.

The most prevalent subtype of diabetes is the Type 2 diabetes mellitus (T2DM) that comprises 95% of this disease. The salient features of T2DM are high levels of blood glucose (hyperglycaemia), hyper-insulinemia, and insulin resistance (Taylor, 2012). Insulin resistance arises due to decreased insulin sensitivity of muscle, liver, and fat cells to insulin. Another prominent feature of T2DM is the formation of human islet amyloid polypeptide that causes pancreatic β-cell dysfunction (Marzban et al., 2003). Both these features ultimately result in a reduced uptake of circulating blood glucose for glycogenesis eventually leading to chronic hyperglycemia as one of the pathological hallmarks of T2DM.

What is the evidence that there is a patho-physiological link between Diabetes and AD?

Evidence From Epidemiological Studies

Epidemiological studies show that T2DM increases the risk of AD by at least 2-fold (Barbagallo and Dominguez, 2014). In a study cohort recruited from Manhattan in 1992–1994 and then in 1999–2001 Cheng et al. demonstrated that T2DM is associated strongly with late-onset AD (LOAD) after adjustment of sex and age. Their findings also suggested that the link between T2DM and LOAD is partly mediated by cerebrovascular pathology (Cheng et al., 2011). Recent studies from Li et al. report that T2DM in an elderly Chinese population with mild cognitive impairment (MCI) influences the progression to AD, while no change is observed in age-matched controls (Li et al., 2016). These data are supported by longitudinal studies conducted by Leibson et al. and Huang et al. in which patients with adult onset diabetes exhibited a significantly higher risk of developing AD than age-matched subjects without T2DM (Leibson et al., 1997; Huang et al., 2014). Epidemiological studies have also examined the association between ApoE4 genotype and diabetes or insulin resistance, although the reports are controversial. For instance, a longitudinal study in Japanese-American men demonstrated that ApoE4 increases the risk of LOAD in individuals with T2DM (Peila et al., 2002). In contrast, population-based studies conducted by Marseglia et al. show an association between T2DM and risk of dementia only in ApoE4 non-carriers (Marseglia et al., 2016).

Evidence From Neuroimaging Studies

The evidence from epidemiological studies has recently been corroborated by findings from neuroimaging studies (PET and MRI) that monitor the structural alterations in brains of patients affected by AD and T2DM. The data from the neuroimaging studies reveals a considerable overlap between the vulnerable brain regions in both patient groups.

AD is generally associated with widespread brain atrophy that initiates in the transentorhinal and entorhinal cortex in the early stages and then spreads to the remaining neocortical areas (Fjell et al., 2015). Neuroimaging studies show that the widespread pattern of neurodegeneration caused by AD in the limbic and neocortical regions correlates closely with cognitive deficits and behavioral patterns that AD patients exhibit. However, determining the early stages of AD pathophysiology still remains a challenge. Recently a comprehensive study based on high-resolution MRI on people with MCI and AD revealed that the earliest signs of AD pathology appeared in the cholinergic cells of the nucleus basalis of Meynert (NbM) in the basal forebrain (Schmitz et al., 2016).

Interestingly, neuroimaging studies of brains in individuals with T2DM also show structural alterations that resemble those seen in AD patients. In an elegant study conducted by Moran et al. 350 people with T2DM and 363 control individuals were assessed for cognitive functions with an MRI scan to identify the regional distribution of brain atrophy to identify the causes of cognitive impairment in T2DM patients (Beckett et al., 2015; Moran et al., 2015). The investigators found that T2DM was associated with more cerebral infarcts and reduced volumes of gray matter, white matter, and hippocampus compared to non-diabetic individuals. It was further observed that in people with T2DM, gray matter loss was most prominent in medial temporal, anterior, cingulate, and medial frontal lobes—the regions maximally vulnerable to AD. Moreover, cognitive functions, and in particular visuo-spatial skills, were markedly affected in the T2DM group. Another study by Roberts et al. examined the associations of T2DM with imaging biomarkers and cognitive abilities in 1,437 elderly individuals without dementia (Roberts et al., 2014). They found that midlife T2DM was associated with reduced hippocampal and whole brain volumes strongly indicating decline of cognitive functions later in life. Wennberg et al. conducted a study on 233 cognitively normal individuals who were assessed for fasting blood glucose and cortical thickness measurements by MRI (Wennberg et al., 2016). This study showed that higher blood glucose was associated with reduced average thickness in the AD vulnerable regions. Based on these observations, the authors conclude that the brain atrophy in T2DM, evident from imaging studies, bears striking resemblance to that seen in preclinical AD.

Shared Pathophysiology Between AD and T2DM

PET and MRI studies show marked impairment of glucose and energy metabolism in both T2DM and AD (Umegaki, 2014). In addition, amyloidogenesis remains a salient feature in both these diseases. Extracellular β-amyloid plaques form one of the characteristic features of AD. Likewise, deposits of amyloidogenic peptide (IAPP) are detected in the pancreatic islets of Langerhans of T2DM patients (Haataja et al., 2008). Interestingly, diabetic mice overexpressing IAPP develop oligomers and fibrils with more severe diabetic trait similar to AD mouse models that overexpress APP (Marzban et al., 2003). Advanced glycation end products (AGE) and their receptors (RAGE) accumulate in the sites of diabetic complications such as kidney, retina, and atherosclerotic plaques under conditions of ER and oxidative stress (Nowotny et al., 2015). Similarly, glycated products of Aβ and tau form in transgenic AD models as well as in post-mortem brains of AD patients under similar stress conditions and form an important component of neurofibrillary tangles (Schedin-Weiss et al., 2014). Moreover, additional traits of synaptic dysfunction, activation of the inflammatory response pathways and impairment of autophagy are pathological features common to both AD and T2DM (De Felice and Ferreira, 2014; Carvalho et al., 2015).

The first section of this review will discuss the impact of brain insulin resistance evident in T2DM on the two hallmarks of AD, Aβ, and tau and describe the possible mechanisms that interconnect AD and T2DM in the areas of synaptic dysfunction, inflammation, and autophagic impairment (**Figure 1**).

ALZHEIMER'S DISEASE: INSULIN RESISTANCE IN THE BRAIN

Brain insulin resistance is a significant, yet often over-looked feature of AD (De Felice et al., 2014). Insulin released from the pancreas is transported to the brain via the blood brain barrier using a receptor-mediated mechanism. While the crucial role of insulin response in the peripheral tissues is well documented, there are very few reports about the function of insulin in the central nervous system. The insulin levels in human and rodent brain tissue are relatively low compared to circulating levels (Talbot, 2014). There are some reports about reduced insulin levels in the AD brains; however, this finding was not significant compared to the age-matched controls (Stanley et al., 2016). Recently several studies have reported reductions of insulin mRNA in AD, however the results of *de novo* insulin synthesis have been controversial (Blázquez et al., 2014). Thus, it is hypothesized that majority of brain insulin comes from the peripheral tissues and the role of insulin produced in the CNS is still unclear.

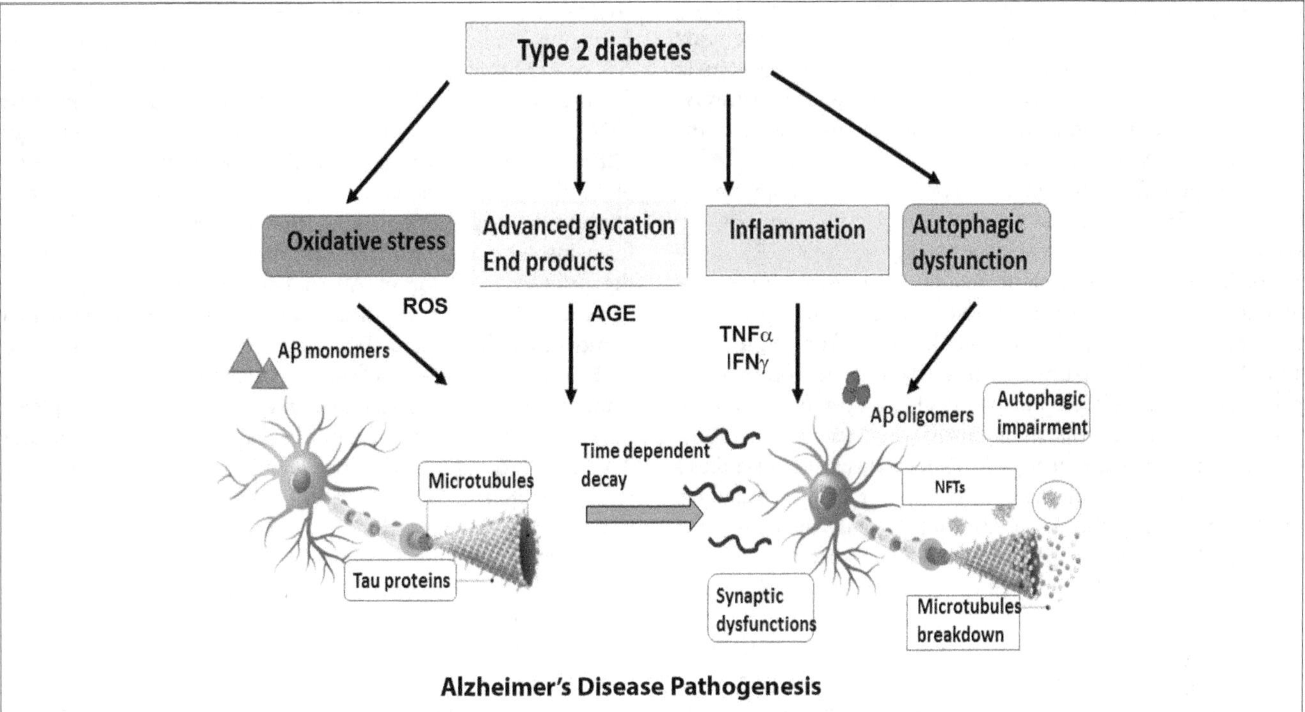

FIGURE 1 | Overview of the diverse mechanisms by which Type 2 Diabetes can cause AD pathogenesis. Type 2 Diabetes accompanied by insulin resistance and hyperglycemia gives rise to metabolic problems in the brain and other target tissues that sets off a cascade of pathogenic processes such as oxidative stress, inflammatory responses, advanced glycation products and autophagic dysfunction. The reactive oxygen species generated by these pathways expedite the process of neuronal death. At the same time, the insulin resistance impairs the downstream signaling pathways and exacerbates the formation of Aβ oligomers and aggregates of hyperphosphorylated tau. The cumulative effect of all these factors expose the neurons to a range of assaults and gradually result in the loss of synapses and neuronal death.

Although, the brain was initially considered a non-insulin target organ; several studies indicate the widespread distribution of insulin receptors (IR) in the brain particularly in the olfactory bulb, cortex, hippocampus, and hypothalamus indicating an intricate "neuroregulatory" role for insulin (Kim and Feldman, 2015). IRs in the brain are enriched in neurons compared to glia, and concentrated at the synapse. However, contrary to the IRs found in the peripheral tissues, the primary function of brain IRs is not glucose transport and metabolism. Instead, the brain IRs perform diverse functions including homeostatic regulation, modulation of synaptic plasticity, and neurotransmission and age related neurodegeneration (Plum et al., 2005).

The crucial function of glucose uptake and utilization in the brain is carried out by Glucose transporter 4 (GLUT4). Insulin activates GLUT4 gene expression and translocation from the cytosol to the plasma membrane to regulate glucose homeostasis in the brain and maintains energy requirements for a variety neuronal functions (Chiang et al., 2001; Reno et al., 2017).

Insulin Signaling in the Brain

A large number of recent studies provide compelling evidence that deficits in insulin signaling, arising due to insulin resistance, occurs in AD (Talbot et al., 2012; Mullins et al., 2017). FDG-PET studies of the brains of "early stage" AD patients have demonstrated reduced glucose uptake leading Suzanne de la Monte and colleagues to classify AD as "Type 3 Diabetes"(de la Monte and Wands, 2008).

In the brain, insulin and IGF signaling mechanisms are crucial for maintaining synaptic plasticity and cognitive functions (Boucher et al., 2014). Once insulin binds to the IR, it is activated by auto-phosphorylation of several tyrosine residues which in turn activates insulin receptor substrates 1 (IRS-1) and 2 that initiate a host of downstream signaling cascades through phosphatidylinositol-3-kinase (PI3K) (**Figure 2**). PI3K then activates AKT, which phosphorylates GSK-3β at serine 9 residue thereby inhibiting its activity and resulting in glycogen synthesis (Avila et al., 2012). There are numerous reports that GSK-3β is one of the key tau kinases playing a central role in AD pathogenesis (Chatterjee et al., 2009; Hernandez et al., 2013). Physiologically GSK-3β is involved in maintaining synaptic plasticity and regulates NMDA receptor-mediated long-term potentiation (LTP) and long-term depression (LTD) effects at the synapses (Bradley et al., 2012). In the disease state however, GSK-3β is hyperactive and phosphorylates tau at pathological epitopes. Hyperphosphorylated tau then aggregates to form neurofibrillary tangles (Avila et al., 2010). GSK-3β is also a key mediator of apoptosis suggesting that it might activate neuronal loss in degenerative diseases with increased production of Aβ (Qu et al., 2014). Emerging data also shows that PI3K/AKT pathway regulates synaptic plasticity by stimulating excitatory and inhibitory cell membrane receptors, enhances neurotransmitter activities and increases cortical glucose metabolism in the brain regions that are important for learning and memory (Farrar et al., 2005). In parallel, insulin activates the MAPK pathways leading to Ras activation at the plasma membrane and the sequential activation of Raf, MEK, and ERK (Zhang et al., 2011) (**Figure 2**). Although a direct role of the components of the MAPK pathway in mediating AD pathology has not yet been deciphered, recent reports indicate that ERK plays a crucial role in synapse formation and learning/memory functions implying that it may have additional neuroprotective functions (Thiels and Klann, 2001). Apart from PI3K/AKT and Ras/Raf/MAPK pathways, less well-defined roles in AD pathogenesis are played by mammalian target of rapamycin (mTOR) and its downstream targets that regulate neuronal survival and nutrient sensing. mTOR regulates protein synthesis by phosphorylating the key substrates of the translational machinery namely the eukaryotic initiation factor 4E-binding protein (4E-BP1) and p70S6 kinase (S6K1). Rapamycin inhibits mTOR *in vivo* and halts cellular growth and proliferation (Showkat et al., 2014).

It is hypothesized that in an insulin-resistant state these downstream signaling pathways are compromised leading to increased levels of Aβ oligomers and hyperphosphorylated tau not only due to a dysregulation of the downstream kinases but also due to an impairment of autophagic clearance that arises as a result of imbalance of the mTOR and autophagy pathways. Autophagic dysfunction, which is an emerging feature of AD causes the progressive accumulation of toxic proteins and eventually leads to neuronal death (Orr and Oddo, 2013).

From the epidemiological and brain neuroimaging studies it is evident that insulin and IGF signaling pathways are important for preservation and maintenance of learning and memory processes that are compromised in AD. Supporting this, intranasal insulin administration improves learning and memory functions in AD patients, emphasizing the shared pathophysiology in both diseases (Benedict et al., 2007).

CROSSTALK OF T2DM AND Aβ PATHOLOGY IN AD

One of the hallmarks of AD pathology is the formation of extracellular amyloid plaques composed of insoluble deposits of amyloid-β protein aggregates. Aβ is generated from the proteolytic cleavage of amyloid precursor protein (APP) by a sequence of enzymatic reactions from BACE-1, β and γ-secretase complex (Vassar, 2004). It is hypothesized that lower concentration of Aβ remains in the soluble form and subject to clearance after degradation, while higher concentrations aggregate into insoluble plaques that are resistant to degradation (Esparza et al., 2016). While there is no evidence that AD brains secrete more soluble Aβ than normal brains, a recent body of evidence suggests that an increased accumulation of insoluble Aβ plaques arise due to impaired clearance of Aβ protein (Wildsmith et al., 2013).

Impact of Hyperinsulinemia on Aβ

Emerging studies indicate that hyperinsulinemia may confer risk of AD by modulating Aβ toxicity. The enzyme responsible for degrading the Aβ protein is Insulin Degrading Enzyme (IDE), which also degrades insulin (Qiu and Folstein, 2006). In T2DM, peripheral hyperinsulinemia increases the concentration of insulin which acts as a competitive substrate for IDE and inhibits the degradation of Aβ that gradually accumulates to form insoluble plaques. IDE has previously been identified as the primary regulator of Aβ in both neurons and glia (Son et al., 2016). In a recent study Farris et al. demonstrated that homozygous deletions of IDE gene (IDE–/–) in mice, resulted in 50% decrease in Aβ clearance in brain homogenates and primary neuronal cultures (Farris et al., 2003). The IDE depleted mice exhibited increased cerebral accumulation of endogenous Aβ, in addition to the hyperinsulinemia and glucose intolerance that characterize T2DM. Hyperinsulinemia also affects APP transport. *In vitro* studies by Gasparini et al. demonstrated that in βAPP overexpressing N2a cells and primary neuronal cultures, insulin decreases the intracellular accumulation of Aβ by promoting the transport of βAPP/Aβ from the trans-golgi network to the plasma membrane (Gasparini et al., 2001). Thus, in addition to inhibiting the degradation of Aβ by IDE, insulin increases the concentration of extracellular Aβ by modulating the trafficking of APP. The investigators also show the involvement of receptor tyrosine kinase/mitogen-activated protein (MAP) kinase pathway in regulating intracellular Aβ transport (Matos et al., 2008).

Impact of Insulin Resistance on Aβ

Studies by Cheignon et al. have shown that inhibition of PI3K leads to reduced Aβ production (Cheignon et al., 2018). When they crossed neuron specific IR knockout mice to APP overexpressing Tg2576 transgenic mice, this study found that loss of insulin signaling in the brain reduced production of Aβ and amyloid plaque deposits. However, the decrease of Aβ burden was not sufficient to rescue the mortality observed in these transgenic mice. Nevertheless, this data provides strong evidence that IRS signaling plays an important role in modulating the Aβ deposition.

Investigating the effect of diet-induced insulin resistance on amyloidosis in Tg2576 AD transgenic mouse models, Ho et al. found that the animals displayed the first signs of memory deficits only at 6 months of age. These animals also maintained normal circulating insulin levels and glucose metabolism till they were 13 months old when there was evidence of plasma hyperinsulinemia. Interestingly, despite high production of Aβ and senile plaques in the brain, these mice showed no evidence of neuronal death and neurofibrillary tangles. However when these mice were reared on a high fat diet they developed non-insulin dependent diabetes mellitus, that led to increased production of Aβ40 and Aβ42, higher activation of γ-secretase as well as GSK-3α and GSK-3β. Biochemical evidence has shown that these mice displayed lower PI3K and AKT activation signals denoting insulin resistance with impaired learning and memory functions (Ho et al., 2004; Chouliaras et al., 2010).

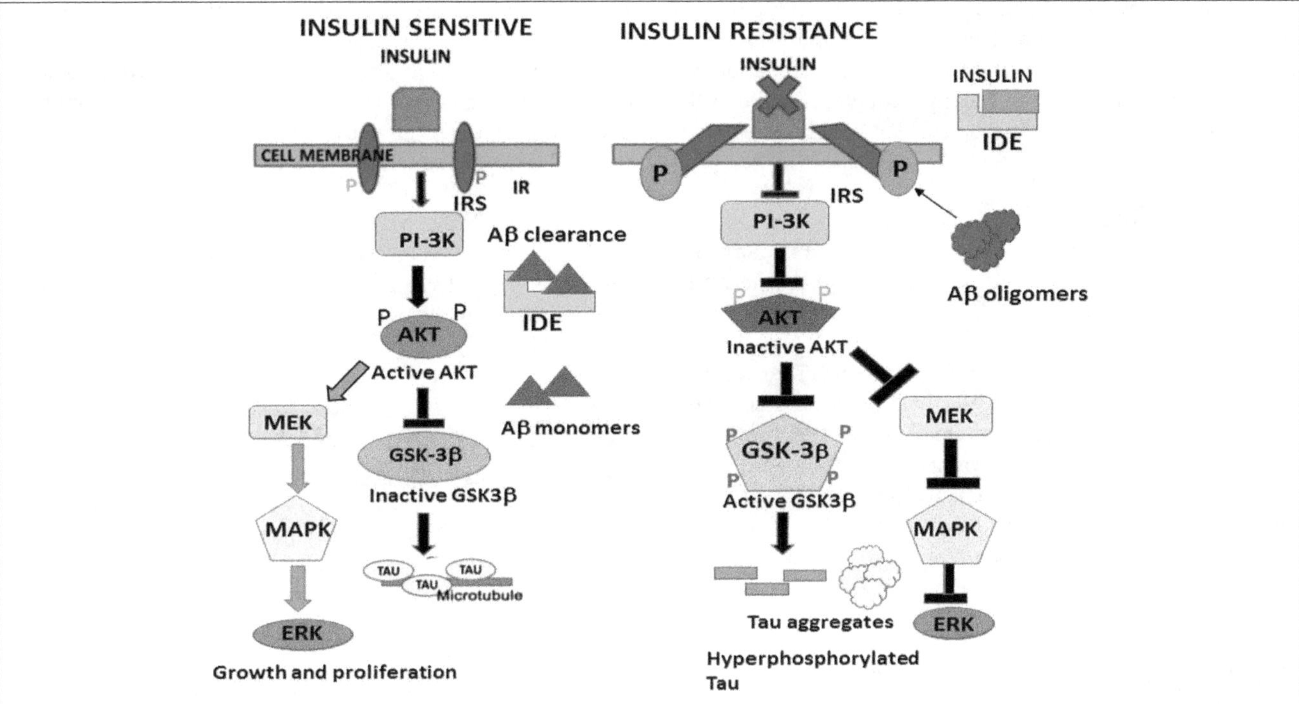

FIGURE 2 | Neuronal signaling mechanisms in a state of insulin sensitivity and insulin resistance. In the insulin sensitive state insulin binds to the receptor and activates the insulin receptor tyrosine kinase that initiates a cascade of phosphorylation events at the IRS/PI3K/AKT and Ras/Raf/ERK pathways. AKT phosphorylates GSK-3β at the inhibitory serine 9 residue and allows tau to maintain its physiological function of binding to microtubules and facilitates normal axonal transport of neuronal vesicles. In a state of insulin resistance, GSK-3β is activated by phosphorylation at Tyrosine 216 residue and hyperphosphorylates tau at pathological epitopes. Hyperphosphorylated tau then detaches from the microtubules and aggregates to form neurofibrillary tangles. Likewise, in the presence of excess insulin, the insulin degrading enzyme (IDE) is unable to degrade and facilitate clearance of Aβ oligomers that act as a competitive substrate for insulin. Thus, insulin resistance facilitates the formation of both Aβ and tau oligomers.

Impact of Hyperglycemia on Aβ

Elevated plasma glucose levels are a common pathological feature of T2DM affected individuals. A compelling link between glucose metabolism and AD was established in a study conducted in transgenic APP/PS1 murine models (Macauley et al., 2015). The researchers observed that the induction of acute hyperglycaemia in young mice increased the production of Aβ and lactate in hippocampal interstitial fluid and this was associated with an increase in neuronal activity (Minkeviciene et al., 2009). These effects worsened in aged AD mice with increased Aβ plaque pathology. These findings suggest that transient hyperglycemia associated with T2DM can initiate the formation of Aβ plaques. In this study, the authors also show that hippocampal ATP sensitive potassium (KATP) channels act as metabolic sensors of the alterations in glucose concentration with changes in electrical activity and extracellular Aβ deposition.

In addition, aberrant glucose metabolism activates glycation reactions that leads to the formation of advanced glycated end products (AGE). Elevated AGE levels in the circulation and in the brain have been associated with cognitive impairments in AD patients (Li et al., 2013). Numerous studies show that there is an increased accumulation of AGE in the brain of diabetic rats implying that AGE products impair the removal of Aβ42 and induce Aβ aggregation in the brain (Moreira et al., 2003).

AGEs enhance the expression of its receptor RAGE, which is also a presumed receptor for Aβ (Srikanth et al., 2011). Recent reports have shown increased RAGE expression in the astrocytes and microglia of AD brains (Solito and Sastre, 2012). Also, studies on triple transgenic model of AD (3xTg AD) expressing 3 dementia-related transgenes, namely APPSWE, PS1M146V, and tauP301L and raised on high-fat diet as well as STZ-induced diabetic APP/PS1 dual transgenic AD mice demonstrate increased RAGE expression in neurons and astrocytes with an activation of pro-inflammatory cytokines and enhanced decline of cognitive and memory functions (Choi et al., 2014). As a consequence of the damaging inflammatory responses, RAGE causes vascular complications in AD and T2DM. Neuron-specific overexpression of dominant negative RAGE results in restoration of cognitive functions and stops the progression of neuropathological changes in AD mice (Liu L. P. et al., 2009). Treatment of transgenic AD mice with RAGE inhibitor decreases microglial activation and Aβ production (Criscuolo et al., 2017). Interestingly, soluble form of RAGE (sRAGE) is neuroprotective (Deane et al., 2012; Lee and Park, 2013).

O-GlcNAcylation is a nucleocytoplasmic post-translational modification that occurs abundantly in neurons and protects against Aβ-mediated neuronal toxicity. Recent studies show that a moderate level of O-GlcNAcylation is neuroprotective and decreases formation of Aβ production by inhibiting γ-secretase activity (Hanover and Wang, 2013). Insulin resistance and hyperglycemia increases the level of O-GlcNAcylation but the amelioration of γ-secretase activity is counterbalanced by the accumulation of glycated end products that are ultimately toxic to neurons.

Impact of Dyslipidemia on Aβ

Insulin plays a crucial role in lipid metabolism and impairments in insulin signaling lead to increased lipolysis and elevated synthesis of free fatty acids (FFA) (Wilson and Binder, 1997). Human brain produces approximately 30% of total body cholesterol, hence slight alterations in lipid metabolism can have profound effects on cognitive function. Recent studies show that the interaction between cholesterol and APP in the plasma membrane is necessary for Aβ synthesis and clearance. Tg2576 AD mice raised on a diet supplemented with high fat and high cholesterol displayed increased production of Aβ. When these animals were treated with cholesterol lowering drugs the brain amyloid levels were reduced by more than 2-fold (Nizari et al., 2016).

Impact of Aβ Oligomers on Insulin Resistance

Soluble oligomers of Aβ42 have been shown to be the most toxic species to the neurons. In the brains of AD patients with MCI, Aβ oligomers have been shown to correlate with rapid cognitive decline (Ferreira et al., 2015). Also, in the brain and CSF of AD patients the level of soluble oligomers ranging from trimer to 24-mer or higher is significantly elevated when compared to levels found in non-demented controls (Jimenez et al., 2014). Studies in human APP overexpressing Tg2576 AD mice show that the onset of memory deficits correlate with production of soluble Aβ oligomers. Small oligomers of Aβ, particularly dimers and trimers that are formed within the neurons *in vitro* are secreted into conditioned medium. The treatment of rat hippocampal slices or live animals with these oligomers showed potent LTP defects and cognitive deficits (Puzzo et al., 2017). Similarly, synaptotoxicity is observed when soluble Aβ oligomers isolated from the brains and CSF of AD patients are applied to brain tissue slices or live animals (Minkeviciene et al., 2009). These, inhibitory effects are blocked by Aβ antibodies and γ-secretase inhibitors (Goure et al., 2014). This LTP blockage is also restored by treatment with 1μM insulin (Sakono and Zako, 2010). These observations were confirmed by other investigators who demonstrated that Aβ42 oligomers were more potent in blocking LTP than monomers and this effect was rescued by insulin by preventing Aβ oligomerization (Selkoe, 2008; Mucke and Selkoe, 2012).

Recent evidence indicates an intimate connection between brain insulin resistance and the formation of Aβ oligomers. In a study by Zhao et al. the scientists found that the treatment of primary hippocampal neurons by soluble Aβ oligomers results in a profound loss of insulin receptors from the neuronal surface. In addition, Aβ oligomers were found to increase the AKT phosphorylation at Serine-473 residue which results in insulin resistance (Zhao and Townsend, 2009). In addition, Aβ oligomers inhibit insulin signaling by phosphorylating IRS1 at inhibitory serine residues via the JNK/TNF alpha pathway (De Felice et al., 2009). Conversely, treating AD patients and transgenic animals with intranasal insulin lowers the concentration of soluble Aβ and improves memory (De Felice et al., 2009). Aβ-induced insulin resistance was also observed in the Familial AD (5XFAD) transgenic mouse models that overexpress high levels of mutant APP and PS1 and display severe amyloid pathology since 2 months of age (Mosconi et al., 2008).

Overall these studies demonstrate a strong impact of insulin resistance, hyperglycemia, dyslipidemia, and other hallmarks of T2DM on the pathological effects of Aβ amyloidogenesis as observed in AD.

CROSSTALK OF T2DM AND TAU PATHOLOGY IN AD

The traditional physiological function of tau protein is to promote assembly and stabilization of microtubules, though newer, atypical functions are now being reported (Sotiropoulos et al., 2017). There are about 80 Ser/Thr and 5 Tyr phosphorylation sites on tau that are phosphorylated by the key tau kinases namely GSK-3β, MARK/PAR1, and CDK5 (Stoothoff and Johnson, 2005; Chatterjee et al., 2009). While in the normal brain, tau contains 2–3 moles of phosphate/mole of tau protein; in abnormal situations as seen in AD brains and other tauopathies, tau becomes hyperphosphorylated with 6–9 moles of phosphate/mole of tau and aggregates to form intracellular neurofibrillary tangles, one of the pathological hallmarks of AD (Iqbal et al., 2010).

A wealth of emerging studies in recent years indicate that the density of the neurofibrillary tau tangles deposited at the neocortex of the brains of MCI patients correlated more strongly with the severity of the disease (Bierer et al., 1995; Nelson et al., 2012). This study showed that learning and memory defects were more acute in patients with higher accumulation of the tangles in the temporal lobe which is the brain region associated with learning and memory. Thus, the post translational modifications of tau (hyperphosphorylation, truncation, acetylation, and glycation) and associated cellular and biochemical changes that cause these abnormal structural alterations are of potential interest for the development of tau targeted therapeutic studies.

Two of the important features of T2DM namely insulin resistance and hyperglycemia are able to influence post translational modifications of tau and exacerbate tau pathology, discussed below:

Impact of Insulin Resistance on Tau Kinases and Phosphatases

Under physiological conditions, a host of kinases and phosphatases regulate the intricate balance between tau phosphorylation and dephosphorylation to maintain neuronal homeostasis. Several protein kinases such as GSK-3β, CDK5, MARK, PKA, PKB/AKT, and MAPK including ERK1/2, c-JUN N terminal kinase (JNK) and p38 are the important kinases that phosphorylate tau (Avila, 2008; Gómez-Sintes et al., 2011).

Among these kinases, AKT and GSK-3β are located downstream of one arm of the insulin signaling pathway while components of the MAPK pathway lie downstream of the other arm (Fröjdö et al., 2009). AKT phosphorylates GSK-3β at the inhibitory Serine-9 residue and maintains GSK-3β in the inactive form. However, under conditions of insulin resistance, GSK-3β is converted to its active form by phosphorylation at Tyrosine-216 residue. Active GSK-3β then hyperphosphorylates tau to generate the pathological epitopes AT8, AT100, and PHF1 which make up the pre-tangles and NFTs in the AD brains (Clodfelder-Miller et al., 2005).

Several other studies have found that p70S6 ribosomal protein kinase—an AKT/mTOR substrate can directly phosphorylate tau and upregulate its synthesis through phosphorylation of S6 (Yoon, 2017).

These key pathways, namely PI3K/AKT, MAPK, and mTOR/p70S6K are regulated by insulin binding to the insulin receptor and trigger downstream phosphorylation events (Fröjdö et al., 2009). Thus, it is not surprising that in an insulin resistant state, insulin is unable to activate these pathways thereby disrupting physiological tau phosphorylation. Additionally, in diabetic brains p38 and JNK activation can cause insulin resistance by inhibiting the insulin receptor substrate and trigger tau hyperphosphorylation and pathological events (Wu et al., 2013).

Tau is also regulated by phosphatases especially PP2A that dephosphorylates it at crucial residues Thr205, Thr212, and Ser 262 that are phospho-epitopes of GSK-3β and MARK/PAR-1. In addition, PP2A dephosphorylates the kinases GSK-3β and p70S6K to maintain tau phosphorylation at a physiological level (Gratuze et al., 2017). Interestingly, several researchers have shown a downregulation of PP2A in both T1DM and T2DM mice suggesting that insulin resistance might exacerbate tau phosphorylation by downregulating PP2A (Qu et al., 2011; Jung et al., 2013).

The impact of isolated CNS-specific insulin resistance on tau phosphorylation was investigated *in vivo* by Schubert et al. using NIRKO mice where the brain/neuron specific IR gene was conditionally inactivated. They found that NIRKO mice displayed a complete loss of insulin-mediated PI3K/AKT signaling resulting in reduced phosphorylation of GSK-3β at Serine-9 and increased tau phosphorylation. However, these animals did not exhibit any change in survival or learning and memory defects or basal brain glucose metabolism (Schubert et al., 2004). In another study modeling peripheral insulin resistance in IRS2 knock out (KO) mice Schubert and colleagues show that neurofibrillary tangles composed of hyperphosphorylated tau aggregates accumulate in the hippocampus of IRS2 KO mice, revealing a direct molecular link between diabetes and Alzheimer's disease (Schubert et al., 2003). Likewise, Cheng et al. in IGF KO mouse brains displayed increased tau phosphorylation at Ser-396 and Ser-202 residues both of which are implicated in neurodegeneration (Cheng et al., 2005). In STZ-induced Type 1 diabetic mouse models, Planel and colleagues observed a robust increase in tau hyperphosphorylation that prevented tau from binding to microtubules (Planel et al., 2007). The scientists further observed that a downregulation in the activity of PP2A in these transgenic models exacerbated tau pathology. Similarly, Yazi and colleagues administered STZ to induce diabetes in pR5 mice expressing P301L mutation. Compared to non-transgenic controls, the pR5 mice displayed massive tau hyper-phosphorylation with the formation of neurofibrillary tangles by 6 months of age (Ke et al., 2009). In addition, other studies show that treatment of STZ-induced diabetic mice with GSK-3β inhibitors improves learning and memory functions (King et al., 2013). All these studies study provide compelling evidence that both Type 1 and Type 2 diabetes can accelerate onset and disease progression in individuals with a predisposition to developing tau pathology.

Impact of Insulin Resistance on Tau Cleavage

In addition to hyperphosphorylation, another abnormal post-translational modification of tau is truncation. Tau is cleaved by a host of proteolytic enzymes including caspases, calpains, thrombins, and puromycin-sensitive amino peptidase. These truncated tau fragments lack both N terminal and C terminal fragments and form the core component of NFTs (Karsten et al., 2006; Zilka et al., 2006).

In AD brains, caspases are activated causing tau protein to be cleaved at several residues. The C-terminal cleavage of tau by caspase-3 gives rise to Asp421 residue that has a higher propensity of aggregation and is found to be associated with neurofibrillary pathology in AD brains. The presence of Asp421 truncated tau in the neurofibrillary aggregates observed in the neurons of double transgenic mice (Tet/GSK-3β/VLW) and in P301S mouse models of tauopathy indicates that the formation of Asp421 cleavage product is an important step toward formation and maturation of tau aggregates (Basurto-Islas et al., 2008; Gendron and Petrucelli, 2009; Gómez-Sintes et al., 2011).

Diabetes has been known to stimulate apoptosis by the activation of caspase-3 in affected tissues (Savu et al., 2013). Using an animal model of T2DM, Kim et al. in their studies demonstrated an increased level of tau phosphorylation and cleavage in the brains of db/db mice which are models for diabetic dyslipidemia (Kim B. et al., 2013). Feldman and colleagues found that hyperglycemia promotes tau cleavage by activation of caspases (Kim et al., 2009). Thus, these studies demonstrate that T2DM enhances the formation of tau truncated fragments by caspase activation that contribute toward an increased risk of AD in diabetic patients.

Impact of Hyperglycemia on Other Posttranslational Modifications of Tau

Acetylation is a post translational modification in which the acetyl group from acetyl CoA is reversibly transferred to lysine ε amino group in the tau protein. This process is modulated by acetyltransferases and deacetylases (Cook et al., 2014). Cohen et al. observed that tau acetylation at the key lysine residues at K/163/280/281/369 was crucial for tau-microtubule binding interactions and microtubule stabilization. Using cellular and transgenic mouse models as well as human brains from a wide spectrum of tauopathies this group has demonstrated that tau acetylation disrupts the tau-microtubule binding interactions and promotes pathological tau aggregation. This group further demonstrated that acetylated tau was associated with the formation of insoluble tau NFTs in tau transgenic mice and human tauopathies indicating "acetylation" as a pathogenic post-translational modification of tau (Cohen et al., 2011).

Protein acetylation plays an important role in intermediary metabolism and metabolic disorders including T2DM. Mass spectrometry on STZ-induced diabetic rats showed high levels of lysine-acetylated proteins in their kidney cells compared to control animals (Kosanam et al., 2014). Also, treatment of murine aorta cells with high glucose or FFA to induce short term diabetes causes increased levels of lysine acetylation (Samuel et al., 2017). Although, there are very few reports, aberrant acetylation of tau in T2DM may interfere with the physiological functions of microtubule binding and assembly predisposing cytoplasmic tau toward the formation of aggregates (Irwin et al., 2013; Trzeciakiewicz et al., 2017).

Glycosylation involves the attachment of oligosachharide moieties to proteins and lipids. O-glycosylation is the linkage of sugar residues to the hydroxyl groups of Serine or Threonine residues while N-glycosylation involves attaching the sugar moieties to the amine group of the aspargine residues in proteins (Wang et al., 1996). Impaired OGlcNAc cycling is implicated in AD. In *post-mortem* AD brains Zhu et al. have demonstrated a significant decrease of O-GlcNAc glycosylation of tau proteins compared to controls (Zhu et al., 2014). Other studies from AD patients show hyperphosphorylated but hypo-O-GlcNAc glycosylated tau implying that phosphorylation and O-glycosylation at Serine and Threonine residues act in opposition (Wang et al., 1996; Iqbal et al., 2010). *In vitro* studies in NMR and Mass spectrometry analysis by Smet-Nocca et al. demonstrated that tau hyper phosphorylation at residues Ser-396 and Ser-404 were reduced by O-glycosylation at Ser-400 (Smet-Nocca et al., 2011). Treatment of mouse models of AD with OGA inhibitor Thiamet-G (that increases the levels of O-GlcNAcylation of tau) was found to decrease the levels of NFT burden and pathological tau species and slow down disease progression (Robertson et al., 2004; Gong et al., 2005; Yuzwa et al., 2012). However, it is interesting that Thiamet-G decreases tau phosphorylation over a short period of time and prolonged OGA inhibition has no effect on phosphorylation. This is probably due to cellular adaptability over time. Compared to O-glycosylation, *in vitro* studies show that N-glycosylated tau isolated from AD brain promotes tau hyperphosphorylaton (Liu Y. et al., 2009). Taken together these studies demonstrate that glycosylation exerts varying effects on tau hyperphosphorylation.

Although it is still speculative, it has been hypothesized that abnormal glucose metabolism in the brain induced by T2DM may lead to decreased brain O-GlcNAc levels. This reflects a failure in the neuroprotective mechanism in the brain and triggers the cascade of tau pathology enabling disease progression.

Impact of Tau on Insulin Resistance

While insulin resistance stimulates tau hyperphosphorylation and aggregation, in a recent study Rodriguez-Rodriguez and colleagues have shown that pathological alterations in tau (hyperphosphorylation and aggregation) accumulates insulin. In this study, the researchers have shown that insulin accumulates in the sarcosyl-insoluble fractions of the AD brain. Moreover, the researchers found increased accumulation of insulin *in vivo* in the brains of tau overexpressing P301S mice and SHSY5Y cells as well as in okadoic acid treated primary neuronal cultures. Both the cells and primary neurons demonstrated increased insulin uptake from the surroundings that eventually led to insulin resistance (Rodriguez-Rodriguez et al., 2017). Another study shows impaired insulin sensitivity in hippocampal slices from tau KO mice compared to litter-mate controls (Marciniak et al., 2017).

These studies suggest a complex relationship between tau and insulin resistance as it is evident that not only insulin resistance can exacerbate tau pathology but pathological tau phosphorylation or absence of tau can affect neuronal insulin resistance.

SYNAPTIC DYSFUNCTIONS AT THE CROSSROADS OF AD AND T2DM

There is widespread neuronal loss and atrophy of the cortex and hippocampus in the brains of AD patients (Sheng et al., 2012). The cognitive failure in AD patients is accompanied by loss in synapses and neuronal cell death with a marked reduction in brain volumes particularly at the entorhinal cortex and hippocampus. Although plaques and tangles characterize the neuropathological features of AD, the closest correlation to the severity of disease progression is the synapse loss that occurs in the disease. There are conflicting reports as to whether the amyloid plaques or NFTs correlate more strongly with disease progression. Some scientists have reported that the spatiotemporal signature of NFTs of tau correlate more severely with the disease pathology (Nelson et al., 2012; Horvath et al., 2013). However, investigating the "neurodegenerative triad" Tackenberg et al. have shown that the loss of dendritic spines and LTP that occurs early in the disease is mediated by Aβ while the late stage cell death mediated by NMDAR requires tau phosphorylation (Tackenberg and Brandt, 2009).

Alterations in synaptic transmission and plasticity are also observed in the hippocampus of diabetic animal models including depletion of synaptic vesicles at presynaptic sites and changes of AMPA and NMDA receptors at the postsynaptic sites. Moreover, diabetes affected the synthesis and release of both inhibitory and excitatory neurotransmitters (Gaspar et al., 2016). All of these factors have the potential to activate synaptic dysfunction and widespread neuronal loss thereby predisposing the diabetic brain to AD. In this section the impact of T2DM on Aβ and tau mediated dysfunctions will be elaborated.

Synaptic Dysfunctions in AD

Recent studies indicate that cognitive ability in AD patients is closely related to the alterations of the density of the presynaptic glutamatergic boutons with an elevation of the glutamatergic synapses in MCI patients and a gradual depletion of the boutons with the progression of AD (Bell et al., 2007).

Aβ and Synaptic Dysfunction

There are numerous reports that show Aβ oligomers can cause synaptic dysfunction and toxicity (LaFerla and Oddo, 2005; Shankar and Walsh, 2009). Under physiological conditions, low concentration of monomeric Aβ is essential for maintaining synaptic plasticity and neuronal survival with the improvement of cognitive abilities. Conversely, in the disease state higher concentration of Aβ together with aging causes synaptic dysfunction followed by neuronal loss as seen in AD. Recent studies show that APP and BACE1 KO mice display pronounced defects in LTP and memory functions (Tyan et al., 2012). Puzzo et al. showed that the treatment of mouse brain hippocampal slices with low concentrations (200 picomoles) of synthetic Aβ42 monomers and oligomers increased the LTP. This study suggests that LTP is mediated by α7-nicotinic acetylcholine receptors indicating a presynaptic role of Aβ. Likewise, treatment with nanomolar concentration of Aβ produced synaptic depression. This indicates that an optimal level of Aβ is needed for synaptic transmission (Puzzo et al., 2017).

Elevated levels of Aβ impairs glutamatergic transmission by decreasing the number of AMPA and NMDA receptors on the surface of the neurons. Moreover, increased concentration of Aβ results in the internalization of NMDA receptors enhancing LTD at the synapses. LTD causes a significant loss of dendritic spines that is associated with early symptoms of AD and disease progression (Palop and Mucke, 2010). EEG recording from cortical and hippocampal networks In human APP overexpressing mouse models shows that high levels of Aβ oligomers elicits epileptic and nonconvulsive seizures (LaFerla and Oddo, 2005). Consistent with these findings, *in vivo* calcium imaging of cortical circuits shows that double transgenic (hAPP/PS1) mice have a greater proportion of hyperactive and hypoactive neurons than nontransgenic control (Palop and Mucke, 2010; Puzzo et al., 2017). AD transgenic mice showed an increased neuronal activity in the hippocampal regions before the formation of insoluble amyloid plaques. On treatment with a γ-secretase inhibitor, soluble Aβ levels were reduced and the neuronal activity decreased implying that this effect was a soluble Aβ-dependent effect (Busche et al., 2012). Although the mechanisms are not completely elucidated, these studies suggest that Aβ-dependent effects on synaptic plasticity and neurotransmission are tightly controlled by the activation of α7-nicotinic acetylcholine receptors or NMDARs and involves downstream effector components including p38 MAPK and GSK-3β (Baglietto-Vargas et al., 2016).

T2DM may trigger Aβ-mediated synaptic dysfunction in multiple ways. Hyperinsulinemia in T2DM promotes the formation of Aβ oligomers that cause synaptotoxicity. Investigators have shown that when Aβ oligomers are applied *in vitro* to rat hippocampal slices or *in vivo* to live animals they blocked LTP and inhibited memory formation (Busche et al., 2012). Interestingly, this effect is overcome by 1μm insulin. A similar result was reported by Li et al. who observed that Aβ monomers were more effective than Aβ oligomers in inhibiting LTP and that insulin prevented Aβ-induced LTP defects by blocking Aβ oligomerization (Balducci et al., 2010; Li et al., 2011). Previous studies have shown that Aβ oligomers are capable of binding to insulin receptors which causes an impairment of receptor functions (Bradley et al., 2012; Uranga et al., 2013). In addition, it has been shown that Aβ oligomers alter GSK-3β phosphorylation state and directly impacts the ERK pathway (Magrane et al., 2006; Reddy, 2013).

Tau and Synaptic Dysfunction

Recent research suggests an emerging role of tau at the synapse (Pooler et al., 2014). Physiologically tau is localized primarily in the axons where it binds and regulates microtubule dynamics in a phosphorylation dependent manner (Janning et al., 2014). However, recent isolation and analysis of AD brain-derived synaptoneurosomes indicate that tau is present in both pre-synaptic and post-synaptic compartments (Tai et al., 2012). There are multiple mechanisms by which tau could mediate synaptic function and neuronal excitability. Recent study has shown that tau binds to the post-synaptic protein complex which includes the PSD-95 through Fyn kinase. The interaction of tau and Fyn appears to be crucial for directing Fyn to the postsynaptic compartments where it can regulate the NMDA receptor by phosphorylating one of its subunits. Abnormal tau phosphorylation can disrupt the tau-Fyn interaction and affect postsynaptic receptor targeting (Haass and Mandelkow, 2010). Thus, neurons from conditionally overexpressing P301L tau mice display impaired targeting of excitatory glutamate receptors to dendritic spines. In addition, biochemical analysis of the synaptosomes from these mice display a marked decrease in the levels of synaptic markers (PSD95, Synapsin, NMDAR1, and GluR1) implying that the loss of functional synapses plays an important role in maintaining postsynaptic integrity (Katsuse et al., 2006; Spires-Jones and Hyman, 2014). Electron microscopy of NFT-carrying motor neurons in P301L mice revealed a significant decrease in the number and size of synaptic boutons compared to nontransgenic controls. These studies point out that loss of synapses occur during neurodegeneration. Evidence for tau involvement in regulating neuronal excitability comes from a study in which a reduction in tau levels reduced hyperexcitability in a mouse model of seizure (Holth et al., 2013; Guerrero-Muñoz et al., 2015). Other studies have found that neurons isolated from transgenic Tg4510 mice overexpressing 0N4R P301L mutation were more excitable than neurons from nontransgenic mice (Kopeikina et al., 2013). However, it is worth noting that the animal models mostly express mutant tau protein and therefore could be more representative of FTDP-17 cases than AD.

Although there are fewer reports, glucotoxicity in T1 and T2DM are capable of influencing tau-mediated synaptic impairments. Investigators have shown synaptic defects and cognitive impairments in STZ-induced diabetic models, where genetically ablating tau ameliorated cognitive defects. (Abbondante et al., 2014). Using a mouse model of tauopathy, scientists have observed that under glucose-deprived conditions as observed in hypometabolic AD brains, transgenic mice had impaired memory and reduced LTP accompanied by tau hyperphosphorylation and apoptosis (Lauretti et al., 2017).

Synaptic Dysfunctions in Diabetes That Influence Neurodegeneration

Other than directly influencing Aβ and tau-mediated synaptic defects, diabetes also affects the synthesis and release of key neurotransmitters that may underlie cognitive defects. For instance under chronic hyperglycemia extracellular brain levels of GABA and glutamate were decreased in STZ-induced diabetic animal models (van Bussel et al., 2016). An imbalance between excitatory and inhibitory neurotransmission impaired the cognitive deficits observed in these animals. Diabetes also affects acetylcholine esterase that plays a crucial role in cognitive processes. Recent studies have shown a reduction of cholinergic transmission in the hippocampus of STZ-induced diabetic animals (Molina et al., 2014). Moreover, in the STZ-induced animals, treatment of hippocampal slices with insulin resulted in a significant decrease in the number of NMDA receptors that consequently affected LTP and decreased postsynaptic densities (van der Heide et al., 2005).

Taken together these results suggest that both Type 1 and Type 2 diabetes are able to directly influence Aβ and tau-mediated synaptic dysfunctions. In addition, both these subtypes cause an imbalance of neurotransmitter release and alterations in synaptic plasticity that ultimately leads to memory impairments. Hence, synaptic dysfunctions form a shared pathological trait between AD and T2DM.

INFLAMMATION: SHARED PATHOPHYSIOLOGY OF AD AND T2DM

Emerging evidence in recent times points toward a compelling link between inflammation and the pathogenesis of Alzheimer's disease since Aβ plaques and NFTs colocalize with glial cells (Serrano-Pozo et al., 2011). T2DM disease pathogenesis in particular involves high levels of ER and oxidative stress response that might trigger the inflammatory cascade (Back and Kaufman, 2012). Additionally, misfolded toxic protein species detected in AD and T2DM may generate oxidative stress and activate inflammatory pathways. In this section, we discuss the role of inflammation in AD and T2DM and how this impacts the shared pathophysiology in both these diseases.

Inflammation and AD Pathology

Recently preclinical, genetic, and bioinformatics studies have shown that the immune system activation accompanies AD pathology. The genome wide association studies (GWAS) between AD and rare mutations in the genes encoding triggering receptor expressed on myeloid cells 2 (TREM2) and myeloid cell surface antigen CD33 provide clear evidence that there is a strong linkage between alterations in the immune system and the progression of AD pathology (Griciuc et al., 2013; Ulrich et al., 2017).

Based on the amyloid cascade hypothesis, the Aβ deposition is followed by immune system activation mediated by glial cells such as microglia and astrocytes. This is supported by electron microscopy studies that show increased accumulation of glial cells surrounding the amyloid plaque deposits in AD brain (Wyss-Coray et al., 2003). However, recent data of cerebrospinal fluid analysis from patients with symptoms of MCI has demonstrated a marked alteration in the inflammatory markers implying their involvement early in the disease pathway (Zotova et al., 2010; Wyss-Coray, 2012). In another significant study, scientists showed that systemic immune challenge elicited by injecting viral mimics of polyriboinosinic-polyribocytidilic acid resulted in "sporadic AD" like features in wild-type mouse models accompanied by Aβ deposition, tau pathology, microglia activation, and reactive gliosis implying that alterations in the immune system can precede AD pathology and drive the disease itself (Michalovicz et al., 2015). In addition, tissue microarrays from patients with neurodegenerative diseases including AD revealed an upregulation of inflammatory components further suggesting an intimate linkage between inflammatory markers and AD, early in the pathogenic cascade (Sekar et al., 2015).

Aβ and Inflammation

In AD brains, microglia and astrocytes have been known to accumulate around neuritic plaques and are associated with the tissue damages that occur in AD. Aβ oligomers and fibrils are capable of binding to receptors expressed by microglia including CD14, CD36, CD47, a6β1 integrin, RAGE, and Toll-like receptors (TLRs) (Doens and Fernandez, 2014). *In vitro* studies have shown that binding of Aβ to RAGE receptors, helps guide microglia to Aβ deposits and this effect is inhibited by anti-RAGE antibodies (Wyss-Coray, 2012). Binding of Aβ to CD36 or TLR4, on the other hand, results in the production of inflammatory chemokines and cytokines that eventually lead to increased neuronal damage in vulnerable regions of the AD brain (Doens and Fernandez, 2014). Besides the secretion of inflammatory cytokines, microglia are found to phagocytose soluble Aβ oligomers via the extracellular proteases such as neprilysin and insulin-degrading enzyme (IDE). However, there are evidences of Aβ dependent impairment of microglial phagocytosis functions in AD mouse models (Koenigsknecht and Landreth, 2004). Recent studies have shown that microglia isolated from AD transgenic mouse models displayed a substantial reduction in the levels of Aβ-binding scavenger receptor and Aβ-degrading enzyme (Zhao et al., 2017). Interestingly, it has been shown that transient depletion of dysfunctional microglia has no impact on Aβ deposition in an animal model of AD (Morimoto et al., 2011). This is because microglial impairment maybe compensated by inflammatory cytokines such as TNF, IL-1, IL-12, and IL-23 suggesting a negative feedback loop, that might exacerbate the AD pathology (Rubio-Perez and Morillas-Ruiz, 2012). In addition, an upregulation in the levels of inflammatory markers has been demonstrated in animal models of AD or in the brains or CSF of AD patients (Moro et al., 2018).

Recently a huge repertoire of GWAS studies show that structural variants of genes encoding immune receptors TREM2, CD33, and CR1, all of which are expressed in the microglia confer higher risk of AD (Tosto and Reitz, 2013). However, the function of TREM2 deficiency in the progression of AD has been controversial. For instance, while TREM2 deficiency in APP/PS1 mice ameliorated hippocampal Aβ accumulation; the 5XFAD mice displayed an opposite result. In these mice the Aβ pathology was found to develop slower than APP/PS1 mice and increased accumulation of hippocampal Aβ was observed in the absence of TREM2 (Bemiller et al., 2017; Jay et al., 2017). Elevated levels of soluble TREM2 was detected in the CSF of early AD patients suggesting a change in microglial activation in response to neuronal death. Although the exact mechanism still remains to be deciphered, these findings show that impaired TREM2 function plays a vital role in Aβ-mediated AD pathogenesis.

The transmembrane protein CD33 is another microglial receptor the structural variants of which has led to increased risk of AD. A significant study from *post mortem* AD brains has shown the upregulation of CD33 compared to age-matched controls (Jiang et al., 2014). Conversely, the expression of a CD33 variant, namely the protective CD33 (SNP) rs3865444 was downregulated in AD brains and reduced insoluble Aβ deposits (Hu et al., 2014; Li et al., 2015b).

Astrocytes too respond to AD pathogenic stimuli by reactive gliosis. In transgenic AD mouse models exhibiting cerebral amyloidosis the activation of astrocytes occur in the early stages of pathogenesis. In these transgenic animals the astrocytes underwent severe atrophy which preceded the Aβ plaque mediated gliosis (Verkhratsky et al., 2010). Conversely, reducing astrocytes in a transgenic Aβ overexpressing mouse model ameliorated AD pathology (Garwood et al., 2017). The involvement of astrocytes in neuroinflammation entails increased production of cytokines that either affect the neurons directly or via microglial activation (Van Eldik et al., 2016). For instance, NFκβ-mediated activation of astrocytes release the complement protein C3 that can bind to neuronal C3aR and trigger neuronal damage. Another astrocyte signaling molecule is the soluble CD40 ligand that binds to microglial cell surface receptor. This binding interaction releases pro-inflammatory tumor necrosis alpha (TNF-α) that has been widely reported to contribute to tissue damage in AD (Van Eldik et al., 2016). Astrocytes also play a neuroprotective role. Recent studies have also shown that reactive astrocytes surrounding the Aβ plaques take up and degrade Aβ. For instance, in Tg2576 transgenic mice this has been shown to be linked to insulin degrading enzyme (IDE) which plays an important role in Aβ degradation. Reportedly, Aβ exposure of IDE enhanced the number of activated astrocytes surrounding the neuritic plaques (Wyss-Coray, 2012). Other studies have shown that treatment of astrocytes with *ex-vivo* Aβ extracts, increase the secretion of Aβ degrading enzymes (Wyss-Coray et al., 2003). Thus, the Aβ pathogenesis in AD may result in alterations of normal astrocyte functions which may be then trigger downstream inflammatory cascades prompting further neuronal damage in AD.

Tau and Inflammation

Although there are fewer reports, *in vitro* studies have shown that microglial cells stimulated by Aβ or LPS release pro-inflammatory cytokines such as interleukin-1β and activate tau phosphorylation at the pathological phospho-epitopes via MAPK pathway. This was confirmed by *in vivo* studies in 3xTg mouse model that displays both Aβ and tau pathologies. When these animals were subjected to high dose of LPS treatment, tau hyperphosphorylation was triggered at the pathological epitopes mediated by GSK-3β, CDK5, JNK, and MAP kinases (Barron et al., 2017). Several other studies have shown that the activation of the key kinases CDK5 and GSK-3β by themselves resulted in microglial activation and secretion of IL-1β implying a close link between tau hyperphosphorylation and pro-inflammatory markers. The gene expression profile analysis in a mouse model of tauopathy (rTg4510) which expresses the P301L mutation, revealed upregulation of pro-inflammatory markers such as complement 4B, glial fibrillary acidic protein (GFAP) and osteopontin (Spp1) on treatment with LPS. This result confirms that neuroinflammation modulates tau pathology in the absence of Aβ plaques (Wes et al., 2014). In addition, TREM2 levels were decreased in these transgenic mouse models indicating an alteration in microglial functions (Maphis et al., 2015). In this landmark study, Bhaskar et al. showed that LPS treatment of hTau mice expressing all 6 non-mutated tau isoforms enhanced microglial activation and accelerated tau pathology. These mice were deficient in microglia-specific fractalkine receptor (CX3CR1) that caused an exacerbation of tau hyperphosphorylation via p38/MAPK pathway. Further, studies in a P301S mutant human tau transgenic mice demonstrated that these animals displayed synaptic pathology and microgliosis before the onset of tangle formation confirming that microglial activation occurs early in the disease pathway. In this study, the researchers have shown that the immunosuppression of young P301S transgenic mice by FK506 significantly diminished tau pathology and increased their lifespan (Yoshiyama et al., 2007). These studies conclude that neuroinflammation accompanies early AD progression and blocking neuroinflammatory pathways might be beneficial in ameliorating tauopathies.

Hence, anti-inflammatory drugs have been used in clinical trials to prevent disease progression in AD. A study of nonsteroidal anti-inflammatory drugs (NSAIDS) in a Netherlands population (Rotterdam study) showed a significantly decreased risk of AD with increasing use of NSAIDS. In this study the short-term use of NSAID showed a relative risk of 0.95 while a long-term use of 24 months or more showed a relative risk of 0.2 with a confidence interval of 0.05–0.83 (In 't Veld et al., 1998). In a similar study reported in 2011 by Breitner et al. administration of NSAID Naproxen over a period of 2–3 years decreased the incidence of AD. These results were enhanced by measuring a marker of neurodegeneration, CSF ratios of tau to Aβ1-42 (Breitner et al., 2011). In contrast, a recent study by Marjerova et al. found that LPS treatment of immortalized microglial cells *in vitro* were capable of removing intracellular and extracellular tau oligomers by phagocytosis. These observations were validated *in vivo* in C57BL/6 mice. When injected with soluble and insoluble human tau aggregates, these mice displayed active microglial phagocytosis of both tau species (Barron et al., 2017). Thus, the suppression of immune system by anti-inflammatory drugs may not prove beneficial to AD treatment in the long run as these might enhance the spread of tau oligomers across healthy neurons.

Inflammation in Type 2 Diabetes That Influence Neurodegeneration

Type 2 Diabetes has been associated with excess immune system activation, which increases the expression of proinflammatory cytokines especially microglia in the brain. It is noteworthy that Swaroop et al. observed elevated levels of TNFα, IL-1β, IL-2, and IL-6 in the hippocampus of diabetic animals (Swaroop et al., 2012). Previous studies have shown that incubation of cells with TNFα or high levels of FFA promotes inhibitory phosphorylation of the serine residues of IRS-1. This impairs the ability of IRS-1 to interact with the insulin receptor and generates an insulin-resistant condition capable of triggering Aβ and tau pathological cascades (Peraldi et al., 1996). It has also been demonstrated that obesity and hyperglycemia in T2DM contributes to ER and mitochondrial stress that generates reactive oxygen species (ROS). Elevated ROS then causes enhanced activation of inflammatory pathways (Kaneto et al., 2010; Back and Kaufman, 2012).

Along with evidences that relate oxidative stress and inflammation to the pathophysiology of diabetes, studies performed in various cellular and animal models suggest NFκβ activation is a key event early in the disease pathobiology and its complications. Several studies have shown that NF-κβ is induced by hyperglycemia and in conditions of neuronal damage (Romeo et al., 2002; Wellen and Hotamisligil, 2005). The activation of NF-κβ is followed by the expression of pro-inflammatory cytokines that jointly trigger brain inflammation and neuronal apoptosis eventually leading to cognitive decline. For instance, in the hippocampus of the STZ-treated rats there is a strong increase of ROS followed by NF-κβ activation (Locke and Anderson, 2011). Activated NF-κβ can induce cytotoxicity, trigger inflammation and promote apoptosis (Jaeschke et al., 2004). In STZ-induced retinopathy rat models, NF-κβ activation has been associated with enhanced expression of caspase 1 (Yin et al., 2017). Recent reports show that NF-κβ might be an important regulator of insulin sensitivity in T2DM by controlling the expression of GLUT2 receptor which is important for glucose secretion and transport in pancreatic beta cells (Patel and Santani, 2009).

Incidentally, the metabolic stresses that promote insulin resistance and T2DM also activate the inflammation and stress-induced kinases Ikβ kinase-β (IKKβ) and JUN N-terminal kinase (JNK) suggesting that these kinases play an important role in disease pathogenesis. Both JNK and IKκβ can phosphorylate the IRS-1 at the inhibitory Serine 307 thereby impairing insulin action (Jaeschke et al., 2004; Morel et al., 2010).

Oxidative stress in insulin resistance generates FFA and AGE products which result in glucotoxicity and impairment of insulin signaling. These ligands act through Toll-like receptors (TLRs) and receptors for advanced glycation end products (RAGE) that are also activated in neurodegenerative diseases (Ozcan et al., 2004). RAGE especially acts as a putative Aβ receptor and plays a significant role in AD pathogenesis. It is therefore predicted that the cumulative effect of these stress factors may lead to neuronal apoptosis and brain inflammation, both of which are prominent features of neurodegenerative diseases including AD.

To investigate whether inflammatory pathways act as a potential link between AD and T2DM, Takeda et al. generated a dual model of AD and T2DM by crossing an APP23 transgenic mice that overexpresses human APP to leptin-deficient ob/ob mice or polygenic NSY mice as a model for diabetes. The APP+/ob/ob dual transgenics showed increased levels of amyloid deposition around brain microvessels and enhanced cerebrovascular inflammation even before the manifestation of cerebral amyloid angiopathy. (Takeda et al., 2010). The authors also report an increased levels of RAGE in blood vessels as well as elevated levels of TNFα and IL-6 in the brain microvasculature of these animals. Progressive cognitive deficits and increased cerebrovascular inflammation were also noted in APP_{+}-NSY dual transgenics raised on high-fat diet compared to NSY mice raised on the same diet. In a study conducted by Knight et al. a similar impact of high-fat diet was observed in 3xTg AD mice that overexpress triple mutations in human APP/MAPT-P301L/PSEN1 and in nontransgenic mice. When raised on a high-fat diet both the transgenics and the control animals displayed considerable weight gain and memory impairments. However, the memory impairments were more severe in the 3xTg mice compared to the controls. It is also interesting that although no significant differences were observed in the amyloid plaques and tau-tangle loads, the brains of 3xTg animals were accompanied by severe microgliosis that was not observed in age-matched controls. This strongly implies the role of neuroinflammation in the development of AD pathogenesis especially when subjected to abnormal dietary conditions (Knight et al., 2014).

Emerging studies have shown that loss of inflammatory mediators prevents insulin resistance, therefore pharmacological targeting of inflammatory pathways improve insulin action. For instance, salicylates activate insulin signaling by inhibiting inflammatory kinases within the cell (Kim M. S. et al., 2013). Similarly, targeting JNK using a synthetic inhibitor has been reported to enhance insulin signaling in obese mice and reduce atherosclerosis in ApoE mutant rodent model (Lee et al., 2003). There are yet other studies which show that thiazolidinediones (TZDs), high-affinity ligands of PPARγ act as insulin sensitizing agents and improve insulin action by activating lipid metabolism as well as by reducing the production of inflammatory molecules like TNFα (Peraldi et al., 1996).

These studies support a significant correlation between hyperglycemia, impaired insulin resistance, oxidative stress, and inflammation. All these factors are capable of directly impacting Aβ and tau pathologies as well as triggering a chain of inflammatory stress responses that might eventually lead to neurodegeneration as observed in AD.

AUTOPHAGIC IMPAIRMENTS IN AD AND T2DM

Intracellular accumulation of misfolded protein aggregates is a salient feature of most neurodegenerative diseases (Frake et al., 2015). Autophagy is the process by which such protein aggregates are cleared from the neurons and is important for maintaining neuronal homeostasis. As neurons age they accumulate toxic intracellular protein aggregates and damaged organelles such as mitochondria that must be immediately cleared for the neuron to function at a physiological level (Lee, 2012; Son et al., 2012). Recent studies show that autophagic machinery is also involved in the pathophysiology of T2DM and it regulates the normal function of pancreatic beta cells. Insulin resistance generates oxidative stress on insulin-responsive tissues, enhanced autophagy in these cases acts as a protective factor (Masini et al., 2009). Other than indirect effects, there are studies that report direct impact of insulin resistance on autophagy by an inhibition of the downstream mTOR signaling pathway (Blagosklonny, 2013). Although, the connection between AD and T2DM pathogenesis in terms of autophagic dysfunction is not well documented, in this section we elaborate on the shared pathophysiologies of autophagy malfunctioning in these diseases and elaborate on the mechanisms by which insulin resistance might impact autophagy impairment and exacerbate AD pathogenesis.

Autophagy Malfunction in AD

Macroautophagy is the most prevalent form of neuronal autophagy (Frake et al., 2015). In this process, cytoplasmic proteins and organelles are sequestered into double membrane bound structures called autophagosomes (**Figure 3**). In the next step, the autophagosomes fuse with the lysosomes to form autolysosomes or alternatively with endosomes to form amphisomes before fusing with lysosomes and finally the contents are degraded.

There is a substantial evidence that autophagy is dysregulated in the brains of AD patients. In 2005, Nixon and colleagues used immunogold labeling and electron microscopy techniques on AD brain biopsies of neocortical regions and detected diverse formations of immature autophagic vacuoles (AVs) in the dystrophic neurites (Nixon, 2007). The same phenomenon was also observed in transgenic animal models of AD. A study in PS-1/APP double transgenic mice showed that AVs were formed in dendrites and soma before the appearance of Aβ plaques compared to age-matched control animals (Nixon et al., 2005). Chen et al. using LC3-EGFP overexpressing 5X FAD mouse models and age-matched controls, observed increased accumulation of autophagosomes in the neurons of FAD-mouse models compared to the controls. This was more prominent under conditions of starvation. Interestingly, the macroautophagy induced by starvation in the transgenic animals was not sufficient to degrade the endogenous Aβ levels which resulted due to increased cellular uptake of extracellular Aβ (Chen et al., 2015). The importance of autophagy in the brain was highlighted in a study demonstrating that neuron-specific loss of autophagy proteins (ATG7 and ATG5) in mice results in neurodegeneration even when other pathological factors are absent (Frake et al., 2015). However, actual mechanisms underlying autophagic dysfunctions in AD has not been fully elucidated. Till date it is a matter of debate as to whether autophagy is the cause or a result of AD.

Presenilins as Autophagy Modulators

Neely et al. has shown that Presenilins play an important role in mediating autophagy as PS-1 has been shown to facilitate N-glycosylation of V0a1 subunit of the lysosomal vacuolar ATPase (v-ATPase) (Neely et al., 2011). FAD-associated mutations in PS-1 and PS-2 leads to an impairment of lysosomal function due to failed acidification of the internal lysosomal contents. This causes an increased accumulation of autophagosomes and a failure to fuse with dysfunctional lysosomes. In their study, Wilson et al. found that in PS-1–/– neurons both α and β synuclein are mislocalized to the lysosomes of the neuronal cell body and not in the presynaptic regions. The increased accumulation of synuclein suggests that PS-1 deficiencies play a crucial role in developing α-syn lesions in neurodegenerative diseases as observed in familial AD and PD (Wilson et al., 2004). Interestingly, Tung et al. found that non-neuronal and neuronal cells lacking PS-1 displayed reduced levels of p62 protein which serves as a "cargo receptor" for tau degradation. Their study suggests a novel mechanism by which the reduction PS-1 or its mutation in FAD impairs p62-dependent tau clearance (Tung et al., 2014).

Aβ as an Autophagy Modulator

There is a complex interplay between Aβ and autophagy. Several studies have shown that autophagy plays a crucial role in Aβ metabolism including Aβ production, secretion, and degradation (Nilsson et al., 2015). Autophagy facilitates the degradation and clearance of APP and all APP cleavage products comprising Aβ and APP-C-terminal-fragments. Deficiency of autophagy protein beclin 1 in cultured neurons and human APP transgenic mice resulted in elevated intraneuronal Aβ and formation of extracellular amyloid plaques. Overexpression of beclin 1 promoted neuronal autophagy, reduced Aβ levels, and ameliorated neurodegeneration (Pickford et al., 2008). Autophagy may also play a role in the secretion of Aβ into extracellular environment where it causes plaque formation. For instance, deletion of ATG7 in APP transgenic mice resulted in less amount of Aβ secretion and plaque formation (Xiong, 2015).

Interestingly, Aβ by itself could also be a regulator of autophagy as intracellular Aβ can activate autophagy by an AKT-dependent pathway or RAGE-CAMKβ-AMPK pathway by induction of mitochondrial ROS generation (Kim et al., 2017). Thus rapamycin, an mTOR inhibitor that upregulates autophagy, is able to reduce both Aβ pathology in AD mouse models and improve cognition (Spilman et al., 2010).

Several studies indicate that insulin resistance in T2DM inhibits the downstream mTOR pathway and activates autophagy. Insulin resistance also causes ER and oxidative

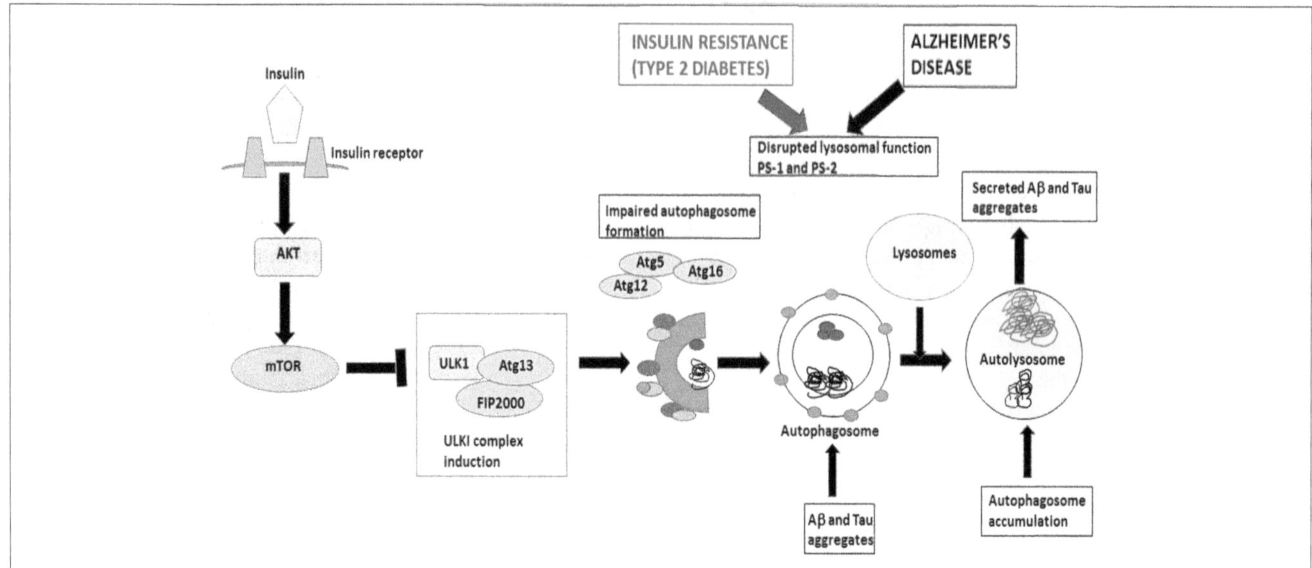

FIGURE 3 | Insulin signaling also controls mTOR pathway that inhibits autophagy. Both insulin resistance in Type 2 Diabetes and Alzheimer's disease impairs the formation of autophagosomes and disrupts lysosomal function. Autophagosomes fuse with lysosomes to form autolysosomes. These autolysosomes have impaired lysosomal function in AD and T2DM and accumulate Aβ and tau aggregates. Undigested toxic aggregates are secreted out of the neurons and propagate toxic oligomers in adjacent neurons.

stress that are capable of inducing autophagy (Quan et al., 2012). Ideally, enhanced autophagy should facilitate Aβ clearance; however, studies in ATG7 mouse models have shown that increased autophagy may also cause an increased secretion of Aβ in the extracellular matrix and enhance the deposition of Aβ plaques (Inoue et al., 2012). Thus, activation of autophagy under conditions of insulin resistance may worsen Aβ-mediated AD pathogenesis.

Tau and Autophagic Dysfunction

Recent studies suggest that autophagy plays a vital role in tau protein degradation and clearance (Inoue et al., 2012). A study in autophagy-impaired Nrf2 KO mice shows that the levels of phosphorylated and sarcosyl-insoluble tau increases (Jo et al., 2014). In ATG7 conditional KO mouse models the loss of ATG7 from the forebrains of transgenic mice leads to an accumulation of phospho-tau resembling pre-tangle formation within neurons (Inoue et al., 2012). On the restoration of autophagy, the levels of phospho-tau was found to be diminished. It has also been shown that the full-length tau (2N4R) and the caspase cleaved version (tauδC) are preferentially degraded by macroautophagy, while the truncated version of tau (taudelta280) is translocated to lysosomes by cell mediated autophagy (CMA) pathway (Dolan and Johnson, 2010).

Recent studies in primary neurons and transgenic P301S mouse models have demonstrated that treatment with autophagy-inducers trehalose and rapamycin reduced insoluble tau levels (Schaeffer et al., 2012; Ozcelik et al., 2013). Conversely, other studies have shown that mammalian target of rapamycin (mTOR) impairs tau clearance by inhibiting autophagy. The TSC1 and TSC2 are negative regulators of mTOR. Consequently, in TSC−/− transgenic mice the elevated levels of endogenous total and phosphorylated tau suggests an impairment of autophagy (Caccamo et al., 2013; Steele et al., 2013).

Under physiological conditions, tau promotes microtubule assembly and regulates microtubule dynamics (Janning et al., 2014). The microtubular arrays provide tracks for retrograde trafficking and maturation of autophagosomes before fusing with lysosomes in the soma (Kononenko, 2017). In the disease state, hyperphosphorylated tau is capable of disassembly and breakdown of microtubules that could subsequently inhibit retrograde trafficking causing the accumulation of immature autophagosomes within the axons (Rodríguez-Martín et al., 2013).

Autophagic Dysfunction in T2DM That Can Trigger AD Pathogenesis

Insulin resistance in T2DM effectively results in increased oxidative stress that causes the production of ROS leading to damage of intracellular organelles such as ER and mitochondria (Jung et al., 2011). These ER and mitochondrial stress factors are the critical upstream events for the induction of downstream autophagic pathways for the removal and clearance of misfolded proteins in the ER lumen and the dysfunctional ER and mitochondria (Quan et al., 2012). However, during prolonged periods of intracellular stress autophagy pathway becomes inefficient leading to increased accumulation of autophagosomes and impaired clearance. *In vivo* studies in pancreatic beta-cell specific ATG7 KO mice have shown a decrease in the number of pancreatic beta-cells, impaired glucose tolerance, and reduction in insulin secretion (Chen et al., 2011). In addition, these cells accumulate large ubiquitinated proteinaceous materials and p62 implying an autophagic impairment. Supporting these observations, Fujitani et al. demonstrated an increased accumulation of autophagosomes in the pancreas of db/db mice (Fujitani et al., 2009). In addition, these ATG7-null beta-cells were found to be apoptotic leading to a decreased beta cell mass. When these ATG7 KO mice were crossed to ob/ob mice (a model for obesity with a mutation in the leptin gene) the progeny displayed severe diabetes suggesting that autophagic impairment in obese animals might make them more susceptible to diabetes (Quan et al., 2012). These studies suggest that autophagy acts as a neuroprotective factor in response to ER and mitochondrial stress generated in T2DM.

To elucidate the autophagic impairments underlying AD and T2DM, Jung et al. compared tau pathology and its associated signaling pathways in diabetic OLEF rats and age-matched non-diabetic controls (Jung et al., 2011). The scientists observed an increased accumulation of total and phospho-tau in the soluble fractions of brain extracts from OLEF rats. Interestingly, the increased accumulation of polyubiquitinated tau protein in the neurons of OLEF rats was accompanied by a decrease in p62 protein levels that is responsible for degradation of ubiquitinated tau by autophagy and proteasomal pathways In a similar study by Carvalho et al. using 3xTgAD and T2DM mouse models, a significant reduction was observed in the levels of autophagy markers ATG7 and LC3-II in the cerebral cortex and hippocampus of both these mice (Carvalho et al., 2015). Pronounced behavioral deficits were observed in these animals that correlated strongly with a reduction of the autophagy markers including the lysosomal marker LAMP1 suggesting an accumulation of autophagosomes and impaired protein clearance in both these models. It can be inferred that the impaired clearance of toxic, soluble aggregates of hyperphosphorylated tau protein is a critical mechanism underlying increased AD-like pathology in T2DM.

Taken together, these results show that firstly insulin resistance in T2DM is capable of inducing prolonged period of oxidative stress which leads to the failure of autophagic machinery and impaired autophagic clearance. This in turn may lead to the progressive build-up of toxic protein aggregates such as Aβ and tau oligomers and trigger AD pathogenesis. Secondly, under abnormal metabolic conditions or aging, autophagic impairment might be a crucial risk factor for T2DM. This could lead to a viscous cycle in which T2DM can promote tau hyperphosphorylation and induce the accumulation of autophagosomes within the neurons. Impaired autophagic clearance then triggers neurodegenerative events that lead to AD pathogenesis. The crucial role played by autophagy in AD and T2DM opens a new chapter in the development of pro-autophagy drugs that would be used as part of combinatorial therapy in targeting both diseases.

CONCLUSION

In this review we have attempted to summarize the growing body of research that depicts the shared pathophysiology of AD and T2DM and elaborated on the underlying mechanistic pathways at the crossroads of these two diseases. However, it should be noted that almost all the animal models of Aβ and tau that have been used for preclinical studies are based on FTDP-17 cases and not on sporadic AD models. Although the mechanistic uderpinnings that link AD and T2DM could be similar, there is a possibility of considerable variation in the development and propagation of the disease pathology in the familial vs. sporadic cases. This is particularly relevant when designing combinatorial therapies.

A growing body of evidence suggests that the structural and functional integrity of the CNS is compromised in T2DM in the presence of excess insulin or under a condition of insulin resistance. In addition, T2DM impairs glucose metabolism and generates oxidative stress in vital cell organelles. Insulin resistance which is a prominent feature of T2DM is capable of increasing the production and secretion of Aβ by decreasing proteolysis by IDE. Also, insulin resistance dysregulates the PI3K/AKT/GSK-3β signaling cascade and generates hyperphosphorylated tau. Insulin resistance leads to loss of synapses, impaired autophagy and increased neuronal apoptosis. These alterations might trigger a cascade of events leading to abnormal Aβ and tau accumulation culminating in Alzheimer's disease pathology. Hence, targeting brain insulin signaling with pharmacological therapies used for treating T2DM is a novel and compelling approach to treat AD (Morris and Burns, 2012). This has given way to "drug-repositioning" strategies in which pre-existing anti-diabetic drugs are subjected to clinical trials to test their efficacy in AD therapeutics (Watson et al., 2005; Chen et al., 2009; Miller et al., 2011; Moore et al., 2013; Yarchoan and Arnold, 2014; Luchsinger et al., 2016; Femminella et al., 2017).

AUTHOR CONTRIBUTIONS

SC researched articles and prepared the manuscript for the review. AM critically revised the draft before submission.

FUNDING

Funded by European Union's Horizon 2020 research and innovation programme under Marie Sklodowska-Curie grant agreement number 705417.

REFERENCES

Abbondante, S., Baglietto-Vargas, D., Rodriguez-Ortiz, C. J., Estrada-Hernandez, T., Medeiros, R., and Laferla, F. M. (2014). Genetic ablation of tau mitigates cognitive impairment induced by type 1 diabetes. *Am. J. Pathol.* 184, 819–826. doi: 10.1016/j.ajpath.2013.11.021

American Diabetes, A. (2009). Diagnosis and classification of diabetes mellitus. *Diabetes Care 32(Suppl.* 1), S62–S67. doi: 10.2337/dc09-S062

Avila, J. (2008). Tau kinases and phosphatases. *J. Cell. Mol. Med.* 12, 258–259. doi: 10.1111/j.1582-4934.2007.00214.x

Avila, J., Leon-Espinosa, G., García, E., García-Escudero, V., Hernández, F., and Defelipe, J. (2012). Tau phosphorylation by GSK3 in different conditions. *Int. J. Alzheimers Dis.* 2012:578373. doi: 10.1155/2012/578373

Avila, J., Wandosell, F., and Hernández, F. (2010). Role of glycogen synthase kinase-3 in Alzheimer's disease pathogenesis and glycogen synthase kinase-3 inhibitors. *Expert. Rev. Neurother.* 10, 703–710. doi: 10.1586/ern.10.40

Back, S. H., and Kaufman, R. J. (2012). Endoplasmic reticulum stress and type 2 diabetes. *Annu. Rev. Biochem.* 81, 767–793. doi: 10.1146/annurev-biochem-072909-095555

Baglietto-Vargas, D., Shi, J., Yaeger, D. M., Ager, R., and LaFerla, F. M. (2016). Diabetes and Alzheimer's disease crosstalk. *Neurosci. Biobehav. Rev.* 64, 272–287. doi: 10.1016/j.neubiorev.2016.03.005

Balducci, C., Beeg, M., Stravalaci, M., Bastone, A., Sclip, A., Biasini, E., et al. (2010). Synthetic amyloid-β oligomers impair long-term memory independently of cellular prion protein. *Proc. Natl. Acad. Sci. U.S.A.* 107, 2295–2300. doi: 10.1073/pnas.0911829107

Barbagallo, M., and Dominguez, L. J. (2014). Type 2 diabetes mellitus and Alzheimer's disease. *World J. Diabetes* 5, 889–893. doi: 10.4239/wjd.v5.i6.889

Barron, H., Hafizi, S., Andreazza, A. C., and Mizrahi, R. (2017). Neuroinflammation and oxidative stress in psychosis and psychosis risk. *Int. J. Mol. Sci.* 18:651. doi: 10.3390/ijms18030651

Basurto-Islas, G., Luna-Munoz, J., Guillozet-Bongaarts, A. L., Binder, L. I., Mena, R., and Garcia-Sierra, F. (2008). Accumulation of aspartic acid421- and glutamic acid391-cleaved tau in neurofibrillary tangles correlates with progression in Alzheimer disease. *J. Neuropathol. Exp. Neurol.* 67, 470–483. doi: 10.1097/NEN.0b013e31817275c7

Beckett, L. A., Donohue, M. C., Wang, C., Aisen, P., Harvey, D. J., Saito, N., et al. (2015). The Alzheimer's disease neuroimaging initiative phase 2: increasing the length, breadth, and depth of our understanding. *Alzheimers Dement.* 11, 823–831. doi: 10.1016/j.jalz.2015.05.004

Bell, K. F., Bennett, D. A., and Cuello, A. C. (2007). Paradoxical upregulation of glutamatergic presynaptic boutons during mild cognitive impairment. *J. Neurosci.* 27, 10810–10817. doi: 10.1523/JNEUROSCI.3269-07.2007

Bemiller, S. M., McCray, T. J., Allan, K., Formica, S. V., Xu, G., Wilson, G., et al. (2017). TREM2 deficiency exacerbates tau pathology through dysregulated kinase signaling in a mouse model of tauopathy. *Mol. Neurodegener.* 12:74. doi: 10.1186/s13024-017-0216-6

Benedict, C., Hallschmid, M., Schultes, B., Born, J., and Kern, W. (2007). Intranasal insulin to improve memory function in humans. *Neuroendocrinology* 86, 136–142. doi: 10.1159/000106378

Bertram, L., and Tanzi, R. E. (2009). Genome-wide association studies in Alzheimer's disease. *Hum. Mol. Genet.* 18, R137–R145. doi: 10.1093/hmg/ddp406

Bierer, L. M., Hof, P. R., Purohit, D. P., Carlin, L., Schmeidler, J., Davis, K. L., et al. (1995). Neocortical neurofibrillary tangles correlate with dementia severity in Alzheimer's disease. *Arch. Neurol.* 52, 81–88. doi: 10.1001/archneur.1995.00540250089017

Blagosklonny, M. V. (2013). TOR-centric view on insulin resistance and diabetic complications: perspective for endocrinologists and gerontologists. *Cell Death Dis.* 4:e964. doi: 10.1038/cddis.2013.506

Blázquez, E., Velazquez, E., Hurtado-Carneiro, V., and Ruiz-Albusac, J. M. (2014). Insulin in the brain: its pathophysiological implications for States related with central insulin resistance, type 2 diabetes and Alzheimer's disease. *Front. Endocrinol.* 5:161. doi: 10.3389/fendo.2014.00161

Boucher, J., Kleinridders, A., and Kahn, C. R. (2014). Insulin receptor signaling in normal and insulin-resistant states. *Cold Spring Harb. Perspect. Biol.* 6:a009191. doi: 10.1101/cshperspect.a009191

Bradley, C. A., Peineau, S., Taghibiglou, C., Nicolas, C. S., Whitcomb, D. J., Bortolotto, Z. A., et al. (2012). A pivotal role of GSK-3 in synaptic plasticity. *Front. Mol. Neurosci.* 5:13. doi: 10.3389/fnmol.2012.00013

Breitner, J. C., Baker, L. D., Montine, T. J., Meinert, C. L., Lyketsos, C. G., Ashe, K. H., et al. (2011). Extended results of the Alzheimer's disease anti-inflammatory prevention trial. *Alzheimers Dement.* 7, 402–411. doi: 10.1016/j.jalz.2010.12.014

Busche, M. A., Chen, X., Henning, H. A., Reichwald, J., Staufenbiel, M., Sakmann, B., et al. (2012). Critical role of soluble amyloid-β for early hippocampal hyperactivity in a mouse model of Alzheimer's disease. *Proc. Natl. Acad. Sci. U.S.A.* 109, 8740–8745. doi: 10.1073/pnas.1206171109

Caccamo, A., Magri, A., Medina, D. X., Wisely, E. V., Lopez-Aranda, M. F., Silva, A. J., et al. (2013). mTOR regulates tau phosphorylation and degradation: implications for Alzheimer's disease and other tauopathies. *Aging Cell* 12, 370–380. doi: 10.1111/acel.12057

Carvalho, C., Santos, M. S., Oliveira, C. R., and Moreira, P. I. (2015). Alzheimer's disease and type 2 diabetes-related alterations in brain mitochondria, autophagy and synaptic markers. *Biochim. Biophys. Acta* 1852, 1665–1675. doi: 10.1016/j.bbadis.2015.05.001

Chatterjee, S., Sang, T. K., Lawless, G. M., and Jackson, G. R. (2009). Dissociation of tau toxicity and phosphorylation: role of GSK-3beta, MARK and Cdk5 in a Drosophila model. *Hum. Mol. Genet.* 18, 164–177. doi: 10.1093/hmg/ddn326

Cheignon, C., Tomas, M., Bonnefont-Rousselot, D., Faller, P., Hureau, C., and Collin, F. (2018). Oxidative stress and the amyloid beta peptide in Alzheimer's disease. *Redox. Biol.* 14, 450–464. doi: 10.1016/j.redox.2017.10.014

Chen, X., Kondo, K., Motoki, K., Homma, H., and Okazawa, H. (2015). Fasting activates macroautophagy in neurons of Alzheimer's disease mouse model but is insufficient to degrade amyloid-β. *Sci. Rep.* 5:12115. doi: 10.1038/srep12115

Chen, Y., Zhou, K., Wang, R., Liu, Y., Kwak, Y. D., Ma, T., et al. (2009). Antidiabetic drug metformin (GlucophageR) increases biogenesis of Alzheimer's amyloid peptides via up-regulating BACE1 transcription. *Proc. Natl. Acad. Sci. U.S.A.* 106, 3907–3912. doi: 10.1073/pnas.0807991106

Chen, Z. F., Li, Y. B., Han, J. Y., Wang, J., Yin, J. J., Li, J. B., et al. (2011). The double-edged effect of autophagy in pancreatic β cells and diabetes. *Autophagy* 7, 12–16. doi: 10.4161/auto.7.1.13607

Cheng, C. M., Tseng, V., Wang, J., Wang, D., Matyakhina, L., and Bondy, C. A. (2005). Tau is hyperphosphorylated in the insulin-like growth factor-I null brain. *Endocrinology* 146:508. doi: 10.1210/en.2005-0063

Cheng, D., Noble, J., Tang, M. X., Schupf, N., Mayeux, R., and Luchsinger, J. A. (2011). Type 2 diabetes and late-onset Alzheimer's disease. *Dement. Geriatr. Cogn. Disord.* 31, 424–430. doi: 10.1159/000324134

Chiang, S. H., Baumann, C. A., Kanzaki, M., Thurmond, D. C., Watson, R. T., Neudauer, C. L., et al. (2001). Insulin-stimulated GLUT4 translocation requires the CAP-dependent activation of TC10. *Nature* 410, 944–948. doi: 10.1038/35073608

Choi, B. R., Cho, W. H., Kim, J., Lee, H. J., Chung, C., Jeon, W. K., et al. (2014). Increased expression of the receptor for advanced glycation end products in neurons and astrocytes in a triple transgenic mouse model of Alzheimer's disease. *Exp. Mol. Med.* 46:e75. doi: 10.1038/emm.2013.147

Chouliaras, L., Sierksma, A. S., Kenis, G., Prickaerts, J., Lemmens, M. A., Brasnjevic, I., et al. (2010). Gene-environment interaction research and transgenic mouse models of Alzheimer's disease. *Int. J. Alzheimers Dis.* 2010:859101. doi: 10.4061/2010/859101

Clodfelder-Miller, B., De Sarno, P., Zmijewska, A. A., Song, L., and Jope, R. S. (2005). Physiological and pathological changes in glucose regulate brain Akt and glycogen synthase kinase-3. *J. Biol. Chem.* 280, 39723–39731. doi: 10.1074/jbc.M508824200

Cohen, T. J., Guo, J. L., Hurtado, D. E., Kwong, L. K., Mills, I. P., Trojanowski, J. Q., et al. (2011). The acetylation of tau inhibits its function and promotes pathological tau aggregation. *Nat. Commun.* 2:252. doi: 10.1038/ncomms1255

Cook, C., Stankowski, J. N., Carlomagno, Y., Stetler, C., and Petrucelli, L. (2014). Acetylation: a new key to unlock tau's role in neurodegeneration. *Alzheimers Res. Ther.* 6:29. doi: 10.1186/alzrt259

Criscuolo, C., Fontebasso, V., Middei, S., Stazi, M., Ammassari-Teule, M., Yan, S. S., et al. (2017). Entorhinal cortex dysfunction can be rescued by inhibition of microglial RAGE in an Alzheimer's disease mouse model. *Sci. Rep.* 7:42370. doi: 10.1038/srep42370

De Felice, F. G., and Ferreira, S. T. (2014). Inflammation, defective insulin signaling, and mitochondrial dysfunction as common molecular denominators connecting type 2 diabetes to Alzheimer disease. *Diabetes* 63, 2262–2272. doi: 10.2337/db13-1954

De Felice, F. G., Lourenco, M. V., and Ferreira, S. T. (2014). How does brain insulin resistance develop in Alzheimer's disease? *Alzheimers Dement.* 10, S26–S32. doi: 10.1016/j.jalz.2013.12.004

De Felice, F. G., Vieira, M. N., Bomfim, T. R., Decker, H., Velasco, P. T., Lambert, M. P., et al. (2009). Protection of synapses against Alzheimer's-linked toxins: insulin signaling prevents the pathogenic binding of Abeta oligomers. *Proc. Natl. Acad. Sci. U.S.A.* 106, 1971–1976. doi: 10.1073/pnas.0809158106 de la Monte, S. M., and Wands, J. R. (2008). Alzheimer's disease is type 3 diabetes-evidence reviewed. *J. Diabetes Sci. Technol.* 2, 1101–1113. doi: 10.1177/193229680800200619

De Strooper, B. (2007). Loss-of-function presenilin mutations in Alzheimer disease. *talking point on the role of presenilin mutations in Alzheimer disease. EMBO Rep.* 8, 141–146. doi: 10.1038/sj.embor.7400897

Deane, R., Singh, I., Sagare, A. P., Bell, R. D., Ross, N. T., LaRue, B., et al. (2012). A multimodal RAGE-specific inhibitor reduces amyloid beta-mediated brain disorder in a mouse model of Alzheimer disease. *J. Clin. Invest.* 122, 1377–1392. doi: 10.1172/JCI58642

Doens, D., and Fernandez, P. L. (2014). Microglia receptors and their implications in the response to amyloid β for Alzheimer's disease pathogenesis. *J. Neuroinflammation* 11:48. doi: 10.1186/1742-2094-11-48

Dolan, P. J., and Johnson, G. V. (2010). A caspase cleaved form of tau is preferentially degraded through the autophagy pathway. *J. Biol. Chem.* 285, 21978–21987. doi: 10.1074/jbc.M110.110940

Dorszewska, J., Prendecki, M., Oczkowska, A., Dezor, M., and Kozubski, W. (2016). Molecular basis of familial and sporadic Alzheimer's disease. *Curr. Alzheimer Res.* 13, 952–963. doi: 10.2174/1567205013666160314150501

Esparza, T. J., Wildburger, N. C., Jiang, H., Gangolli, M., Cairns, N. J., Bateman, R. J., et al. (2016). Soluble amyloid-beta aggregates from human Alzheimer's disease brains. *Sci. Rep.* 6:38187. doi: 10.1038/srep38187

Farrar, C., Houser, C. R., and Clarke, S. (2005). Activation of the PI3K/Akt signal transduction pathway and increased levels of insulin receptor in protein repair-deficient mice. *Aging Cell* 4, 1–12. doi: 10.1111/j.1474-9728.2004.00136.x

Farris, W., Mansourian, S., Chang, Y., Lindsley, L., Eckman, E. A., Frosch, M. P., et al. (2003). Insulin-degrading enzyme regulates the levels of insulin, amyloid beta-protein, and the beta-amyloid precursor protein intracellular domain *in vivo*. *Proc. Natl. Acad. Sci. U.S.A.* 100, 4162–4167. doi: 10.1073/pnas.0230450100

Femminella, G. D., Bencivenga, L., Petraglia, L., Visaggi, L., Gioia, L., Grieco, F. V., et al. (2017). Antidiabetic drugs in Alzheimer's Disease: mechanisms of action and future perspectives. *J. Diabetes Res.* 2017:7420796. doi: 10.1155/2017/7420796

Ferreira, S. T., Lourenco, M. V., Oliveira, M. M., and De Felice, F. G. (2015). Soluble amyloid-beta oligomers as synaptotoxins leading to cognitive impairment in Alzheimer's disease. *Front. Cell. Neurosci.* 9:191. doi: 10.3389/fncel.2015.00191

Fjell, A. M., Amlien, I. K., Sneve, M. H., Grydeland, H., Tamnes, C. K., Chaplin, T. A., et al. (2015). The roots of Alzheimer's disease: are high-expanding cortical areas preferentially targeted?dagger. *Cereb. Cortex* 25, 2556–2565. doi: 10.1093/cercor/bhu055

Frake, R. A., Ricketts, T., Menzies, F. M., and Rubinsztein, D. C. (2015). Autophagy and neurodegeneration. *J. Clin. Invest.* 125, 65–74. doi: 10.1172/JCI73944

Fröjdö, S., Vidal, H., and Pirola, L. (2009). Alterations of insulin signaling in type 2 diabetes: a review of the current evidence from humans. *Biochim. Biophys. Acta* 1792, 83–92. doi: 10.1016/j.bbadis.2008.10.019

Fujitani, Y., Kawamori, R., and Watada, H. (2009). The role of autophagy in pancreatic β-cell and diabetes. *Autophagy* 5, 280–282. doi: 10.4161/auto.5.2.7656

Garwood, C. J., Ratcliffe, L. E., Simpson, J. E., Heath, P. R., Ince, P. G., and Wharton, S. B. (2017). Review: Astrocytes in Alzheimer's disease and other age-associated dementias: a supporting player with a central role. *Neuropathol. Appl. Neurobiol.* 43, 281–298. doi: 10.1111/nan.12338

Gaspar, J. M., Baptista, F. I., Macedo, M. P., and Ambrosio, A. F. (2016). Inside the diabetic brain: role of different players involved in cognitive decline. *ACS Chem. Neurosci.* 7, 131–142. doi: 10.1021/acschemneuro.5b00240

Gasparini, L., Gouras, G. K., Wang, R., Gross, R. S., Beal, M. F., Greengard, P., et al. (2001). Stimulation of beta-amyloid precursor protein trafficking by insulin reduces intraneuronal beta-amyloid and requires mitogen-activated protein kinase signaling. *J. Neurosci.* 21, 2561–2570. doi: 10.1523/JNEUROSCI.21-08-02561.2001

Gendron, T. F., and Petrucelli, L. (2009). The role of tau in neurodegeneration. *Mol. Neurodegener.* 4:13. doi: 10.1186/1750-1326-4-13

Gilley, J., Ando, K., Seereeram, A., Rodriguez-Martin, T., Pooler, A. M., Sturdee, L., et al. (2016). Mislocalization of neuronal tau in the absence of tangle pathology in phosphomutant tau knockin mice. *Neurobiol. Aging* 39, 1–18. doi: 10.1016/j.neurobiolaging.2015.11.028

Gómez-Sintes, R., Hernandez, F., Lucas, J. J., and Avila, J. (2011). GSK-3 mouse models to study neuronal apoptosis and neurodegeneration. *Front. Mol. Neurosci.* 4:45. doi: 10.3389/fnmol.2011.00045

Gong, C. X., Liu, F., Grundke-Iqbal, I., and Iqbal, K. (2005). Post-translational modifications of tau protein in Alzheimer's disease. *J. Neural Transm.* 112, 813–838. doi: 10.1007/s00702-004-0221-0

Goure, W. F., Krafft, G. A., Jerecic, J., and Hefti, F. (2014). Targeting the proper amyloid-beta neuronal toxins: a path forward for Alzheimer's disease immunotherapeutics. *Alzheimers Res. Ther.* 6:42. doi: 10.1186/alzrt272

Gratuze, M., Julien, J., Petry, F. R., Morin, F., and Planel, E. (2017). Insulin deprivation induces PP2A inhibition and tau hyperphosphorylation in hTau mice, a model of Alzheimer's disease-like tau pathology. *Sci. Rep.* 7:46359. doi: 10.1038/srep46359

Griciuc, A., Serrano-Pozo, A., Parrado, A. R., Lesinski, A. N., Asselin, C. N., Mullin, K., et al. (2013). Alzheimer's disease risk gene CD33 inhibits microglial uptake of amyloid β. *Neuron* 78, 631–643. doi: 10.1016/j.neuron.2013.04.014

Guerrero-Muñoz, M. J., Gerson, J., and Castillo-Carranza, D. L. (2015). Tau oligomers: the toxic player at Synapses in Alzheimer's Disease. *Front. Cell. Neurosci.* 9:464. doi: 10.3389/fncel.2015.00464

Haass, C., and Mandelkow, E. (2010). Fyn-tau-amyloid: a toxic triad. *Cell* 142, 356–358. doi: 10.1016/j.cell.2010.07.032

Haataja, L., Gurlo, T., Huang, C. J., and Butler, P. C. (2008). Islet amyloid in type 2 diabetes, and the toxic oligomer hypothesis. *Endocr. Rev.* 29, 303–316. doi: 10.1210/er.2007-0037

Hanover, J. A., and Wang, P. (2013). O-GlcNAc cycling shows neuroprotective potential in C. *elegans models of neurodegenerative disease. Worm* 2:e27043. doi: 10.4161/worm.27043

Hernandez, F., Lucas, J. J., and Avila, J. (2013). GSK3 and tau: two convergence points in Alzheimer's disease. *J. Alzheimers Dis.* 33(Suppl. 1), S141–S144. doi: 10.3233/JAD-2012-129025

Ho, L., Qin, W., Pompl, P. N., Xiang, Z., Wang, J., Zhao, Z., et al. (2004). Diet-induced insulin resistance promotes amyloidosis in a transgenic mouse model of Alzheimer's disease. *FASEB J.* 18, 902–904. doi: 10.1096/fj.03-0978fje

Holth, J. K., Bomben, V. C., Reed, J. G., Inoue, T., Younkin, L., Younkin, S. G., et al. (2013). Tau loss attenuates neuronal network hyperexcitability in mouse and Drosophila genetic models of epilepsy. *J. Neurosci.* 33, 1651–1659. doi: 10.1523/JNEUROSCI.3191-12.2013

Horvath, J., Herrmann, F. R., Burkhard, P. R., Bouras, C., and Kovari, E. (2013). Neuropathology of dementia in a large cohort of patients with Parkinson's disease. *Parkinsonism Relat. Disord. 19*, 864–868. doi: 10.1016/j.parkreldis.2013.05.010

Hu, N., Tan, M. S., Sun, L., Jiang, T., Wang, Y. L., Tan, L., et al. (2014). Decreased expression of CD33 in peripheral mononuclear cells of Alzheimer's disease patients. *Neurosci. Lett.* 563, 51–54. doi: 10.1016/j.neulet.2014.01.004

Huang, C. C., Chung, C. M., Leu, H. B., Lin, L. Y., Chiu, C. C., Hsu, C. Y., et al. (2014). Diabetes mellitus and the risk of Alzheimer's disease: a nationwide population-based study. *PLoS ONE* 9:e87095. doi: 10.1371/journal.pone.0087095

Huda, M. N., Erdene-Ochir, E., and Pan, C. H. (2017). Assay for phosphorylation and microtubule binding along with localization of tau protein in colorectal cancer cells. *J. Vis. Exp.* doi: 10.3791/55932

In 't Veld, B. A., Launer, L. J., Hoes, A. W., Ott, A., Hofman, A., Breteler, M. M., et al. (1998). NSAIDs and incident Alzheimer's disease. *The Rotterdam Study. Neurobiol. Aging* 19, 607–611. doi: 10.1016/S0197-4580(98)00096-7

Inoue, K., Rispoli, J., Kaphzan, H., Klann, E., Chen, E. I., Kim, J., et al. (2012). Macroautophagy deficiency mediates age-dependent neurodegeneration through a phospho-tau pathway. *Mol. Neurodegener.* 7:48. doi: 10.1186/1750-1326-7-48

Iqbal, K., Liu, F., Gong, C. X., and Grundke-Iqbal, I. (2010). Tau in Alzheimer disease and related tauopathies. *Curr. Alzheimer Res.* 7, 656–664. doi: 10.2174/156720510793611592

Irwin, D. J., Cohen, T. J., Grossman, M., Arnold, S. E., McCarty-Wood, E., Van Deerlin, V. M., et al. (2013). Acetylated tau neuropathology in sporadic and hereditary tauopathies. *Am. J. Pathol.* 183, 344–351. doi: 10.1016/j.ajpath.2013.04.025

Jaeschke, A., Czech, M. P., and Davis, R. J. (2004). An essential role of the JIP1 scaffold protein for JNK activation in adipose tissue. *Genes Dev.* 18, 1976–1980. doi: 10.1101/gad.1216504

James, B. D., Leurgans, S. E., Hebert, L. E., Scherr, P. A., Yaffe, K., and Bennett, D. A. (2014). Contribution of Alzheimer disease to mortality in the United States. *Neurology* 82, 1045–1050. doi: 10.1212/WNL.0000000000000240

Janning, D., Igaev, M., Sundermann, F., Bruhmann, J., Beutel, O., Heinisch, J. J., et al. (2014). Single-molecule tracking of tau reveals fast kiss-and-hop interaction with microtubules in living neurons. *Mol. Biol. Cell* 25, 3541–3551. doi: 10.1091/mbc.e14-06-1099

Jay, T. R., Hirsch, A. M., Broihier, M. L., Miller, C. M., Neilson, L. E., Ransohoff, R. M., et al. (2017). Disease progression-dependent effects of TREM2 deficiency in a mouse model of Alzheimer's disease. *J. Neurosci.* 37, 637–647. doi: 10.1523/JNEUROSCI.2110-16.2016

Jiang, T., Yu, J. T., Hu, N., Tan, M. S., Zhu, X. C., and Tan, L. (2014). CD33 in Alzheimer's disease. *Mol. Neurobiol.* 49, 529–535. doi: 10.1007/s12035-013-8536-1

Jimenez, S., Navarro, V., Moyano, J., Sanchez-Mico, M., Torres, M., Davila, J. C., et al. (2014). Disruption of amyloid plaques integrity affects the soluble oligomers content from Alzheimer disease brains. *PLoS ONE* 9:e114041. doi: 10.1371/journal.pone.0114041

Jo, C., Gundemir, S., Pritchard, S., Jin, Y. N., Rahman, I., and Johnson, G. V. (2014). Nrf2 reduces levels of phosphorylated tau protein by inducing autophagy adaptor protein NDP52. *Nat. Commun.* 5:3496. doi: 10.1038/ncomms4496

Jung, H. J., Kim, Y. J., Eggert, S., Chung, K. C., Choi, K. S., and Park, S. A. (2013). Age-dependent increases in tau phosphorylation in the brains of type 2 diabetic rats correlate with a reduced expression of p62. *Exp. Neurol.* 248, 441–450. doi: 10.1016/j.expneurol.2013.07.013

Jung, H. J., Park, S. S., Mok, J. O., Lee, T. K., Park, C. S., and Park, S. A. (2011). Increased expression of three-repeat isoforms of tau contributes to tau pathology in a rat model of chronic type 2 diabetes. *Exp. Neurol.* 228, 232–241. doi: 10.1016/j.expneurol.2011.01.012

Kadavath, H., Hofele, R. V., Biernat, J., Kumar, S., Tepper, K., Urlaub, H., et al. (2015). Tau stabilizes microtubules by binding at the interface between tubulin heterodimers. *Proc. Natl. Acad. Sci. U.S.A.* 112, 7501–7506. doi: 10.1073/pnas.1504081112

Kaneto, H., Katakami, N., Matsuhisa, M., and Matsuoka, T. A. (2010). Role of reactive oxygen species in the progression of type 2 diabetes and atherosclerosis. *Mediators Inflamm.* 2010:453892. doi: 10.1155/2010/453892

Karsten, S. L., Sang, T. K., Gehman, L. T., Chatterjee, S., Liu, J., Lawless, G. M., et al. (2006). A genomic screen for modifiers of tauopathy identifies puromycin-sensitive aminopeptidase as an inhibitor of tau-induced neurodegeneration. *Neuron* 51, 549–560. doi: 10.1016/j.neuron.2006.07.019

Katsuse, O., Lin, W. L., Lewis, J., Hutton, M. L., and Dickson, D. W. (2006). Neurofibrillary tangle-related synaptic alterations of spinal motor neurons of P301L tau transgenic mice. *Neurosci. Lett.* 409, 95–99. doi: 10.1016/j.neulet.2006.09.021

Ke, Y. D., Delerue, F., Gladbach, A., Gotz, J., and Ittner, L. M. (2009). Experimental diabetes mellitus exacerbates tau pathology in a transgenic mouse model of Alzheimer's disease. *PLoS ONE* 4:e7917. doi: 10.1371/journal.pone.0007917

Kim, B., and Feldman, E. L. (2015). Insulin resistance as a key link for the increased risk of cognitive impairment in the metabolic syndrome. *Exp. Mol. Med.* 47:e149. doi: 10.1038/emm.2015.3

Kim, B., Backus, C., Oh, S., and Feldman, E. L. (2013). Hyperglycemia-induced tau cleavage *in vitro* and *in vivo*: a possible link between diabetes and Alzheimer's disease. *J. Alzheimers Dis.* 34, 727–739. doi: 10.3233/JAD-121669

Kim, B., Backus, C., Oh, S., Hayes, J. M., and Feldman, E. L. (2009). Increased tau phosphorylation and cleavage in mouse models of type 1 and type 2 diabetes. *Endocrinology* 150, 5294–5301. doi: 10.1210/en.2009-0695

Kim, I., Lee, K. O., Yun, Y. J., Jeong, J. Y., Kim, E. H., Cheong, H., et al. (2017). Biophysical characterization of $Ca^{(2+)}$-binding of S100A5 and Ca(2+)-induced interaction with RAGE. *Biochem. Biophys. Res. Commun.* 483, 332–338. doi: 10.1016/j.bbrc.2016.12.143

Kim, M. S., Yamamoto, Y., Kim, K., Kamei, N., Shimada, T., Liu, L., et al. (2013). Regulation of diet-induced adipose tissue and systemic inflammation by salicylates and pioglitazone. *PLoS ONE* 8:e82847. doi: 10.1371/journal.pone.0082847

King, M. R., Anderson, N. J., Guernsey, L. S., and Jolivalt, C. G. (2013). Glycogen synthase kinase-3 inhibition prevents learning deficits in diabetic mice. *J. Neurosci. Res.* 91, 506–514. doi: 10.1002/jnr.23192

Knight, E. M., Martins, I. V., Gumusgoz, S., Allan, S. M., and Lawrence, C. B. (2014). High-fat diet-induced memory impairment in triple-transgenic Alzheimer's disease (3xTgAD) mice is independent of changes in amyloid and tau pathology. *Neurobiol. Aging* 35, 1821–1832. doi: 10.1016/j.neurobiolaging.2014.02.010

Koenigsknecht, J., and Landreth, G. (2004). Microglial phagocytosis of fibrillar β-amyloid through a beta1 integrin-dependent mechanism. *J. Neurosci.* 24, 9838–9846. doi: 10.1523/JNEUROSCI.2557-04.2004

Kononenko, N. L. (2017). Lysosomes convene to keep the synapse clean. *J Cell Biol.* 216:2251. doi: 10.1083/jcb.201707070

Kopeikina, K. J., Polydoro, M., Tai, H. C., Yaeger, E., Carlson, G. A., Pitstick, R., et al. (2013). Synaptic alterations in the rTg4510 mouse model of tauopathy. *J. Comp. Neurol.* 521, 1334–1353. doi: 10.1002/cne.23234

Kosanam, H., Thai, K., Zhang, Y., Advani, A., Connelly, K. A., Diamandis, E. P., et al. (2014). Diabetes induces lysine acetylation of intermediary metabolism enzymes in the kidney. *Diabetes* 63, 2432–2439. doi: 10.2337/db12-1770

LaFerla, F. M., and Oddo, S. (2005). Alzheimer's disease: Aβ, tau and synaptic dysfunction. *Trends Mol. Med.* 11, 170–176. doi: 10.1016/j.molmed.2005.02.009

Lathuilière, A., Valdes, P., Papin, S., Cacquevel, M., Maclachlan, C., Knott, G. W., et al. (2017). Motifs in the tau protein that control binding to microtubules and aggregation determine pathological effects. *Sci. Rep.* 7:13556. doi: 10.1038/s41598-017-13786-2

Lauretti, E., Li, J. G., Di Meco, A., and Pratico, D. (2017). Glucose deficit triggers tau pathology and synaptic dysfunction in a tauopathy mouse model. *Transl. Psychiatry* 7:e1020. doi: 10.1038/tp.2016.296

Lee, E. J., and Park, J. H. (2013). Receptor for advanced glycation endproducts (RAGE), its ligands, and soluble RAGE: potential biomarkers for diagnosis and therapeutic targets for human renal diseases. *Genomics Inform.* 11, 224–229. doi: 10.5808/GI.2013.11.4.224

Lee, J. A. (2012). Neuronal autophagy: a housekeeper or a fighter in neuronal cell survival? *Exp. Neurobiol.* 21, 1–8. doi: 10.5607/en.2012.21.1.1

Lee, Y. H., Giraud, J., Davis, R. J., and White, M. F. (2003). c-Jun N-terminal kinase (JNK) mediates feedback inhibition of the insulin signaling cascade. *J. Biol. Chem.* 278, 2896–2902. doi: 10.1074/jbc.M208359200

Leibson, C. L., Rocca, W. A., Hanson, V. A., Cha, R., Kokmen, E., O'Brien, P. C., et al. (1997). The risk of dementia among persons with diabetes mellitus: a population-based cohort study. *Ann. N. Y. Acad. Sci.* 826, 422–427. doi: 10.1111/j.1749-6632.1997.tb48496.x

Li, S., Jin, M., Koeglsperger, T., Shepardson, N. E., Shankar, G. M., and Selkoe, D. J. (2011). Soluble Aβ oligomers inhibit long-term potentiation through a mechanism involving excessive activation of extrasynaptic NR2B-containing NMDA receptors. *J. Neurosci.* 31, 6627–6638. doi: 10.1523/JNEUROSCI.0203-11.2011

Li, W., Wang, T., and Xiao, S. (2016). Type 2 diabetes mellitus might be a risk factor for mild cognitive impairment progressing to Alzheimer's disease. *Neuropsychiatr. Dis. Treat.* 12, 2489–2495. doi: 10.2147/NDT.S111298

Li, X. H., Du, L. L., Cheng, X. S., Jiang, X., Zhang, Y., Lv, B. L., et al. (2013). Glycation exacerbates the neuronal toxicity of beta-amyloid. *Cell Death Dis.* 4:e673. doi: 10.1038/cddis.2013.180

Li, X., Shen, N., Zhang, S., Liu, J., Jiang, Q., Liao, M., et al. (2015b). CD33 rs3865444 polymorphism contributes to alzheimer's disease susceptibility in Chinese, European, and North American Populations. *Mol. Neurobiol.* 52, 414–421. doi: 10.1007/s12035-014-8880-9

Li, X., Song, D., and Leng, S. X. (2015a). Link between type 2 diabetes and Alzheimer's disease: from epidemiology to mechanism and treatment. *Clin. Interv. Aging* 10, 549–560. doi: 10.2147/CIA.S74042

Liu, L. P., Hong, H., Liao, J. M., Wang, T. S., Wu, J., Chen, S. S., et al. (2009). Upregulation of RAGE at the blood-brain barrier in streptozotocin-induced diabetic mice. *Synapse* 63, 636–642. doi: 10.1002/syn.20644

Liu, Y., Liu, F., Grundke-Iqbal, I., Iqbal, K., and Gong, C. X. (2009). Brain glucose transporters, O-GlcNAcylation and phosphorylation of tau in diabetes and Alzheimer's disease. *J. Neurochem.* 111, 242–249. doi: 10.1111/j.1471-4159.2009.06320.x

Locke, M., and Anderson, J. (2011). NF-kappaB activation in organs from STZ-treated rats. *Appl. Physiol. Nutr. Metab.* 36, 121–127. doi: 10.1139/H10-094

Luchsinger, J. A., Perez, T., Chang, H., Mehta, P., Steffener, J., Pradabhan, G., et al. (2016). Metformin in amnestic mild cognitive impairment: results of a pilot randomized placebo controlled clinical trial. *J. Alzheimers Dis.* 51, 501–514. doi: 10.3233/JAD-150493

Macauley, S. L., Stanley, M., Caesar, E. E., Yamada, S. A., Raichle, M. E., Perez, R., et al. (2015). Hyperglycemia modulates extracellular amyloid-beta concentrations and neuronal activity *in vivo*. *J. Clin. Invest.* 125, 2463–2467. doi: 10.1172/JCI79742

Magrane, J., Christensen, R. A., Rosen, K. M., , Veereshwarayya, V., and Querfurth, H. W. (2006). Dissociation of ERK and Akt signaling in endothelial cell angiogenic responses to beta-amyloid. *Exp. Cell Res.* 312, 996–1010. doi: 10.1016/j.yexcr.2005.12.009

Mandelkow, E., and Mandelkow, E. M. (1995). Microtubules and microtubule-associated proteins. *Curr. Opin. Cell Biol.* 7, 72–81. doi: 10.1016/0955-0674(95)80047-6

Maphis, N., Xu, G., Kokiko-Cochran, O. N., Jiang, S., Cardona, A., Ransohoff, R. M., et al. (2015). Reactive microglia drive tau pathology and contribute to the spreading of pathological tau in the brain. *Brain 138*, 1738–1755. doi: 10.1093/brain/awv081

Marciniak, E., Leboucher, A., Caron, E., Ahmed, T., Tailleux, A., Dumont, J., et al. (2017). Tau deletion promotes brain insulin resistance. *J. Exp. Med.* 214, 2257–2269. doi: 10.1084/jem.20161731

Marseglia, A., Fratiglioni, L., Laukka, E. J., Santoni, G., Pedersen, N. L., Backman, L., et al. (2016). Early cognitive deficits in Type 2 Diabetes: a population-based study. *J. Alzheimers Dis.* 53, 1069–1078. doi: 10.3233/JAD-160266

Marzban, L., Park, K., and Verchere, C. B. (2003). Islet amyloid polypeptide and type 2 diabetes. *Exp. Gerontol.* 38, 347–351. doi: 10.1016/S0531-5565(03)00004-4

Masini, M., Bugliani, M., Lupi, R., del Guerra, S., Boggi, U., Filipponi, F., et al. (2009). Autophagy in human type 2 diabetes pancreatic β cells. *Diabetologia* 52, 1083–1086. doi: 10.1007/s00125-009-1347-2

Matos, M., Augusto, E., Oliveira, C. R., and Agostinho, P. (2008). Amyloid-beta peptide decreases glutamate uptake in cultured astrocytes: involvement of oxidative stress and mitogen-activated protein kinase cascades. *Neuroscience* 156, 898–910. doi: 10.1016/j.neuroscience.2008.08.022

Michalovicz, L. T., Lally, B., and Konat, G. W. (2015). Peripheral challenge with a viral mimic upregulates expression of the complement genes in the hippocampus. *J. Neuroimmunol.* 285, 137–142. doi: 10.1016/j.jneuroim.2015.06.003

Miller, B. W., Willett, K. C., and Desilets, A. R. (2011). Rosiglitazone and pioglitazone for the treatment of Alzheimer's disease. *Ann. Pharmacother.* 45, 1416–1424. doi: 10.1345/aph.1Q238

Minkeviciene, R., Rheims, S., Dobszay, M. B., Zilberter, M., Hartikainen, J., Fulop, L., et al. (2009). Amyloid β-induced neuronal hyperexcitability triggers progressive epilepsy. *J. Neurosci.* 29, 3453–3462. doi: 10.1523/JNEUROSCI.5215-08.2009

Molina, J., Rodriguez-Diaz, R., Fachado, A., Jacques-Silva, M. C., Berggren, P. O., and Caicedo, A. (2014). Control of insulin secretion by cholinergic signaling in the human pancreatic islet. *Diabetes* 63, 2714–2726. doi: 10.2337/db13-1371

Moore, E. M., Mander, A. G., Ames, D., Kotowicz, M. A., Carne, R. P., Brodaty, H., et al. (2013). Increased risk of cognitive impairment in patients with diabetes is associated with metformin. *Diabetes Care* 36, 2981–2987. doi: 10.2337/dc13-0229

Moro, M., Phillips, A. S., Gaimster, K., Paul, C., Mudher, A., Nicoll, J., et al. (2018). Pyroglutamate and isoaspartate modified amyloid-beta in ageing and Alzheimer's disease. *Acta Neuropathol. Commun.* 6:3. doi: 10.1186/s40478-017-0505-x

Moran, C., Beare, R., Phan, T. G., Bruce, D. G., Callisaya, M. L., Srikanth, V., et al. (2015). Type 2 diabetes mellitus and biomarkers of neurodegeneration. *Neurology* 85, 1123–1130. doi: 10.1212/WNL.0000000000001982

Moreira, P. I., Santos, M. S., Moreno, A. M., Seica, R., and Oliveira, C. R. (2003). Increased vulnerability of brain mitochondria in diabetic (Goto-Kakizaki) rats with aging and amyloid-beta exposure. *Diabetes* 52, 1449–1456. doi: 10.2337/diabetes.52.6.1449

Morel, C., Standen, C. L., Jung, D. Y., Gray, S., Ong, H., Flavell, R. A., et al. (2010). Requirement of JIP1-mediated c-Jun N-terminal kinase activation for obesity-induced insulin resistance. *Mol. Cell Biol.* 30, 4616–4625. doi: 10.1128/MCB.00585-10

Morimoto, K., Horio, J., Satoh, H., Sue, L., Beach, T., Arita, S., et al. (2011). Expression profiles of cytokines in the brains of Alzheimer's disease (AD) patients compared to the brains of non-demented patients with and without increasing AD pathology. *J. Alzheimers Dis.* 25, 59–76. doi: 10.3233/JAD-2011-101815

Morris, J. K., and Burns, J. M. (2012). Insulin: an emerging treatment for Alzheimer's disease dementia? *Curr. Neurol. Neurosci. Rep.* 12, 520–527. doi: 10.1007/s11910-012-0297-0

Mosconi, L., Pupi, A., and De Leon, M. J. (2008). Brain glucose hypometabolism and oxidative stress in preclinical Alzheimer's disease. *Ann. N. Y. Acad. Sci.* 1147, 180–195. doi: 10.1196/annals.1427.007

Mucke, L., and Selkoe, D. J. (2012). Neurotoxicity of amyloid beta-protein: synaptic and network dysfunction. *Cold Spring Harb. Perspect. Med.* 2:a006338. doi: 10.1101/cshperspect.a006338

Mudher, A., Shepherd, D., Newman, T. A., Mildren, P., Jukes, J. P., Squire, A., et al. (2004). GSK-3beta inhibition reverses axonal transport defects and behavioural phenotypes in Drosophila. *Mol. Psychiatry* 9, 522–530. doi: 10.1038/sj.mp.4001483

Mullins, R. J., Diehl, T. C., Chia, C. W., and Kapogiannis, D. (2017). Insulin resistance as a link between amyloid-beta and tau pathologies in Alzheimer's disease. *Front. Aging Neurosci.* 9:118. doi: 10.3389/fnagi.2017.00118

Neely, K. M., Green, K. N., and LaFerla, F. M. (2011). Presenilin is necessary for efficient proteolysis through the autophagy-lysosome system in a gamma-secretase-independent manner. *J. Neurosci.* 31, 2781–2791. doi: 10.1523/JNEUROSCI.5156-10.2010

Nelson, P. T., Alafuzoff, I., Bigio, E. H., Bouras, C., Braak, H., Cairns, N. J., et al. (2012). Correlation of Alzheimer disease neuropathologic changes with cognitive status: a review of the literature. *J. Neuropathol. Exp. Neurol.* 71, 362–381. doi: 10.1097/NEN.0b013e31825018f7

Niewidok, B., Igaev, M., Sundermann, F., Janning, D., Bakota, L., and Brandt, R. (2016). Presence of a carboxy-terminal pseudorepeat and disease-like pseudohyperphosphorylation critically influence tau's interaction with microtubules in axon-like processes. *Mol. Biol. Cell* 27, 3537–3549. doi: 10.1091/mbc.e16-06-0402

Nilsson, P., Sekiguchi, M., Akagi, T., Izumi, S., Komori, T., Hui, K., et al. (2015). Autophagy-related protein 7 deficiency in amyloid β (Abeta) precursor protein transgenic mice decreases Abeta in the multivesicular bodies and induces Abeta accumulation in the Golgi. *Am. J. Pathol.* 185, 305–313. doi: 10.1016/j.ajpath.2014.10.011

Nixon, R. A. (2007). Autophagy, amyloidogenesis and Alzheimer disease. *J. Cell. Sci. 120(Pt* 23), 4081–4091. doi: 10.1242/jcs.019265

Nixon, R. A., Wegiel, J., Kumar, A., Yu, W. H., Peterhoff, C., Cataldo, A., et al. (2005). Extensive involvement of autophagy in Alzheimer disease: an immuno-electron microscopy study. *J. Neuropathol. Exp. Neurol.* 64, 113–122. doi: 10.1093/jnen/64.2.113

Nizari, S., Carare, R. O., and Hawkes, C. A. (2016). Increased Abeta pathology in aged Tg2576 mice born to mothers fed a high fat diet. *Sci. Rep.* 6:21981. doi: 10.1038/srep21981

Nowotny, K., Jung, T., Hohn, A., Weber, D., and Grune, T. (2015). Advanced glycation end products and oxidative stress in type 2 diabetes mellitus. *Biomolecules* 5, 194–222. doi: 10.3390/biom5010194

Orr, M. E., and Oddo, S. (2013). Autophagic/lysosomal dysfunction in Alzheimer's disease. *Alzheimers Res. Ther.* 5:53. doi: 10.1186/alzrt217

Ozcan, U., Cao, Q., Yilmaz, E., Lee, A. H., Iwakoshi, N. N., Ozdelen, E., et al. (2004). Endoplasmic reticulum stress links obesity, insulin action, and type 2 diabetes. *Science* 306, 457–461. doi: 10.1126/science.1103160

Ozcelik, S., Fraser, G., Castets, P., Schaeffer, V., Skachokova, Z., Breu, K., et al. (2013). Rapamycin attenuates the progression of tau pathology in P301S tau transgenic mice. *PLoS ONE* 8:e62459. doi: 10.1371/journal.pone.0062459

Palop, J. J., and Mucke, L. (2010). Amyloid-β-induced neuronal dysfunction in Alzheimer's disease: from synapses toward neural networks. *Nat. Neurosci.* 13, 812–818. doi: 10.1038/nn.2583

Patel, S., and Santani, D. (2009). Role of NF-kappa B in the pathogenesis of diabetes and its associated complications. *Pharmacol. Rep.* 61, 595–603. doi: 10.1016/S1734-1140(09)70111-2

Peila, R., Rodriguez, B. L., Launer, L. J., and Honolulu-Asia Aging Study. (2002). Type 2 diabetes, APOE gene, and the risk for dementia and related pathologies: the honolulu-asia aging study. *Diabetes* 51, 1256–1262. doi: 10.2337/diabetes.51.4.1256

Peraldi, P., Hotamisligil, G. S., Buurman, W. A., White, M. F., and Spiegelman, B. M. (1996). Tumor necrosis factor (TNF)-α inhibits insulin signaling through stimulation of the p55 TNF receptor and activation of sphingomyelinase. *J. Biol. Chem.* 271, 13018–13022. doi: 10.1074/jbc.271.22.13018

Pickford, F., Masliah, E., Britschgi, M., Lucin, K., Narasimhan, R., Jaeger, P. A., et al. (2008). The autophagy-related protein beclin 1 shows reduced expression in early Alzheimer disease and regulates amyloid beta accumulation in mice. *J. Clin. Invest.* 118, 2190–2199. doi: 10.1172/JCI33585

Planel, E., Tatebayashi, Y., Miyasaka, T., Liu, L., Wang, L., Herman, M., et al. (2007). Insulin dysfunction induces *in vivo* tau hyperphosphorylation through distinct mechanisms. *J. Neurosci. 27*, 13635–13648. doi: 10.1523/JNEUROSCI.3949-07.2007

Plum, L., Schubert, M., and Bruning, J. C. (2005). The role of insulin receptor signaling in the brain. *Trends Endocrinol. Metab.* 16, 59–65. doi: 10.1016/j.tem.2005.01.008

Pooler, A. M., Noble, W., and Hanger, D. P. (2014). A role for tau at the synapse in Alzheimer's disease pathogenesis. Neuropharmacology 76(Pt A), 1–8. doi: 10.1016/j.neuropharm.2013.09.018

Puzzo, D., Piacentini, R., Fa, M., Gulisano, W., Li Puma, D. D., Staniszewski, A., et al. (2017). LTP and memory impairment caused by extracellular Aβ and Tau oligomers is APP-dependent. *Elife* 6:e26991. doi: 10.7554/eLife.26991

Qiu, W. Q., and Folstein, M. F. (2006). Insulin, insulin-degrading enzyme and amyloid-beta peptide in Alzheimer's disease: review and hypothesis. *Neurobiol. Aging* 27, 190–198. doi: 10.1016/j.neurobiolaging.2005.01.004

Qu, Z. S., Li, L., Sun, X. J., Zhao, Y. W., Zhang, J., Geng, Z., et al. (2014). Glycogen synthase kinase-3 regulates production of amyloid-β peptides and tau phosphorylation in diabetic rat brain. *ScientificWorldJournal* 2014:878123. doi: 10.1155/2014/878123

Qu, Z., Jiao, Z., Sun, X., Zhao, Y., Ren, J., and Xu, G. (2011). Effects of streptozotocin-induced diabetes on tau phosphorylation in the rat brain. *Brain Res.* 1383, 300–306. doi: 10.1016/j.brainres.2011.01.084

Quan, W., Lim, Y. M., and Lee, M. S. (2012). Role of autophagy in diabetes and endoplasmic reticulum stress of pancreatic β-cells. *Exp. Mol. Med.* 44, 81–88. doi: 10.3858/emm.2012.44.2.030

Quraishe, S., Cowan, C. M., and Mudher, A. (2013). NAP (davunetide) rescues neuronal dysfunction in a Drosophila model of tauopathy. *Mol. Psychiatry* 18, 834–842. doi: 10.1038/mp.2013.32

Reddy, P. H. (2013). Amyloid beta-induced glycogen synthase kinase 3β phosphorylated VDAC1 in Alzheimer's disease: implications for synaptic dysfunction and neuronal damage. *Biochim. Biophys. Acta* 1832, 1913–1921. doi: 10.1016/j.bbadis.2013.06.012

Reno, C. M., Puente, E. C., Sheng, Z., Daphna-Iken, D., Bree, A. J., Routh, V. H., et al. (2017). Brain GLUT4 knockout mice have impaired glucose tolerance, decreased insulin sensitivity, and impaired hypoglycemic counterregulation. *Diabetes* 66, 587–597. doi: 10.2337/db16-0917

Roberts, R. O., Knopman, D. S., Przybelski, S. A., Mielke, M. M., Kantarci, K., Preboske, G. M., et al. (2014). Association of type 2 diabetes with brain atrophy and cognitive impairment. *Neurology* 82, 1132–1141. doi: 10.1212/WNL.0000000000000269

Robertson, L. A., Moya, K. L., and Breen, K. C. (2004). The potential role of tau protein O-glycosylation in Alzheimer's disease. *J. Alzheimers Dis.* 6, 489–495. doi: 10.3233/JAD-2004-6505

Rodríguez-Martín, T., Cuchillo-Ibanez, I., Noble, W., Nyenya, F., Anderton, B. H., and Hanger, D. P. (2013). Tau phosphorylation affects its axonal transport and degradation. *Neurobiol. Aging* 34, 2146–2157. doi: 10.1016/j.neurobiolaging.2013.03.015

Rodriguez-Rodriguez, P., Sandebring-Matton, A., Merino-Serrais, P., Parrado-Fernandez, C., Rabano, A., Winblad, B., et al. (2017). Tau hyperphosphorylation induces oligomeric insulin accumulation and insulin resistance in neurons. *Brain* 140, 3269–3285. doi: 10.1093/brain/awx256

Romeo, G., Liu, W. H., Asnaghi, V., Kern, T. S., and Lorenzi, M. (2002). Activation of nuclear factor-kappaB induced by diabetes and high glucose regulates a proapoptotic program in retinal pericytes. *Diabetes* 51, 2241–2248. doi: 10.2337/diabetes.51.7.2241

Rubio-Perez, J. M., and Morillas-Ruiz, J. M. (2012). A review: inflammatory process in Alzheimer's disease, role of cytokines. *ScientificWorldJournal* 2012:756357. doi: 10.1100/2012/756357

Sakono, M., and Zako, T. (2010). Amyloid oligomers: formation and toxicity of Abeta oligomers. *FEBS J.* 277, 1348–1358. doi: 10.1111/j.1742-4658.2010.07568.x

Samuel, S., Zhang, K., Tang, Y. D., Gerdes, A. M., and Carrillo-Sepulveda, M. A. (2017). Triiodothyronine potentiates vasorelaxation via PKG/VASP signaling in vascular smooth muscle cells. *Cell. Physiol. Biochem.* 41, 1894–1904. doi: 10.1159/000471938

Savu, O., Bradescu, O. M., Serafinceanu, C., Iosif, L., Tirgoviste, C. I., and Stoian, I. (2013). Erythrocyte caspase-3 and antioxidant defense is activated in red blood cells and plasma of type 2 diabetes patients at first clinical onset. *Redox Rep.* 18, 56–62. doi: 10.1179/1351000213Y.0000000040

Schaeffer, V., Lavenir, I., Ozcelik, S., Tolnay, M., Winkler, D. T., and Goedert, M. (2012). Stimulation of autophagy reduces neurodegeneration in a mouse model of human tauopathy. *Brain* 135, 2169–2177. doi: 10.1093/brain/aws143

Schedin-Weiss, S., Winblad, B., and Tjernberg, L. O. (2014). The role of protein glycosylation in Alzheimer disease. *FEBS J.* 281, 46–62. doi: 10.1111/febs.12590

Schmitz, T. W., Nathan Spreng, R., and Alzheimer's Disease Neuroimaging Initiative. (2016). Basal forebrain degeneration precedes and predicts the cortical spread of Alzheimer's pathology. *Nat. Commun.* 7:13249. doi: 10.1038/ncomms13249

Schubert, M., Brazil, D. P., Burks, D. J., Kushner, J. A., Ye, J., Flint, C. L., et al. (2003). Insulin receptor substrate-2 deficiency impairs brain growth and promotes tau phosphorylation. *J. Neurosci.* 23, 7084–7092. doi: 10.1523/JNEUROSCI.23-18-07084.2003

Schubert, M., Gautam, D., Surjo, D., Ueki, K., Baudler, S., Schubert, D., et al. (2004). Role for neuronal insulin resistance in neurodegenerative diseases. *Proc. Natl. Acad. Sci. U.S.A.* 101, 3100–3105. doi: 10.1073/pnas.0308724101

Sekar, S., McDonald, J., Cuyugan, L., Aldrich, J., Kurdoglu, A., Adkins, J., et al. (2015). Alzheimer's disease is associated with altered expression of genes involved in immune response and mitochondrial processes in astrocytes. *Neurobiol. Aging* 36, 583–591. doi: 10.1016/j.neurobiolaging.2014.09.027

Selkoe, D. J. (2008). Soluble oligomers of the amyloid beta-protein impair synaptic plasticity and behavior. *Behav. Brain Res.* 192, 106–113. doi: 10.1016/j.bbr.2008.02.016

Serpell, L. C., Blake, C. C., and Fraser, P. E. (2000). Molecular structure of a fibrillar Alzheimer's A beta fragment. *Biochemistry* 39, 13269–13275. doi: 10.1021/bi000637v

Serrano-Pozo, A., Frosch, M. P., Masliah, E., and Hyman, B. T. (2011). Neuropathological alterations in Alzheimer disease. *Cold Spring Harb. Perspect. Med.* 1:a006189. doi: 10.1101/cshperspect.a006189

Shankar, G. M., and Walsh, D. M. (2009). Alzheimer's disease: synaptic dysfunction and Abeta. *Mol. Neurodegener.* 4:48. doi: 10.1186/1750-1326-4-48

Sheng, M., Sabatini, B. L., and Sudhof, T. C. (2012). Synapses and Alzheimer's disease. *Cold Spring Harb. Perspect. Biol.* 4:a005777 doi: 10.1101/cshperspect.a005777

Showkat, M., Beigh, M. A., and Andrabi, K. I. (2014). mTOR signaling in protein translation regulation: implications in cancer genesis and therapeutic interventions. *Mol. Biol. Int.* 2014:686984. doi: 10.1155/2014/686984

Smet-Nocca, C., Broncel, M., Wieruszeski, J. M., Tokarski, C., Hanoulle, X., Leroy, A., et al. (2011). Identification of O-GlcNAc sites within peptides of the Tau protein and their impact on phosphorylation. *Mol. Biosyst.* 7, 1420–1429. doi: 10.1039/c0mb00337a

Solito, E., and Sastre, M. (2012). Microglia function in Alzheimer's disease. *Front. Pharmacol.* 3:14. doi: 10.3389/fphar.2012.00014

Son, J. H., Shim, J. H., Kim, K. H., Ha, J. Y., and Han, J. Y. (2012). Neuronal autophagy and neurodegenerative diseases. *Exp. Mol. Med.* 44, 89–98. doi: 10.3858/emm.2012.44.2.031

Son, S. M., Cha, M. Y., Choi, H., Kang, S., Choi, H., Lee, M. S., et al. (2016). Insulin-degrading enzyme secretion from astrocytes is mediated by an autophagy-based unconventional secretory pathway in Alzheimer disease. *Autophagy* 12, 784–800. doi: 10.1080/15548627.2016.1159375

Sotiropoulos, I., Galas, M. C., Silva, J. M., Skoulakis, E., Wegmann, S., Maina, M. B., et al. (2017). Atypical, non-standard functions of the microtubule associated Tau protein. *Acta Neuropathol. Commun.* 5:91. doi: 10.1186/s40478-017-0489-6

Spilman, P., Podlutskaya, N., Hart, M. J., Debnath, J., Gorostiza, O., Bredesen, D., et al. (2010). Inhibition of mTOR by rapamycin abolishes cognitive deficits and reduces amyloid-β levels in a mouse model of Alzheimer's disease. *PLoS ONE* 5:e9979. doi: 10.1371/journal.pone.0009979

Spires-Jones, T. L., and Hyman, B. T. (2014). The intersection of amyloid beta and tau at synapses in Alzheimer's disease. *Neuron* 82, 756–771. doi: 10.1016/j.neuron.2014.05.004

Srikanth, V., Maczurek, A., Phan, T., Steele, M., Westcott, B., Juskiw, D., et al. (2011). Advanced glycation endproducts and their receptor RAGE in Alzheimer's disease. *Neurobiol. Aging* 32, 763–777. doi: 10.1016/j.neurobiolaging.2009.04.016

Stanley, M., Macauley, S. L., and Holtzman, D. M. (2016). Changes in insulin and insulin signaling in Alzheimer's disease: cause or consequence? *J. Exp. Med.* 213, 1375–1385. doi: 10.1084/jem.20160493

Steele, J. W., Fan, E., Kelahmetoglu, Y., Tian, Y., and Bustos, V. (2013). Modulation of Autophagy as a Therapeutic Target for Alzheimer's Disease. *Postdoc J* 1, 21–34.

Stoothoff, W. H., and Johnson, G. V. (2005). Tau phosphorylation, physiological and pathological consequences. *Biochim. Biophys. Acta* 1739, 280–297. doi: 10.1016/j.bbadis.2004.06.017

Swaroop, J. J., Rajarajeswari, D., and Naidu, J. N. (2012). Association of TNF-α with insulin resistance in type 2 diabetes mellitus. *Indian J. Med. Res.* 135, 127–130. doi: 10.4103/0971-5916.93435

Tackenberg, C., and Brandt, R. (2009). Divergent pathways mediate spine alterations and cell death induced by amyloid-β, wild-type tau, and R406W tau. *J. Neurosci.* 29, 14439–14450. doi: 10.1523/JNEUROSCI.3590-09.2009

Tai, H. C., Serrano-Pozo, A., Hashimoto, T., Frosch, M. P., Spires-Jones, T. L., and Hyman, B. T. (2012). The synaptic accumulation of hyperphosphorylated tau oligomers in Alzheimer disease is associated with dysfunction of the ubiquitin-proteasome system. *Am. J. Pathol.* 181, 1426–1435. doi: 10.1016/j.ajpath.2012.06.033

Takeda, S., Sato, N., Uchio-Yamada, K., Sawada, K., Kunieda, T., Takeuchi, D., et al. (2010). Diabetes-accelerated memory dysfunction via cerebrovascular inflammation and Abeta deposition in an Alzheimer mouse model with diabetes. *Proc. Natl. Acad. Sci. U.S.A.* 107, 7036–7041. doi: 10.1073/pnas.1000645107

Talbot, K. (2014). Brain insulin resistance in Alzheimer's disease and its potential treatment with GLP-1 analogs. *Neurodegener. Dis. Manag.* 4, 31–40. doi: 10.2217/nmt.13.73

Talbot, K., Wang, H. Y., Kazi, H., Han, L. Y., Bakshi, K. P., Stucky, A., et al. (2012). Demonstrated brain insulin resistance in Alzheimer's disease patients is associated with IGF-1 resistance, IRS-1 dysregulation, and cognitive decline. *J. Clin. Invest.* 122, 1316–1338. doi: 10.1172/JCI59903

Taylor, R. (2012). Insulin resistance and type 2 diabetes. *Diabetes* 61, 778–779. doi: 10.2337/db12-0073

Thiels, E., and Klann, E. (2001). Extracellular signal-regulated kinase, synaptic plasticity, and memory. *Rev. Neurosci.* 12, 327–345. doi: 10.1515/REVNEURO.2001.12.4.327

Tosto, G., and Reitz, C. (2013). Genome-wide association studies in Alzheimer's disease: a review. *Curr. Neurol. Neurosci. Rep.* 13:381. doi: 10.1007/s11910-013-0381-0

Trzeciakiewicz, H., Tseng, J. H., Wander, C. M., Madden, V., Tripathy, A., Yuan, C. X., et al. (2017). A dual pathogenic mechanism links tau acetylation to sporadic tauopathy. *Sci. Rep.* 7:44102. doi: 10.1038/srep44102

Tung, Y. T., Wang, B. J., Hsu, W. M., Hu, M. K., Her, G. M., Huang, W. P., et al. (2014). Presenilin-1 regulates the expression of p62 to govern p62-dependent tau degradation. *Mol. Neurobiol.* 49, 10–27. doi: 10.1007/s12035-013-8482-y

Tyan, S. H., Shih, A. Y., Walsh, J. J., Maruyama, H., Sarsoza, F., Ku, L., et al. (2012). Amyloid precursor protein (APP) regulates synaptic structure and function. *Mol. Cell Neurosci.* 51, 43–52. doi: 10.1016/j.mcn.2012.07.009

Ulrich, J. D., Ulland, T. K., Colonna, M., and Holtzman, D. M. (2017). Elucidating the role of TREM2 in Alzheimer's Disease. *Neuron* 94, 237–248. doi: 10.1016/j.neuron.2017.02.042

Umegaki, H. (2014). Type 2 diabetes as a risk factor for cognitive impairment: current insights. *Clin. Interv. Aging* 9, 1011–1019. doi: 10.2147/CIA.S48926

Uranga, R. M., Katz, S., and Salvador, G. A. (2013). Enhanced phosphatidylinositol 3-kinase (PI3K)/Akt signaling has pleiotropic targets in hippocampal neurons exposed to iron-induced oxidative stress. *J Biol Chem* 288, 19773–19784. doi: 10.1074/jbc.M113.457622

van Bussel, F. C., Backes, W. H., Hofman, P. A., Puts, N. A., Edden, R. A., van Boxtel, M. P., et al. (2016). Increased GABA concentrations in type 2 diabetes mellitus are related to lower cognitive functioning. *Medicine* 95:e4803. doi: 10.1097/MD.0000000000004803

van der Flier, W. M., and Scheltens, P. (2005). Epidemiology and risk factors of dementia. *J. Neurol. Neurosurg. Psychiatry. 76 (Suppl.* 5), v2–v7. doi: 10.1136/jnnp.2005.082867

van der Heide, L. P., Kamal, A., Artola, A., Gispen, W. H., and Ramakers, G. M. (2005). Insulin modulates hippocampal activity-dependent synaptic plasticity in a N-methyl-d-aspartate receptor and phosphatidyl-inositol-3-kinase-dependent manner. *J. Neurochem.* 94, 1158–1166. doi: 10.1111/j.1471-4159.2005.03269.x

Van Eldik, L. J., Carrillo, M. C., Cole, P. E., Feuerbach, D., Greenberg, B. D., Hendrix, J. A., et al. (2016). The roles of inflammation and immune mechanisms in Alzheimer's disease. *Alzheimers Dement.* 2, 99–109. doi: 10.1016/j.trci.2016.05.001

Vassar, R. (2004). BACE1: the beta-secretase enzyme in Alzheimer's disease. *J. Mol. Neurosci.* 23, 105–114. doi: 10.1385/JMN:23:1-2:105

Verkhratsky, A., Olabarria, M., Noristani, H. N., Yeh, C. Y., and Rodriguez, J. J. (2010). Astrocytes in Alzheimer's disease. *Neurotherapeutics* 7, 399–412. doi: 10.1016/j.nurt.2010.05.017

Vlassenko, A. G., Benzinger, T. L., and Morris, J. C. (2012). PET amyloid-beta imaging in preclinical Alzheimer's disease. *Biochim. Biophys. Acta* 1822, 370–379. doi: 10.1016/j.bbadis.2011.11.005

Wang, J. Z., Grundke-Iqbal, I., and Iqbal, K. (1996). Glycosylation of microtubule-associated protein tau: an abnormal posttranslational modification in Alzheimer's disease. *Nat. Med.* 2, 871–875. doi: 10.1038/nm0896-871

Watson, G. S., Cholerton, B. A., Reger, M. A., Baker, L. D., Plymate, S. R., Asthana, S., et al. (2005). Preserved cognition in patients with early Alzheimer disease and amnestic mild cognitive impairment during treatment with rosiglitazone: a preliminary study. *Am. J. Geriatr. Psychiatry* 13, 950–958. doi: 10.1176/appi.ajgp.13.11.950

Wellen, K. E., and Hotamisligil, G. S. (2005). Inflammation, stress, and diabetes. *J. Clin. Invest.* 115, 1111–1119. doi: 10.1172/JCI25102

Wennberg, A. M., Spira, A. P., Pettigrew, C., Soldan, A., Zipunnikov, V., Rebok, G. W., et al. (2016). Blood glucose levels and cortical thinning in cognitively normal, middle-aged adults. *J. Neurol. Sci.* 365, 89–95. doi: 10.1016/j.jns.2016.04.017

Wes, P. D., Easton, A., Corradi, J., Barten, D. M., Devidze, N., DeCarr, L. B., et al. (2014). Tau overexpression impacts a neuroinflammation gene expression network perturbed in Alzheimer's disease. *PLoS ONE* 9:e106050. doi: 10.1371/journal.pone.0106050

Wildsmith, K. R., Holley, M., Savage, J. C., Skerrett, R., and Landreth, G. E. (2013). Evidence for impaired amyloid beta clearance in Alzheimer's disease. *Alzheimers Res. Ther.* 5:33. doi: 10.1186/alzrt187

Wilson, C. A., Murphy, D. D., Giasson, B. I., Zhang, B., Trojanowski, J. Q., and Lee, V. M. (2004). Degradative organelles containing mislocalized α-and α-synuclein proliferate in presenilin-1 null neurons. *J. Cell Biol.* 165, 335–346. doi: 10.1083/jcb.200403061

Wilson, D. M., and Binder, L. I. (1997). Free fatty acids stimulate the polymerization of tau and amyloid beta peptides, *in vitro* evidence for a common effector of pathogenesis in Alzheimer's disease. *Am. J. Pathol.* 150, 2181–2195.

Wu, J., Nie, S. D., and Wang, S. (2013). Tau pathology in diabetes mellitus. *Pharmazie* 68, 649–652.

Wyss-Coray, T., Loike, J. D., Brionne, T. C., Lu, E., Anankov, R., Yan, F., et al. (2003). Adult mouse astrocytes degrade amyloid-β *in vitro* and *in situ*. *Nat. Med.* 9, 453–457. doi: 10.1038/nm838

Wyss-Coray, T., and Rogers, J. (2012). Inflammation in Alzheimer disease-a brief review of the basic science and clinical literature. *Cold Spring Harb. Perspect. Med.* 2:a006346. doi: 10.1101/cshperspect.a006346

Xiong, J. (2015). Atg7 in development and disease: panacea or Pandora's Box? *Protein Cell* 6, 722–734. doi: 10.1007/s13238-015-0195-8

Yarchoan, M., and Arnold, S. E. (2014). Repurposing diabetes drugs for brain insulin resistance in Alzheimer disease. *Diabetes* 63, 2253–2261. doi: 10.2337/db14-0287

Yiannopoulou, K. G., and Papageorgiou, S. G. (2013). Current and future treatments for Alzheimer's disease. *Ther. Adv. Neurol. Disord.* 6, 19–33. doi: 10.1177/1756285612461679

Yin, Y., Chen, F., Wang, W., Wang, H., and Zhang, X. (2017). Resolvin D1 inhibits inflammatory response in STZ-induced diabetic retinopathy rats: possible involvement of NLRP3 inflammasome and NF-kappaB signaling pathway. *Mol. Vis.* 23, 242–250.

Yoon, M. S. (2017). The role of mammalian target of rapamycin (mTOR) in insulin signaling. *Nutrients* 9:E1176. doi: 10.3390/nu9111176

Yoshiyama, Y., Higuchi, M., Zhang, B., Huang, S. M., Iwata, N., Saido, T. C., et al. (2007). Synapse loss and microglial activation precede tangles in a P301S tauopathy mouse model. *Neuron* 53, 337–351. doi: 10.1016/j.neuron.2007.01.010

Yuzwa, S. A., Shan, X., Macauley, M. S., Clark, T., Skorobogatko, Y., Vosseller, K., et al. (2012). Increasing O-GlcNAc slows neurodegeneration and stabilizes tau against aggregation. *Nat. Chem. Biol.* 8, 393–399. doi: 10.1038/nchembio.797

Zhang, W., Thompson, B. J., Hietakangas, V., and Cohen, S. M. (2011). MAPK/ERK signaling regulates insulin sensitivity to control glucose metabolism in Drosophila. *PLoS Genet.* 7:e1002429. doi: 10.1371/journal.pgen.1002429

Zhao, R., Hu, W., Tsai, J., Li, W., and Gan, W. B. (2017). Microglia limit the expansion of beta-amyloid plaques in a mouse model of Alzheimer's disease. *Mol. Neurodegener.* 12:47. doi: 10.1186/s13024-017-0188-6

Zhao, W. Q., and Townsend, M. (2009). Insulin resistance and amyloidogenesis as common molecular foundation for type 2 diabetes and Alzheimer's disease. *Biochim. Biophys. Acta* 1792, 482–496. doi: 10.1016/j.bbadis.2008.10.014

Zhu, Y., Shan, X., Yuzwa, S. A., and Vocadlo, D. J. (2014). The emerging link between O-GlcNAc and Alzheimer disease. *J. Biol. Chem.* 289, 34472–34481. doi: 10.1074/jbc.R114.601351

Zilka, N., Filipcik, P., Koson, P., Fialova, L., Skrabana, R., Zilkova, M., et al. (2006). Truncated tau from sporadic Alzheimer's disease suffices to drive neurofibrillary degeneration *in vivo*. *FEBS Lett.* 580, 3582–3588. doi: 10.1016/j.febslet.2006.05.029

Zotova, E., Nicoll, J. A., Kalaria, R., Holmes, C., and Boche, D. (2010). Inflammation in Alzheimer's disease: relevance to pathogenesis and therapy. *Alzheimers Res. Ther.* 2:1. doi: 10.1186/alzrt24

3

Perspective Insights into Disease Progression, Diagnostics and Therapeutic Approaches in Alzheimer's Disease: A Judicious Update

Arif Tasleem Jan[1†‡], *Mudsser Azam*[2‡], *Safikur Rahman*[1], *Angham M. S. Almigeiti*[1], *Duk Hwan Choi*[1], *Eun Ju Lee*[1], *Qazi Mohd Rizwanul Haq*[2] *and Inho Choi*[1*]

[1] *Department of Medical Biotechnology, Yeungnam University, Gyeongsan, South Korea,* [2] *Department of Biosciences, Jamia Millia Islamia, New Delhi, India*

Correspondence:
Inho Choi
inhochoi@ynu.ac.kr

Alzheimer's disease (AD) is a neurodegenerative disorder characterized by the progressive accumulation of β-amyloid fibrils and abnormal tau proteins in and outside of neurons. Representing a common form of dementia, aggravation of AD with age increases the morbidity rate among the elderly. Although, mutations in the ApoE4 act as potent risk factors for sporadic AD, familial AD arises through malfunctioning of APP, PSEN-1, and−2 genes. AD progresses through accumulation of amyloid plaques (Aβ) and neurofibrillary tangles (NFTs) in brain, which interfere with neuronal communication. Cellular stress that arises through mitochondrial dysfunction, endoplasmic reticulum malfunction, and autophagy contributes significantly to the pathogenesis of AD. With high accuracy in disease diagnostics, Aβ deposition and phosphorylated tau (p-tau) are useful core biomarkers in the cerebrospinal fluid (CSF) of AD patients. Although five drugs are approved for treatment in AD, their failures in achieving complete disease cure has shifted studies toward a series of molecules capable of acting against Aβ and p-tau. Failure of biologics or compounds to cross the blood-brain barrier (BBB) in most cases advocates development of an efficient drug delivery system. Though liposomes and polymeric nanoparticles are widely adopted for drug delivery modules, their use in delivering drugs across the BBB has been overtaken by exosomes, owing to their promising results in reducing disease progression.

Keywords: Alzheimer's disease, diagnostics, drugs, neurodegeneration, therapeutics

INTRODUCTION

Alzheimer's disease (AD) is recognized as a disease of neurons and neuronal circuits. It arises as a result of progressive accumulation of β-amyloid fibrils (β-amyloid plaques) and abnormal forms of tau (tau tangles) within and outside of neurons (Jucker and Walker, 2013; Jaunmuktane et al., 2015). Approximately 46.8 million people over the age of 60 years have been diagnosed with AD worldwide (Prince et al., 2016). Though occurrence of the early onset of dementia is <1% per 4,000 individuals, the projected figure is estimated to be 131.5 million in 2050 (Prince et al., 2016). The projected increase in the prevalence of dementia is substantially higher in developing countries than in the USA and Europe, which already have a high proportion of older individuals in their populations. The Alzheimer's Association presented an estimate of 5.5 million people suffering from AD in the USA, and the incidence of AD in the USA is projected to be 7.7 millions in 2030 and 11–16 millions in 2050 (ADFF, 2016).

The pathology of AD begins well before symptom manifestation, with intracellular accumulation of neurofibrillary tangles that arise via abnormal tau protein phosphorylation and extracellular deposition of Aβ-plaques (Selkoe, 1994, 2001a,b). Interfering with neuronal communication, deposition of β-amyloid plaques causes neuronal death, while tau tangles Blocks transport of essentials into interior of the neurons. Characterized by progressive memory loss and cognitive impairment, advanced stage AD patients show symptoms ranging from neuron inflammation to neuron death. Various risk factors promote pathological changes well before the onset of clinical symptoms of AD. In addition to cardiovascular risk, studies suggest a significant contribution of lifestyle related factors such as obesity, diabetes, depression, smoking, and insufficient diet in dementia. This review presents an overview of AD with recent updates on epidemiology, factors that aggravate the disease, and a prospective insight into diagnostic markers and therapeutic options for disease treatment.

GENETIC SUSCEPTIBILITY

AD represents one of the greatest health-care challenges of the twenty-first century. Its dependence on age and genetic background has resulted in its classification as either familial (FAD; showing early onset), which is observed in 5% of AD cases, or sporadic (SAD; showing late disease onset), which shows a high disease incidence rate. Though ApoE4 is a well-characterized risk factor in SAD, disease etiology in FAD is attributed to mutations of *amyloid precursor protein* (APP), *presenilin*1 (PS1), and *presenilin* 2 (PS2) genes (Goate et al., 1991; Levy-Lahad et al., 1995; Rogaev et al., 1995; Sherrington et al., 1996; Selkoe, 2001b). Accounting for 15% of total ApoE, APOE4 interferes with the clearance of Aβ from brain. Differing in amino acid substitutions at 112 and 158 positions, ApoE4 carries two arginines, while ApoE3 have two cysteines and ApoE2 has arginine and cysteine at these positions (Mahley and Huang, 2009). Attribution of APOE4 to AD is 50% in homozygous (Apo E4/E4) and 20–30% in heterozygous condition with APOE3 (Genin et al., 2011).

Over the time, substantial evidences regarding accumulation of misfolded Aβ and tau tangles (so-called seeds of pathological consequences) in the brain of patients suffering from AD have been established (Karran et al., 2011). Evidential support of Aβ and tau involvement comes from FAD studies that report mutations in APP (Aβ precursor) and PS1&2 (catalytic γ-secretase subunit; Karch and Goate, 2015; Ahmad et al., 2016). Having a critical role in the multi-causality of dementia (Boyle et al., 2013), mutations in APP enhance aggregation, while PSEN1&2 mutations cause less efficient APP processing, leading to longer and more hydrophobic Aβs (Scheuner et al., 1996; Chávez-Gutiérrez et al., 2012; Wong et al., 2013; **Table 1**). Though mutations in APP and PS1&2 accelerate generation of disease seeds, decreased Aβ clearance (Mawuenyega et al., 2010) and increased Aβ accumulation (Wahlster et al., 2013) enhances SAD.

MITOCHONDRIAL STRESS IN AD

Performing vital biochemical functions, mitochondrial dysfunction significantly affects progression in the pathogenesis of AD (Swerdlow et al., 2014). Associated with the regulation of cellular metabolism, functional impairment of metabolic enzymes, in particular enzymes of the TCA cycle, causes reduction in the energy metabolism in brain (Huang et al., 2003; Bubber et al., 2005). Studies of the AD brain have revealed significant impairment in the functioning of pyruvate dehydrogenase complex (PDHC) and α-ketoglutarate dehydrogenase complex (KGDHC) enzymes, followed by impairment of isocitrate dehydrogenase (Huang et al., 2003; Bubber et al., 2005). Although, increased activity of succinate and malate dehydrogenases was observed, activities of the remaining four enzymes remains unaltered. Considering the high energy demand of neurons, a role of mitochondrial oxidative stress leading to energy imbalance appears to have a considerable effect on neurodegeneration.

Mitochondrial dysfunction, observed as altered mitochondrial DNA and increased cytochrome oxidase (COX) levels, indicates oxidative damage to the neurons of AD patients (Hirai et al., 2001; Nunomura et al., 2001; Moreira et al., 2006, 2007, 2009; Su et al., 2008). In concert with the amyloid hypothesis, altered APP processing increases Aβ deposition (Furukawa et al., 1996), whose aggregation causes oxidative stress through an increase in the production of H_2O_2 (Readnower et al., 2011). Inhibition of the mitochondrial electron transport chain (ETC) causes increased ROS production, which damages proteins, lipids, and nucleic acids, observed as increases in 8-hydroxy-2-deoxyguanosine (8-OHdG) and nitrotyrosine levels (Wang et al., 2005). Accumulation of Aβ in the synaptic mitochondria makes them susceptible to changes in synaptic Ca^{2+} as they have high levels of cyclophilin D (CypD; Sayre et al., 2005). Being a component of the mitochondrial permeability transition pore (mPTP), CypD translocation from matrix to mPTP increases interaction of CypD-mPTP with adenine nucleotide translocase resulting in opening of the pore and as such collapse of membrane potential, which ultimately leads to neuronal death (Juhaszova et al., 2004). An increase in the oxidative burden of mitochondria mediates activation of FoxO transcription factor (Kops et al., 2002; Fu and Tindall, 2008), which is associated with induction of SOD and catalase activity, as well as causing cell cycle arrest and cell death (Castellani et al., 2002). Increased ROS attenuation of the antioxidant arsenal of mitochondria alters the cellular redox state. Increased ROS levels act as an autophagy trigger and subjects mitochondria to mitophagy (Scherz-Shouval and Elazar, 2011).

TABLE 1 | Summary of mutations predicted in genes that have been associated with the occurrence of AD.

S. No	Gene	No. of mutations	Mutation type	Representation	Location	Effect
1.	APP	52	Point, Missense, Silent, Deletion	Both coding & non-coding	Exon 5 = 1 Exon 6 = 3 Exon 7 = 2 Exon 11 = 2 Exon 12 = 2 Exon 13 = 2 Exon 14 = 4 Exon 16 = 10 Exon 17 = 25 Non-coding = 1	Pathogenic = 1 Not-pathogenic = 15 Unclear pathogenicity = 9 Protective = 1
2.	MAPT	15	Point, Missense, Deletion	Both coding & non-coding	Exon 1 = 2 Exon 3 = 1 Exon 4a = 5 Exon 6 = 1 Exon 7 = 1 Exon 8 = 1 Exon 10 = 2 Non-coding = 1 *In silico* = 1	Pathogenic = 0 Not-pathogenic = 5 Unclear pathogenicity = 10 Risk modifier = 1
3.	PSEN1	241	Point, Missense, Insertion, Deletion, Complex	Both coding & non-coding (Intron)	Exon 4 = 22 Exon 5 = 46 Exon 6 = 27 Exon 7 = 56 Exon 8 = 36 Exon 9 = 7 Exon 10 = 7 Exon 11 = 22 Exon 12 = 17 Intron = 1	Pathogenic = 223 Not-pathogenic = 3 Unclear pathogenicity = 16
4.	PSEN 2	45	Point, Missense, Insertion, Deletion	Coding	Exon 3 = 2 Exon 4 = 8 Exon 5 = 12 Exon 6 = 3 Exon 7 = 11 Exon 8 = 1 Exon 9 = 1 Exon 10 = 3 Exon 11 = 2 Exon 12 = 2	Pathogenic = 18 Not-pathogenic = 12 Unclear pathogenicity = 15

ENDOPLASMIC RETICULUM (ER) STRESS IN AD

Acting as a site of protein synthesis, disruption in the proteostasis causes accumulation of unfolded proteins in the ER lumen (Wu and Kaufman, 2006; Ron and Walter, 2007). To reduce abnormal protein aggregation, unfolded proteins are translocated to cytoplasm for degradation; a process referred as ER-associated protein degradation (ERAD; Hetz et al., 2011; Walter and Ron, 2011). Attainment of saturation in the ER's protein-folding capacity elicits a dynamic signaling response referred as unfolded protein response (UPR; Lee, 2001; Ledoux et al., 2003). Recognition of unfolded proteins by stress sensors such as inositol requiring protein 1 (IRE1), protein kinase RNA (PKR) like ER kinase (PERK), and activating transcription factor 6 (ATF6) triggers downstream signaling via transcription factors (Hetz and Mollereau, 2014). PERK induces rapid translational attenuation by inhibition of the eukaryotic translational initiation factor 2α (eIF2α). PERK-mediated phosphorylation of eIF2α also favors translation of transcription factor ATF4, which is capable of controlling expression of genes related to amino acid metabolism, autophagy, and apoptosis. Increased phosphorylation of eIF2α in PS1 mutant knockout mice confirmed the inhibition of eIF2α phosphorylation by PS1 (Milhavet et al., 2002). Additionally, PS1-mediated abnormal processing of IRE1 disturbs UPR by interfering with the ER stress. Activation of IRE1 signaling induces splicing of X-box binding protein 1 (XBP-1), which controls the expression of lipid synthesis, ER protein translocation, protein folding, and ERAD genes (Hetz et al., 2011; Walter and Ron, 2011). Polymorphism in the promoter region of XBP-1, which reduces its transcription, is considered as a risk factor for AD (Liu et al., 2013). Expression of GPR78 and GPR94 associated with the refolding of unfolded proteins attenuated in PS2-expressed cells is attributed to impaired IRE1 phosphorylation. Though protection against Aβ toxicity through enforced *Xbp1* expression in a *Drosophila melanogaster* AD model is attributed to reduction in the release of Ca^{2+} from ER (Casas-Tinto et al., 2011), a similar effect in *Caenorhabditis elegans* AD model is correlated with augmented stress levels and enhanced autophagy (Safra et al., 2013). Nuclear translocation of ATF6 following protease cleavage activates ERAD genes and XBP-1. Moreover, ATF4, ATF6, and XBP-1 stimulate C/EBP homologous protein (CHOP) and its target growth arrest and DNA damage inducible 34 (GADD34), as well as pro-apoptotic components of the B cell lymphoma-2 (BCL2) family of proteins (Xu et al., 2005). Neurons expressing p-tau show enhanced UPR activation (Hoozemans et al., 2009; Abisambra et al., 2013). Excessive adaptive capacity of UPR triggers pro-apoptotic events through upregulation of the cell death genes such as caspase-12 (Szegezdi et al., 2003).

AUTOPHAGY IN AD

Degradation of non-essential cellular components, such as misfolded and aggregated proteins, occurs through the autophagy-lysosomal system (ALS; Li et al., 2010; Murrow and Debnath, 2013). Activated by oxidative stress, nutrient starvation, etc., clearance of unwanted entities helps in restoring substrates for cellular remodeling (Ichimura and Komatsu, 2010; Li et al., 2010; Murrow and Debnath, 2013). Abundance of growth factors and cellular nutrients activates mTOR kinase, whereas a starvation state exerts inhibitory effect on mTOR kinase activity. The mTOR kinase-mediated phosphorylation of ATG13 prevents its association to Unc-51 like kinase (ULK), and recruitment of focal adhesion kinase family interacting protein of 200 kD (FIP200) inhibits autophagy, whereas inhibition of mTOR activates phosphatases that cause dephosphorylation of ATG13 (Kundu, 2011; Lee et al., 2012), thereby promotes autophagy. Although mTOR-dependent autophagy is prominent, there are reports of mTOR-independent autophagy mediated by (1) ATG5 and ATG7 via microtubule associated light chain 3-II (LC3-II; Nishida et al., 2009); (2) autophagic proteins Beclin1, Bcl-2, and ULK1 (Nishida et al., 2009; Shimizu et al., 2010); and (3) non-canonical signaling events involving Ca^{2+}. In addition, Ca^{2+} has a prominent role in both canonical and non-canonical mTOR-independent autophagy (Cárdenas and Foskett, 2012; Decuypere et al., 2013). Deletion of Beclin-1 in AD mouse models has resulted in increased Aβ accumulation, while its overexpression leads to reduction in amyloid pathology (Pickford et al., 2008; Jaeger and Wyss-Coray, 2010). Though IP3 receptor-mediated Ca^{2+} signaling inhibits autophagy, an increase in the cytosolic Ca^{2+} level promotes autophagy (Criollo et al., 2007; Wang et al., 2008; Khan and Joseph, 2010; Vingtdeux et al., 2010). Some studies have linked PS mutation in FAD with neuronal dysfunction and apoptosis via Ca^{2+} dysfunction (Del Prete et al., 2014; Duggan and McCarthy, 2016).

Despite entrapping non-selective molecules, selective trapping of various molecules occurs through interaction of LC3-II with cargo-receptors such as nuclear dot protein-52 (NDP52), p62, and neighbor of BRAC1 (NRB1; Bjørkøy et al., 2005; Kirkin et al., 2009; Jo et al., 2014). Acting as an autophagic adaptor for degradation of toll/IL-1 receptor homology domain containing adaptor including IFN-β (TRIF) and tumor receptor associated factor-6 (TRAF6), a role of NDP-52 in docking of autophagosomes to T6BP, myosin VI, and optineurin for maturation has been reported (Inomata et al., 2012; Tumbarello et al., 2012). Interaction of NBR1 and p62 with ubiquitinated misfolded proteins and members of the ATG8 family makes them critical for autophagosome formation (Kabeya et al., 2000; Bjørkøy et al., 2005; Pankiv et al., 2007; Kirkin et al., 2009). PS1 mutations that cause a loss of lysosomal acidification ultimately lead to loss of lysosomal proteolytic activity (Lee et al., 2010). Disruption in the lysosomal function causes accumulation of autophagosomes containing protein aggregates, as observed in the AD brain. Studies indicate involvement of NDP-52 as a downstream facilitator of nuclear factor erythroid-2 related factor 2 (Nrf2)-mediated tau (phosphorylated) degradation (Jo et al., 2014). Reduction in the autophagy-aggravated AD pathology underlines the critical role of autophagy in the removal of Aβ aggregates (Cai et al., 2012; Di Domenico et al., 2014).

BIOMARKERS OF AD

Cortical amyloid deposition of Aβ and phosphorylated tau (p-tau) are core biomarkers of AD in CSF (Blennow et al., 2010). With high accuracy diagnostics, specificity of the core repertoire of biomarkers is in the 80–90% range in the mild cognitive impairment stage of AD (Shaw et al., 2009; Visser et al., 2009). Despite this, assessment of the sensitivity of disease biomarkers reflects an imperfect criterion in the gold standard of clinical diagnosis of the disease because it fails to distinguish pathological changes such as plaque count between cognitively normal elderly persons and those with AD (Coart et al., 2015; Curtis et al., 2015). Changes in α-synuclein (α-syn), TDP43, and several vascular indicators, are other pathological markers in patients suffering from AD (Kovacs et al., 2013).

A step to increase the specificity and sensitivity of biomarkers has led to the screening of several different entities for use in the diagnosis of AD. One such biomarker involves Aβ oligomers (toxic forms of Aβ), which are associated with synaptic dysfunction (Overk and Masliah, 2014). Though increases in the Aβ oligomers are observed in AD, their limited occurrence in the CSF hinders their reliability in the diagnosis of AD (Hölttä et al., 2013; Yang et al., 2013). Neurogranin, a dendritic protein, is another synaptic biomarker candidate (Díez-Guerra, 2010). Increased amount of neurogranin in CSF of AD patients is correlated with the progression of mild cognitive impairment (Kvartsberg et al., 2015). Additionally, an increase in the level of presynaptic protein SNAP25 might indicate AD diagnosis (Brinkmalm et al., 2014). Of the other biomarkers, screening of CNS-specific protein candidates in blood also seems suitable; when sampling populations for AD. Combinations of proteins, lipids, and other molecules have been used in the assessment of AD (Henriksen et al., 2014; Mapstone et al., 2014). However, as they may be secreted in low amounts and are prone to degradation by plasma proteases, their suitability as biomarkers for AD is uncertain. Similarly, tau-imaging, which is commonly employed in drug trials to determine delay in the progression of AD may be another potentially suitable option for AD diagnosis.

THERAPEUTIC APPROACHES TO COMBAT AD

The fact that critical care provides patients a better quality of life family care is considered as the mainstay in the treatment of AD. At present, efforts are being made on two fronts; toward developing disease modifying therapies that can uphold progression of the disease, and; developing drugs that can act as disease pathway blockers. As Aβ and tau hyper-phosphorylation are well-recognized hallmarks of AD (Lee et al., 2005; Querfurth and Laferla, 2010; Ahmad et al., 2017), current drug approaches are aimed at:

Improved APP Processing via Inhibition and/or Activation of Enzymatic Machinery

To date, only five drugs have been approved by the USA FDA for treatment of cognitive manifestations of AD (**Table 2**). Of the different drug regimes, glutamate agonist memantine, and acetylcholine esterase (AchE) inhibitors such as rivastigmine, donepezil, and galantamine are employed in the treatment of the dementia phase of AD (Raina et al., 2008). Blocking the pathological stimulation of NMDA receptors, memantine protects neural cells from glutamate-mediated excitoxicity. AchE inhibitors cause temporary slowdown in cognitive function by decreasing activity of cholinesterase, leading to enhanced acetylcholine (Ach) levels and, thereby, brain functions (Godyn et al., 2016). As disruption of AchE has a direct correlation with NFT and Aβ deposits (Tavitian et al., 1993), AchE inhibitors stabilize cognitive performance and daily functioning in early dementia stages, whereas application of memantine provides benefits to patients suffering from moderate to severe dementia (Godyn et al., 2016). The fifth drug, tacrine is less prescribed due to its hepatotoxicity. Although these drugs provide symptomatic improvement in AD, benefits are generally short lived and with no effect on the pathogenic mechanism or on disease progression. Research into potential strategies is currently directed at screening bioactive compounds for their effect on enzyme inhibition, aggregation, prevention of Aβ formation, and upregulation in the removal of toxic Aβ.

Immunotherapeutic Approaches to Existing Amyloids

Currently, the most attractive Aβ-directed approach, immunotherapy enlists both active (immune stimulation by vaccine for antibody production) and passive (injection of pre-prepared antibodies) immunization. Engaging both the cellular and humoral immune systems, active immunization is cost effective and ensures long-term high antibody titers. An active vaccination journey begins with AN1792, a full-length $A\beta_{1-42}$ peptide injected with the immune stimulant adjuvant QS21 (Panza et al., 2014). However, on observing meningoencephalitis among 6% of the enrolled AD patients, the phase II AN1792 trial was halted in 2002. Taking strong cognizance of AN1792 trials, larger studies were directed at testing passive immunotherapy by using human anti-Aβ monoclonal antibodies. At present various 2nd generation active Aβ vaccines are undergoing clinical trials; of particular note are CAD106 ($A\beta_{1-6}$; Novartis), ACC001 ($A\beta_{1-6}$; Janssen and Pfizer), ACI-24, V-950, and AD-02 ($A\beta_{1-6}$; Alzforum, 2016). Compared to active immunization that leads to a polyclonal antibody response, target specificity (specific against monomeric Aβ, Aβ fibrils, and their carrier and transport proteins) in passive immunization has advantages both in preventing Aβ-aggregation and in promoting Aβ-clearance in anti-Aβ immunotherapy. The first monoclonal antibody was bapineuzumab directed against $A\beta_{1-5}$ (Abushouk et al., 2017; Xing et al., 2017). Although it reduced Aβ in brain during phase II trials, it failed to achieve significant benefit in a phase III trial, leading to its termination in 2012. This was followed by trials of mAb m266, which showed enhanced Aβ clearance from brain to blood (Demattos et al., 2001; Dodart et al., 2002). Using am266 precursor, Solanezumab directed against mid-domain $A\beta_{16-24}$ revealed dose-dependent increases in plasma Aβ, suggesting cleavage of insoluble species from senile plaques (Farlow et al., 2012; Han and Mook-Jung, 2014). Other Abs undergoing clinical trials include gantenerumab (showing binding specificity for Aβ plaques), crenezumab IgG4 mAb (showing binding specificity for Aβ oligomers, plaques, and fibrils that inhibit aggregation), GSK933766, and BAN2401 mAb (Alzforum, 2016). Reduction in Aβ production is also achieved by using inhibitors against secretases such as NIC5-15, Bryostatin-1, AZD3293, MK8931, and E2609 (Alzforum, 2016).

Tau Centric Therapies

Tau centric therapies include the use of putative tau kinase inhibitors, microtubule stabilizers, and tau immunotherapy. Glycogen synthase kinase-3β (GSK-3β), the primary enzyme involved in tau phosphorylation, is considered the primary target for disease modification (Jaworski et al., 2011). As Aβ promotes GSK-3β activity, studies of GSK-3β inhibitors such as tideglusib and AZD1080 were pursued (King et al., 2014; Lovestone et al., 2015). Clinical trials of AZD1080 revealed nephrotoxicity (Eldar-Finkelman and Martinez, 2011), while the trials for tideglusib showed diminished clinical benefits. Microtubule stabilizers inhibit tau aggregation (Bulic et al., 2010). LMTC, a methylthionium chloride (MTC) derivative prevents tau interactions, thereby facilitating its clearance from the brain (Wischik et al., 2015). Other microtubule stabilizers include TPI207 and BMS241027 (epothilone-D). Immunotherapy for tau protein is directed toward prevention of NFT formation. Both AADvacl (a synthetic tau derived peptide) and ACI-35 (liposome formulated based tau protein) are currently being evaluated for their effects on avoiding tau aggregation (Alzforum, 2016).

TABLE 2 | Summary of therapeutic options available in the treatment of AD.

S. No	Therapy type (categorization)	Phase 1/2	Phase 3	Phase 4		Approval for treatment			
		Number	Name	Name (synonyms)	Target	Name	Synonyms	Target	Approved for
1.	Small molecules	50	LMTM, AGB101, ALZT-OP1, AVP-786, AZD3293, Aripiprazole, Azeliragon, Brexpiprazole, Elenbecestat, ITI-007, Idalopirdine, Intepirdine, Masitinib, Nilvadipine, Pioglitazone, Verubecestat	AVP-923 (Nuedexta, Zenvia)	Other Neurotransmitters	Donepezil	Aricept™, Donepezil hydrochloride, Eranz®, E 2020	Cholinergic system	Alzheimer's disease
				Carvedilol (Coreg, Artist, Aucardic, Dilatrend, Kredex)	Unknown	Galantamine	Razadyne™, Reminyl™, Nivalin®	Cholinergic system	Mild to Moderate Alzheimer's disease
				Prazosin (Prazosin hydrochloride, Minipress, VasoflexHypovase,)	Other Neurotransmitters	Memantine	Ebixa™, Memary®, Axura®, Akatinol®, Namenda™,	Other neurotransmitters	Alzheimer's disease
				Resveratrol (trans-3,4′,5-trihydroxystilbene)	Other	Rivastigmine	Exelon™, Rivastigmine tartrate, Rivastach® Patch, Prometax®, SDZ ENA 713	Cholinergic system	Mild to moderate Alzheimer's disease
				Simvastatin (Zocor®, Denan®, Lipovas® Lipex®)	Cholesterol	Tacrine	Cognex™	Cholinergic system	Alzheimer's disease
2.	Dietary Supplement	4	Alpha-Tocopherol (Vitamin E)	Docosahexaenoic acid (DHA; Omega 3 fatty acid)	Others (reduction of amyloid, tau)	–	–	–	–
				Ketasyn (Axona, Caprylic Acid, AC-1202)	Others	–	–	–	–
				Resveratrol (trans-3,4′,5-trihydroxystilbene)	Others (prevention of amyloid deposition, induction of sirtuin-1 gene)	–	–	–	–
3.	Immunotherapy (active)	8	–	–	–	–	–	–	–
4.	Immunotherapy (passive)	11	Aducanumab (BIIB037), Crenezumab (MABT5102A, RG7412), Gantenerumab (RO4909832, RG1450), Solanezumab (LY2062430)	–	–	–	–	–	–
5.	Procedural intervention	2	Continuous Positive Airway Pressure (CPAP)	–	–	–	–	–	–

http://www.alzforum.org/therapeutics

Therapies to Combat Oxidative Stress

Oxidative stress due to reactive oxygen species (ROS), being a major player in neurodegeneration strategies, are currently being devised to combat its emergence at mitochondria (Federico et al., 2012; Yan et al., 2013; Kim et al., 2015). On the forefront, ferulic acid (FA), epigallocatechin-3-gallate, and nano formulation of naturally occurring curcumin were found exerting strong antioxidant, anti-inflammatory and amyloid disintegration properties (Rezai-Zadeh et al., 2005; Yang et al., 2005; Cheng et al., 2013; Sgarbossa et al., 2015; Cascella et al., 2017). Alleviating mitochondrial dysfunction under diseased conditions, peptide based strategies complemented with different drug molecules have shown positive results in overcoming the inefficiency of low antioxidant levels (Kumar and Singh, 2015). Of them, Szeto-Schiller (SS) peptides displaying a sequence motif that directs its accumulation inside mitochondria inhibit lipid peroxidation. Accumulation of SS31 on inner mitochondrial membrane prevents release of cyt-C (Szeto, 2008; Kumar and Singh, 2015). Similarly, accumulation of drugs such as MitoQ inside mitochondria increases its potential to neutralize free radicals several 100-folds than that attributed by natural antioxidants (Tauskela, 2007; Ross et al., 2008). Probucol, a drug that helps establishment of balance of mitochondal fission-fusion processes, also maintains AD mitochondria induced extracellular signal regulated kinase (ERK) activation (Champagne et al., 2003; Gan et al., 2014).

Autophagy Enhancer Therapy

As accumulation of the aggregated proteins enhances neurodegeneration, enhancement in the degenerative capacity via, autophagy inducers seems a good therapeutic approach. Their mode of action involves prevention in the accumulation of Aβ plaques and tau tangles via degradation of the aggregates. Of the available drugs, rapamycin acting as mTOR inhibitor was found ameliorating Aβ and tau pathies in AD mouse model (Caccamo et al., 2010; Rubinsztein et al., 2012). Latrepirdine stimulation of autophagy reduces Aβ neuropathy in mouse brain (Steele and Gandy, 2013). Metformin, a PP2A agonist, inhibition of TORC1 prevents hyperphosphorylation of tau protein (Kickstein et al., 2010). Other authophagy enhancers include reservatol and its analogs, RSVA314 and RSVA405, virally packaged BECN1 and its mimetics, nicotinamide, etc (Vingtdeux et al., 2010; Shoji-Kawata et al., 2013). Though, Beclin1 deficiency increases APP and Aβ levels, its over-expression in cultured neurons cause significant reduction in Aβ accumulation (Pickford et al., 2008). Additionally, PS1 and PS2 serving as a catalytic subunit of γ-secretase was found acting as autophagy modulators (Lee et al., 2010). Associated with the substrate cleavage, their knockdown was found exhibiting inefficiency in the clearance of protein aggregates. Cells deficient in PS1 was found having reduced levels of cargo shuttle protein p62, associated with the degradation of abnormal tau (Tung et al., 2014; Caccamo et al., 2017).

Failure of biologics that target amyloids to cross the blood-brain barrier (BBB) indicates the necessity of development of an efficient drug delivery system. Liposomes and polymeric nanoparticles have shown promising results in delivering drugs and other therapeutic molecules (Ha et al., 2016); however, their use as a means to deliver drugs across the BBB has encountered roadblocks associated with biocompatibility and long-term safety. Persistent problems with low biocompatibility, restricted immune escape, circulation stability, and toxicity have led to a gradual shift of research toward the use of exosomes. Their long circulatory half-life, host biocompatibility, target-specific drug delivery ability, and low toxicity have increased the interest in using exosomes to deliver drugs in several neurodegenerative diseases (Lai and Breakefield, 2012; Liu et al., 2016). As drug delivery through exosomes has shown promising results in the ongoing studies, their utilization in reducing disease progression may indicate their suitability in reducing progression of AD.

CONCLUSION

AD progresses via aggregation and accumulation in the extracellular milieu of amyloid plaques and intraneuronal neurofibrillary tangles produced by p-tau. Although malfunctioning APP, PS-1 &-2 genes are considered the main culprits behind AD, mitochondrial dysfunction, ER stress and mitophagy significantly increase progression of the disease. Current research provides useful information on new targets and their utilization in designing novel inhibitors or drugs as part of attempts to achieve successful treatment of AD. It also studies different entities for employment as potent biomarkers in disease diagnosis and provides information on therapeutic suitability in the treatment of AD. Further studies on the use of exosomes as drug delivery vehicles are needed in order to reveal and reduce safety and ethical concerns. With increases in newly identified targets, studies pertaining to the design of drugs and other potent therapeutic molecules are needed in order to combat the progression of AD.

AUTHOR CONTRIBUTIONS

IC, QH, and AJ: conceived the idea; AJ and MA: contributed to writing of the manuscript; AJ, SR, AA, DC, and EL: contributed to upgrading the contents and preparing the tables.

ACKNOWLEDGMENTS

Authors extend their thanks to colleagues for their criticism, which helped to improve the quality of this paper's contents and broaden its perspective to reach a broader audience. This work was supported by the Creative Economy Leading Technology Development Program through the Gyeongsangbuk-Do and Gyeongbuk Science & Technology Promotion Center of Korea (SF316001A).

REFERENCES

Abisambra, J. F., Jinwal, U. K., Blair, L. J., O'leary, J. C., Li, Q., Brady, S., et al. (2013). Tau accumulation activates the unfolded protein response by impairing endoplasmic reticulum-associated degradation. *J. Neurosci.* 33, 9498–9507. doi: 10.1523/JNEUROSCI.5397-12.2013

Abushouk, A. I., Elmaraezy, A., Aglan, A., Salama, R., Fouda, S., Fouda, R., et al. (2017). Bapineuzumab for mild to moderate Alzheimer's disease: a meta-analysis of randomized controlled trials. *BMC Neurol* 17:66. doi: 10.1186/s12883-017-0850-1

ADFF (2016). Alzheimer's disease facts and figures. *Alzheimers Dement.* 12, 459–509. doi: 10.1016/j.jalz.2016.03.001

Ahmad, K., Baig, M. H., Gupta, G. K., Kamal, M. A., Pathak, N., and Choi, I. (2016). Identification of common therapeutic targets for selected neurodegenerative disorders: an *in silico* approach. *J. Comput. Sci.* 17, 292–306. doi: 10.1016/j.jocs.2016.03.007

Ahmad, K., Baig, M. H., Mushtaq, G., Kamal, M. A., Greig, N. H., and Choi, I. (2017). Commonalities in biological pathways, genetics, and cellular mechanism between Alzheimer Disease and other neurodegenerative diseases: an *in silico*-updated overview. *Curr Alzheimer Res.* 14, 1190–1197. doi: 10.2174/1567205014666170203141151

Alzforum (2016). *Therapeutics for Alzheimers Disease.* Available online at: http://www.alzforum.org/therapeutics.

Bjørkøy, G., Lamark, T., Brech, A., Outzen, H., Perander, M., Overvatn, A., et al. (2005). p62/SQSTM1 forms protein aggregates degraded by autophagy and has a protective effect on huntingtin-induced cell death. *J. Cell. Biol.* 171, 603–614. doi: 10.1083/jcb.200507002

Blennow, K., Hampel, H., Weiner, M., and Zetterberg, H. (2010). Cerebrospinal fluid and plasma biomarkers in Alzheimer disease. *Nat. Rev. Neurol.* 6, 131–144. doi: 10.1038/nrneurol.2010.4

Boyle, P. A., Wilson, R. S., Yu, L., Barr, A. M., Honer, W. G., Schneider, J. A., et al. (2013). Much of late life cognitive decline is not due to common neurodegenerative pathologies. *Ann. Neurol.* 74, 478–489. doi: 10.1002/ana.23964

Brinkmalm, A., Brinkmalm, G., Honer, W. G., Frölich, L., Hausner, L., Minthon, L., et al. (2014). SNAP-25 is a promising novel cerebrospinal fluid biomarker for synapse degeneration in Alzheimer's disease. *Mol. Neurodegener.* 9:53. doi: 10.1186/1750-1326-9-53

Bubber, P., Haroutunian, V., Fisch, G., Blass, J. P., and Gibson, G. E. (2005). Mitochondrial abnormalities in Alzheimer brain: mechanistic implications. *Ann. Neurol.* 57, 695–703. doi: 10.1002/ana.20474

Bulic, B., Pickhardt, M., Mandelkow, E. M., and Mandelkow, E. (2010). Tau protein and tau aggregation inhibitors. *Neuropharmacology* 59, 276–289. doi: 10.1016/j.neuropharm.2010.01.016

Caccamo, A., Ferreira, E., Branca, C., and Oddo, S. (2017). p62 improves AD-like pathology by increasing autophagy. *Mol. Psychiatry* 22, 865–873. doi: 10.1038/mp.2016.139

Caccamo, A., Majumder, S., Richardson, A., Strong, R., and Oddo, S. (2010). Molecular interplay between mammalian target of rapamycin (mTOR), amyloid-beta, and Tau: effects on cognitive impairments. *J. Biol. Chem.* 285, 13107–13120. doi: 10.1074/jbc.M110.100420

Cai, Z., Zhao, B., Li, K., Zhang, L., Li, C., Quazi, S. H., et al. (2012). Mammalian target of rapamycin: a valid therapeutic target through the autophagy pathway for Alzheimer's disease? *J. Neurosci. Res.* 90, 1105–1118. doi: 10.1002/jnr.23011

Cárdenas, C., and Foskett, J. K. (2012). Mitochondrial Ca(2+) signals in autophagy. *Cell Calcium* 52, 44–51. doi: 10.1016/j.ceca.2012.03.001

Casas-Tinto, S., Zhang, Y., Sanchez-Garcia, J., Gomez-Velazquez, M., Rincon-Limas, D. E., and Fernandez-Funez, P. (2011). The ER stress factor XBP1s prevents amyloid-beta neurotoxicity. *Hum. Mol. Genet.* 20, 2144–2160. doi: 10.1093/hmg/ddr100

Cascella, M., Bimonte, S., Muzio, M. R., Schiavone, V., and Cuomo, A. (2017). The efficacy of Epigallocatechin-3-gallate (green tea) in the treatment of Alzheimer's disease: an overview of pre-clinical studies and translational perspectives in clinical practice. *Infect. Agent Cancer* 12:36. doi: 10.1186/s13027-017-0145-6

Castellani, R., Hirai, K., Aliev, G., Drew, K. L., Nunomura, A., Takeda, A., et al. (2002). Role of mitochondrial dysfunction in Alzheimer's disease. *J. Neurosci. Res.* 70, 357–360. doi: 10.1002/jnr.10389

Champagne, D., Pearson, D., Dea, D., Rochford, J., and Poirier, J. (2003). The cholesterol-lowering drug Probucol increases apolipoprotein e production in the hippocampus of aged rats: implications for Alzheimer's disease. *Neuroscience* 121, 99–110. doi: 10.1016/S0306-4522(03)00361-0

Chávez-Gutiérrez, L., Bammens, L., Benilova, I., Vandersteen, A., Benurwar, M., Borgers, M., et al. (2012). The mechanism of gamma-Secretase dysfunction in familial Alzheimer disease. *EMBO J.* 31, 2261–2274. doi: 10.1038/emboj.2012.79

Cheng, K. K., Yeung, C. F., Ho, S. W., Chow, S. F., Chow, A. H., and Baum, L. (2013). Highly stabilized curcumin nanoparticles tested in an *in vitro* blood-brain barrier model and in Alzheimer's disease Tg2576 mice. *AAPS J.* 15, 324–336. doi: 10.1208/s12248-012-9444-4

Coart, E., Barrado, L. G., Duits, F. H., Scheltens, P., van der Flier, W. M., Teunissen, C. E., et al. (2015). Correcting for the absence of a gold standard improves diagnostic accuracy of biomarkers in Alzheimer's Disease. *J Alzheimers Dis.* 46, 889–899. doi: 10.3233/JAD-142886

Criollo, A., Maiuri, M. C., Tasdemir, E., Vitale, I., Fiebig, A. A., Andrews, D., et al. (2007). Regulation of autophagy by the inositol trisphosphate receptor. *Cell Death Differ* 14, 1029–1039. doi: 10.1038/sj.cdd.4402099

Curtis, C., Gamez, J. E., Singh, U., Sadowsky, C. H., Villena, T., Sabbagh, M. N., et al. (2015). Phase 3 trial of flutemetamol labeled with radioactive fluorine 18 imaging and neuritic plaque density. *JAMA Neurol.* 72, 287–294. doi: 10.1001/jamaneurol.2014.4144

Decuypere, J. P., Kindt, D., Luyten, T., Welkenhuyzen, K., Missiaen, L., De Smedt, H., et al. (2013). mTOR-controlled autophagy requires intracellular Ca(2+) signaling. *PLoS ONE* 8:e61020. doi: 10.1371/journal.pone.0061020

Del Prete, D., Checler, F., and Chami, M. (2014). Ryanodine receptors: physiological function and deregulation in Alzheimer disease. *Mol. Neurodegener.* 9, 21–29. doi: 10.1186/1750-1326-9-21

Demattos, R. B., Bales, K. R., Cummins, D. J., Dodart, J. C., Paul, S. M., and Holtzman, D. M. (2001). Peripheral anti-A beta antibody alters CNS and plasma A beta clearance and decreases brain A beta burden in a mouse model of Alzheimer's disease. *Proc. Natl. Acad. Sci. U.S.A.* 98, 8850–8855. doi: 10.1073/pnas.151261398

Di Domenico, F., Head, E., Butterfield, D. A., and Perluigi, M. (2014). Oxidative stress and proteostasis network: culprit and casualty of Alzheimer's- like Neurodegeneration. *Adv. Geriatr.* 2014:14. doi: 10.1155/2014/527518

Díez-Guerra, F. J. (2010). Neurogranin, a link between calcium/calmodulin and protein kinase C signaling in synaptic plasticity. *IUBMB Life* 62, 597–606. doi: 10.1002/iub.357

Dodart, J. C., Bales, K. R., Gannon, K. S., Greene, S. J., Demattos, R. B., Mathis, C., et al. (2002). Immunization reverses memory deficits without reducing brain Abeta burden in Alzheimer's disease model. *Nat. Neurosci.* 5, 452–457. doi: 10.1038/nn842

Duggan, S. P., and McCarthy, J. V. (2016). Beyond gamma-secretase activity: the multifunctional nature of presenilins in cell signalling pathways. *Cell Signal* 28, 1–11. doi: 10.1016/j.cellsig.2015.10.006

Eldar-Finkelman, H., and Martinez, A. (2011). GSK-3 Inhibitors: preclinical and clinical focus on CNS. *Front. Mol. Neurosci.* 4:32. doi: 10.3389/fnmol.2011.00032

Farlow, M., Arnold, S. E., Van Dyck, C. H., Aisen, P. S., Snider, B. J., Porsteinsson, A. P., et al. (2012). Safety and biomarker effects of solanezumab in patients with Alzheimer's disease. *Alzheimers Dement.* 8, 261–271. doi: 10.1016/j.jalz.2011.09.224

Federico, A., Cardaioli, E., Da Pozzo, P., Formichi, P., Gallus, G. N., and Radi, E. (2012). Mitochondria, oxidative stress and neurodegeneration. *J. Neurol. Sci.* 322, 254–262. doi: 10.1016/j.jns.2012.05.030

Fu, Z., and Tindall, D. J. (2008). FOXOs, cancer and regulation of apoptosis. *Oncogene* 27, 2312–2319. doi: 10.1038/onc.2008.24

Furukawa, K., Sopher, B. L., Rydel, R. E., Begley, J. G., Pham, D. G., Martin, G. M., et al. (1996). Increased activity-regulating and neuroprotective efficacy of alpha-secretase-derived secreted amyloid precursor protein conferred by a C-terminal heparin-binding domain. *J. Neurochem.* 67, 1882–1896. doi: 10.1046/j.1471-4159.1996.67051882.x

Gan, X., Huang, S., Wu, L., Wang, Y., Hu, G., Li, G., et al. (2014). Inhibition of ERK-DLP1 signaling and mitochondrial division alleviates mitochondrial dysfunction in Alzheimer's disease cybrid cell. *Biochim. Biophys. Acta* 1842, 220–231. doi: 10.1016/j.bbadis.2013.11.009

Genin, E., Hannequin, D., Wallon, D., Sleegers, K., Hiltunen, M., Combarros, O., et al. (2011). APOE and Alzheimer disease: a major gene with semi-dominant inheritance. *Mol. Psychiatry* 16, 903–907. doi: 10.1038/mp.2011.52

Goate, A., Chartier-Harlin, M. C., Mullan, M., Brown, J., Crawford, F., Fidani, L., et al. (1991). Segregation of a missense mutation in the amyloid precursor protein gene with familial Alzheimer's disease. *Nature* 349, 704–706. doi: 10.1038/349704a0

Godyn, J., Jonczyk, J., Panek, D., and Malawska, B. (2016). Therapeutic strategies for Alzheimer's disease in clinical trials. *Pharmacol. Rep.* 68, 127–138. doi: 10.1016/j.pharep.2015.07.006

Ha, D., Yang, N., and Nadithe, V. (2016). Exosomes as therapeutic drug carriers and delivery vehicles across biological membranes: current perspectives and future challenges. *Acta Pharm. Sin. B* 6, 287–296. doi: 10.1016/j.apsb.2016.02.001

Han, S. H., and Mook-Jung, I. (2014). Diverse molecular targets for therapeutic strategies in Alzheimer's disease. *J. Korean Med. Sci.* 29, 893–902. doi: 10.3346/jkms.2014.29.7.893

Henriksen, K., O'Bryant, S. E., Hampel, H., Trojanowski, J. Q., Montine, T. J., Jeromin, A., et al. (2014). The future of blood-based biomarkers for Alzheimer's disease. *Alzheimers Dement.* 10, 115–131. doi: 10.1016/j.jalz.2013.01.013

Hetz, C., and Mollereau, B. (2014). Disturbance of endoplasmic reticulum proteostasis in neurodegenerative diseases. *Nat. Rev. Neurosci.* 15, 233–249. doi: 10.1038/nrn3689

Hetz, C., Martinon, F., Rodriguez, D., and Glimcher, L. H. (2011). The unfolded protein response: integrating stress signals through the stress sensor IRE1alpha. *Physiol. Rev.* 91, 1219–1243. doi: 10.1152/physrev.00001.2011

Hirai, K., Aliev, G., Nunomura, A., Fujioka, H., Russell, R. L., Atwood, C. S., et al. (2001). Mitochondrial abnormalities in Alzheimer's disease. *J. Neurosci.* 21, 3017–3023.

Hölttä, M., Hansson, O., Andreasson, U., Hertze, J., Minthon, L., Nägga, K., et al. (2013). Evaluating amyloid-beta oligomers in cerebrospinal fluid as a biomarker for Alzheimer's disease. *PLoS ONE* 8:e66381. doi: 10.1371/journal.pone.0066381

Hoozemans, J. J., Van Haastert, E. S., Nijholt, D. A., Rozemuller, A. J., Eikelenboom, P., and Scheper, W. (2009). The unfolded protein response is activated in pretangle neurons in Alzheimer's disease hippocampus. *Am. J. Pathol.* 174, 1241–1251. doi: 10.2353/ajpath.2009.080814

Huang, H. M., Ou, H. C., Xu, H., Chen, H. L., Fowler, C., and Gibson, G. E. (2003). Inhibition of alpha-ketoglutarate dehydrogenase complex promotes cytochrome c release from mitochondria, caspase-3 activation, and necrotic cell death. *J. Neurosci. Res.* 74, 309–317. doi: 10.1002/jnr.10756

Ichimura, Y., and Komatsu, M. (2010). Selective degradation of p62 by autophagy. *Semin. Immunopathol.* 32, 431–436. doi: 10.1007/s00281-010-0220-1

Inomata, M., Niida, S., Shibata, K., and Into, T. (2012). Regulation of Toll-like receptor signaling by NDP52-mediated selective autophagy is normally inactivated by A20. *Cell. Mol. Life Sci.* 69, 963–979. doi: 10.1007/s00018-011-0819-y

Jaeger, P. A., and Wyss-Coray, T. (2010). Beclin 1 complex in autophagy and Alzheimer disease. *Arch. Neurol.* 67, 1181–1184. doi: 10.1001/archneurol.2010.258

Jaunmuktane, Z., Mead, S., Ellis, M., Wadsworth, J. D., Nicoll, A. J., Kenny, J., et al. (2015). Evidence for human transmission of amyloid-beta pathology and cerebral amyloid angiopathy. *Nature* 525, 247–250. doi: 10.1038/nature 15369

Jaworski, T., Dewachter, I., Lechat, B., Gees, M., Kremer, A., Demedts, D., et al. (2011). GSK-3alpha/beta kinases and amyloid production *in vivo*. *Nature* 480, E4–E5; discussion: E6. doi: 10.1038/nature10615

Jo, C., Gundemir, S., Pritchard, S., Jin, Y. N., Rahman, I., and Johnson, G. V. (2014). Nrf2 reduces levels of phosphorylated tau protein by inducing autophagy adaptor protein NDP52. *Nat. Commun.* 5:3496. doi: 10.1038/ncomms4496

Jucker, M., and Walker, L. C. (2013). Self-propagation of pathogenic protein aggregates in neurodegenerative diseases. *Nature* 501, 45–51. doi: 10.1038/nature12481

Juhaszova, M., Zorov, D. B., Kim, S. H., Pepe, S., Fu, Q., Fishbein, K. W., et al. (2004). Glycogen synthase kinase-3beta mediates convergence of protection signaling to inhibit the mitochondrial permeability transition pore. *J. Clin. Invest.* 113, 1535–1549. doi: 10.1172/JCI19906

Kabeya, Y., Mizushima, N., Ueno, T., Yamamoto, A., Kirisako, T., Noda, T., et al. (2000). LC3, a mammalian homologue of yeast Apg8p, is localized in autophagosome membranes after processing. *EMBO J.* 19, 5720–5728. doi: 10.1093/emboj/19.21.5720

Karch, C. M., and Goate, A. M. (2015). Alzheimer's disease risk genes and mechanisms of disease pathogenesis. *Biol. Psychiatry* 77, 43–51. doi: 10.1016/j.biopsych.2014.05.006

Karran, E., Mercken, M., and De Strooper, B. (2011). The amyloid cascade hypothesis for Alzheimer's disease: an appraisal for the development of therapeutics. *Nat. Rev. Drug Discov.* 10, 698–712. doi: 10.1038/nrd3505

Khan, M. T., and Joseph, S. K. (2010). Role of inositol trisphosphate receptors in autophagy in DT40 cells. *J. Biol. Chem.* 285, 16912–16920. doi: 10.1074/jbc.M110.114207

Kickstein, E., Krauss, S., Thornhill, P., Rutschow, D., Zeller, R., Sharkey, J., et al. (2010). Biguanide metformin acts on tau phosphorylation via mTOR/protein phosphatase 2A (PP2A) signaling. *Proc. Natl. Acad. Sci. U.S.A.* 107, 21830–21835. doi: 10.1073/pnas.0912793107

Kim, G. H., Kim, J. E., Rhie, S. J., and Yoon, S. (2015). The role of oxidative stress in neurodegenerative diseases. *Exp. Neurobiol.* 24, 325–340. doi: 10.5607/en.2015.24.4.325

King, M. K., Pardo, M., Cheng, Y., Downey, K., Jope, R. S., and Beurel, E. (2014). Glycogen synthase kinase-3 inhibitors: rescuers of cognitive impairments. *Pharmacol. Ther.* 141, 1–12. doi: 10.1016/j.pharmthera.2013.07.010

Kirkin, V., Lamark, T., Sou, Y. S., Bjørkøy, G., Nunn, J. L., Bruun, J. A., et al. (2009). A role for NBR1 in autophagosomal degradation of ubiquitinated substrates. *Mol. Cell* 33, 505–516. doi: 10.1016/j.molcel.2009.01.020

Kops, G. J., Dansen, T. B., Polderman, P. E., Saarloos, I., Wirtz, K. W., Coffer, P. J., et al. (2002). Forkhead transcription factor FOXO3a protects quiescent cells from oxidative stress. *Nature* 419, 316–321. doi: 10.1038/nature01036

Kovacs, G. G., Milenkovic, I., Wöhrer, A., Höftberger, R., Gelpi, E., Haberler, C., et al. (2013). Non-Alzheimer neurodegenerative pathologies and their combinations are more frequent than commonly believed in the elderly brain: a community-based autopsy series. *Acta Neuropathol.* 126, 365–384. doi: 10.1007/s00401-013-1157-y

Kumar, A., and Singh, A. (2015). A review on mitochondrial restorative mechanism of antioxidants in Alzheimer's disease and other neurological conditions. *Front. Pharmacol.* 6:206. doi: 10.3389/fphar.2015.00206

Kundu, M. (2011). ULK1, mammalian target of rapamycin, and mitochondria: linking nutrient availability and autophagy. *Antioxid. Redox Signal.* 14, 1953–1958. doi: 10.1089/ars.2010.3809

Kvartsberg, H., Duits, F. H., Ingelsson, M., Andreasen, N., Ohrfelt, A., Andersson, K., et al. (2015). Cerebrospinal fluid levels of the synaptic protein neurogranin correlates with cognitive decline in prodromal Alzheimer's disease. *Alzheimers Dement.* 11, 1180–1190. doi: 10.1016/j.jalz.2014.10.009

Lai, C., and Breakefield, X. (2012). Role of exosomes/microvesicles in the nervous system and use in emerging therapies. *Front. Physiol.* 3:228. doi: 10.3389/fphys.2012.00228

Ledoux, S., Yang, R., Friedlander, G., and Laouari, D. (2003). Glucose depletion enhances P-glycoprotein expression in hepatoma cells: role of endoplasmic reticulum stress response. *Cancer Res.* 63, 7284–7290.

Lee, A. S. (2001). The glucose-regulated proteins: stress induction and clinical applications. *Trends Biochem. Sci.* 26, 504–510. doi: 10.1016/S0968-0004(01)01908-9

Lee, H. G., Perry, G., Moreira, P. I., Garrett, M. R., Liu, Q., Zhu, X., et al. (2005). Tau phosphorylation in Alzheimer's disease: pathogen or protector? *Trends Mol. Med.* 11, 164–169. doi: 10.1016/j.molmed.2005.02.008

Lee, J. H., Yu, W. H., Kumar, A., Lee, S., Mohan, P. S., Peterhoff, C. M., et al. (2010). Lysosomal proteolysis and autophagy require presenilin 1 and are disrupted by Alzheimer-related PS1 mutations. *Cell* 141, 1146–1158. doi: 10.1016/j.cell.2010.05.008

Lee, J., Giordano, S., and Zhang, J. (2012). Autophagy, mitochondria and oxidative stress: cross-talk and redox signalling. *Biochem. J.* 441, 523–540. doi: 10.1042/BJ20111451

Levy-Lahad, E., Wasco, W., Poorkaj, P., Romano, D. M., Oshima, J., Pettingell, W. H., et al. (1995). Candidate gene for the chromosome 1 familial Alzheimer's disease locus. *Science* 269, 973–977. doi: 10.1126/science.7638622

Li, L., Zhang, X., and Le, W. (2010). Autophagy dysfunction in Alzheimer's disease. *Neurodegener. Dis.* 7, 265–271. doi: 10.1159/000276710

Liu, D., Yang, F., Xiong, F., and Gu, N. (2016). The smart drug delivery system and its clinical potential. *Theranostics* 6, 1306–1323. doi: 10.7150/thno.14858

Liu, S. Y., Wang, W., Cai, Z. Y., Yao, L. F., Chen, Z. W., Wang, C. Y., et al. (2013). Polymorphism−116C/G of human X-box-binding protein 1 promoter is associated with risk of Alzheimer's disease. *CNS Neurosci. Ther.* 19, 229–234. doi: 10.1111/cns.12064

Lovestone, S., Boada, M., Dubois, B., Hull, M., Rinne, J. O., Huppertz, H. J., et al. (2015). A phase II trial of tideglusib in Alzheimer's disease. *J. Alzheimers Dis.* 45, 75–88. doi: 10.3233/JAD-141959

Mahley, R. W., and Huang, Y. (2009). Alzheimer disease: multiple causes, multiple effects of apolipoprotein E4, and multiple therapeutic approaches. *Ann. Neurol.* 65, 623–625. doi: 10.1002/ana.21736

Mapstone, M., Cheema, A. K., Fiandaca, M. S., Zhong, X., Mhyre, T. R., Macarthur, L. H., et al. (2014). Plasma phospholipids identify antecedent memory impairment in older adults. *Nat. Med.* 20, 415–418. doi: 10.1038/nm.3466

Mawuenyega, K. G., Sigurdson, W., Ovod, V., Munsell, L., Kasten, T., Morris, J. C., et al. (2010). Decreased clearance of CNS beta-amyloid in Alzheimer's disease. *Science* 330:1774. doi: 10.1126/science.1197623

Milhavet, O., Martindale, J. L., Camandola, S., Chan, S. L., Gary, D. S., Cheng, A., et al. (2002). Involvement of Gadd153 in the pathogenic action of presenilin-1 mutations. *J. Neurochem.* 83, 673–681. doi: 10.1046/j.1471-4159.2002.01165.x

Moreira, P. I., Cardoso, S. M., Santos, M. S., and Oliveira, C. R. (2006). The key role of mitochondria in Alzheimer's disease. *J. Alzheimers Dis.* 9, 101–110. doi: 10.3233/JAD-2006-9202

Moreira, P. I., Duarte, A. I., Santos, M. S., Rego, A. C., and Oliveira, C. R. (2009). An integrative view of the role of oxidative stress, mitochondria and insulin in Alzheimer's disease. *J. Alzheimers Dis.* 16, 741–761. doi: 10.3233/JAD-2009-0972

Moreira, P. I., Santos, M. S., and Oliveira, C. R. (2007). Alzheimer's disease: a lesson from mitochondrial dysfunction. *Antioxid. Redox Signal.* 9, 1621–1630. doi: 10.1089/ars.2007.1703

Murrow, L., and Debnath, J. (2013). Autophagy as a stress-response and quality-control mechanism: implications for cell injury and human disease. *Annu. Rev. Pathol.* 8, 105–137. doi: 10.1146/annurev-pathol-020712-163918

Nishida, Y., Arakawa, S., Fujitani, K., Yamaguchi, H., Mizuta, T., Kanaseki, T., et al. (2009). Discovery of Atg5/Atg7-independent alternative macroautophagy. *Nature* 461, 654–658. doi: 10.1038/nature08455

Nunomura, A., Perry, G., Aliev, G., Hirai, K., Takeda, A., Balraj, E. K., et al. (2001). Oxidative damage is the earliest event in Alzheimer disease. *J. Neuropathol. Exp. Neurol.* 60, 759–767. doi: 10.1093/jnen/60.8.759

Overk, C. R., and Masliah, E. (2014). Pathogenesis of synaptic degeneration in Alzheimer's disease and Lewy body disease. *Biochem. Pharmacol.* 88, 508–516. doi: 10.1016/j.bcp.2014.01.015

Pankiv, S., Clausen, T. H., Lamark, T., Brech, A., Bruun, J. A., Outzen, H., et al. (2007). p62/SQSTM1 binds directly to Atg8/LC3 to facilitate degradation of ubiquitinated protein aggregates by autophagy. *J. Biol. Chem.* 282, 24131–24145. doi: 10.1074/jbc.M702824200

Panza, F., Logroscino, G., Imbimbo, B. P., and Solfrizzi, V. (2014). Is there still any hope for amyloid-based immunotherapy for Alzheimer's disease? *Curr. Opin. Psychiatry* 27, 128–137. doi: 10.1097/YCO.0000000000000041

Pickford, F., Masliah, E., Britschgi, M., Lucin, K., Narasimhan, R., Jaeger, P. A., et al. (2008). The autophagy-related protein beclin 1 shows reduced expression in early Alzheimer disease and regulates amyloid beta accumulation in mice. *J. Clin. Invest.* 118, 2190–2199. doi: 10.1172/JCI33585

Prince, M., Comas-Herrera, A., Knapp, M., Guerchet, M., and Karagiannidou, M. (2016). *World Alzheimer Report.* Alzheimers Disease International.

Querfurth, H. W., and Laferla, F. M. (2010). Alzheimer's disease. *N. Engl. J. Med.* 362, 329–344. doi: 10.1056/NEJMra0909142

Raina, P., Santaguida, P., Ismaila, A., Patterson, C., Cowan, D., Levine, M., et al. (2008). Effectiveness of cholinesterase inhibitors and memantine for treating dementia: evidence review for a clinical practice guideline. *Ann. Intern. Med.* 148, 379–397. doi: 10.7326/0003-4819-148-5-200803040-00009

Readnower, R. D., Sauerbeck, A. D., and Sullivan, P. G. (2011). Mitochondria, amyloid beta, and Alzheimer's Disease. *Int. J. Alzheimers Dis.* 2011:104545. doi: 10.4061/2011/104545

Rezai-Zadeh, K., Shytle, D., Sun, N., Mori, T., Hou, H., Jeanniton, D., et al. (2005). Green Tea Epigallocatechin-3-Gallate (EGCG) modulates amyloid precursor protein cleavage and reduces cerebral amyloidosis in alzheimer transgenic mice. *J. Neurosci.* 25:8807. doi: 10.1523/JNEUROSCI.1521-05.2005

Rogaev, E. I., Sherrington, R., Rogaeva, E. A., Levesque, G., Ikeda, M., Liang, Y., et al. (1995). Familial Alzheimer's disease in kindreds with missense mutations in a gene on chromosome 1 related to the Alzheimer's disease type 3 gene. *Nature* 376, 775–778. doi: 10.1038/376775a0

Ron, D., and Walter, P. (2007). Signal integration in the endoplasmic reticulum unfolded protein response. *Nat. Rev. Mol. Cell Biol.* 8, 519–529. doi: 10.1038/nrm2199

Ross, M. F., Prime, T. A., Abakumova, I., James, A. M., Porteous, C. M., Smith, R. A., et al. (2008). Rapid and extensive uptake and activation of hydrophobic triphenylphosphonium cations within cells. *Biochem. J.* 411, 633–645. doi: 10.1042/BJ20080063

Rubinsztein, D. C., Codogno, P., and Levine, B. (2012). Autophagy modulation as a potential therapeutic target for diverse diseases. *Nat. Rev. Drug Discov.* 11, 709–730. doi: 10.1038/nrd3802

Safra, M., Ben-Hamo, S., Kenyon, C., and Henis-Korenblit, S. (2013). The ire-1 ER stress-response pathway is required for normal secretory-protein metabolism in *C. elegans*. *J. Cell. Sci.* 126, 4136–4146. doi: 10.1242/jcs.123000

Sayre, L. M., Moreira, P. I., Smith, M. A., and Perry, G. (2005). Metal ions and oxidative protein modification in neurological disease. *Ann. Ist. Super. Sanita* 41, 143–164.

Scherz-Shouval, R., and Elazar, Z. (2011). Regulation of autophagy by ROS: physiology and pathology. *Trends Biochem. Sci.* 36, 30–38. doi: 10.1016/j.tibs.2010.07.007

Scheuner, D., Eckman, C., Jensen, M., Song, X., Citron, M., Suzuki, N., et al. (1996). Secreted amyloid beta-protein similar to that in the senile plaques of Alzheimer's disease is increased *in vivo* by the presenilin 1 and 2 and APP mutations linked to familial Alzheimer's disease. *Nat. Med.* 2, 864–870. doi: 10.1038/nm0896-864

Selkoe, D. J. (1994). Amyloid beta-protein precursor: new clues to the genesis of Alzheimer's disease. *Curr. Opin. Neurobiol.* 4, 708–716. doi: 10.1016/0959-4388(94)90014-0

Selkoe, D. J. (2001a). Alzheimer's disease results from the cerebral accumulation and cytotoxicity of amyloid beta-protein. *J. Alzheimers Dis.* 3, 75–80. doi: 10.3233/JAD-2001-3111

Selkoe, D. J. (2001b). Presenilin, Notch, and the genesis and treatment of Alzheimer's disease. *Proc. Natl. Acad. Sci. U.S.A.* 98, 11039–11041. doi: 10.1073/pnas.211352598

Sgarbossa, A., Giacomazza, D., and Di Carlo, M. (2015). Ferulic acid: a hope for Alzheimer's Disease therapy from plants. *Nutrients* 7, 5764–5782. doi: 10.3390/nu7075246

Shaw, L. M., Vanderstichele, H., Knapik-Czajka, M., Clark, C. M., Aisen, P. S., Petersen, R. C., et al. (2009). Cerebrospinal fluid biomarker signature in Alzheimer's disease neuroimaging initiative subjects. *Ann. Neurol.* 65, 403–413. doi: 10.1002/ana.21610

Sherrington, R., Froelich, S., Sorbi, S., Campion, D., Chi, H., Rogaeva, E. A., et al. (1996). Alzheimer's disease associated with mutations in presenilin 2 is rare and variably penetrant. *Hum. Mol. Genet.* 5, 985–988. doi: 10.1093/hmg/5.7.985

Shimizu, S., Arakawa, S., and Nishida, Y. (2010). Autophagy takes an alternative pathway. *Autophagy* 6, 290–291. doi: 10.4161/auto.6.2.11127

Shoji-Kawata, S., Sumpter, R., Leveno, M., Campbell, G. R., Zou, Z., Kinch, L., et al. (2013). Identification of a candidate therapeutic autophagy-inducing peptide. *Nature* 494, 201–206. doi: 10.1038/nature11866

Steele, J. W., and Gandy, S. (2013). Latrepirdine (Dimebon®), a potential Alzheimer therapeutic, regulates autophagy and neuropathology in an Alzheimer mouse model. *Autophagy* 9, 617–618. doi: 10.4161/auto.23487

Su, B., Wang, X., Nunomura, A., Moreira, P. I., Lee, H. G., Perry, G., et al. (2008). Oxidative stress signaling in Alzheimer's disease. *Curr. Alzheimer Res.* 5, 525–532. doi: 10.2174/156720508786898451

Swerdlow, R. H., Burns, J. M., and Khan, S. M. (2014). The Alzheimer's disease mitochondrial cascade hypothesis: progress and perspectives. *Biochim. Biophys. Acta* 1842, 1219–1231. doi: 10.1016/j.bbadis.2013.09.010

Szegezdi, E., Fitzgerald, U., and Samali, A. (2003). Caspase-12 and ER-stress-mediated apoptosis: the story so far. *Ann. N.Y. Acad. Sci.* 1010, 186–194. doi: 10.1196/annals.1299.032

Szeto, H. H. (2008). Mitochondria-targeted cytoprotective peptides for ischemia-reperfusion injury. *Antioxid. Redox Signal.* 10, 601–619. doi: 10.1089/ars.2007.1892

Tauskela, J. S. (2007). MitoQ–a mitochondria-targeted antioxidant. *IDrugs* 10, 399–412.

Tavitian, B., Pappata, S., Bonnot-Lours, S., Prenant, C., Jobert, A., Crouzel, C., et al. (1993). Positron emission tomography study of [11C]methyl-tetrahydroaminoacridine (methyl-tacrine) in baboon brain. *Eur. J. Pharmacol.* 236, 229–238. doi: 10.1016/0014-2999(93)90593-7

Tumbarello, D. A., Waxse, B. J., Arden, S. D., Bright, N. A., Kendrick-Jones, J., and Buss, F. (2012). Autophagy receptors link myosin VI to autophagosomes to mediate Tom1-dependent autophagosome maturation and fusion with the lysosome. *Nat. Cell Biol.* 14, 1024–1035. doi: 10.1038/ncb2589

Tung, Y. T., Wang, B. J., Hsu, W. M., Hu, M. K., Her, G. M., Huang, W. P., et al. (2014). Presenilin-1 regulates the expression of p62 to govern p62-dependent tau degradation. *Mol. Neurobiol.* 49, 10–27. doi: 10.1007/s12035-013-8482-y

Vingtdeux, V., Giliberto, L., Zhao, H., Chandakkar, P., Wu, Q., Simon, J. E., et al. (2010). AMP-activated protein kinase signaling activation by resveratrol modulates amyloid-beta peptide metabolism. *J. Biol. Chem.* 285, 9100–9113. doi: 10.1074/jbc.M109.060061

Visser, P. J., Verhey, F., Knol, D. L., Scheltens, P., Wahlund, L. O., Freund-Levi, Y., et al. (2009). Prevalence and prognostic value of CSF markers of Alzheimer's disease pathology in patients with subjective cognitive impairment or mild cognitive impairment in the DESCRIPA study: a prospective cohort study. *Lancet Neurol.* 8, 619–627. doi: 10.1016/S1474-4422(09)70139-5

Wahlster, L., Arimon, M., Nasser-Ghodsi, N., Post, K. L., Serrano-Pozo, A., Uemura, K., et al. (2013). Presenilin-1 adopts pathogenic conformation in normal aging and in sporadic Alzheimer's disease. *Acta Neuropathol.* 125, 187–199. doi: 10.1007/s00401-012-1065-6

Walter, P., and Ron, D. (2011). The unfolded protein response: from stress pathway to homeostatic regulation. *Science* 334, 1081–1086. doi: 10.1126/science.1209038

Wang, J., Xiong, S., Xie, C., Markesbery, W. R., and Lovell, M. A. (2005). Increased oxidative damage in nuclear and mitochondrial DNA in Alzheimer's disease. *J. Neurochem.* 93, 953–962. doi: 10.1111/j.1471-4159.2005.03053.x

Wang, S. H., Shih, Y. L., Ko, W. C., Wei, Y. H., and Shih, C. M. (2008). Cadmium-induced autophagy and apoptosis are mediated by a calcium signaling pathway. *Cell Mol. Life Sci.* 65, 3640–3652. doi: 10.1007/s00018-008-8383-9

Wischik, C. M., Staff, R. T., Wischik, D. J., Bentham, P., Murray, A. D., Storey, J. M., et al. (2015). Tau aggregation inhibitor therapy: an exploratory phase 2 study in mild or moderate Alzheimer's disease. *J. Alzheimers Dis.* 44, 705–720. doi: 10.3233/JAD-142874

Wong, H. K., Veremeyko, T., Patel, N., Lemere, C. A., Walsh, D. M., Esau, C., et al. (2013). De-repression of FOXO3a death axis by microRNA-132 and−212 causes neuronal apoptosis in Alzheimer's disease. *Hum. Mol. Genet.* 22, 3077–3092. doi: 10.1093/hmg/ddt164

Wu, J., and Kaufman, R. J. (2006). From acute ER stress to physiological roles of the unfolded protein response. *Cell Death Differ.* 13, 374–384. doi: 10.1038/sj.cdd.4401840

Xing, H. Y., Li, B., Peng, D., Wang, C. Y., Wang, G. Y., Li, P., et al. (2017). A novel monoclonal antibody against the N-terminus of Abeta1-42 reduces plaques and improves cognition in a mouse model of Alzheimer's disease. *PLoS ONE* 12:e0180076. doi: 10.1371/journal.pone.0180076

Xu, C., Bailly-Maitre, B., and Reed, J. C. (2005). Endoplasmic reticulum stress: cell life and death decisions. *J. Clin. Invest.* 115, 2656–2664. doi: 10.1172/JCI26373

Yan, J. J., Jung, J. S., Kim, T. K., Hasan, A., Hong, C. W., Nam, J. S., et al. (2013). Protective effects of ferulic acid in amyloid precursor protein plus presenilin-1 transgenic mouse model of Alzheimer disease. *Biol. Pharm. Bull.* 36, 140–143. doi: 10.1248/bpb.b12-00798

Yang, F., Lim, G. P., Begum, A. N., Ubeda, O. J., Simmons, M. R., Ambegaokar, S. S., et al. (2005). Curcumin inhibits formation of amyloid beta oligomers and fibrils, binds plaques, and reduces amyloid *in vivo*. *J. Biol. Chem.* 280, 5892–5901. doi: 10.1074/jbc.M404751200

Yang, T., Hong, S., O'malley, T., Sperling, R. A., Walsh, D. M., and Selkoe, D. J. (2013). New ELISAs with high specificity for soluble oligomers of amyloid beta-protein detect natural Abeta oligomers in human brain but not CSF. *Alzheimers Dement.* 9, 99–112. doi: 10.1016/j.jalz.2012.11.005

4

Autophagy and Alzheimer's Disease: From Molecular Mechanisms to Therapeutic Implications

Md. Sahab Uddin[1], Anna Stachowiak[2], Abdullah Al Mamun[1], Nikolay T. Tzvetkov[3], Shinya Takeda[4], Atanas G. Atanasov[5,6], Leandro B. Bergantin[7], Mohamed M. Abdel-Daim[8,9] and Adrian M. Stankiewicz[5]**

[1] Department of Pharmacy, Southeast University, Dhaka, Bangladesh, [2] Department of Experimental Embryology, Institute of Genetics and Animal Breeding, Polish Academy of Sciences, Magdalenka, Poland, [3] Department of Molecular Biology and Biochemical Pharmacology, Institute of Molecular Biology "Roumen Tsanev", Bulgarian Academy of Sciences, Sofia, Bulgaria, [4] Department of Clinical Psychology, Tottori University Graduate School of Medical Sciences, Tottori, Japan, [5] Department of Molecular Biology, Institute of Genetics and Animal Breeding, Polish Academy of Sciences, Magdalenka, Poland, [6] Department of Pharmacognosy, University of Vienna, Vienna, Austria, [7] Department of Pharmacology, Federal University of São Paulo, São Paulo, Brazil, [8] Department of Pharmacology, Suez Canal University, Ismailia, Egypt, [9] Department of Ophthalmology and Micro-technology, Yokohama City University, Yokohama, Japan

***Correspondence:**
Adrian M. Stankiewicz
adrianstankiewicz85@gmail.com
Atanas G. Atanasov
a.atanasov@ighz.pl

Alzheimer's disease (AD) is the most common cause of progressive dementia in the elderly. It is characterized by a progressive and irreversible loss of cognitive abilities and formation of senile plaques, composed mainly of amyloid β (Aβ), and neurofibrillary tangles (NFTs), composed of tau protein, in the hippocampus and cortex of afflicted humans. In brains of AD patients the metabolism of Aβ is dysregulated, which leads to the accumulation and aggregation of Aβ. Metabolism of Aβ and tau proteins is crucially influenced by autophagy. Autophagy is a lysosome-dependent, homeostatic process, in which organelles and proteins are degraded and recycled into energy. Thus, dysfunction of autophagy is suggested to lead to the accretion of noxious proteins in the AD brain. In the present review, we describe the process of autophagy and its importance in AD. Additionally, we discuss mechanisms and genes linking autophagy and AD, i.e., the mTOR pathway, neuroinflammation, endocannabinoid system, *ATG7, BCL2, BECN1, CDK5, CLU, CTSD, FOXO1, GFAP, ITPR1, MAPT, PSEN1, SNCA, UBQLN1*, and *UCHL1*. We also present pharmacological agents acting via modulation of autophagy that may show promise in AD therapy. This review updates our knowledge on autophagy mechanisms proposing novel therapeutic targets for the treatment of AD.

Keywords: autophagy, Alzheimer's disease, amyloid beta, tau

INTRODUCTION

Introduced to biology in 1963 by Belgian biochemist Christian de Duve (De Duve and Wattiaux, 1966) autophagy (from Greek "self-eating") is an intracellular self-degradative process that is responsible for the systematic degradation and recycling of cellular components such as misfolded or accumulated proteins and damaged organelles (Glick et al., 2010). In 2016, the Japanese cell

---

Abbreviations: Aβ, Amyloid β; AD, Alzheimer's disease; CSF, cerebrospinal fluid; MAPT, microtubule-associated protein tau; NFTs, neurofibrillary tangles.

biologist Yoshinori Ohsumi was awarded Nobel Prize in Physiology or Medicine for identification of autophagy-related genes and the discovery of the mechanisms of autophagy (Nobelprize.org, 2017).

Autophagy has been classified into three categories based on the mechanism by which intracellular constituents are supplied into lysosome for degradation: microautophagy, chaperone-mediated autophagy, and macroautophagy. In microautophagy, the cytoplasmic material is absorbed into lysosome by direct invagination of the lysosomal membrane (Marzella et al., 1981). The chaperone-mediated autophagy facilitates the degradation of cytosolic proteins by directly targeting them to lysosomes and into the lysosomal lumen (Kaushik and Cuervo, 2012). In macroautophagy, degradable contents of cytoplasm are encapsulated in subcellular double-membrane structures named "autophagosomes". Autophagosomes transport the cell "waste" to the lysosomes for degradation (Settembre et al., 2013). Macroautophagy is the most predominant form of autophagy and will be denoted as such in this review.

Healthy mammalian cells show a low basal level of autophagy (Funderburk et al., 2010). This basal autophagic activity plays a dominant role in the intracellular homeostatic turnover of proteins and organelles (Funderburk et al., 2010). Basal activity of autophagy is essential in post-mitotic neuronal cells, possibly due to their inability to dilute noxious components through cell division (Funderburk et al., 2010). Autophagic activity is enhanced by diverse stresses such as nutrient starvation, hypoxia or inflammation (Melendez and Neufeld, 2008; Francois et al., 2013). Enhanced autophagy participates in various physiological processes and pathological conditions, including cell death, removal of microorganisms invading the cell, and tumor suppression (Glick et al., 2010). On the other hand, reduced autophagic potential is associated with aging (Rubinsztein et al., 2011). During autophagy, proteins are degraded into amino acids, which provide an energy source and are likely used as building blocks for protein synthesis (Onodera and Ohsumi, 2005; Meijer et al., 2015). Thus, dysregulated autophagy may result in accumulation of proteins inside the cell. Various autophagy dysfunctions may contribute to neurodegeneration or neurodegeneration-like symptoms, for example inhibition of the fusion of an autophagosome with a lysosome (Boland et al., 2008), reduction of lysosomal acidification (Shen and Mizushima, 2014) or accumulation of proteins in cells (Garcia-Arencibia et al., 2010).

Alzheimer's disease is the most predominant type of dementia diagnosed in the aged people (Uddin et al., 2016). It is characterized by a chronic, irreversible, and progressive neuronal degradation in the human brain caused by complex pathophysiological processes, including oxidative stress, neuroinflammation, excitotoxicity, mitochondrial dysfunction, proteolytic stress, and more (Jellinger, 2010). Formation of intracellular NFTs and extracellular senile plaques in the brain are two common hallmarks of AD (Armstrong, 2009). NFTs consist of aggregated, abnormally hyperphosphorylated MAPT (Iqbal et al., 2010). Senile plaques are primarily composed of insoluble and toxic amyloid-β (Aβ) peptides and of dysfunctional dystrophic neurites, which include abnormally large amounts of neurofilament, tau, or chromogranin A proteins (Dickson et al., 1999; Armstrong, 2009).

Despite the accumulated wealth of knowledge, AD remains incurable. The significance of autophagy in pathophysiology of AD is now appreciated due to the discoveries of molecular mechanisms for autophagy. The objective of this review is to introduce an outline of the discovery of autophagy and describe the relationship between autophagy and AD.

Please consider, that in the present review the names of genes are written in italic, while names of proteins are written in standard font. Names of human or *Saccharomyces* sp. genes/proteins are written in all capital letters. Names of rodent genes/proteins are written in capital letter followed by small letters.

HISTORY OF AUTOPHAGY RESEARCH

Lysosome

In the mid 1950's researchers explored a novel specialized cellular substructure (organelle), encapsulating enzymes that digest macromolecules such as proteins and lipids (Xu and Ren, 2015). This compartment was named "lysosome" (de Duve, 2005). The lysosome was discovered by the Belgian cytologist and biochemist Christian de Duve. For this achievement de Duve was awarded the 1974 Nobel Prize in Physiology or Medicine (Blobel, 2013).

The lysosome is generally 100–1500 nanometers in diameter and enclosed by a typical lipid bilayer membrane (Xu and Ren, 2015). Lysosomes contain more than 60 different hydrolase enzymes such as proteases and lipases (Xu and Ren, 2015). The lysosomal enzymes are the most active in acidic environment, such as this in the lumen of a lysosome (pH of approximately 4.6) (Xu and Ren, 2015). This characteristic of lysosomal enzymes provides protection against unrestrained, pathological digestion of the constituents of the cell, as cytosol pH is almost neutral (pH 7.2) (Alberts et al., 2002). Hence, even if lysosomal membrane would become damaged and the enzymes were to leak into the cytosol, harm to the cell itself would be minimal (Alberts et al., 2002).

Lysosomes serve as an intracellular digestive system protecting the cell from its unused and/or noxious constituents (Huber and Teis, 2016). Furthermore, lysosomes are involved in various cell processes, including secretion, cell membrane repair, cell signaling and energy metabolism (Settembre et al., 2013). Mutations in the genes involved in the synthesis of lysosomal proteins have been linked to over 40 human genetic diseases (lysosomal storage diseases) (Parenti et al., 2013).

Proteasome

Like autophagy, the ubiquitin-proteasome system is another degradation pathway for cellular proteins. During the 1970's and 1980's, researchers began to study second system of cell protein degradation, namely the "proteasome". The significance of intracellular proteolytic degradation and the contribution of ubiquitin-proteasome system to the proteolytic pathways (i.e., discovery of ubiquitin-mediated proteolysis) was acknowledged with the award of the Nobel Prize in Chemistry in 2004 to the Israeli biologist Aaron Ciechanover; the Hungarian-born Israeli biochemist Avram Hershko and the American biologist Irwin Rose (Karigar and Murthy, 2005).

Proteasomes are large, multisubunit protease complexes that are responsible for the degradation of unnecessary or damaged proteins by proteolysis (Tanaka et al., 2004). Proteasomal degradation produces amino acids, which may be subsequently used in generation of new proteins (Rogel et al., 2010). Proteins are labeled for degradation with a 76-amino acid protein called "ubiquitin" (Weissman, 2001). Single labeling event leads to a cascade, resulting in the formation of polyubiquitin chain, which binds to the proteasome for proteolysis (Ciechanover and Schwartz, 1998; Li and Ye, 2008).

The proteasomal degradation pathway plays an important role in numerous cellular processes, for example cell cycle and immune response (Ciechanover and Schwartz, 1998). Improper ubiquitin-mediated protein degradation has been linked to several neurodegenerative disorders including AD, Parkinson's disease, Huntington's disease and amyotrophic lateral sclerosis (Atkin and Paulson, 2014).

Recent studies showed the existence of cross-talk between proteasomal and autophagy pathways (Lilienbaum, 2013). Both processes share protein degradation signaling network molecules, may be recruited by ubiquitinated substrates, and under specific conditions display compensatory functions to maintain cellular homeostasis (Lilienbaum, 2013).

Autophagosome

Additional biochemical and microscopic investigations identified a new type of vesicles carrying cellular cargo to the lysosome for degradation. Christian de Duve, the discoverer of the lysosome, introduced the term "autophagy" to define this process (Klionsky, 2008). The new vesicles were named autophagosomes (Klionsky, 2008). Autophagy research was kick-started in 1990s with studies performed by Yoshinori Ohsumi, for which he was awarded the 2016 Nobel Prize in Physiology or Medicine (Nobelprize.org, 2017).

He studied autophagy using as a model organism the budding yeast (Takeshige et al., 1992), whose vacuole is functionally similar to the mammalian lysosome (Li and Kane, 2009). His group has shown that starved yeast devoid of some of the functional vacuolar proteases developed spherical bodies inside the vacuoles (Takeshige et al., 1992). These bodies were encompassed by a membrane and contained constituents of cytosol such as cytoplasmic ribosomes, mitochondria, rough endoplasmic reticulum fragments, glycogen, etc. The constituents would be normally degraded in yeast cultured on the nutrient-poor medium to facilitate adaptation to adverse environment. Without functional proteases the degradation could not commence, and so the spherical bodies remained easily perceivable. These spherical structures were named "autophagic bodies".

In 1993, Ohsumi's group published research, in which they identified 15 genes (*APG1-15)* that are essential for the activation of autophagy in yeast cells (Tsukada and Ohsumi, 1993). Later, as a result of efforts of the scientific community to standardize the gene names, the *APG* genes were renamed to *ATG* (Klionsky et al., 2003). Afterward, Ohsumi's group cloned numerous *ATG* genes and identified the function of their protein products (e.g., Funakoshi et al., 1997; Matsuura et al., 1997). Further studies established the interactions between these products providing the basis for autophagy mechanisms (see **Figure 1**). They found that the ATG1 protein (now: ULK1) combines with the product of the *ATG13* gene to form autophagic complex (Kamada et al., 2000). This process is controlled by target of rapamycin (TOR) kinase (Kamada et al., 2000). Further, Ohsumi's group established that for proper activation the ATG1 protein needs to form complex not only with ATG13, but also with ATG17 (RB1CC1/FIP200) (**Figure 1**) (Ohsumi, 2014). As shown in **Figure 1**, the formation of this complex is the first stage in autophagosome genesis (The Nobel Assembly at Karolinska Institutet, 2016). The phosphatidylinositol-3 kinase (PI3K) complex that is composed of PIK3C3 (VPS34), PIK3R4 (VPS15), BECN1, and ATG14 (Barkor) proteins (Ohsumi, 2014), produces phosphatidylinositol-3 phosphate (PtdIns3P or PI3P), which facilitates binding of further effector proteins to the membrane of the autophagosome (Ohsumi, 2014).

In the late 1990', Ohsumi's group discovered two ubiquitin-like conjugation systems involved in the autophagosome formation (**Figure 1**) (Ohsumi, 2014). First conjugation system results in a formation of an ATG12-ATG5 complex, while the second one results in the formation of a conjugate of ATG8 (MAP1LC3A/GABARAPL2/LC3) with a membrane phospholipid, phosphatidylethanolamine (Ohsumi, 2014). The formation of both conjugates is mediated by the ATG7 protein (Ohsumi, 2014). ATG12-related system regulates ATG8 lipidation and lipidated ATG8 is a crucial participant in the processes of autophagosome elongation (Nakatogawa et al., 2007; Nakatogawa, 2013). These two conjugation systems are evolutionary conserved among yeast and mammals (Ohsumi, 2014). Actually, fluorescently labeled product of the mammalian homologue of yeast gene *ATG8* is used as an indicator of the formation of autophagosome in mammalian systems (Kabeya et al., 2000; Mizushima et al., 2004).

The *ATG* genes proved to play crucial roles in mammalian organisms. For example, mice with knock-out of *ATG5* gene die in the first days of life due to their inability to cope with the post-labor starvation period (Kuma et al., 2004). In this life period, functional autophagy allows the neonate to keep the steady energy supply before milk feeding starts (Kuma et al., 2004). Further studies on knockout mouse models lacking functional versions of autophagy-related genes have established the functions of the autophagy

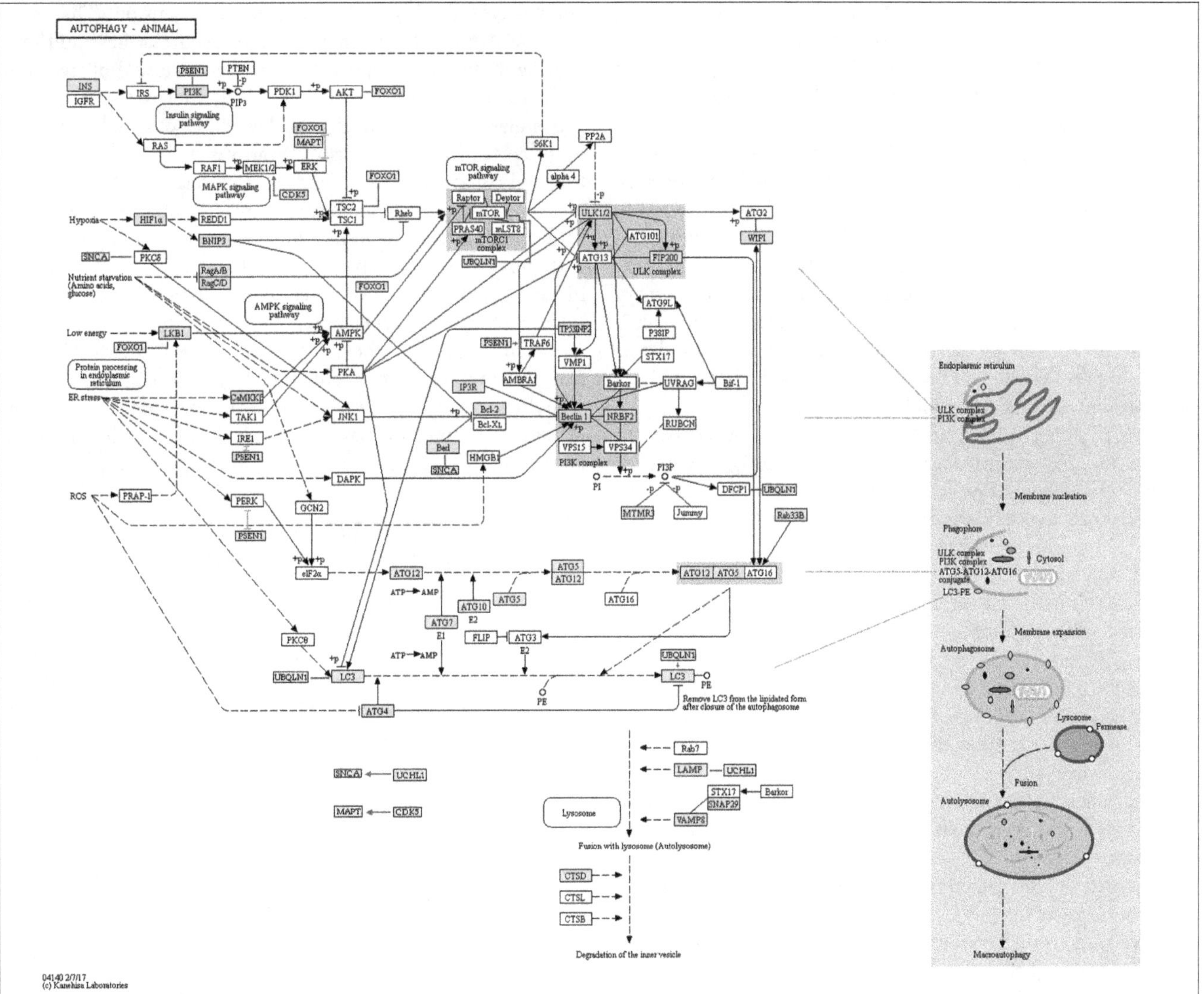

FIGURE 1 | Representation of proteins and protein complexes involved in the "Autophagy – animal" KEGG pathway. This figure was taken from the KEGG database (http://www.genome.jp/kegg-bin/show_pathway?ko04140) and modified. Blue boxes mark the proteins that are associated with AD. Orange boxes mark additional proteins that are not originally included in the pathway. These genes are associated with both AD and autophagy, and are discussed in the present review. Red, blue, and violet lines mark partners with which the additional proteins interact (red color means activation, blue color means inhibition, and violet color means unspecified or complex (e.g., both inhibitory and stimulatory effect) according to STRING database). The interactions data were extracted from the STRING database (http://string-db.org). To assure that the presented data is reliable, we have included only interactions that showed at least medium STRING confidence score and were either identified in an experiment or are annotated in manually curated databases. Additionally, we have added interaction between GFAP and LAMP, which was not included in STRING database but was found by manual literature search. Permission to use KEGG figure was granted.

in different mammalian tissues (Mizushima and Komatsu, 2011).

BIOLOGICAL MECHANISMS LINKING AUTOPHAGY AND AD

Aβ Metabolism and the Autophagy

Alzheimer's disease is a progressive neurodegenerative disorder, which pathophysiology includes formation of Aβ aggregates (Oddo et al., 2006). In a healthy human central nervous system the production rate of Aβ peptides is generally lower than their rate of clearance, at 7.6 and 8.3% per hour, respectively (Bateman et al., 2006).

Autophagy is a key regulator of Aβ generation and clearance (Nilsson and Saido, 2014). Aβ peptides are produced through cleavage of amyloid precursor protein (APP) in the autophagosomes during autophagic turnover of APP-rich organelles (Nixon, 2007; Steele et al., 2013). In AD the maturation of autophagolysosomes (i.e., autophagosomes that have undergone fusion with lysosomes) and their retrograde passage toward the neuronal body are hindered (Nixon, 2007). This contributes to an immense accretion of autophagic vacuoles in neurons. Such accretion may be related to dysfunction of the ESCRT-III complex. This dysfunction is associated with neurodegeneration (Lee et al., 2007; Yamazaki et al., 2010) and may affect autophagosome maturation by disrupting fusion of autophagosomes with the endolysosomal system (Rusten and Stenmark, 2009).

There are two pathways for disposing Aβ peptides. Firstly, they can be simply degraded by various Aβ-degrading proteases, including BACE1 and CTSD (Saido and Leissring, 2012). Secondly, Aβ peptides can accumulate in autophagosomes of dystrophic neurites (i.e., main constituents of neuritic senile plaques in AD), thus being incorporated into primary intracellular reservoir of toxic peptides (Nixon et al., 2005; Yu et al., 2005). The second recycling path of Aβ peptides is especially prevalent in the brains of people suffering from AD (Nilsson et al., 2013; Nilsson and Saido, 2014).

A paper published by Nilsson et al. (2013) shows that Aβ peptides are released from neurons in an autophagy-dependent manner and suggests that the accumulation of intracellular Aβ plaques is toxic to brain cells leading to AD pathology. To explore the role of autophagy in Aβ pathology *in vivo*, Nilsson et al. (2013) crossed *App* transgenic mice, carrying Swedish mutation, with mice lacking functional autophagy mechanisms in the forebrain neurons due to conditional knockout of *Atg7*. They observed that the offspring had far fewer extracellular Aβ plaques than the mice with functional autophagy. The decrease of extracellular Aβ plaque content reported by Nilsson et al. (2013) was caused by inability of cells with disrupted autophagy to secrete Aβ peptides. Indeed, they report that in the autophagy deficient mice, reduction in Aβ peptides secretion co-occur with accumulation of Aβ inside the brain cells (Nilsson et al., 2013). Moreover, in the autophagy deficient mice, intracellular aggregation of Aβ likely caused neurodegeneration and, together with amyloidosis, memory impairment (Nilsson et al., 2013). These findings are in agreement with previous reports that intracellular Aβ is neurotoxic (Zhang et al., 2002).

Summing up, impaired autophagy is a well-established participating mechanism in the pathology of Aβ metabolism of AD.

Neuroinflammation

Present knowledge suggests that inflammation, autophagy and AD are connected processes. A study by Francois et al. (2013) provided an example of cross-talk between them. They showed that Aβ42 influences the expression and activation of some proteins involved in autophagy (p62, p70S6K) *in vitro* (Francois et al., 2013). They also showed that the processes of inflammation and autophagy interact within brain cells, as severe inflammation induced by IL-1β activated autophagy in microglia grown in tri- or mono-cultures (Francois et al., 2013). Although the role of IL-1β itself in AD is unclear, we do know how the neuroinflammation contributes to AD pathogenesis (Zhang and Jiang, 2015), and why IL-1β is a key mediator of neuroinflammation (Basu et al., 2004). Hence, one could speculate that IL-1β may play role in pathogenesis of AD by eliciting both neuroinflammation and autophagy. It seems viable that during the course of AD, immune signals induce autophagy. Indeed, it was shown that neuroinflammation might influence autophagy following stress-induced hypertension (Du et al., 2017). Correspondingly, another study reported that adult mice bearing mutations of *App* and *Psen1* genes showed higher brain levels of inflammatory mediators (including Il-1β) along with accumulation of autophagic vesicles within dystrophic neurons in the cortex and hippocampus (Francois et al., 2014). Moreover, the levels of inflammatory mediators correlated with expression of key autophagy regulators such as mTOR and Becn1 (Francois et al., 2014). On the other hand, Ye et al. (2017) suggest, that inhibition of autophagy may enhance microglia activity, including secretion of cytokines such as Il-1β and generation of toxic reactive oxygen species (ROS) *in vitro*.

Taken together, these studies suggest that AD and neuroinflammation feed autophagy (and each other), while autophagy decreases inflammation in the brain. Thus, the increase in autophagy may play some protective role during the course of AD via interaction with the immune system.

Mechanistic Target of Rapamycin (mTOR) Pathway

Mechanistic target of rapamycin signaling pathway is initiated by nutrients and growth factors and regulates autophagy (Jung et al., 2010). Human studies suggest participation of mTOR signaling in AD (Sun et al., 2014). It has been shown that mTOR signaling is inhibited in cortex and hippocampus of adult AD model mice (Francois et al., 2014). Decreased mTOR signaling leads to reduction in levels of Aβ (Spilman et al., 2010; Caccamo et al., 2014) and protects memory of AD model mice from deterioration (Caccamo et al., 2014). A study performed by Spilman et al. (2010) on mouse model of AD reported that blocking the mTOR signaling with rapamycin relieves cognitive deficits and reduces amyloid pathology, likely by activating autophagy in brain cells. Correspondingly, studies show that diet enriched with rapamycin prolongs lifespan of animals (Harrison et al., 2009). This may be relevant to AD research, because age is a major factor in the pathogenesis of AD (Guerreiro and Bras, 2015). Moreover, studies on human cells have shown that mTOR mediates intra- and extra-cellular distribution of tau (Tang et al., 2015), its phosphorylation and accumulation as well as resulting behavioral effects of tau pathology (Caccamo et al., 2013). Finally, multiple compounds tested for their efficacy as AD medication impose their beneficial effect by inducing mTOR-depending autophagy (see below).

Summarizing, mTOR pathway is currently one of the most promising targets for autophagy-related AD therapy.

Endocannabinoids

Recently published reports highlight the role of the endocannabinoid system in neurodegenerative diseases and autophagy (Maroof et al., 2013; Shao et al., 2014; Bedse et al., 2015). Endocannabinoids are lipophilic molecules that, when released, activate the cannabinoid receptors CNR1 and CNR2 (cannabinoid receptor 1 and 2) (Katona and Freund, 2012).

Mice with a *Cnr1* deletion have shown a pathological accumulation of some proteins, which are not degradable by lysosomal enzymes through autophagy (Piyanova et al., 2013).

Knockdown of CNR1 expression by siRNA results in both mTOR- and BECN1-independent increase of autophagic vesicle formation (Hiebel et al., 2014).

In a human AD frontal cortex, expression of the CNR1 receptor was significantly reduced (Ramirez et al., 2005; Solas et al., 2013). In an AD mouse model Cnr1 was decreased in dorsal hippocampus and basolateral amygdala complex (Bedse et al., 2014). It seems that in frontal cortex and hippocampus the activity of the CNR1 receptor depends on the progression of AD. While in early AD the activity is increased, it shifts to attenuation in later AD stages (Manuel et al., 2014). Additionally, the expression levels of the CNR2 receptor were increased in microglia cells of an AD patient's in the hippocampus, entorhinal cortex and frontal cortex (Benito et al., 2003; Solas et al., 2013). The high expression of CNR2 receptor was correlated with the Aβ42 levels and senile plaque burden (Solas et al., 2013).

All these findings suggest that there is a non-trivial connection between endocannabinoids, autophagy, and AD. A further investigation is required to fully understand the mechanisms involved.

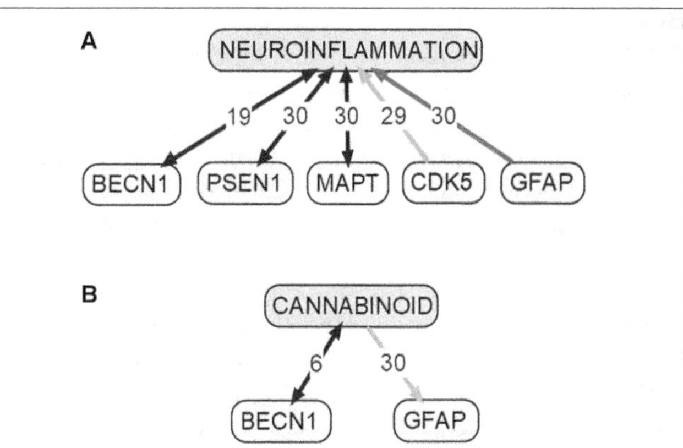

FIGURE 2 | Connections between genes discussed in the "Genes Common to Autophagy and AD" section and **(A)** neuroinflammation as well as **(B)** cannabinoids. This figure was drawn based on data obtained using the Chilibot tool. Black arrows mark relationships that are neither obviously stimulatory nor inhibitory. Orange arrow marks both stimulatory and inhibitory relationship. Red arrow marks inhibitory relationship. Green arrow mark stimulatory relationship. The respective numbers mark the weight of the relationship according to the Chilibot tool.

Genes Common to Autophagy and AD

To identify the genes that may mediate cross-talk between molecular mechanisms of autophagy and AD, we have compared two groups of genes: (1) genes involved in autophagy, defined as being included either in Gene Ontology term "autophagy" (GO:0006914, *Homo sapiens*) or in KEGG Pathway (Kanehisa et al., 2017) "autophagy-animal" (ko04140), and (2) genes involved in AD, defined as being included either in databases AlzBase (Bai et al., 2016) or AlzGene (Bertram et al., 2007), or related to AD as shown by the text-mining tool GLAD4U (Jourquin et al., 2012). AlzBase provides data on "gene dysregulation in AD and closely related processes/diseases such as aging and neurological disorders" (Bai et al., 2016), while AlzGene provides data on "genetic association studies in the field of AD" (Bertram et al., 2007). AlzGene can be treated as a comprehensive database of genes that were associated with AD before year 2011, when it was last updated. Unfortunately, currently there is no other database that collects such information. Finally, GLAD4U is a prioritization tool querying PubMed for given phrase and returning associated genes (Jourquin et al., 2012). The genes that are common to both groups' are summarized in Supplementary Table S1. For detailed discussion we selected genes, which met following requirements: (1) reported to be involved in both autophagy and AD according to the PubMed database, AND (2) constituted top five results from either AlzBase, AlzGene or GLAD4U. Additionally, we arbitrarily selected five genes involved in KEGG Pathway "autophagy-animal" for further discussion. Gene hierarchy was established for AlzBase and AlzGene based on the total number of entries into database and for GLAD4U as a confidence score provided by the tool. Generally, selected genes showed strong (weight > 5) relationship with neuroinflammation, as detected by Chilibot (Chen and Sharp, 2004), especially BECN1, PSEN1, MAPT, GFAP, and CDK5 (see **Figure 2A**). Simultaneously, the genes were not significantly related to the endocannabinoid system (queried in Chilibot via keyword "cannabinoid"), with only BECN1 and GFAP showing strong interaction (see **Figure 2B**). The genes described below were also added to **Figure 1** along with their known interactions with other molecules of the pathway (see also Supplementary Table S2), as extracted from STRING database (organism: *Homo sapiens*) (Szklarczyk et al., 2017).

Autophagy-Related 7 (*ATG7*)

As stated previously, *ATG7* is a key gene regulating autophagic conjugation systems (Ohsumi, 2014). *ATG7* is involved in memory functions as evident from a study, in which forebrain-specific *Atg7* knockout mouse have shown memory deficits (Inoue et al., 2012). We have found two studies connecting dysregulated expression of ATG7 protein and AD-like pathology. Decreased levels of the Atg7 protein were found in cerebral cortex and hippocampus of mouse model of AD (Carvalho et al., 2015). On the other hand, no dysregulation of protein expression of ATG7 was found in temporal cortices of AD patients (Crews et al., 2010).

Atg7 mediates the transport of Aβ peptides to the multivesicular body and their secretion in mouse neurons (Nilsson et al., 2015). Inhibition of *ATG7* expression using siRNA partially protected against increase in production and secretion of Aβ40 *in vitro* (Cho et al., 2015). On the other hand, intra-hippocampal infusion of Aβ is able to increase the expression of the Atg7 protein in hippocampus of rats while reducing their memory performance (Mohammadi et al., 2016).

ATG7 seems to be involved in degradation of tau. Forebrain-specific *Atg7* knockout in mice resulted in an accumulation of phosphorylated tau protein in hippocampus and cerebral cortex, as well as neurodegeneration evident in loss of hippocampal neurons and memory dysfunction (Inoue et al., 2012).

BCL2

BCL2 is an anti-apoptotic factor that interacts with BECN1 to regulate autophagy (Decuypere et al., 2012).

Overexpression of neuronal *Bcl2* improved place recognition memory in mice (Rohn et al., 2008). Contrary, negative correlation between the cortical BLC2 protein expression and memory (immediate recall) was established in AD patients (Perez et al., 2015). Upregulation of the BCL2 protein was found in precuneus (cortex) of AD patients (Perez et al., 2015).

Aβ treatment decreases the BCL2 expression *in vitro* (Clementi et al., 2006), while *APP* mutation (Swedish) mediates similar effect *in vitro* during starvation (Yang et al., 2009). Overexpression of Bcl2 protects against Aβ-related death of neuronal cells *in vitro* (Ferreiro et al., 2007). Rohn et al. (2008) reported that AD model mice engineered to overexpress Bcl2 protein showed decreased processing of App and number of extracellular deposits of Aβ, as compared to base strain (3xTg-AD).

The overexpression of Bcl2 affects also tau processing, reducing the number of NFTs (Rohn et al., 2008).

Beclin 1 (*BECN1/ATG6*)

BECN1 protein mediates the initiation of autophagy and genesis of autophagosomes. Becn1 heterozygotic mice (Becn1+/−) show decreased autophagy in neurons (Pickford et al., 2008).

Several reports suggest, that BECN1 is involved in the pathophysiology of AD. Postmortem midfrontal cortex and isolated microglia of AD patients show reduced content of BECN1 protein (Pickford et al., 2008; Lucin et al., 2013). Similarly, reduced Becn1 expression was found in cortex and hippocampus of adult mouse model of AD (Francois et al., 2014). BECN1 may protect against AD-associated cellular death. Xue et al. (2013) report that expression of Becn1 correlates with viability of cells treated with toxic Aβ42. Interestingly, Becn1 activity seems to be regulated by Aβ42 (Nah et al., 2013).

A study performed on the frontoparietal cortex and the hippocampus of mice showed that decreasing of Becn1 expression leads to increased levels of Aβ (Pickford et al., 2008). Becn1-mediated decrease in autophagy leads to accretion of Aβ peptides and, finally, to neurodegeneration (Pickford et al., 2008).

BECN1 is also involved in neuroinflammation and cannabinoid system activity. Inhibition of Becn1 expression increases microglia inflammatory response (Zhou et al., 2011). Chronic LPS-induced inflammation decreases hippocampal Becn1 expression (Jiang et al., 2017). On the other hand, *Cb2r* deletion decreases Becn1 expression in the spinal cord of mice (Shao et al., 2014).

Cyclin Dependent Kinase 5 (CDK5)

CDK5 is an autophagy-regulating kinase (Wong et al., 2011), which expression is enriched in central nervous system as shown in Human Protein Atlas (HPA) (Uhlen et al., 2015).

Cdk5 modulates various cognition-related biological processes such as neurogenesis in adult hippocampus (Crews et al., 2011) and synaptic functions (Sheng et al., 2016). Silencing of hippocampal Cdk5 expression using RNAi resulted in improved memory performance in AD model mice (Posada-Duque et al., 2015). Study connected *CDK5*-associated polymorphisms with increased risk of AD (Rademakers et al., 2005). CDK5 protein expression is enhanced in frontal cortices of AD patients (Sadleir and Vassar, 2012). On the contrary, CDK5 protein expression is decreased in cerebrospinal fluid (CSF) of AD patients (Olah et al., 2015).

CDK5 influences the metabolism and effects of Aβ. CDK5 may regulate BACE1 protein expression (Sadleir and Vassar, 2012) as well as activity (Song W.J. et al., 2015). *BACE1* gene encodes β-secretase, which is a crucial enzyme involved in APP metabolism (Cai et al., 2015). Furthermore, Cdk5 participates in cytotoxic activity of Aβ42 in primary cortical neurons (Chang et al., 2012), mediates Aβ peptide-induced dendritic spine loss (Qu et al., 2011) and APP phosphorylation (Iijima et al., 2000). On the other hand, Aβ increases Cdk5 activity in primary cortical neurons (Seyb et al., 2007).

CDK5 is similarly involved in tau metabolism. Cdk5 binds to tau *in vitro* and is co-localized with it in rat cortex (Li et al., 2006). Cdk5 participates in tau phosphorylation (Noble et al., 2003), although whether this may lead to formation of NFTs is disputed (Bian et al., 2002; Noble et al., 2003). Prevention of Cdk5 hyperactivity in the mouse model of AD protects against tau hyperphosphorylation, Aβ accumulation, memory loss, and enhanced neuroinflammation (Shukla et al., 2013).

Clusterin (*CLU/APOJ*)

CLU is a chaperone protein that participates in autophagosome biogenesis via interaction with ATG8E (MAP1LC3A) (Zhang F. et al., 2014).

CLU is one of the top AD candidate genes with the third lowest *p*-value of the association ($p = 3.37E\text{-}23$) according to the meta-analysis included in AlzGene database (Bertram et al., 2007). Meta-analyses showed the involvement of *CLU*-related mutations in AD pathogenesis (Liu et al., 2014; Shuai et al., 2015). *CLU* mutations that are suggested as causal for AD affect hippocampal connectivity (Zhang et al., 2015), white matter integrity in several brain regions (Braskie et al., 2011), cortical gray matter volume (Stevens et al., 2014), as well as working memory (Stevens et al., 2014) and episodic memory performance (Barral et al., 2012). *CLU* mRNA is upregulated in hippocampi of AD patients (May et al., 1990). According to Miners et al. (2017) CLU protein rises in several brain regions, including frontal cortex, of AD patients in correlation with noxious Aβ40/42 levels. Results of study by Baig et al. (2012) did not confirm these findings. The CLU protein is upregulated in CSF of AD patients (Deming et al., 2016). The content of CLU protein in the blood plasma of AD patients was reported to be dysregulated in some studies (Mullan et al., 2013), while others did not confirm this finding (Deming et al., 2016).

Moreover, CLU protein interacts with Aβ, reduces its aggregation and protects against its toxic effects (Beeg et al., 2016). CLU decreases the Aβ intake by human primary glia cells (Mulder et al., 2014).

The interaction between tau and CLU is less studied (Zhou et al., 2014). However, Zhou et al. (2014) reported that the Clu protein is upregulated in a tau-overexpressing mouse model of AD. Furthermore, the AD-associated *CLU* polymorphism rs11136000 regulates the levels of tau protein in CSF in AD patients (Zhou et al., 2014).

Cathepsin D (*CTSD*)

Cathepsin D is a lysosomal protease (Dean, 1975) that is involved in degradation of the APP protein (Letronne et al., 2016).

Two meta-analyses on the influence of *CTSD* mutation rs17571 on AD yielded contrary results (Schuur et al., 2011; Mo et al., 2014). Similar discrepancy is also reported for another *CTSD* mutation (Ala224Val) (Ntais et al., 2004; Paz-Y-Miño et al., 2015). Directionality of the change of *CTSD* gene expression seems to depend on studied tissue. CTSD level was decreased in bone marrow-derived monocytes isolated from AD patients (Tian et al., 2014). *CTSD* mRNA expression was upregulated in whole blood of AD patients (Bai et al., 2014). On the other hand, *CTSD* is downregulated on both mRNA and protein levels in skin fibroblasts from AD patients (Urbanelli et al., 2008).

Cathepsin D participates in processing of Aβ peptides (McDermott and Gibson, 1996) and clearance of amyloid plaques *in vitro* (Tian et al., 2014). Nevertheless, Aβ processing mechanisms are fairly resistant to modest (38%) changes in expression of *Ctsd*, at least in cerebral cortex of mouse model of AD (Cheng et al., 2017).

Cathepsin D also interacts with tau protein. Previously mentioned rs17571 mutation causes changes in processing of tau, but not of APP (Riemenschneider et al., 2006).

Forkhead Box O1 (*FOXO1*)

FOXO1 gene encodes transcription factor that plays a role in autophagy modulation in neurons (Xu et al., 2011). *FOXO1* mutation rs7981045 was associated with response of AD patients to a treatment based on acetylcholinesterase inhibitors (Paroni et al., 2014)

Glial Fibrillary Acidic Protein (*GFAP*)

GFAP is a cytoskeletal intermediate filament-III and a marker of astrocytes (Sofroniew and Vinters, 2010; Yang and Wang, 2015). GFAP binds with LAMP2A (**Figure 1**) (Bandyopadhyay et al., 2010). Multiple studies found increased levels of GFAP in tissues of AD patients. GFAP levels are increased in the frontal cortices, hippocampi (Korolainen et al., 2005; Kamphuis et al., 2014), and the CSF of AD patients (Ishiki et al., 2016). Moreover, *Gfap* expression is modulated by cannabinoid receptor 1 (Cnr1) in the hypothalamus of mice (Higuchi et al., 2010) and neuroinflammation regulates astrogliosis (abnormal increase in the number of astrocytes) (Carson et al., 2006).

Inositol 1,4,5-Trisphosphate Receptor Type 1 (*ITPR1/IP3R1*)

ITPR1 gene encodes intracellular receptor mediating calcium release from the endoplasmic reticulum (Santulli and Marks, 2015) and also plays a role in inducing autophagy (Messai et al., 2014). Engineered downregulation of *Itpr1* expression protected AD model mice from Aβ accumulation, tau hyperphosphorylation, as well as from dysfunction of memory and hippocampal LTP (Shilling et al., 2014).

Microtubule Associated Protein Tau (*MAPT/TAU*)

MAPT gene encodes tau protein, which pathology is one of the most well-recognized markers of AD. Autophagy is a main pathway of degradation of tauDeltaC, which is a form of the protein found in the brains of AD patients (Dolan and Johnson, 2010). Autophagy dysfunction plays important role in tau aggregation (Inoue et al., 2012). Tau may also regulate autophagy (Pacheco et al., 2009), likely via inhibition of HDAC6 activity (Perez et al., 2009). Finally, Mapt deficiency reduces neuroinflammation (Maphis et al., 2015), while neuroinflammation in turn induces Mapt phosphorylation (Bhaskar et al., 2010).

Presenilin 1 (*PSEN1*)

PSEN1 protein is a regulator of the APP-cleaving γ-secretase complex (De Strooper et al., 1998), and autophagic proteolysis (Neely and Green, 2011).

PSEN1 gene mutations contribute to the pathogenesis of early onset AD (Karch and Goate, 2015), and this effect may be mediated by loss of stability and hydrophobicity of the proteins encoded by the mutated variants (Somavarapu and Kepp, 2016). CSF of AD patients with *PSEN1* mutations showed lower levels of Aβ than AD patients without *PSEN1* mutation (Ikeda et al., 2013). This may suggest that the proteins are retained in the brain cells due to dysregulated autophagy. Cataldo et al. (2004) compared brains of AD patients with mutation of presenilin 1 with brains of sporadic AD patients. They concluded that *PSEN1* mutation is associated with higher prevalence of lysosomal pathology in neurons of AD patients (Cataldo et al., 2004). This corresponds to report by Lee et al. (2010), where the authors show that *Psen1* is crucial for modulating lysosome acidification and proteolysis during autophagy. Dysregulated lysosomal proteolysis may lead to accumulation of proteins and cell death (Lee et al., 2010). Additionally, PSEN1 is hypothesized to be involved in brain immune response as *Psen1/2* knock-out changes the expression of neuroinflammation-related genes (Mirnics et al., 2008).

Alpha-Synuclein (*SNCA/PARK1/NACP*)

Expression of *SNCA* is enriched in brain according to Human Protein Atlas (Uhlen et al., 2015). SNCA regulates autophagosome formation (Yan et al., 2014), but it is also negatively regulated by autophagy (Colasanti et al., 2014).

SNCA mutations are connected to the risk of AD (Matsubara et al., 2001; Wang et al., 2016). Changes in expression of SNCA proteins were also reported in some brain regions of AD patients (Quinn et al., 2012). Dysregulated levels of SNCA in CSF are associated with cognitive performance (Korff et al., 2013). Effect of Snca protein expression on memory was also reported in mice (Larson et al., 2012).

SNCA is an important component of Aβ plaques (Ueda et al., 1993). Snca induces expression of Aβ peptides and vice versa (Majd et al., 2013). SNCA also likely regulates APP processing by modulating the activity of BACE1 (Roberts et al., 2017), binds Aβ peptides and promotes their aggregation (Yoshimoto et al., 1995).

There are also reports of Snca inhibiting Aβ plaque formation (Bachhuber et al., 2015). On the other hand, Aβ40 decreases SNCA uptake by neurons (Chan et al., 2016).

Similarly to interaction of SNCA with Aβ peptides, SNCA and tau also induce each other fibrillization (Giasson et al., 2003). SNCA binds, phosphorylates, and inhibits microtubule assembly activity of tau (Oksman et al., 2013; Oikawa et al., 2016).

Ubiquilin 1 (*UBQLN1*)

UBQLN1 gene encodes ubiquitin-like protein involved in autophagosome–lysosome fusion (N'Diaye et al., 2009) likely by interacting with ATG8E (MAP1LC3A) (Rothenberg et al., 2010).

There is a strong evidence for involvement of *UBQLN1* in AD pathology. UBQ-8i polymorphism of *UBQLN1* was associated with increased risk of AD in two separate meta-analyses (Zhang and Jia, 2014; Yue et al., 2015). In hippocampi of AD patients UBQLN1 protein localizes to dystrophic neurites (Satoh et al., 2013). Expression of UBQLN1 protein is reduced in temporal and frontal cortices of AD patients (Stieren et al., 2011; Natunen et al., 2016). This decrease may cause enhanced processing and intracellular trafficking of APP (Hiltunen et al., 2006; Stieren et al., 2011), and secretion of Aβ40/42 (Hiltunen et al., 2006).

Moreover, UBQLN1 interacts with BACE1, which is a key APP processing protein. Ubqln1 overexpression causes an increase of Bace1 in neuron-microglia co-cultures, though this effect did not reach significance in the brains of mice (Natunen et al., 2016).

Ubiquitin C-Terminal Hydrolase L1 (*UCHL1*)

UCHL1 is a brain-enriched ubiquitin-specific hydrolase (Uhlen et al., 2015). It influences autophagy by interaction with LAMP2 (**Figure 1**), which modulates autophagosome-lysosome fusion (Costes et al., 2014; Hubert et al., 2016).

Uchl1 plays an important role in synaptic functions and memory as shown in mouse model of AD (Gong et al., 2006). This effect may be related to the Uchl1 ability to restore Bdnf signaling, which is disrupted by Aβ (Poon et al., 2013). BDNF is one of the most critical mediators of brain functions (Lu et al., 2014). Several publications have reported either effect or lack of effect of *UCHL1* mutations on AD (Xue and Jia, 2006; Shibata et al., 2012). Similarly, there is some discrepancy in the directionality of changes in expression of *UCHL1* gene between different studies performed on AD patients. In frontal cortices the UCHL1 protein was upregulated (Donovan et al., 2012). On the other hand, downregulation of UCHL1 was reported in hippocampi (Poon et al., 2013) and in unspecified brain area (Choi et al., 2004).

Co-immunoprecipitation assay showed that Uchl1 interacts with App (Zhang M. et al., 2014). The Uchl1 overexpression, induced by intracranial injection of *Uchl1*-expressing virus, decreases the Aβ production and protects AD model mice against memory impairment (Zhang M. et al., 2014). Decreased expression and activity of UCHL1 protein is associated with Aβ treatment *in vitro* (Guglielmotto et al., 2012). Similarly, decreased expression of UCHL1 protein is found in the cerebral cortex of AD patients (Guglielmotto et al., 2012). Additionally, the cortical UCHL1 protein levels seem to be inversely correlated to the number of NFT in AD patients (Chen et al., 2013). Moreover, UCHL1 is involved in lysosomal degradation of BACE1 (Guglielmotto et al., 2012).

UCHL1 protein co-localizes with NFTs in AD brains (Choi et al., 2004). The Uchl1 expression and activity negatively influence the levels of phosphorylated tau and aggregation of tau protein in mouse neuroblastoma cells (Xie et al., 2016). Tau induces mitochondrial degradation, synaptic deterioration, and cellular death by recruiting UCHL1 *in vitro* (Corsetti et al., 2015).

THERAPEUTIC IMPLICATIONS OF THE INTERPLAY OF ALZHEIMER'S DISEASE AND AUTOPHAGY

The protein aggregates, e.g., Aβ and tau proteins, participating in the pathology of neurodegenerative disorders cause neuronal damage and synaptic dysfunction (Irvine et al., 2008; Bloom, 2014). Their removal or inhibition of their formation are proposed as potential therapeutic approaches for the treatment of neurodegenerative disorders (Nowacek et al., 2009). Autophagy is one of the main mechanisms by which the cell degrades abnormal proteins. Thus, elimination of such protein aggregates may be achieved utilizing mechanisms of autophagy (Metcalf et al., 2012). Several autophagy-stimulating drugs have already demonstrated considerable therapeutic potential for AD treatment in clinical trials. We shortly discuss some of them below.

Carbamazepine (CBZ)

Carbamazepine was primarily developed as a drug used in the treatment of epilepsy (Okuma and Kishimoto, 1998). In the past, scientists studied therapeutic effect of CBZ on AD-related agitation (Xiao et al., 2010). Recently two publications have shown that carbamazepine-induced autophagy also protected against memory dysfunction and increase in Aβ content in brains of mouse model of AD (Li et al., 2013; Zhang et al., 2017).

Latrepirdine

Latrepirdine stimulates mTOR- and Atg5- dependent autophagy and reduces intracellular content of App metabolites, including Aβ peptides, in the brain of mouse (Steele and Gandy, 2013). Recent meta-analysis has shown no adverse effects and small improvement in dementia-related behaviors by latrepirdine in AD patients (Chau et al., 2015). Nevertheless, as Chau et al. (2015) themselves admit, the analyzed literature was not comprehensive enough to allow for more confident conclusions.

Lithium

Clinical trials have shown that lithium may ameliorate AD and this effect may be related to its mTOR-independent autophagy-inducing activity (Sarkar et al., 2005; Forlenza et al., 2012). In meta-analysis of clinical studies on AD, lithium significantly decreased cognitive decline compared to placebo, while showing no significant adverse effects (Matsunaga et al., 2015a).

Memantine

The NMDA (*N*-methyl-D-aspartate) receptors antagonist memantine is widely used for treatment of moderate-to-severe AD. According to recent meta-analysis it shows good tolerance and some efficacy in AD treatment (Matsunaga et al., 2015b). This effect may be in some extent mediated by memantine ability to influence autophagy in either mTOR-dependent or mTOR-independent manner (Song G. et al., 2015).

Nicotinamide

Liu et al. (2013) reported that long-term treatment with nicotinamide (Vitamin B3/PP) reduces Aβ and tau pathologies as well as cognitive decline in a mouse model of AD. The effect of nicotinamide is likely mediated by enhancement of the acidification of lysosome or autophagolysosome, leading to reduced autophagosome accretion (Liu et al., 2013). Gong et al. (2013) have shown that nicotinamide activity depends also on its ability to induce degradation of Bace1. Recently published clinical trials showed safety, but no effect of nicotinamide on cognitive function of AD patients (Phelan et al., 2017). Despite this, nicotinamide anti-AD activity is still studied and further trial is currently ongoing (Grill, 2017).

Protein Phosphatase 2A Agonists

Clinical trials have suggested that protein phosphatase 2A agonists, such as metformin, can inhibit the hyperphosphorylation of tau (Kickstein et al., 2010). Similar results were obtained from a study on mice (Li et al., 2012). Hyperphosphorylation of tau is a key step in generation of NFTs in AD patients (Iqbal et al., 2010). On the other hand, metformin did not protect diabetic mice from AD-like memory dysfunction (Li et al., 2012).

Rapamycin

Rapamycin, a selective inhibitor of target-of-rapamycin complex 1 (TORC1) and thus modulator of the mTOR pathway activity, improved learning and memory and reduced Aβ and tau pathology in the brains of AD mouse model (Caccamo et al., 2010; Spilman et al., 2010). Rapamycin also increased viability of cells treated with Aβ42 (Xue et al., 2013). Rapamycin prodrug, temsirolimus was shown to induce autophagy-dependent Aβ clearance and to improve memory in mouse model of AD (Jiang et al., 2014). Temsirolimus also lowered tau accumulation and rescued motor dysfunctions in tau mutant mice (Frederick et al., 2015). SMER28, a small molecule-based enhancer of rapamycin, increases autophagy via Atg5-dependent pathway while reducing the levels of Aβ peptide in a γ-secretase-independent manner (Tian et al., 2011). Recent rapamycin clinical trial showed non-significant decrease in expression of the cellular senescence marker beta galactosidase (Singh et al., 2016).

Resveratrol

Resveratrol, a grape-derived polyphenol, and its derivatives decreased extracellular Aβ peptide accumulation by activating autophagy via AMPK signaling pathway (**Figure 1**) (Vingtdeux et al., 2010). Recently published clinical trials studying the efficacy of resveratrol for AD treatment showed that resveratrol is well-tolerated but, surprisingly, AD biomarkers, such as plasma Aβ40 level, were present in treated group at even higher levels than in a placebo group (Turner et al., 2015). On the other hand, long-term resveratrol treatment rescued memory loss and Aβ levels in the brain of AD mouse model (Porquet et al., 2014). Hence, viability of this compound as a medication for AD is unclear.

Other Autophagy-Regulating Substances That Have Shown Relevant Results Only in Animal AD Models

Arctigenin

Arctigenin, a polyphenol extracted from *Arctium lappa*, was found to inhibit Aβ production and memory impairment in mouse model of AD (Zhu et al., 2013). The effect was mediated by mTOR- and AMPK-dependent autophagy (Zhu et al., 2013).

β-Asarone

β-asarone is an ether found, e.g., in *Acori graminei* (Liu et al., 2016). β-asarone treatment decreases Aβ42 levels in hippocampus and improves memory in a mouse model of AD, probably through mTOR-dependent autophagy (Deng et al., 2016).

GTM-1

It was shown that administration of GTM-1, a derivative of quinolone, rescues cognitive dysfunction and Aβ pathologies in mouse model of AD by activating mTOR-independent autophagy (Chu et al., 2013; Zhang et al., 2017).

Oleuropein Aglycone

Oleuropein aglycone is a polyphenol, which is present in plants of *Oleaceae* family and induces autophagy via mTOR pathway (Grossi et al., 2013; Luccarini et al., 2015). According to a recent review (Martorell et al., 2016), regulation of autophagy is one of the mechanisms via which oleuropein aglycone counteracts amyloid aggregation and toxicity.

Tetrahydrohyperforin

Tetrahydrohyperforin is a derivative of hyperforin, which is an active component of St. John's Wort plant (*Hypericum perforatum*). In AD model mice tetrahydrohyperforin prevented memory impairment and physiological dysfunctions such as tau hyperphosphorylation or turnover of amyloid plaques (Cerpa et al., 2010; Inestrosa et al., 2011). At least one of its beneficial effects is mediated by its autophagy-related activity, that is clearance of APP via ATG5-dependent pathway (Cavieres et al., 2015).

Trehalose

The disaccharide trehalose, an inducer of mTOR-independent autophagy (Sarkar et al., 2007), inhibits the aggregation of both Aβ40 and tau, and reduces their cytotoxicity *in vitro* (Liu et al., 2005; Kruger et al., 2012). Similarly, in two separate studies utilizing mouse models of AD, trehalose protected against cognitive dysfunction (Du et al., 2013; Portbury et al., 2017).

Interestingly, one of these studies also reported effect of trehalose on hippocampal Aβ levels (Du et al., 2013), while the other one reported a lack of this effect (Portbury et al., 2017).

Summarizing, scientific community puts a significant effort into developing autophagy-related therapeutics for AD. Several agents, such as rapamycin and latrepirdine, have already been tested on AD patients and show promising results. However, many more potential therapeutics showing efficacy for treatment of cognitive dysfunctions in animal models of AD await for more comprehensive studies and trials on humans.

CONCLUSION

Despite much of the data presented in the review being acquired in studies performed on animal models, we propose that properly functioning autophagy is crucial for the normal aging of neurons. Malfunction in neuronal autophagy is one of the key factors influencing the development of neurodegenerative disorders, including AD. The autophagy plays a key role in the metabolism of Aβ and tau protein, the mTOR pathway, neuroinflammation, and in the endocannabinoid system, all of which may mediate its effect on AD. Accordingly, autophagy-targeted therapeutic approaches may lead to the development of novel therapeutic strategies for the management of AD.

AUTHOR CONTRIBUTIONS

This work was carried out in collaboration between all authors. MU, AMS, AS, and AM have written the first draft of the manuscript. NT, ST, AA, LB, and MA-D revised and improved the first draft. All authors have seen and agreed on the finally submitted version of the manuscript.

FUNDING

The authors acknowledge the support by the Polish KNOW (Leading National Research Centre) Scientific Consortium "Healthy Animal—Safe Food" decision of Ministry of Science and Higher Education No. 05-1/KNOW2/2015.

ACKNOWLEDGMENTS

The authors are grateful to the Department of Pharmacy, Southeast University, Dhaka, Bangladesh.

REFERENCES

Alberts, B., Johnson, A., Lewis, J., Raff, M., Roberts, K., and Walter, P. (2002). *Transport from the Trans Golgi Network to Lysosomes*. New York, NY: Garland Science.

Armstrong, R. A. (2009). The molecular biology of senile plaques and neurofibrillary tangles in Alzheimer's disease. *Folia Neuropathol.* 47, 289–299.

Atkin, G., and Paulson, H. (2014). Ubiquitin pathways in neurodegenerative disease. *Front. Mol. Neurosci.* 7:63. doi: 10.3389/fnmol.2014.00063

Bachhuber, T., Katzmarski, N., Mccarter, J. F., Loreth, D., Tahirovic, S., Kamp, F., et al. (2015). Inhibition of amyloid-beta plaque formation by alpha-synuclein. *Nat. Med.* 21, 802–807. doi: 10.1038/nm.3885

Bai, Z., Han, G., Xie, B., Wang, J., Song, F., Peng, X., et al. (2016). AlzBase: an integrative database for gene dysregulation in Alzheimer's disease. *Mol. Neurobiol.* 53, 310–319. doi: 10.1007/s12035-014-9011-3

Bai, Z., Stamova, B., Xu, H., Ander, B. P., Wang, J., Jickling, G. C., et al. (2014). Distinctive RNA expression profiles in blood associated with Alzheimer disease after accounting for white matter hyperintensities. *Alzheimer Dis. Assoc. Disord.* 28, 226–233. doi: 10.1097/WAD.0000000000000022

Baig, S., Palmer, L. E., Owen, M. J., Williams, J., Kehoe, P. G., and Love, S. (2012). Clusterin mRNA and protein in Alzheimer's disease. *J. Alzheimers Dis.* 28, 337–344. doi: 10.3233/JAD-2011-110473

Bandyopadhyay, U., Sridhar, S., Kaushik, S., Kiffin, R., and Cuervo, A. M. (2010). Identification of regulators of chaperone-mediated autophagy. *Mol. Cell* 39, 535–547. doi: 10.1016/j.molcel.2010.08.004

Barral, S., Bird, T., Goate, A., Farlow, M. R., Diaz-Arrastia, R., Bennett, D. A., et al. (2012). Genotype patterns at PICALM, CR1, BIN1, CLU, and APOE genes are associated with episodic memory. *Neurology* 78, 1464–1471. doi: 10.1212/WNL.0b013e3182553c48

Basu, A., Krady, J. K., and Levison, S. W. (2004). Interleukin-1: a master regulator of neuroinflammation. *J. Neurosci. Res.* 78, 151–156. doi: 10.1002/jnr.20266

Bateman, R. J., Munsell, L. Y., Morris, J. C., Swarm, R., Yarasheski, K. E., and Holtzman, D. M. (2006). Human amyloid-beta synthesis and clearance rates as measured in cerebrospinal fluid *in vivo*. *Nat. Med.* 12, 856–861. doi: 10.1038/nm1438

Bedse, G., Romano, A., Cianci, S., Lavecchia, A. M., Lorenzo, P., Elphick, M. R., et al. (2014). Altered expression of the CB1 cannabinoid receptor in the triple transgenic mouse model of Alzheimer's disease. *J. Alzheimers Dis.* 40, 701–712. doi: 10.3233/JAD-131910

Bedse, G., Romano, A., Lavecchia, A. M., Cassano, T., and Gaetani, S. (2015). The role of endocannabinoid signaling in the molecular mechanisms of neurodegeneration in Alzheimer's disease. *J. Alzheimers Dis.* 43, 1115–1136. doi: 10.3233/JAD-141635

Beeg, M., Stravalaci, M., Romeo, M., Carra, A. D., Cagnotto, A., Rossi, A., et al. (2016). Clusterin binds to Abeta1-42 oligomers with high affinity and interferes with peptide aggregation by inhibiting primary and secondary nucleation. *J. Biol. Chem.* 291, 6958–6966. doi: 10.1074/jbc.M115.689539

Benito, C., Nunez, E., Tolon, R. M., Carrier, E. J., Rabano, A., Hillard, C. J., et al. (2003). Cannabinoid CB2 receptors and fatty acid amide hydrolase are selectively overexpressed in neuritic plaque-associated glia in Alzheimer's disease brains. *J. Neurosci.* 23, 11136–11141.

Bertram, L., Mcqueen, M. B., Mullin, K., Blacker, D., and Tanzi, R. E. (2007). Systematic meta-analyses of Alzheimer disease genetic association studies: the AlzGene database. *Nat. Genet.* 39, 17–23. doi: 10.1038/ng1934

Bhaskar, K., Konerth, M., Kokiko-Cochran, O. N., Cardona, A., Ransohoff, R. M., and Lamb, B. T. (2010). Regulation of tau pathology by the microglial fractalkine receptor. *Neuron* 68, 19–31. doi: 10.1016/j.neuron.2010.08.023

Bian, F., Nath, R., Sobocinski, G., Booher, R. N., Lipinski, W. J., Callahan, M. J., et al. (2002). Axonopathy, tau abnormalities, and dyskinesia, but no neurofibrillary tangles in p25-transgenic mice. *J. Comp. Neurol.* 446, 257–266. doi: 10.1002/cne.10186

Blobel, G. (2013). Christian de Duve (1917-2013). *Nature* 498:300. doi: 10.1038/498300a

Bloom, G. S. (2014). Amyloid-beta and tau: the trigger and bullet in Alzheimer disease pathogenesis. *JAMA Neurol.* 71, 505–508. doi: 10.1001/jamaneurol.2013.5847

Boland, B., Kumar, A., Lee, S., Platt, F. M., Wegiel, J., Yu, W. H., et al. (2008). Autophagy induction and autophagosome clearance in neurons: relationship to autophagic pathology in Alzheimer's disease. *J. Neurosci.* 28, 6926–6937. doi: 10.1523/JNEUROSCI.0800-08.2008

Braskie, M. N., Jahanshad, N., Stein, J. L., Barysheva, M., Mcmahon, K. L., De Zubicaray, G. I., et al. (2011). Common Alzheimer's disease risk variant within the CLU gene affects white matter microstructure in young adults. *J. Neurosci.* 31, 6764–6770. doi: 10.1523/JNEUROSCI.5794-10.2011

Caccamo, A., De Pinto, V., Messina, A., Branca, C., and Oddo, S. (2014). Genetic reduction of mammalian target of rapamycin ameliorates Alzheimer's disease-like cognitive and pathological deficits by restoring hippocampal gene expression signature. *J. Neurosci.* 34, 7988–7998. doi: 10.1523/JNEUROSCI.0777-14.2014

Caccamo, A., Magri, A., Medina, D. X., Wisely, E. V., Lopez-Aranda, M. F., Silva, A. J., et al. (2013). mTOR regulates tau phosphorylation and degradation: implications for Alzheimer's disease and other tauopathies. *Aging Cell* 12, 370–380. doi: 10.1111/acel.12057

Caccamo, A., Majumder, S., Richardson, A., Strong, R., and Oddo, S. (2010). Molecular interplay between mammalian target of rapamycin (mTOR), amyloid-beta, and Tau: effects on cognitive impairments. *J. Biol. Chem.* 285, 13107–13120. doi: 10.1074/jbc.M110.100420

Cai, Z., Zhou, Y., Liu, Z., Ke, Z., and Zhao, B. (2015). Autophagy dysfunction upregulates beta-amyloid peptides via enhancing the activity of gamma-secretase complex. *Neuropsychiatr. Dis. Treat.* 11, 2091–2099. doi: 10.2147/NDT.S84755

Carson, M. J., Thrash, J. C., and Walter, B. (2006). The cellular response in neuroinflammation: the role of leukocytes, microglia and astrocytes in neuronal death and survival. *Clin. Neurosci. Res.* 6, 237–245. doi: 10.1016/j.cnr.2006.09.004

Carvalho, C., Santos, M. S., Oliveira, C. R., and Moreira, P. I. (2015). Alzheimer's disease and type 2 diabetes-related alterations in brain mitochondria, autophagy and synaptic markers. *Biochim. Biophys. Acta* 1852, 1665–1675. doi: 10.1016/j.bbadis.2015.05.001

Cataldo, A. M., Peterhoff, C. M., Schmidt, S. D., Terio, N. B., Duff, K., Beard, M., et al. (2004). Presenilin mutations in familial Alzheimer disease and transgenic mouse models accelerate neuronal lysosomal pathology. *J. Neuropathol. Exp. Neurol.* 63, 821–830. doi: 10.1093/jnen/63.8.821

Cavieres, V. A., Gonzalez, A., Munoz, V. C., Yefi, C. P., Bustamante, H. A., Barraza, R. R., et al. (2015). Tetrahydrohyperforin inhibits the proteolytic processing of amyloid precursor protein and enhances its degradation by Atg5-dependent autophagy. *PLOS ONE* 10:e0136313. doi: 10.1371/journal.pone.0136313

Cerpa, W., Hancke, J. L., Morazzoni, P., Bombardelli, E., Riva, A., Marin, P. P., et al. (2010). The hyperforin derivative IDN5706 occludes spatial memory impairments and neuropathological changes in a double transgenic Alzheimer's mouse model. *Curr. Alzheimer Res.* 7, 126–133. doi: 10.2174/156720510790691218

Chan, D. K., Braidy, N., Xu, Y. H., Chataway, T., Guo, F., Guillemin, G. J., et al. (2016). Interference of alpha-synuclein uptake by monomeric beta-Amyloid1-40 and potential core acting site of the interference. *Neurotox. Res.* 30, 479–485. doi: 10.1007/s12640-016-9644-2

Chang, K. H., Vincent, F., and Shah, K. (2012). Deregulated Cdk5 triggers aberrant activation of cell cycle kinases and phosphatases inducing neuronal death. *J. Cell Sci.* 125, 5124–5137. doi: 10.1242/jcs.108183

Chau, S., Herrmann, N., Ruthirakuhan, M. T., Chen, J. J., and Lanctot, K. L. (2015). Latrepirdine for Alzheimer's disease. *Cochrane Database Syst. Rev.* 4:CD009524. doi: 10.1002/14651858.CD009524.pub2

Chen, H., and Sharp, B. M. (2004). Content-rich biological network constructed by mining PubMed abstracts. *BMC Bioinformatics* 5:147. doi: 10.1186/1471-2105-5-147

Chen, J., Huang, R. Y., and Turko, I. V. (2013). Mass spectrometry assessment of ubiquitin carboxyl-terminal hydrolase L1 partitioning between soluble and particulate brain homogenate fractions. *Anal. Chem.* 85, 6011–6017. doi: 10.1021/ac400831z

Cheng, S., Wani, W. Y., Hottman, D. A., Jeong, A., Cao, D., Leblanc, K. J., et al. (2017). Haplodeficiency of Cathepsin D does not affect cerebral amyloidosis and autophagy in APP/PS1 transgenic mice. *J. Neurochem.* 142, 297–304. doi: 10.1111/jnc.14048

Cho, S. J., Yun, S. M., Jo, C., Lee, D. H., Choi, K. J., Song, J. C., et al. (2015). SUMO1 promotes Abeta production via the modulation of autophagy. *Autophagy* 11, 100–112. doi: 10.4161/15548627.2014.984283

Choi, J., Levey, A. I., Weintraub, S. T., Rees, H. D., Gearing, M., Chin, L. S., et al. (2004). Oxidative modifications and down-regulation of ubiquitin carboxyl-terminal hydrolase L1 associated with idiopathic Parkinson's and Alzheimer's diseases. *J. Biol. Chem.* 279, 13256–13264. doi: 10.1074/jbc.M314124200

Chu, C., Zhang, X., Ma, W., Li, L., Wang, W., Shang, L., et al. (2013). Induction of autophagy by a novel small molecule improves a beta pathology and ameliorates cognitive deficits. *PLOS ONE* 8:e65367. doi: 10.1371/journal.pone.0065367

Ciechanover, A., and Schwartz, A. L. (1998). The ubiquitin-proteasome pathway: the complexity and myriad functions of proteins death. *Proc. Natl. Acad. Sci. U.S.A.* 95, 2727–2730. doi: 10.1073/pnas.95.6.2727

Clementi, M. E., Pezzotti, M., Orsini, F., Sampaolese, B., Mezzogori, D., Grassi, C., et al. (2006). Alzheimer's amyloid beta-peptide (1-42) induces cell death in human neuroblastoma via bax/bcl-2 ratio increase: an intriguing role for methionine 35. *Biochem. Biophys. Res. Commun.* 342, 206–213. doi: 10.1016/j.bbrc.2006.01.137

Colasanti, T., Vomero, M., Alessandri, C., Barbati, C., Maselli, A., Camperio, C., et al. (2014). Role of alpha-synuclein in autophagy modulation of primary human T lymphocytes. *Cell Death Dis.* 5:e1265. doi: 10.1038/cddis.2014.211

Corsetti, V., Florenzano, F., Atlante, A., Bobba, A., Ciotti, M. T., Natale, F., et al. (2015). NH2-truncated human tau induces deregulated mitophagy in neurons by aberrant recruitment of Parkin and UCHL-1: implications in Alzheimer's disease. *Hum. Mol. Genet.* 24, 3058–3081. doi: 10.1093/hmg/ddv059

Costes, S., Gurlo, T., Rivera, J. F., and Butler, P. C. (2014). UCHL1 deficiency exacerbates human islet amyloid polypeptide toxicity in beta-cells: evidence of interplay between the ubiquitin/proteasome system and autophagy. *Autophagy* 10, 1004–1014. doi: 10.4161/auto.28478

Crews, L., Patrick, C., Adame, A., Rockenstein, E., and Masliah, E. (2011). Modulation of aberrant CDK5 signaling rescues impaired neurogenesis in models of Alzheimer's disease. *Cell Death Dis.* 2:e120. doi: 10.1038/cddis.2011.2

Crews, L., Spencer, B., Desplats, P., Patrick, C., Paulino, A., Rockenstein, E., et al. (2010). Selective molecular alterations in the autophagy pathway in patients with Lewy body disease and in models of alpha-synucleinopathy. *PLOS ONE* 5:e9313. doi: 10.1371/journal.pone.0009313

de Duve, C. (2005). The lysosome turns fifty. *Nat. Cell Biol.* 7, 847–849. doi: 10.1038/ncb0905-847

De Duve, C., and Wattiaux, R. (1966). Functions of lysosomes. *Annu. Rev. Physiol.* 28, 435–492. doi: 10.1146/annurev.ph.28.030166.002251

De Strooper, B., Saftig, P., Craessaerts, K., Vanderstichele, H., Guhde, G., Annaert, W., et al. (1998). Deficiency of presenilin-1 inhibits the normal cleavage of amyloid precursor protein. *Nature* 391, 387–390. doi: 10.1038/34910

Dean, R. T. (1975). Direct evidence of importance of lysosomes in degradation of intracellular proteins. *Nature* 257, 414–416. doi: 10.1038/257414a0

Decuypere, J. P., Parys, J. B., and Bultynck, G. (2012). Regulation of the autophagic bcl-2/beclin 1 interaction. *Cells* 1, 284–312. doi: 10.3390/cells1030284

Deming, Y., Xia, J., Cai, Y., Lord, J., Holmans, P., Bertelsen, S., et al. (2016). A potential endophenotype for Alzheimer's disease: cerebrospinal fluid clusterin. *Neurobiol. Aging* 37, 208.e1–208.e209. doi: 10.1016/j.neurobiolaging.2015.09.009

Deng, M., Huang, L., Ning, B., Wang, N., Zhang, Q., Zhu, C., et al. (2016). beta-asarone improves learning and memory and reduces Acetyl Cholinesterase and Beta-amyloid 42 levels in APP/PS1 transgenic mice by regulating Beclin-1-dependent autophagy. *Brain Res.* 1652, 188–194. doi: 10.1016/j.brainres.2016.10.008

Dickson, T. C., King, C. E., Mccormack, G. H., and Vickers, J. C. (1999). Neurochemical diversity of dystrophic neurites in the early and late stages of Alzheimer's disease. *Exp. Neurol.* 156, 100–110. doi: 10.1006/exnr.1998.7010

Dolan, P. J., and Johnson, G. V. (2010). A caspase cleaved form of tau is preferentially degraded through the autophagy pathway. *J. Biol. Chem.* 285, 21978–21987. doi: 10.1074/jbc.M110.110940

Donovan, L. E., Higginbotham, L., Dammer, E. B., Gearing, M., Rees, H. D., Xia, Q., et al. (2012). Analysis of a membrane-enriched proteome from postmortem human brain tissue in Alzheimer's disease. *Proteomics Clin. Appl.* 6, 201–211. doi: 10.1002/prca.201100068

Du, D., Hu, L., Wu, J., Wu, Q., Cheng, W., Guo, Y., et al. (2017). Neuroinflammation contributes to autophagy flux blockage in the neurons of rostral ventrolateral medulla in stress-induced hypertension rats. *J. Neuroinflammation* 14:169. doi: 10.1186/s12974-017-0942-2

Du, J., Liang, Y., Xu, F., Sun, B., and Wang, Z. (2013). Trehalose rescues Alzheimer's disease phenotypes in APP/PS1 transgenic mice. *J. Pharm. Pharmacol.* 65, 1753–1756. doi: 10.1111/jphp.12108

Ferreiro, E., Eufrasio, A., Pereira, C., Oliveira, C. R., and Rego, A. C. (2007). Bcl-2 overexpression protects against amyloid-beta and prion toxicity in GT1-7 neural cells. *J. Alzheimers Dis.* 12, 223–228. doi: 10.3233/JAD-2007-12303

Forlenza, O. V., De Paula, V. J., Machado-Vieira, R., Diniz, B. S., and Gattaz, W. F. (2012). Does lithium prevent Alzheimer's disease? *Drugs Aging* 29, 335–342. doi: 10.2165/11599180-000000000-00000

Francois, A., Rioux Bilan, A., Quellard, N., Fernandez, B., Janet, T., Chassaing, D., et al. (2014). Longitudinal follow-up of autophagy and inflammation in brain of APPswePS1dE9 transgenic mice. *J. Neuroinflammation* 11:139. doi: 10.1186/s12974-014-0139-x

Francois, A., Terro, F., Janet, T., Rioux Bilan, A., Paccalin, M., and Page, G. (2013). Involvement of interleukin-1beta in the autophagic process of microglia: relevance to Alzheimer's disease. *J. Neuroinflammation* 10:151. doi: 10.1186/1742-2094-10-151

Frederick, C., Ando, K., Leroy, K., Heraud, C., Suain, V., Buee, L., et al. (2015). Rapamycin ester analog CCI-779/Temsirolimus alleviates tau pathology and improves motor deficit in mutant tau transgenic mice. *J. Alzheimers Dis.* 44, 1145–1156. doi: 10.3233/JAD-142097

Funakoshi, T., Matsuura, A., Noda, T., and Ohsumi, Y. (1997). Analyses of APG13 gene involved in autophagy in yeast, *Saccharomyces cerevisiae*. *Gene* 192, 207–213. doi: 10.1016/S0378-1119(97)00031-0

Funderburk, S. F., Marcellino, B. K., and Yue, Z. (2010). Cell "self-eating" (autophagy) mechanism in Alzheimer's disease. *Mt. Sinai J. Med.* 77, 59–68. doi: 10.1002/msj.20161

Garcia-Arencibia, M., Hochfeld, W. E., Toh, P. P., and Rubinsztein, D. C. (2010). Autophagy, a guardian against neurodegeneration. *Semin. Cell Dev. Biol.* 21, 691–698. doi: 10.1016/j.semcdb.2010.02.008

Giasson, B. I., Forman, M. S., Higuchi, M., Golbe, L. I., Graves, C. L., Kotzbauer, P. T., et al. (2003). Initiation and synergistic fibrillization of tau and alpha-synuclein. *Science* 300, 636–640. doi: 10.1126/science.1082324

Glick, D., Barth, S., and Macleod, K. F. (2010). Autophagy: cellular and molecular mechanisms. *J. Pathol.* 221, 3–12. doi: 10.1002/path.2697

Gong, B., Cao, Z., Zheng, P., Vitolo, O. V., Liu, S., Staniszewski, A., et al. (2006). Ubiquitin hydrolase Uch-L1 rescues beta-amyloid-induced decreases in synaptic function and contextual memory. *Cell* 126, 775–788. doi: 10.1016/j.cell.2006.06.046

Gong, B., Pan, Y., Vempati, P., Zhao, W., Knable, L., Ho, L., et al. (2013). Nicotinamide riboside restores cognition through an upregulation of proliferator-activated receptor-gamma coactivator 1alpha regulated beta-secretase 1 degradation and mitochondrial gene expression in Alzheimer's mouse models. *Neurobiol. Aging* 34, 1581–1588. doi: 10.1016/j.neurobiolaging.2012.12.005

Grill, J. (2017). *Nicotinamide as an Early Alzheimer's Disease Treatment (NEAT).* Bethesda, MD: National Library of Medicine.

Grossi, C., Rigacci, S., Ambrosini, S., Dami, T., Luccarini, I., Traini, C., et al. (eds) (2013). The polyphenol oleuropein aglycone protects TgCRND8 mice against Ass plaque pathology. *PLOS ONE* 8:e71702. doi: 10.1371/journal.pone.0071702

Guerreiro, R., and Bras, J. (2015). The age factor in Alzheimer's disease. *Genome Med.* 7:106. doi: 10.1186/s13073-015-0232-5

Guglielmotto, M., Monteleone, D., Boido, M., Piras, A., Giliberto, L., Borghi, R., et al. (2012). Abeta1-42-mediated down-regulation of Uch-L1 is dependent on NF-kappaB activation and impaired BACE1 lysosomal degradation. *Aging Cell* 11, 834–844. doi: 10.1111/j.1474-9726.2012.00854.x

Harrison, D. E., Strong, R., Sharp, Z. D., Nelson, J. F., Astle, C. M., Flurkey, K., et al. (2009). Rapamycin fed late in life extends lifespan in genetically heterogeneous mice. *Nature* 460, 392–395. doi: 10.1038/nature08221

Hiebel, C., Kromm, T., Stark, M., and Behl, C. (2014). Cannabinoid receptor 1 modulates the autophagic flux independent of mTOR- and BECLIN1-complex. *J. Neurochem.* 131, 484–497. doi: 10.1111/jnc.12839

Higuchi, S., Irie, K., Mishima, S., Araki, M., Ohji, M., Shirakawa, A., et al. (2010). The cannabinoid 1-receptor silent antagonist O-2050 attenuates preference for high-fat diet and activated astrocytes in mice. *J. Pharmacol. Sci.* 112, 369–372. doi: 10.1254/jphs.09326SC

Hiltunen, M., Lu, A., Thomas, A. V., Romano, D. M., Kim, M., Jones, P. B., et al. (2006). Ubiquilin 1 modulates amyloid precursor protein trafficking and Abeta secretion. *J. Biol. Chem.* 281, 32240–32253. doi: 10.1074/jbc.M603106200

Huber, L. A., and Teis, D. (2016). Lysosomal signaling in control of degradation pathways. *Curr. Opin. Cell Biol.* 39, 8–14. doi: 10.1016/j.ceb.2016.01.006

Hubert, V., Peschel, A., Langer, B., Groger, M., Rees, A., and Kain, R. (2016). LAMP-2 is required for incorporating syntaxin-17 into autophagosomes and for their fusion with lysosomes. *Biol. Open* 5, 1516–1529. doi: 10.1242/bio.018648

Iijima, K., Ando, K., Takeda, S., Satoh, Y., Seki, T., Itohara, S., et al. (2000). Neuron-specific phosphorylation of Alzheimer's beta-amyloid precursor protein by cyclin-dependent kinase 5. *J. Neurochem.* 75, 1085–1091. doi: 10.1046/j.1471-4159.2000.0751085.x

Ikeda, M., Yonemura, K., Kakuda, S., Tashiro, Y., Fujita, Y., Takai, E., et al. (2013). Cerebrospinal fluid levels of phosphorylated tau and Abeta1-38/Abeta1-40/Abeta1-42 in Alzheimer's disease with PS1 mutations. *Amyloid* 20, 107–112. doi: 10.3109/13506129.2013.790810

Inestrosa, N. C., Tapia-Rojas, C., Griffith, T. N., Carvajal, F. J., Benito, M. J., Rivera-Dictter, A., et al. (2011). Tetrahydrohyperforin prevents cognitive deficit, A beta deposition, tau phosphorylation and synaptotoxicity in the APPswe/PSEN1DeltaE9 model of Alzheimer's disease: a possible effect on APP processing. *Transl. Psychiatry* 1:e20. doi: 10.1038/tp.2011.19

Inoue, K., Rispoli, J., Kaphzan, H., Klann, E., Chen, E. I., Kim, J., et al. (2012). Macroautophagy deficiency mediates age-dependent neurodegeneration through a phospho-tau pathway. *Mol. Neurodegener.* 7:48. doi: 10.1186/1750-1326-7-48

Iqbal, K., Liu, F., Gong, C. X., and Grundke-Iqbal, I. (2010). Tau in Alzheimer disease and related tauopathies. *Curr. Alzheimer Res.* 7, 656–664. doi: 10.2174/156720510793611592

Irvine, G. B., El-Agnaf, O. M., Shankar, G. M., and Walsh, D. M. (2008). Protein aggregation in the brain: the molecular basis for Alzheimer's and Parkinson's diseases. *Mol. Med.* 14, 451–464. doi: 10.2119/2007-00100.Irvine

Ishiki, A., Kamada, M., Kawamura, Y., Terao, C., Shimoda, F., Tomita, N., et al. (2016). Glial fibrillar acidic protein in the cerebrospinal fluid of Alzheimer's disease, dementia with Lewy bodies, and frontotemporal lobar degeneration. *J. Neurochem.* 136, 258–261. doi: 10.1111/jnc.13399

Jellinger, K. A. (2010). Basic mechanisms of neurodegeneration: a critical update. *J. Cell Mol. Med.* 14, 457–487. doi: 10.1111/j.1582-4934.2010.01010.x

Jiang, P., Guo, Y., Dang, R., Yang, M., Liao, D., Li, H., et al. (2017). Salvianolic acid B protects against lipopolysaccharide-induced behavioral deficits and neuroinflammatory response: involvement of autophagy and NLRP3 inflammasome. *J. Neuroinflammation* 14:239. doi: 10.1186/s12974-017-1013-4

Jiang, T., Yu, J. T., Zhu, X. C., Tan, M. S., Wang, H. F., Cao, L., et al. (2014). Temsirolimus promotes autophagic clearance of amyloid-beta and provides protective effects in cellular and animal models of Alzheimer's disease. *Pharmacol. Res.* 81, 54–63. doi: 10.1016/j.phrs.2014.02.008

Jourquin, J., Duncan, D., Shi, Z., and Zhang, B. (2012). GLAD4U: deriving and prioritizing gene lists from PubMed literature. *BMC Genomics* 13(Suppl. 8):S20. doi: 10.1186/1471-2164-13-S8-S20

Jung, C. H., Ro, S. H., Cao, J., Otto, N. M., and Kim, D. H. (2010). mTOR regulation of autophagy. *FEBS Lett.* 584, 1287–1295. doi: 10.1016/j.febslet.2010.01.017

Kabeya, Y., Mizushima, N., Ueno, T., Yamamoto, A., Kirisako, T., Noda, T., et al. (2000). LC3, a mammalian homologue of yeast Apg8p, is localized in autophagosome membranes after processing. *EMBO J.* 19, 5720–5728. doi: 10.1093/emboj/19.21.5720

Kamada, Y., Funakoshi, T., Shintani, T., Nagano, K., Ohsumi, M., and Ohsumi, Y. (2000). Tor-mediated induction of autophagy via an Apg1 protein kinase complex. *J. Cell Biol.* 150, 1507–1513. doi: 10.1083/jcb.150.6.1507

Kamphuis, W., Middeldorp, J., Kooijman, L., Sluijs, J. A., Kooi, E. J., Moeton, M., et al. (2014). Glial fibrillary acidic protein isoform expression in plaque related astrogliosis in Alzheimer's disease. *Neurobiol. Aging* 35, 492–510. doi: 10.1016/j.neurobiolaging.2013.09.035

Kanehisa, M., Furumichi, M., Tanabe, M., Sato, Y., and Morishima, K. (2017). KEGG: new perspectives on genomes, pathways, diseases and drugs. *Nucleic Acids Res.* 45, D353–D361. doi: 10.1093/nar/gkw1092

Karch, C. M., and Goate, A. M. (2015). Alzheimer's disease risk genes and mechanisms of disease pathogenesis. *Biol. Psychiatry* 77, 43–51. doi: 10.1016/j.biopsych.2014.05.006

Karigar, C., and Murthy, K. R. S. (2005). The Nobel Prize in Chemistry 2004. *Resonance* 10, 41–49. doi: 10.1007/BF02835891

Katona, I., and Freund, T. F. (2012). Multiple functions of endocannabinoid signaling in the brain. *Annu. Rev. Neurosci.* 35, 529–558. doi: 10.1146/annurev-neuro-062111-150420

Kaushik, S., and Cuervo, A. M. (2012). Chaperone-mediated autophagy: a unique way to enter the lysosome world. *Trends Cell Biol.* 22, 407–417. doi: 10.1016/j.tcb.2012.05.006

Kickstein, E., Krauss, S., Thornhill, P., Rutschow, D., Zeller, R., Sharkey, J., et al. (2010). Biguanide metformin acts on tau phosphorylation via mTOR/protein phosphatase 2A (PP2A) signaling. *Proc. Natl. Acad. Sci. U.S.A.* 107, 21830–21835. doi: 10.1073/pnas.0912793107

Klionsky, D. J. (2008). Autophagy revisited: a conversation with Christian de Duve. *Autophagy* 4, 740–743. doi: 10.4161/auto.6398

Klionsky, D. J., Cregg, J. M., Dunn, W. A. Jr., Emr, S. D., Sakai, Y., Sandoval, I. V., et al. (2003). A unified nomenclature for yeast autophagy-related genes. *Dev. Cell* 5, 539–545. doi: 10.1016/S1534-5807(03)00296-X

Korff, A., Liu, C., Ginghina, C., Shi, M., Zhang, J., and Alzheimer's Disease Neuroimaging Initiative. (2013). alpha-Synuclein in cerebrospinal fluid of Alzheimer's disease and mild cognitive impairment. *J. Alzheimers Dis.* 36, 679–688. doi: 10.3233/JAD-130458

Korolainen, M. A., Auriola, S., Nyman, T. A., Alafuzoff, I., and Pirttila, T. (2005). Proteomic analysis of glial fibrillary acidic protein in Alzheimer's disease and aging brain. *Neurobiol. Dis.* 20, 858–870. doi: 10.1016/j.nbd.2005.05.021

Kruger, U., Wang, Y., Kumar, S., and Mandelkow, E. M. (2012). Autophagic degradation of tau in primary neurons and its enhancement by trehalose. *Neurobiol. Aging* 33, 2291–2305. doi: 10.1016/j.neurobiolaging.2011.11.009

Kuma, A., Hatano, M., Matsui, M., Yamamoto, A., Nakaya, H., Yoshimori, T., et al. (2004). The role of autophagy during the early neonatal starvation period. *Nature* 432, 1032–1036. doi: 10.1038/nature03029

Larson, M. E., Sherman, M. A., Greimel, S., Kuskowski, M., Schneider, J. A., Bennett, D. A., et al. (2012). Soluble alpha-synuclein is a novel modulator of Alzheimer's disease pathophysiology. *J. Neurosci.* 32, 10253–10266. doi: 10.1523/JNEUROSCI.0581-12.2012

Lee, J. A., Beigneux, A., Ahmad, S. T., Young, S. G., and Gao, F. B. (2007). ESCRT-III dysfunction causes autophagosome accumulation and neurodegeneration. *Curr. Biol.* 17, 1561–1567. doi: 10.1016/j.cub.2007.07.029

Lee, J. H., Yu, W. H., Kumar, A., Lee, S., Mohan, P. S., Peterhoff, C. M., et al. (2010). Lysosomal proteolysis and autophagy require presenilin 1 and are disrupted by Alzheimer-related PS1 mutations. *Cell* 141, 1146–1158. doi: 10.1016/j.cell.2010.05.008

Letronne, F., Laumet, G., Ayral, A. M., Chapuis, J., Demiautte, F., Laga, M., et al. (2016). ADAM30 downregulates APP-linked defects through cathepsin D activation in Alzheimer's disease. *EBioMedicine* 9, 278–292. doi: 10.1016/j.ebiom.2016.06.002

Li, J., Deng, J., Sheng, W., and Zuo, Z. (2012). Metformin attenuates Alzheimer's disease-like neuropathology in obese, leptin-resistant mice. *Pharmacol. Biochem. Behav.* 101, 564–574. doi: 10.1016/j.pbb.2012.03.002

Li, L., Zhang, S., Zhang, X., Li, T., Tang, Y., Liu, H., et al. (2013). Autophagy enhancer carbamazepine alleviates memory deficits and cerebral amyloid-beta pathology in a mouse model of Alzheimer's disease. *Curr. Alzheimer Res.* 10, 433–441. doi: 10.2174/1567205011310040008

Li, S. C., and Kane, P. M. (2009). The yeast lysosome-like vacuole: endpoint and crossroads. *Biochim. Biophys. Acta* 1793, 650–663. doi: 10.1016/j.bbamcr.2008.08.003

Li, T., Hawkes, C., Qureshi, H. Y., Kar, S., and Paudel, H. K. (2006). Cyclin-dependent protein kinase 5 primes microtubule-associated protein tau site-specifically for glycogen synthase kinase 3beta. *Biochemistry* 45, 3134–3145. doi: 10.1021/bi051635j

Li, W., and Ye, Y. (2008). Polyubiquitin chains: functions, structures, and mechanisms. *Cell Mol. Life. Sci.* 65, 2397–2406. doi: 10.1007/s00018-008-8090-6

Lilienbaum, A. (2013). Relationship between the proteasomal system and autophagy. *Int. J. Biochem. Mol. Biol.* 4, 1–26.

Liu, D., Pitta, M., Jiang, H., Lee, J. H., Zhang, G., Chen, X., et al. (2013). Nicotinamide forestalls pathology and cognitive decline in Alzheimer mice: evidence for improved neuronal bioenergetics and autophagy procession. *Neurobiol. Aging* 34, 1564–1580. doi: 10.1016/j.neurobiolaging.2012.11.020

Liu, G., Wang, H., Liu, J., Li, J., Li, H., Ma, G., et al. (2014). The CLU gene rs11136000 variant is significantly associated with Alzheimer's disease in Caucasian and Asian populations. *Neuromolecular Med.* 16, 52–60. doi: 10.1007/s12017-013-8250-1

Liu, R., Barkhordarian, H., Emadi, S., Park, C. B., and Sierks, M. R. (2005). Trehalose differentially inhibits aggregation and neurotoxicity of beta-amyloid 40 and 42. *Neurobiol. Dis.* 20, 74–81. doi: 10.1016/j.nbd.2005.02.003

Liu, S. J., Yang, C., Zhang, Y., Su, R. Y., Chen, J. L., Jiao, M. M., et al. (2016). Neuroprotective effect of beta-asarone against Alzheimer's disease: regulation of synaptic plasticity by increased expression of SYP and GluR1. *Drug Des. Devel. Ther.* 10, 1461–1469. doi: 10.2147/DDDT.S93559

Lu, B., Nagappan, G., and Lu, Y. (2014). BDNF and synaptic plasticity, cognitive function, and dysfunction. *Handb. Exp. Pharmacol.* 220, 223–250. doi: 10.1007/978-3-642-45106-5_9

Luccarini, I., Grossi, C., Rigacci, S., Coppi, E., Pugliese, A. M., Pantano, D., et al. (2015). Oleuropein aglycone protects against pyroglutamylated-3 amyloid-ss toxicity: biochemical, epigenetic and functional correlates. *Neurobiol. Aging* 36, 648–663. doi: 10.1016/j.neurobiolaging.2014.08.029

Lucin, K. M., O'brien, C. E., Bieri, G., Czirr, E., Mosher, K. I., Abbey, R. J., et al. (2013). Microglial beclin 1 regulates retromer trafficking and phagocytosis and is impaired in Alzheimer's disease. *Neuron* 79, 873–886. doi: 10.1016/j.neuron.2013.06.046

Majd, S., Chegini, F., Chataway, T., Zhou, X. F., and Gai, W. (2013). Reciprocal induction between alpha-synuclein and beta-amyloid in adult rat neurons. *Neurotox. Res.* 23, 69–78. doi: 10.1007/s12640-012-9330-y

Manuel, I., Gonzalez De San Roman, E., Giralt, M. T., Ferrer, I., and Rodriguez-Puertas, R. (2014). Type-1 cannabinoid receptor activity during Alzheimer's disease progression. *J. Alzheimers Dis.* 42, 761–766. doi: 10.3233/JAD-140492

Maphis, N., Xu, G., Kokiko-Cochran, O. N., Cardona, A. E., Ransohoff, R. M., Lamb, B. T., et al. (2015). Loss of tau rescues inflammation-mediated neurodegeneration. *Front. Neurosci.* 9:196. doi: 10.3389/fnins.2015.00196

Maroof, N., Pardon, M. C., and Kendall, D. A. (2013). Endocannabinoid signalling in Alzheimer's disease. *Biochem. Soc. Trans.* 41, 1583–1587. doi: 10.1042/BST20130140

Martorell, M., Forman, K., Castro, N., Capo, X., Tejada, S., and Sureda, A. (2016). Potential therapeutic effects of oleuropein aglycone in Alzheimer's disease. *Curr. Pharm. Biotechnol.* 17, 994–1001. doi: 10.2174/1389201017666160725120656

Marzella, L., Ahlberg, J., and Glaumann, H. (1981). Autophagy, heterophagy, microautophagy and crinophagy as the means for intracellular degradation. *Virchows Arch. B Cell Pathol. Incl. Mol. Pathol.* 36, 219–234.

Matsubara, M., Yamagata, H., Kamino, K., Nomura, T., Kohara, K., Kondo, I., et al. (2001). Genetic association between Alzheimer disease and the alpha-synuclein gene. *Dement. Geriatr. Cogn. Disord.* 12, 106–109. doi: 10.1159/000051243

Matsunaga, S., Kishi, T., Annas, P., Basun, H., Hampel, H., and Iwata, N. (2015a). Lithium as a treatment for Alzheimer's disease: a systematic review and meta-analysis. *J. Alzheimers Dis.* 48, 403–410. doi: 10.3233/JAD-150437

Matsunaga, S., Kishi, T., and Iwata, N. (2015b). Memantine monotherapy for Alzheimer's disease: a systematic review and meta-analysis. *PLOS ONE* 10:e0123289. doi: 10.1371/journal.pone.0123289

Matsuura, A., Tsukada, M., Wada, Y., and Ohsumi, Y. (1997). Apg1p, a novel protein kinase required for the autophagic process in *Saccharomyces cerevisiae*. *Gene* 192, 245–250. doi: 10.1016/S0378-1119(97)00084-X

May, P. C., Lampert-Etchells, M., Johnson, S. A., Poirier, J., Masters, J. N., and Finch, C. E. (1990). Dynamics of gene expression for a hippocampal glycoprotein elevated in Alzheimer's disease and in response to experimental lesions in rat. *Neuron* 5, 831–839. doi: 10.1016/0896-6273(90)90342-D

McDermott, J. R., and Gibson, A. M. (1996). Degradation of Alzheimer's beta-amyloid protein by human cathepsin D. *Neuroreport* 7, 2163–2166. doi: 10.1097/00001756-199609020-00021

Meijer, A. J., Lorin, S., Blommaart, E. F., and Codogno, P. (2015). Regulation of autophagy by amino acids and MTOR-dependent signal transduction. *Amino Acids* 47, 2037–2063. doi: 10.1007/s00726-014-1765-4

Melendez, A., and Neufeld, T. P. (2008). The cell biology of autophagy in metazoans: a developing story. *Development* 135, 2347–2360. doi: 10.1242/dev.016105

Messai, Y., Noman, M. Z., Hasmim, M., Janji, B., Tittarelli, A., Boutet, M., et al. (2014). ITPR1 protects renal cancer cells against natural killer cells by inducing autophagy. *Cancer Res.* 74, 6820–6832. doi: 10.1158/0008-5472.CAN-14-0303

Metcalf, D. J., Garcia-Arencibia, M., Hochfeld, W. E., and Rubinsztein, D. C. (2012). Autophagy and misfolded proteins in neurodegeneration. *Exp. Neurol.* 238, 22–28. doi: 10.1016/j.expneurol.2010.11.003

Miners, J. S., Clarke, P., and Love, S. (2017). Clusterin levels are increased in Alzheimer's disease and influence the regional distribution of Abeta. *Brain Pathol.* 27, 305–313. doi: 10.1111/bpa.12392

Mirnics, K., Norstrom, E. M., Garbett, K., Choi, S. H., Zhang, X., Ebert, P., et al. (2008). Molecular signatures of neurodegeneration in the cortex of PS1/PS2 double knockout mice. *Mol. Neurodegener.* 3:14. doi: 10.1186/1750-1326-3-14

Mizushima, N., and Komatsu, M. (2011). Autophagy: renovation of cells and tissues. *Cell* 147, 728–741. doi: 10.1016/j.cell.2011.10.026

Mizushima, N., Yamamoto, A., Matsui, M., Yoshimori, T., and Ohsumi, Y. (2004). *In vivo* analysis of autophagy in response to nutrient starvation using transgenic mice expressing a fluorescent autophagosome marker. *Mol. Biol. Cell* 15, 1101–1111. doi: 10.1091/mbc.E03-09-0704

Mo, C., Peng, Q., Sui, J., Wang, J., Deng, Y., Xie, L., et al. (2014). Lack of association between cathepsin D C224T polymorphism and Alzheimer's disease risk: an update meta-analysis. *BMC Neurol.* 14:13. doi: 10.1186/1471-2377-14-13

Mohammadi, M., Guan, J., Khodagholi, F., Yans, A., Khalaj, S., Gholami, M., et al. (2016). Reduction of autophagy markers mediated protective effects of JNK inhibitor and bucladesine on memory deficit induced by A beta in rats. *Naunyn Schmiedebergs Arch. Pharmacol.* 389, 501–510. doi: 10.1007/s00210-016-1222-x

Mulder, S. D., Nielsen, H. M., Blankenstein, M. A., Eikelenboom, P., and Veerhuis, R. (2014). Apolipoproteins E and J interfere with amyloid-beta uptake by primary human astrocytes and microglia *in vitro*. *Glia* 62, 493–503. doi: 10.1002/glia.22619

Mullan, G. M., Mceneny, J., Fuchs, M., Mcmaster, C., Todd, S., Mcguinness, B., et al. (2013). Plasma clusterin levels and the rs11136000 genotype in individuals with mild cognitive impairment and Alzheimer's disease. *Curr. Alzheimer Res.* 10, 973–978. doi: 10.2174/15672050113106660162

Nah, J., Pyo, J. O., Jung, S., Yoo, S. M., Kam, T. I., Chang, J., et al. (2013). BECN1/Beclin 1 is recruited into lipid rafts by prion to activate autophagy in response to amyloid beta 42. *Autophagy* 9, 2009–2021. doi: 10.4161/auto.26118

Nakatogawa, H. (2013). Two ubiquitin-like conjugation systems that mediate membrane formation during autophagy. *Essays Biochem.* 55, 39–50. doi: 10.1042/bse0550039

Nakatogawa, H., Ichimura, Y., and Ohsumi, Y. (2007). Atg8, a ubiquitin-like protein required for autophagosome formation, mediates membrane tethering and hemifusion. *Cell* 130, 165–178. doi: 10.1016/j.cell.2007.05.021

Natunen, T., Takalo, M., Kemppainen, S., Leskela, S., Marttinen, M., Kurkinen, K. M. A., et al. (2016). Relationship between ubiquilin-1 and BACE1 in human Alzheimer's disease and APdE9 transgenic mouse brain and cell-based models. *Neurobiol. Dis.* 85, 187–205. doi: 10.1016/j.nbd.2015.11.005

N'Diaye, E. N., Kajihara, K. K., Hsieh, I., Morisaki, H., Debnath, J., and Brown, E. J. (2009). PLIC proteins or ubiquilins regulate autophagy-dependent cell survival during nutrient starvation. *EMBO Rep.* 10, 173–179. doi: 10.1038/embor.2008.238

Neely, K. M., and Green, K. N. (2011). Presenilins mediate efficient proteolysis via the autophagosome-lysosome system. *Autophagy* 7, 664–665. doi: 10.4161/auto.7.6.15448

Nilsson, P., Loganathan, K., Sekiguchi, M., Matsuba, Y., Hui, K., Tsubuki, S., et al. (2013). A beta secretion and plaque formation depend on autophagy. *Cell Rep.* 5, 61–69. doi: 10.1016/j.celrep.2013.08.042

Nilsson, P., and Saido, T. C. (2014). Dual roles for autophagy: degradation and secretion of Alzheimer's disease Abeta peptide. *Bioessays* 36, 570–578. doi: 10.1002/bies.201400002

Nilsson, P., Sekiguchi, M., Akagi, T., Izumi, S., Komori, T., Hui, K., et al. (2015). Autophagy-related protein 7 deficiency in amyloid beta (A beta) precursor protein transgenic mice decreases Abeta in the multivesicular bodies and induces Abeta accumulation in the Golgi. *Am. J. Pathol.* 185, 305–313. doi: 10.1016/j.ajpath.2014.10.011

Nixon, R. A. (2007). Autophagy, amyloidogenesis and Alzheimer disease. *J. Cell Sci.* 120, 4081–4091. doi: 10.1242/jcs.019265

Nixon, R. A., Wegiel, J., Kumar, A., Yu, W. H., Peterhoff, C., Cataldo, A., et al. (2005). Extensive involvement of autophagy in Alzheimer disease: an immuno-electron microscopy study. *J. Neuropathol. Exp. Neurol.* 64, 113–122. doi: 10.1093/jnen/64.2.113

Nobelprize.org (2017). *The Nobel Prize in Physiology or Medicine 2016 [Online]. Nobel Media AB 2014.* Available at: https://www.nobelprize.org/nobel_prizes/medicine/laureates/2016/

Noble, W., Olm, V., Takata, K., Casey, E., Mary, O., Meyerson, J., et al. (2003). Cdk5 is a key factor in tau aggregation and tangle formation *in vivo*. *Neuron* 38, 555–565. doi: 10.1016/S0896-6273(03)00259-9

Nowacek, A., Kosloski, L. M., and Gendelman, H. E. (2009). Neurodegenerative disorders and nanoformulated drug development. *Nanomedicine (Lond)* 4, 541–555. doi: 10.2217/nnm.09.37

Ntais, C., Polycarpou, A., and Ioannidis, J. P. (2004). Meta-analysis of the association of the cathepsin D Ala224Val gene polymorphism with the risk of Alzheimer's disease: a HuGE gene-disease association review. *Am. J. Epidemiol.* 159, 527–536. doi: 10.1093/aje/kwh069

Oddo, S., Caccamo, A., Smith, I. F., Green, K. N., and Laferla, F. M. (2006). A dynamic relationship between intracellular and extracellular pools of Abeta. *Am. J. Pathol.* 168, 184–194. doi: 10.2353/ajpath.2006.050593

Ohsumi, Y. (2014). Historical landmarks of autophagy research. *Cell Res.* 24, 9–23. doi: 10.1038/cr.2013.169

Oikawa, T., Nonaka, T., Terada, M., Tamaoka, A., Hisanaga, S., and Hasegawa, M. (2016). alpha-Synuclein fibrils exhibit gain of toxic function, promoting tau aggregation and inhibiting microtubule assembly. *J. Biol. Chem.* 291, 15046–15056. doi: 10.1074/jbc.M116.736355

Oksman, M., Wisman, L. A., Jiang, H., Miettinen, P., Kirik, D., and Tanila, H. (2013). Transduced wild-type but not P301S mutated human tau shows hyperphosphorylation in transgenic mice overexpressing A30P mutated human alpha-synuclein. *Neurodegener. Dis.* 12, 91–102. doi: 10.1159/000341596

Okuma, T., and Kishimoto, A. (1998). A history of investigation on the mood stabilizing effect of carbamazepine in Japan. *Psychiatry Clin. Neurosci.* 52, 3–12. doi: 10.1111/j.1440-1819.1998.tb00966.x

Olah, Z., Kalman, J., Toth, M. E., Zvara, A., Santha, M., Ivitz, E., et al. (2015). Proteomic analysis of cerebrospinal fluid in Alzheimer's disease: wanted dead or alive. *J. Alzheimers Dis.* 44, 1303–1312. doi: 10.3233/JAD-140141

Onodera, J., and Ohsumi, Y. (2005). Autophagy is required for maintenance of amino acid levels and protein synthesis under nitrogen starvation. *J. Biol. Chem.* 280, 31582–31586. doi: 10.1074/jbc.M506736200

Pacheco, C. D., Elrick, M. J., and Lieberman, A. P. (2009). Tau deletion exacerbates the phenotype of Niemann-Pick type C mice and implicates autophagy in pathogenesis. *Hum. Mol. Genet.* 18, 956–965. doi: 10.1093/hmg/ddn423

Parenti, G., Pignata, C., Vajro, P., and Salerno, M. (2013). New strategies for the treatment of lysosomal storage diseases (review). *Int. J. Mol. Med.* 31, 11–20. doi: 10.3892/ijmm.2012.1187

Paroni, G., Seripa, D., Fontana, A., D'onofrio, G., Gravina, C., Urbano, M., et al. (2014). FOXO1 locus and acetylcholinesterase inhibitors in elderly patients with Alzheimer's disease. *Clin. Interv. Aging* 9, 1783–1791. doi: 10.2147/CIA.S64758

Paz-Y-Miño, C. A., Garcia-Cardenas, J. M., Lopez-Cortes, A., Salazar, C., Serrano, M., and Leone, P. E. (2015). Positive association of the cathepsin D Ala224Val gene polymorphism with the risk of Alzheimer's disease. *Am. J. Med. Sci.* 350, 296–301. doi: 10.1097/MAJ.0000000000000555

Perez, M., Santa-Maria, I., Gomez De Barreda, E., Zhu, X., Cuadros, R., Cabrero, J. R., et al. (2009). Tau–an inhibitor of deacetylase HDAC6 function. *J. Neurochem.* 109, 1756–1766. doi: 10.1111/j.1471-4159.2009.06102.x

Perez, S. E., He, B., Nadeem, M., Wuu, J., Scheff, S. W., Abrahamson, E. E., et al. (2015). Resilience of precuneus neurotrophic signaling pathways despite amyloid pathology in prodromal Alzheimer's disease. *Biol. Psychiatry* 77, 693–703. doi: 10.1016/j.biopsych.2013.12.016

Phelan, M. J., Mulnard, R. A., Gillen, D. L., and Schreiber, S. S. (2017). Phase II clinical trial of nicotinamide for the treatment of mild to moderate Alzheimer's disease. *J. Geriatr. Med. Gerontol.* 3:021.

Pickford, F., Masliah, E., Britschgi, M., Lucin, K., Narasimhan, R., Jaeger, P. A., et al. (2008). The autophagy-related protein beclin 1 shows reduced expression in early Alzheimer disease and regulates amyloid beta accumulation in mice. *J. Clin. Invest.* 118, 2190–2199. doi: 10.1172/JCI33585

Piyanova, A., Albayram, O., Rossi, C. A., Farwanah, H., Michel, K., Nicotera, P., et al. (2013). Loss of CB1 receptors leads to decreased cathepsin D levels and accelerated lipofuscin accumulation in the hippocampus. *Mech. Ageing Dev.* 134, 391–399. doi: 10.1016/j.mad.2013.08.001

Poon, W. W., Carlos, A. J., Aguilar, B. L., Berchtold, N. C., Kawano, C. K., Zograbyan, V., et al. (2013). beta-Amyloid (A beta) oligomers impair brain-derived neurotrophic factor retrograde trafficking by down-regulating ubiquitin C-terminal hydrolase, UCH-L1. *J. Biol. Chem.* 288, 16937–16948. doi: 10.1074/jbc.M113.463711

Porquet, D., Grinan-Ferre, C., Ferrer, I., Camins, A., Sanfeliu, C., Del Valle, J., et al. (2014). Neuroprotective role of trans-resveratrol in a murine model of familial Alzheimer's disease. *J. Alzheimers Dis.* 42, 1209–1220. doi: 10.3233/JAD-140444

Portbury, S. D., Hare, D. J., Sgambelloni, C., Perronnes, K., Portbury, A. J., Finkelstein, D. I., et al. (2017). Trehalose improves cognition in the transgenic Tg2576 mouse model of Alzheimer's disease. *J. Alzheimers Dis.* 60, 549–560. doi: 10.3233/JAD-170322

Posada-Duque, R. A., Lopez-Tobon, A., Piedrahita, D., Gonzalez-Billault, C., and Cardona-Gomez, G. P. (2015). p35 and Rac1 underlie the neuroprotection and cognitive improvement induced by CDK5 silencing. *J. Neurochem.* 134, 354–370. doi: 10.1111/jnc.13127

Qu, J., Nakamura, T., Cao, G., Holland, E. A., Mckercher, S. R., and Lipton, S. A. (2011). S-Nitrosylation activates Cdk5 and contributes to synaptic spine loss induced by beta-amyloid peptide. *Proc. Natl. Acad. Sci. U.S.A.* 108, 14330–14335. doi: 10.1073/pnas.1105172108

Quinn, J. G., Coulson, D. T., Brockbank, S., Beyer, N., Ravid, R., Hellemans, J., et al. (2012). alpha-Synuclein mRNA and soluble alpha-synuclein protein levels in post-mortem brain from patients with Parkinson's disease, dementia with Lewy bodies, and Alzheimer's disease. *Brain Res.* 1459, 71–80. doi: 10.1016/j.brainres.2012.04.018

Rademakers, R., Sleegers, K., Theuns, J., Van Den Broeck, M., Bel Kacem, S., Nilsson, L. G., et al. (2005). Association of cyclin-dependent kinase 5 and neuronal activators p35 and p39 complex in early-onset Alzheimer's disease. *Neurobiol. Aging* 26, 1145–1151. doi: 10.1016/j.neurobiolaging.2004.10.003

Ramirez, B. G., Blazquez, C., Gomez Del Pulgar, T., Guzman, M., and De Ceballos, M. L. (2005). Prevention of Alzheimer's disease pathology by cannabinoids: neuroprotection mediated by blockade of microglial activation. *J. Neurosci.* 25, 1904–1913. doi: 10.1523/JNEUROSCI.4540-04.2005

Riemenschneider, M., Blennow, K., Wagenpfeil, S., Andreasen, N., Prince, J. A., Laws, S. M., et al. (2006). The cathepsin D rs17571 polymorphism: effects on CSF tau concentrations in Alzheimer disease. *Hum. Mutat.* 27, 532–537. doi: 10.1002/humu.20326

Roberts, H. L., Schneider, B. L., and Brown, D. R. (2017). alpha-Synuclein increases beta-amyloid secretion by promoting beta-/gamma-secretase processing of APP. *PLOS ONE* 12:e0171925. doi: 10.1371/journal.pone.0171925

Rogel, M. R., Jaitovich, A., and Ridge, K. M. (2010). The role of the ubiquitin proteasome pathway in keratin intermediate filament protein degradation. *Proc. Am. Thorac. Soc.* 7, 71–76. doi: 10.1513/pats.200908-089JS

Rohn, T. T., Vyas, V., Hernandez-Estrada, T., Nichol, K. E., Christie, L. A., and Head, E. (2008). Lack of pathology in a triple transgenic mouse model of Alzheimer's disease after overexpression of the anti-apoptotic protein Bcl-2. *J. Neurosci.* 28, 3051–3059. doi: 10.1523/JNEUROSCI.5620-07.2008

Rothenberg, C., Srinivasan, D., Mah, L., Kaushik, S., Peterhoff, C. M., Ugolino, J., et al. (2010). Ubiquilin functions in autophagy and is degraded by chaperone-mediated autophagy. *Hum. Mol. Genet.* 19, 3219–3232. doi: 10.1093/hmg/ddq231

Rubinsztein, D. C., Marino, G., and Kroemer, G. (2011). Autophagy and aging. *Cell* 146, 682–695. doi: 10.1016/j.cell.2011.07.030

Rusten, T. E., and Stenmark, H. (2009). How do ESCRT proteins control autophagy? *J. Cell Sci.* 122, 2179–2183. doi: 10.1242/jcs.050021

Sadleir, K. R., and Vassar, R. (2012). Cdk5 protein inhibition and Abeta42 increase BACE1 protein level in primary neurons by a post-transcriptional mechanism: implications of CDK5 as a therapeutic target for Alzheimer disease. *J. Biol. Chem.* 287, 7224–7235. doi: 10.1074/jbc.M111.333914

Saido, T., and Leissring, M. A. (2012). Proteolytic degradation of amyloid beta-protein. *Cold Spring Harb. Perspect. Med.* 2:a006379. doi: 10.1101/cshperspect.a006379

Santulli, G., and Marks, A. R. (2015). Essential roles of intracellular calcium release channels in muscle, brain, metabolism, and aging. *Curr. Mol. Pharmacol.* 8, 206–222. doi: 10.2174/1874467208666150507105105

Sarkar, S., Davies, J. E., Huang, Z., Tunnacliffe, A., and Rubinsztein, D. C. (2007). Trehalose, a novel mTOR-independent autophagy enhancer, accelerates the clearance of mutant huntingtin and alpha-synuclein. *J. Biol. Chem.* 282, 5641–5652. doi: 10.1074/jbc.M609532200

Sarkar, S., Floto, R. A., Berger, Z., Imarisio, S., Cordenier, A., Pasco, M., et al. (2005). Lithium induces autophagy by inhibiting inositol monophosphatase. *J. Cell Biol.* 170, 1101–1111. doi: 10.1083/jcb.200504035

Satoh, J., Tabunoki, H., Ishida, T., Saito, Y., and Arima, K. (2013). Ubiquilin-1 immunoreactivity is concentrated on Hirano bodies and dystrophic neurites in Alzheimer's disease brains. *Neuropathol. Appl. Neurobiol.* 39, 817–830. doi: 10.1111/nan.12036

Schuur, M., Ikram, M. A., Van Swieten, J. C., Isaacs, A., Vergeer-Drop, J. M., Hofman, A., et al. (2011). Cathepsin D gene and the risk of Alzheimer's disease: a population-based study and meta-analysis. *Neurobiol. Aging* 32, 1607–1614. doi: 10.1016/j.neurobiolaging.2009.10.011

Settembre, C., Fraldi, A., Medina, D. L., and Ballabio, A. (2013). Signals from the lysosome: a control centre for cellular clearance and energy metabolism. *Nat. Rev. Mol. Cell Biol.* 14, 283–296. doi: 10.1038/nrm3565

Seyb, K. I., Ansar, S., Li, G., Bean, J., Michaelis, M. L., and Dobrowsky, R. T. (2007). p35/Cyclin-dependent kinase 5 is required for protection against beta-amyloid-induced cell death but not tau phosphorylation by ceramide. *J. Mol. Neurosci.* 31, 23–35. doi: 10.1007/BF02686115

Shao, B. Z., Wei, W., Ke, P., Xu, Z. Q., Zhou, J. X., and Liu, C. (2014). Activating cannabinoid receptor 2 alleviates pathogenesis of experimental autoimmune encephalomyelitis via activation of autophagy and inhibiting NLRP3 inflammasome. *CNS Neurosci. Ther.* 20, 1021–1028. doi: 10.1111/cns.12349

Shen, H. M., and Mizushima, N. (2014). At the end of the autophagic road: an emerging understanding of lysosomal functions in autophagy. *Trends Biochem. Sci.* 39, 61–71. doi: 10.1016/j.tibs.2013.12.001

Sheng, Y., Zhang, L., Su, S. C., Tsai, L. H., and Julius Zhu, J. (2016). Cdk5 is a new rapid synaptic homeostasis regulator capable of initiating the early Alzheimer-like pathology. *Cereb. Cortex* 26, 2937–2951. doi: 10.1093/cercor/bhv032

Shibata, N., Motoi, Y., Tomiyama, H., Ohnuma, T., Kuerban, B., Tomson, K., et al. (2012). Lack of genetic association of the UCHL1 gene with Alzheimer's disease and Parkinson's disease with dementia. *Dement. Geriatr. Cogn. Disord.* 33, 250–254. doi: 10.1159/000339357

Shilling, D., Muller, M., Takano, H., Mak, D. O., Abel, T., Coulter, D. A., et al. (2014). Suppression of InsP3 receptor-mediated Ca2+ signaling alleviates mutant presenilin-linked familial Alzheimer's disease pathogenesis. *J. Neurosci.* 34, 6910–6923. doi: 10.1523/JNEUROSCI.5441-13.2014

Shuai, P., Liu, Y., Lu, W., Liu, Q., Li, T., and Gong, B. (2015). Genetic associations of CLU rs9331888 polymorphism with Alzheimer's disease: a meta-analysis. *Neurosci. Lett.* 591, 160–165. doi: 10.1016/j.neulet.2015.02.040

Shukla, V., Zheng, Y. L., Mishra, S. K., Amin, N. D., Steiner, J., Grant, P., et al. (2013). A truncated peptide from p35, a Cdk5 activator, prevents Alzheimer's disease phenotypes in model mice. *FASEB J.* 27, 174–186. doi: 10.1096/fj.12-217497

Singh, M., Jensen, M. D., Lerman, A., Kushwaha, S., Rihal, C. S., Gersh, B. J., et al. (2016). Effect of low-dose rapamycin on senescence markers and physical functioning in older adults with coronary artery disease: results of a pilot study. *J Frailty Aging* 5, 204–207.

Sofroniew, M. V., and Vinters, H. V. (2010). Astrocytes: biology and pathology. *Acta Neuropathol.* 119, 7–35. doi: 10.1007/s00401-009-0619-8

Solas, M., Francis, P. T., Franco, R., and Ramirez, M. J. (2013). CB2 receptor and amyloid pathology in frontal cortex of Alzheimer's disease patients. *Neurobiol. Aging* 34, 805–808. doi: 10.1016/j.neurobiolaging.2012.06.005

Somavarapu, A. K., and Kepp, K. P. (2016). Loss of stability and hydrophobicity of presenilin 1 mutations causing Alzheimer's disease. *J. Neurochem.* 137, 101–111. doi: 10.1111/jnc.13535

Song, G., Li, Y., Lin, L., and Cao, Y. (2015). Anti-autophagic and anti-apoptotic effects of memantine in a SH-SY5Y cell model of Alzheimer's disease via mammalian target of rapamycin-dependent and -independent pathways. *Mol. Med. Rep.* 12, 7615–7622. doi: 10.3892/mmr.2015.4382

Song, W. J., Son, M. Y., Lee, H. W., Seo, H., Kim, J. H., and Chung, S. H. (2015). Enhancement of BACE1 activity by p25/Cdk5-mediated phosphorylation in Alzheimer's disease. *PLOS ONE* 10:e0136950. doi: 10.1371/journal.pone.0136950

Spilman, P., Podlutskaya, N., Hart, M. J., Debnath, J., Gorostiza, O., Bredesen, D., et al. (2010). Inhibition of mTOR by rapamycin abolishes cognitive deficits and reduces amyloid-beta levels in a mouse model of Alzheimer's disease. *PLOS ONE* 5:e9979. doi: 10.1371/journal.pone.0009979

Steele, J. W., Fan, E., Kelahmetoglu, Y., Tian, Y., and Bustos, V. (2013). Modulation of autophagy as a therapeutic target for Alzheimer's disease. *Postdoc. J.* 1, 21–34. doi: 10.14304/SURYA.JPR.V1N2.3

Steele, J. W., and Gandy, S. (2013). Latrepirdine (Dimebon(R)), a potential Alzheimer therapeutic, regulates autophagy and neuropathology in an Alzheimer mouse model. *Autophagy* 9, 617–618. doi: 10.4161/auto.23487

Stevens, B. W., Dibattista, A. M., William Rebeck, G., and Green, A. E. (2014). A gene-brain-cognition pathway for the effect of an Alzheimers risk gene on working memory in young adults. *Neuropsychologia* 61, 143–149. doi: 10.1016/j.neuropsychologia.2014.06.021

Stieren, E. S., El Ayadi, A., Xiao, Y., Siller, E., Landsverk, M. L., Oberhauser, A. F., et al. (2011). Ubiquilin-1 is a molecular chaperone for the amyloid precursor protein. *J. Biol. Chem.* 286, 35689–35698. doi: 10.1074/jbc.M111.243147

Sun, Y. X., Ji, X., Mao, X., Xie, L., Jia, J., Galvan, V., et al. (2014). Differential activation of mTOR complex 1 signaling in human brain with mild to severe Alzheimer's disease. *J. Alzheimers Dis.* 38, 437–444. doi: 10.3233/JAD-131124

Szklarczyk, D., Morris, J. H., Cook, H., Kuhn, M., Wyder, S., Simonovic, M., et al. (2017). The STRING database in 2017: quality-controlled protein-protein association networks, made broadly accessible. *Nucleic Acids Res.* 45, D362–D368. doi: 10.1093/nar/gkw937

Takeshige, K., Baba, M., Tsuboi, S., Noda, T., and Ohsumi, Y. (1992). Autophagy in yeast demonstrated with proteinase-deficient mutants and conditions for its induction. *J. Cell Biol.* 119, 301–311. doi: 10.1083/jcb.119.2.301

Tanaka, K., Suzuki, T., Hattori, N., and Mizuno, Y. (2004). Ubiquitin, proteasome and parkin. *Biochim. Biophys. Acta* 1695, 235–247. doi: 10.1016/j.bbamcr.2004.09.026

Tang, Z., Ioja, E., Bereczki, E., Hultenby, K., Li, C., Guan, Z., et al. (2015). mTor mediates tau localization and secretion: Implication for Alzheimer's disease. *Biochim. Biophys. Acta* 1853, 1646–1657. doi: 10.1016/j.bbamcr.2015.03.003

The Nobel Assembly at Karolinska Institutet (2016). *Scientific Background Discoveries of Mechanisms for Autophagy*. Stockholm: The Nobel Assembly at Karolinska Institutet.

Tian, L., Zhang, K., Tian, Z. Y., Wang, T., Shang, D. S., Li, B., et al. (2014). Decreased expression of cathepsin D in monocytes is related to the defective degradation of amyloid-beta in Alzheimer's disease. *J. Alzheimers Dis.* 42, 511–520. doi: 10.3233/JAD-132192

Tian, Y., Bustos, V., Flajolet, M., and Greengard, P. (2011). A small-molecule enhancer of autophagy decreases levels of A beta and APP-CTF via Atg5-dependent autophagy pathway. *FASEB J.* 25, 1934–1942. doi: 10.1096/fj.10-175158

Tsukada, M., and Ohsumi, Y. (1993). Isolation and characterization of autophagy-defective mutants of *Saccharomyces cerevisiae*. *FEBS Lett.* 333, 169–174. doi: 10.1016/0014-5793(93)80398-E

Turner, R. S., Thomas, R. G., Craft, S., Van Dyck, C. H., Mintzer, J., Reynolds, B. A., et al. (2015). A randomized, double-blind, placebo-controlled trial of resveratrol for Alzheimer disease. *Neurology* 85, 1383–1391. doi: 10.1212/WNL.0000000000002035

Uddin, M. S., Mamun, A. A., Hossain, M. S., Asaduzzaman, M., Noor, M. A. A., Hossain, M. S., et al. (2016). Neuroprotective effect of *Phyllanthus acidus* L. on learning and memory impairment in a scopolamine-induced animal model of dementia and oxidative stress: natural wonder for regulating the development and progression of Alzheimer's disease. *Adv. Alzheimers Dis.* 5, 53–72. doi: 10.4236/aad.2016.52005

Ueda, K., Fukushima, H., Masliah, E., Xia, Y., Iwai, A., Yoshimoto, M., et al. (1993). Molecular cloning of cDNA encoding an unrecognized component of amyloid in Alzheimer disease. *Proc. Natl. Acad. Sci. U.S.A.* 90, 11282–11286. doi: 10.1073/pnas.90.23.11282

Uhlen, M., Fagerberg, L., Hallstrom, B. M., Lindskog, C., Oksvold, P., Mardinoglu, A., et al. (2015). Proteomics. Tissue-based map of the human proteome. *Science* 347:1260419. doi: 10.1126/science.1260419

Urbanelli, L., Emiliani, C., Massini, C., Persichetti, E., Orlacchio, A., Pelicci, G., et al. (2008). Cathepsin D expression is decreased in Alzheimer's disease fibroblasts. *Neurobiol. Aging* 29, 12–22. doi: 10.1016/j.neurobiolaging.2006.09.005

Vingtdeux, V., Giliberto, L., Zhao, H., Chandakkar, P., Wu, Q., Simon, J. E., et al. (2010). AMP-activated protein kinase signaling activation by resveratrol modulates amyloid-beta peptide metabolism. *J. Biol. Chem.* 285, 9100–9113. doi: 10.1074/jbc.M109.060061

Wang, Q., Tian, Q., Song, X., Liu, Y., and Li, W. (2016). SNCA gene polymorphism may contribute to an increased risk of Alzheimer's disease. *J. Clin. Lab. Anal.* 30, 1092–1099. doi: 10.1002/jcla.21986

Weissman, A. M. (2001). Themes and variations on ubiquitylation. *Nat. Rev. Mol. Cell Biol.* 2, 169–178. doi: 10.1038/35056563

Wong, A. S., Lee, R. H., Cheung, A. Y., Yeung, P. K., Chung, S. K., Cheung, Z. H., et al. (2011). Cdk5-mediated phosphorylation of endophilin B1 is required for induced autophagy in models of Parkinson's disease. *Nat. Cell Biol.* 13, 568–579. doi: 10.1038/ncb2217

Xiao, H., Su, Y., Cao, X., Sun, S., and Liang, Z. (2010). A meta-analysis of mood stabilizers for Alzheimer's disease. *J. Huazhong Univ. Sci. Technol. Med. Sci.* 30, 652–658. doi: 10.1007/s11596-010-0559-5

Xie, M., Han, Y., Yu, Q., Wang, X., Wang, S., and Liao, X. (2016). UCH-L1 inhibition decreases the microtubule-binding function of tau protein. *J. Alzheimers Dis.* 49, 353–363. doi: 10.3233/JAD-150032

Xu, H., and Ren, D. (2015). Lysosomal physiology. *Annu. Rev. Physiol.* 77, 57–80. doi: 10.1146/annurev-physiol-021014-071649

Xu, P., Das, M., Reilly, J., and Davis, R. J. (2011). JNK regulates FoxO-dependent autophagy in neurons. *Genes Dev.* 25, 310–322. doi: 10.1101/gad.1984311

Xue, S., and Jia, J. (2006). Genetic association between Ubiquitin Carboxy-terminal Hydrolase-L1 gene S18Y polymorphism and sporadic Alzheimer's disease in a Chinese Han population. *Brain Res.* 1087, 28–32. doi: 10.1016/j.brainres.2006.02.121

Xue, Z., Zhang, S., Huang, L., He, Y., Fang, R., and Fang, Y. (2013). Upexpression of Beclin-1-dependent autophagy protects against beta-amyloid-induced cell injury in PC12 cells. *J. Mol. Neurosci.* 51, 180–186. doi: 10.1007/s12031-013-9974-y

Yamazaki, Y., Takahashi, T., Hiji, M., Kurashige, T., Izumi, Y., Yamawaki, T., et al. (2010). Immunopositivity for ESCRT-III subunit CHMP2B in granulovacuolar degeneration of neurons in the Alzheimer's disease hippocampus. *Neurosci. Lett.* 477, 86–90. doi: 10.1016/j.neulet.2010.04.038

Yan, J. Q., Yuan, Y. H., Gao, Y. N., Huang, J. Y., Ma, K. L., Gao, Y., et al. (2014). Overexpression of human E46K mutant alpha-synuclein impairs macroautophagy via inactivation of JNK1-Bcl-2 pathway. *Mol. Neurobiol.* 50, 685–701. doi: 10.1007/s12035-014-8738-1

Yang, T. T., Hsu, C. T., and Kuo, Y. M. (2009). Amyloid precursor protein, heat-shock proteins, and Bcl-2 form a complex in mitochondria and modulate mitochondria function and apoptosis in N2a cells. *Mech. Ageing Dev.* 130, 592–601. doi: 10.1016/j.mad.2009.07.002

Yang, Z., and Wang, K. K. (2015). Glial fibrillary acidic protein: from intermediate filament assembly and gliosis to neurobiomarker. *Trends Neurosci.* 38, 364–374. doi: 10.1016/j.tins.2015.04.003

Ye, J., Jiang, Z., Chen, X., Liu, M., Li, J., and Liu, N. (2017). The role of autophagy in pro-inflammatory responses of microglia activation via mitochondrial reactive oxygen species *in vitro*. *J. Neurochem.* 142, 215–230. doi: 10.1111/jnc.14042

Yoshimoto, M., Iwai, A., Kang, D., Otero, D. A., Xia, Y., and Saitoh, T. (1995). NACP, the precursor protein of the non-amyloid beta/A4 protein (A beta)

component of Alzheimer disease amyloid, binds A beta and stimulates A beta aggregation. *Proc. Natl. Acad. Sci. U.S.A.* 92, 9141–9145. doi: 10.1073/pnas.92.20.9141

Yu, W. H., Cuervo, A. M., Kumar, A., Peterhoff, C. M., Schmidt, S. D., Lee, J. H., et al. (2005). Macroautophagy–a novel Beta-amyloid peptide-generating pathway activated in Alzheimer's disease. *J. Cell Biol.* 171, 87–98. doi: 10.1083/jcb.200505082

Yue, Z., Wang, S., Yan, W., and Zhu, F. (2015). Association of UBQ-8i polymorphism with Alzheimer's disease in Caucasians: a meta-analysis. *Int. J. Neurosci.* 125, 395–401. doi: 10.3109/00207454.2014.943369

Zhang, F., and Jiang, L. (2015). Neuroinflammation in Alzheimer's disease. *Neuropsychiatr. Dis. Treat.* 11, 243–256. doi: 10.2147/NDT.S75546

Zhang, F., Kumano, M., Beraldi, E., Fazli, L., Du, C., Moore, S., et al. (2014). Clusterin facilitates stress-induced lipidation of LC3 and autophagosome biogenesis to enhance cancer cell survival. *Nat. Commun.* 5:5775. doi: 10.1038/ncomms6775

Zhang, L., Wang, L., Wang, R., Gao, Y., Che, H., Pan, Y., et al. (2017). Evaluating the effectiveness of GTM-1, rapamycin, and carbamazepine on autophagy and Alzheimer disease. *Med. Sci. Monit.* 23, 801–808. doi: 10.12659/MSM.898679

Zhang, M., Cai, F., Zhang, S., and Song, W. (2014). Overexpression of ubiquitin carboxyl-terminal hydrolase L1 (UCHL1) delays Alzheimer's progression *in vivo*. *Sci. Rep.* 4:7298. doi: 10.1038/srep07298

Zhang, P., Qin, W., Wang, D., Liu, B., Zhang, Y., Jiang, T., et al. (2015). Impacts of PICALM and CLU variants associated with Alzheimer's disease on the functional connectivity of the hippocampus in healthy young adults. *Brain Struct. Funct.* 220, 1463–1475. doi: 10.1007/s00429-014-0738-4

Zhang, T., and Jia, Y. (2014). Meta-analysis of Ubiquilin1 gene polymorphism and Alzheimer's disease risk. *Med. Sci. Monit.* 20, 2250–2255. doi: 10.12659/MSM.891030

Zhang, Y., Mclaughlin, R., Goodyer, C., and Leblanc, A. (2002). Selective cytotoxicity of intracellular amyloid beta peptide1-42 through p53 and Bax in cultured primary human neurons. *J. Cell Biol.* 156, 519–529. doi: 10.1083/jcb.200110119

Zhou, X., Zhou, J., Li, X., Guo, C., Fang, T., and Chen, Z. (2011). GSK-3beta inhibitors suppressed neuroinflammation in rat cortex by activating autophagy in ischemic brain injury. *Biochem. Biophys. Res. Commun.* 411, 271–275. doi: 10.1016/j.bbrc.2011.06.117

Zhou, Y., Hayashi, I., Wong, J., Tugusheva, K., Renger, J. J., and Zerbinatti, C. (2014). Intracellular clusterin interacts with brain isoforms of the bridging integrator 1 and with the microtubule-associated protein Tau in Alzheimer's disease. *PLOS ONE* 9:e103187. doi: 10.1371/journal.pone.0103187

Zhu, Z., Yan, J., Jiang, W., Yao, X. G., Chen, J., Chen, L., et al. (2013). Arctigenin effectively ameliorates memory impairment in Alzheimer's disease model mice targeting both beta-amyloid production and clearance. *J. Neurosci.* 33, 13138–13149. doi: 10.1523/JNEUROSCI.4790-12.2013

5

Fighting the Cause of Alzheimer's and GNE Myopathy

Shreedarshanee Devi, Rashmi Yadav, Pratibha Chanana and Ranjana Arya*

School of Biotechnology, Jawaharlal Nehru University, New Delhi, India

***Correspondence:**
Ranjana Arya
arya.ranjana24@gmail.com;
ranjanaa@jnu.ac.in

Age is the common risk factor for both neurodegenerative and neuromuscular diseases. Alzheimer disease (AD), a neurodegenerative disorder, causes dementia with age progression while GNE myopathy (GNEM), a neuromuscular disorder, causes muscle degeneration and loss of muscle motor movement with age. Individuals with mutations in presenilin or amyloid precursor protein (APP) gene develop AD while mutations in GNE (UDP *N*-acetylglucosamine 2 epimerase/*N*-acetyl Mannosamine kinase), key sialic acid biosynthesis enzyme, cause GNEM. Although GNEM is characterized with degeneration of muscle cells, it is shown to have similar disease hallmarks like aggregation of Aβ and accumulation of phosphorylated tau and other misfolded proteins in muscle cell similar to AD. Similar impairment in cellular functions have been reported in both disorders such as disruption of cytoskeletal network, changes in glycosylation pattern, mitochondrial dysfunction, oxidative stress, upregulation of chaperones, unfolded protein response in ER, autophagic vacuoles, cell death, and apoptosis. Interestingly, AD and GNEM are the two diseases with similar phenotypic condition affecting neuron and muscle, respectively, resulting in entirely different pathology. This review represents a comparative outlook of AD and GNEM that could lead to target common mechanism to find a plausible therapeutic for both the diseases.

Keywords: amyloid β, NFT, GNE, hyposialylation, sialic acid, ER stress, apoptosis, autophagy

INTRODUCTION

Aging is the process, which initiates with subclinical changes at molecular level including accumulation of mutations, telomere attrition, epigenetic alterations resulting in genome instability (López-Otín et al., 2013). These changes multiply at a very fast rate, ultimately leading to the morphological and functional deterioration of brain by progressive loss of the neurons, reduction in the levels of neurotransmitters at the synaptic junction and disruption of integrity of the brain (Sibille, 2013). In addition to neurons, muscle cells are also affected with age. Loss of muscle mass, reduction in muscle fiber size and number is observed in muscles with age that decreases muscle strength (Narici and Maffulli, 2010; Siparsky et al., 2014). Thus, age is a common risk factor for both neurodegenerative and neuromuscular diseases, that progress with time.

The neurodegenerative disorders like Alzheimer's disease (AD), Parkinson's disease, Huntington's disease and amyotrophic lateral sclerosis (ALS) share similar pattern of brain alterations and relate to each other at sub-cellular levels in numerous studies (Garden and La Spada, 2012; Montie and Durcan, 2013). Oxidative stress and altered Ca^{2+} and mitochondrial

Abbreviations: Aβ, β amyloid; AD, Alzheimer's disease; GNE, UDP-GlcNAc 2-epimerase/ManNAc kinase; GNEM, GNE myopathy; NFT, neurofibrillary tangles.

dysfunctions cause neuronal damage with age (Thibault et al., 1998, 2001). Further, neurons do not divide (with rare exceptions), thus cellular damage tend to accumulate with age (Sibille, 2013). Similarly neuromuscular disorders such as multiple sclerosis, muscular dystrophy, GNE related myopathy, Myasthenia gravis, Spinal muscular atrophy and ALS show subcellular damage in muscle cells where oxidative stress and altered calcium/mitochondrial, and ER stress are observed (Kanekura et al., 2009; Roussel et al., 2013; Stone and Lin, 2015; Xiang et al., 2017). Muscle cells are also among the least dividing cells with average lifespan of 15 years or sometimes reaching four decades. Due to its long life span like neurons, the cellular damage in muscle also accumulates in due course of time. As the age progresses, the satellite cells of muscle decline reducing the regeneration capacity of healthy muscle in place of affected cells (Narici and Maffulli, 2010). Whether there is any correlation of cellular damage in neurons versus muscle cells that can be a common therapeutic target is not known.

Indeed some disorders such as ALS can be placed in either of the two disorders as it affects both neurons and muscle cells. Several neuromuscular disorders, which include muscular dystrophies have reported degeneration of neurons in brain and affect the cognitive function leading to memory loss (Anderson et al., 2002; Ricotti et al., 2011). In ALS, loss of motor neurons affect the movement of various muscles of body leading to muscle wasting and paralysis, along with cognitive impairment (Taylor et al., 2016). Interestingly, a novel missense mutation (histidine to arginine at 705 amino acid) in GNE gene (UDP *N*-acetylglucosamine 2 epimerase/*N*-acetyl Mannosamine kinase) was observed in familial ALS patient (Köroğlu et al., 2017). Mutation in GNE gene causes GNEM, a rare neuromuscular disorder with completely different pathology compared to ALS (Huizing and Krasnewich, 2009). This raises a possibility of a missing link between the two disorders where the pathomechanisms might merge at a common target.

In this review, we have correlated and compared Alzheimer's disease, a neurodegenerative disorder with GNEM, a neuromuscular disorder and put forth how these diseases share common pathological events like aggregation of misfolded proteins, oxidative stress, mitochondrial dysfunction, autophagy and cellular death. This will help us to find a common therapeutic approach for the treatment of these diseases.

EPIDEMIOLOGY

Among various neurological disorders, Alzheimer's disease is the most common form of dementia accounting for 60–80% of all the cases of dementia, with worldwide prevalence above 45 million[1]. It is more prevalent in the Western European and North American population. On the other hand, GNEM is a rare genetic neuromuscular disorder with worldwide prevalence of 1–9 in a millionth population (Orphanet[2]). GNEM has been reported in the Irish, Jewish, Japanese and Indian populations. Also, there are reports of GNEM from North America, European (United Kingdom and Scotland) and other Asian country like Thailand (Bhattacharya et al., 2018).

[1]www.alzheimers.net

[2]http://www.orpha.net/

CAUSES, CHARACTERISTICS AND GENETIC PREDISPOSITION

AD is a multifactorial disease without any single cause. The main characteristic features of AD are senile plaques, composed mainly of extracellular amyloid-β (Aβ) peptides, and Neurofibrillary Tangles (NFTs) formed after accumulation of intracellular hyperphosphorylated tau (Serrano-Pozo et al., 2011). GNEM is caused by autosomal recessive mutation in GNE gene responsible for sialic acid biosynthesis. The characteristic features for GNEM involves weakness in the distal muscles, sparing the quadriceps, presence of rimmed vacuoles in muscle fibers and tubulofilamentous inclusions of aggregated proteins such as Aβ and phosphorylated tau (Jay et al., 2009). Despite the differences in tissues that are affected in the two diseases, accumulation of aggregates of amyloid-β and tau are common characteristics of both the diseases.

Initial symptom of AD is gradual loss in ability of the person to remember new information (Souchay and Moulin, 2009). The greatest risk factor for the development of AD is age as its pathological features increase exponentially with age (doubling every 5 years after the attainment of 65 years of age) (Querfurth and LaFerla, 2010). In GNEM, the initial symptoms include foot drop and weakness in the distal muscles, which gradually worsen with age toward wheel-chair dependence of patients. In GNEM, unlike AD, the brain function has been reported as normal (Anada et al., 2014). The onset of AD is late adulthood while GNEM onset is early adulthood during the second or third decade of life. How aging leads to sudden onset of GNEM is not known.

Beside aging, AD is caused due to mutation in either the presenilin genes or in Amyloid Precursor Protein (APP) gene (Goate et al., 1991; Hutton and Hardy, 1997; Holtzman et al., 2011). There is also an increased risk of AD in individuals suffering from Down's syndrome because chromosome 21 includes a gene encoding the production of APP (Wiseman et al., 2015). The epsilon four allele of the apolipoprotein E gene (APOE) located on chromosome 19 is found to be a risk factor for AD (Reiman et al., 2005). People with a history of diabetes, hypertension, obesity, smoking, head injury leading to memory loss and a family history of AD in close relatives are at a greater risk of AD (Barnes and Yaffe, 2011). The prevalence of AD is higher in women and less educated masses (Letenneur et al., 2000).

On the other hand, GNEM is caused due to mutation in GNE (UDP-GlcNAc 2-epimerase/ManNAc kinase) gene that catalyzes the first two rate limiting steps in the biosynthesis of sialic acid (Jay et al., 2009). Whether hyposialylation is the only cause of GNEM is still unknown. GNEM is a genetic disorder and not known to be associated with lifestyle disease. No gender bias has been reported for GNEM. A complete comparison of characteristics of both AD and GNEM has been described in **Table 1**.

DISEASE PATHOLOGY

In normal condition, neuronal cells release soluble Aβ after cleavage of a cell surface receptor called APP. In case of AD, the cleavage is abnormal leading to the precipitation of Aβ into dense beta sheets and formation of senile plaques (Zhang et al., 2011). To clear the amyloid aggregates, an inflammatory response is generated by astrocytes and microglia leading to the destruction of adjacent neurons and their neuritis (Norfray and Provenzale, 2004; Querfurth and LaFerla, 2010).

The tau protein is a microtubule stabilizing protein and has a role in intracellular transport (both axonal and vesicular). In its abnormally hyper-phosphorylated form, tau form intracellular aggregates called the NFTs or senile plaques, interfering with normal axonal transport of molecules along microtubules (Norfray and Provenzale, 2004).

In GNEM, main pathological feature includes formation of rimmed vacuoles, which is comprised of aggregated proteins such as Aβ and tau (Nalini et al., 2010). Cytoplasmic and nuclear inclusion bodies have also been observed by electron microscopy in muscle biopsies, which contain degradative products from the membrane, cytoplasmic tubulofilaments and mitochondria with irregular size and shape (Huizing and Krasnewich, 2009). However, since GNE is a key sialic acid biosynthetic enzyme, mutation in GNE affects the sialylation of proteins (Noguchi et al., 2004). The immunohistochemistry of GNEM muscle samples revealed upregulation of αβ-crystallin, NCAM, MHC-1, and iNOS levels (Fischer et al., 2013). NCAM was hyposialylated in GNEM and proposed as diagnostic marker for GNEM (Ricci et al., 2006). In aging brain and AD, the expression and function of NCAM and MHC-1 was altered that may result in synaptic and cognitive loss (Aisa et al., 2010). Also, reduced polysialated-NCAM load was reported in entorhinal cortex causing AD (Murray et al., 2016). Thus, NCAM sialylation can be a common target in the pathology of AD and GNEM in addition to Aβ and tau accumulation.

DIAGNOSIS

Medical and family history of individuals, which include psychiatric history, changes in behavior and cognitive functions, help in the diagnosis of AD. Amyloid plaques, presence of NFT's and distribution in the brain are used to establish the disease by an autopsy based pathological evaluation. The clinical diagnosis of AD is about 70–90% accurate relative to the pathological diagnosis (Beach et al., 2012).

GNEM is clinically characterized by weakness in tibialis anterior muscles with a unique sparing of the quadriceps leading to foot drop, gait abnormalities, mild or no elevation in serum creatine kinase levels with no involvement of cardiac muscles, usually in the second or third decade of life (Nalini et al., 2013). Pathologically, GNEM is characterized by presence of rimmed vacuoles in muscle biopsies, without inflammation (Argov and Yarom, 1984). The confirmation of GNEM mainly relies on identification of bi-allelic mutation in GNE gene. As more than 190 mutations in GNE have been identified worldwide, complete

TABLE 1 | Comparison of the characteristics of AD and GNEM.

	Characteristics of AD and GNEM	
	AD	**GNEM**
Disease type	Neurodegenerative	Neuromuscular
Onset of the disease	Early (5%) and late onset (>95%)	Early adulthood
Age	Mainly above 65 years of age	20–30 years of age
Prevalence	45 Million and above	~1–9 in one Million
Demographics	Worldwide but common in Western Europe and North American population	Jewish, Japanese and Indian population
Initial signs	Loss in memory	Foot drop
Gender biasness	Higher in women	Not found
Mutation	FAD-autosomally dominant	Autosomal recessive
Genetic defects	Mutations in Presenilin genes, APOE gene	Mutations in GNE gene
Symptoms	Memory loss, agitation, sleeplessness, and delusions	Foot drop, weakness in distal muscles, and difficulty in walking
Progressiveness	Fast	Slow
Brain function	Affected	Not affected
Pathological effect	Damage to limbic system and neocortical region, Senile plaques and NFTs, aggregation of proteins	Rimmed vacuole of aggregated proteins tubulofilaments and small fibers, cytoplasmic and nuclear inclusion bodies, aggregation of proteins
Diagnosis	Medical history, pathological diagnosis of plaques and NFTs, MRI and CT scan of brain lesions, levels of serum B12, TSH, T4 etc.	Time of disease onset, Gait study, walking pattern, pathological study of rimmed vacuoles and other factors, biallelic mutations in GNE gene through sequencing
Treatment	Acetylcholinesterase (Ach esterase) inhibitors, drugs targeting Aβ and tau protein accumulation	Supplementation with sialic acid and its precursor molecules, IVIG administration, gene therapy

sequencing of the GNE is necessary for diagnosis of GNE myopathy.

COMPARATIVE ANALYSIS OF MOLECULAR MECHANISMS AFFECTING AD AND GNEM

Effect of Glycosylation, Particularly Sialylation, in AD and GNEM

Glycosylation is the process of incorporation of glycan, either monosaccharides or oligosaccharides, unit to proteins and lipid moieties (Spiro, 2002). The role of glycosylation in case of AD was first reported when impaired glucose metabolism increased toxicity from Aβ and affected glycosylation pattern (Ott et al., 1999; Peila et al., 2002; Chornenkyy et al., 2018). Several key proteins involved in Aβ deposition cascade such as APP, BACE-1 (β secretase), γ-secretase, nicastrin, neprisilin (NEP) undergo altered glycosylation in AD (Kizuka et al., 2017). Deletion of N-glycosylation of APP protein results in its reduced secretion (Schedin-Weiss et al., 2014). APP trafficking from trans-Golgi network to plasma membrane and non-amyloidogenic processing is enhanced by O-GlcNAcylation of APP (Chun et al., 2015). Interestingly, enhanced sialylation of APP increased APP secretion and Aβ production (Nakagawa et al., 2006). Defect in sialic acid biosynthesis due to mutation in GNE affects sialylation of glycoproteins in GNEM. Several proteins such as neural cell adhesion molecule (NCAM), α-dystroglycan, integrin, IGF-1R, and other proteins have been found with altered sialylation in absence of functional GNE (Huizing et al., 2004; Ricci et al., 2006; Grover and Arya, 2014; Singh et al., 2018). However, changes in glycosylation pattern of APP or Aβ are not studied in GNEM despite elevated levels of APP reported in ALS and GNEM (Koistinen et al., 2006; Fischer et al., 2013). Thus, there is a need to investigate whether hyposialylation of muscle cells, as effect of mutation in GNE, affects the glycosylation pattern and sialylation of accumulated glycoproteins and proteins like Aβ, presenilin-1 etc.

Proper glycosylation of nicastrin (a subunit of γ-secretase) affects its trafficking to Golgi apparatus and proper binding to presenilin-1, thereby, inhibiting APP processing and γ-secretase substrate preference (Yang et al., 2002; Xie et al., 2014; Moniruzzaman et al., 2018). Expression of glycosylated NEP, protein involved in Aβ clearance, is also reduced in AD (Reilly, 2001). Interestingly, in GNEM also, the glycosylation and sialylation of neprilysin is dramatically reduced, affecting its expression and normal enzymatic activity (Broccolini et al., 2008). The effect of reduced activity in NEP in GNEM may lead to its failure of clearance of Aβ from muscle. Additionally, it has also been reported that enzyme GNE undergoes O-GlcNAcylation thereby, modulating its enzymatic activity (Bennmann et al., 2016). Thus, it would be of interest to study effect of altered sialylation due to GNE mutation on glycosylation pattern of aggregating proteins.

Several reports indicate alteration of protein sialylation to be a leading cause of AD (Wang, 2009; Schnaar et al., 2014). Binding of Aβ to cells is sialic acid dependent as its binding to surface is mediated through sialylated gangliosides, glycolipids, and glycoproteins (Ariga et al., 2001). The levels of sialyltransferase reduce with age that may contribute to altered sialic acid levels (Maguire et al., 1994; Maguire and Breen, 1995). In addition, clearance of Aβ by microglia is enhanced in absence of sialylated immunoglobulin, CD33 (siglec-33) (Jiang et al., 2014; Siddiqui et al., 2017). This suggests that sialylation is important for Aβ uptake and accumulation.

Interestingly, altered levels of sialyltransferases ST3Gal5 and ST8Sia1 were reported in HEKAD293 cells overexpressing wild type recombinant GNE resulting in increased levels of gangliosides GM3 and GD3 (Wang et al., 2006). Thus, GNE may affect sialyltransferases with an unknown mechanism. Molecules affecting sialyltransferase levels may influence Aβ uptake in both GNEM as well as AD. Thus, changes in the sialylation pattern of Aβ deposition cascade proteins in muscle cells may affect rimmed vacuole formation in GNEM and offer new therapeutic approach.

Role of Cytoskeleton Network in AD and GNEM

Cytoskeletal proteins are important functional proteins in both neuronal and muscle cells. In muscle, they help in conducting contraction and movement, while in neurons, they have a vital role in neuronal plasticity that is important for learning and memory process. Cytoskeletal proteins include different proteins like actin, tubulin, and lamin that provide mechanical support to the cell and modulate their dynamics inside the cell.

Tau, the first microtubule associated protein to be identified, was found to be one of the important hallmarks of AD along with Aβ. Tau directly helps in self-assembly of microtubule from tubulin. In AD, tau is found to be hyperphosphorylated at different site than normal (Gong et al., 2005; Hanger et al., 2007). The extent of tau aggregation is correlated with amount of phosphorylation at different sites (Iqbal et al., 2008). Also increased auto-antibodies of tubulin and tau were found in the serum of AD patients indicating a robust target for disease diagnosis (Salama et al., 2018). In GNEM, phosphorylated tau has been observed to accumulate in rimmed vacuoles (Nogalska et al., 2015), but whether aggregated tau is hyperphosphorylated from the normal form is not yet studied.

Actin dynamics and modulation of G-actin and F-actin is an important feature for neuronal plasticity and memory developments (Penzes and Rafalovich, 2012). Impaired cognitive function has been reported in AD pathology where cofilin-1, an actin depolymerizer, was found to be inactive (Barone et al., 2014). Inactivation of cofilin 1 contributes to actin dependent impairment of synaptic plasticity and thus, learning (Rust, 2015). Further, cofilin-1 inactivation is γ-secretase dependent, which controls Aβ peptide production. Also, cofilin-actin rods result in synaptic loss in AD (Bamburg et al., 2010). Small GTPases like RhoA, Rac1, and Cdc42 regulate APP, formation of Aβ and neurotoxicity (Boo et al., 2008; Wang et al., 2009). Phosphorylation of collapsin mediator response protein-2 (CRMP-2) in AD disrupts its binding with kinesin hampering axonal transport and resulting in neuronal defect (Mokhtar et al., 2018). RhoGTPases also play important role in muscle differentiation and muscle contraction (DeHart and Jones, 2004; Zhang et al., 2012). Interestingly, GNE has been shown to interact with CRMP-1, α-actinin-1, and α-actinin-2, key cytoskeletal regulatory proteins (Weidemann et al., 2006; Amsili et al., 2008; Harazi et al., 2017). Being an actin binding protein, binding of α-actinin-1 and α-actinin-2 with GNE raises a possibility of impaired actin function in GNEM. Differential cytoskeletal protein expression was observed in muscle biopsy samples of GNEM patients (Sela et al., 2011). Upstream of actin, FAK (focal adhesion complex) and integrin (extracellular matrix protein) function was affected in mutant GNE cells (Grover and Arya, 2014). It has also been reported that induction of Aβ led to the increased expression of FAK and autophosphorylation at Tyr397 (Han et al., 2013). However, role of RhoA, actin, cofilin needs to be further elucidated in GNEM. Taken together these studies indicate cytoskeletal proteins to be a common target that regulate Aβ production and need therapeutic intervention to explore effective molecules.

Mitochondrial Dysfunction in AD and GNEM

Mitochondria are self-dividing organelles undergoing fission and fusion inside a cell. It is the power house of a cell that provides energy by oxidative phosphorylation during TCA cycle. Neurons and muscle cells have higher demand for mitochondria for their neuronal processes and muscle contraction, respectively. It has been reported that different cytoskeletal proteins help in motility of mitochondria in the cytoplasm (Lackner, 2013). Accumulation of Aβ and increased cellular death has been reported upon dissection of brains of AD patients (Cha et al., 2012). Further, Aβ accumulation in mitochondria precedes amyloid plaque, indicative of an early stage AD (Ankarcrona et al., 2010). In the early stages of AD, the number of mitochondria in the affected neurons is highly reduced leading to decreased glucose metabolism and impaired TCA cycle enzyme activity (Bubber et al., 2005; Mosconi, 2005). Additionally, elevated level of oxidative damage and significant increase in mutation of mtDNA and cytochrome c oxidase has been reported in AD patients (Castellani et al., 2002). Further, impaired mitochondrial trafficking has been observed in rat hippocampal neurons upon exposure to sub-cytotoxic levels of Aβ (Rui et al., 2006). Altered calcium homeostasis affects ATP generation and cause mitochondrial dysfunction (Supnet and Bezprozvanny, 2010; Swerdlow, 2018).

In GNEM, upregulation of a number of mitochondrial genes and transcript encoding mitochondrial proteins like COX, Cytochrome C Oxidase, ATPases, NADH dehydrogenase etc., have been reported in GNEM patient muscle biopsies (Eisenberg et al., 2008). Vacuolar and swollen mitochondria indicative of structure and functional dysfunction have been observed in HEK cells with mutated GNE (Eisenberg et al., 2008). Since function of mitochondria is dependent on its structure, increased branching of mitochondria observed in cells of GNEM patients could lead to oxidative stress (Eisenberg et al., 2008). Thus, both GNEM and AD show mitochondrial dysfunction. It would be of interest to determine the stage at which mitochondria are affected in GNEM and whether any Aβ accumulation occurs in mitochondria besides rimmed vacuoles.

In AD mouse study, COX gene knock out reduced oxidative stress by reducing Aβ plaque formation (Fukui et al., 2007). Inhibition of COX2 function results in protection of neurons and reduces the accumulation of Aβ in neurons of AD transgenic mice (Woodling et al., 2016). In GNEM, COX7A protein is reported to be upregulated (Eisenberg et al., 2008). Thus, inhibiting COX gene in GNEM may reduce mitochondrial oxidative stress and inhibit Aβ aggregate formation in GNE deficient cells and could serve as an important therapeutic target.

Effect of Oxidative Stress in AD and GNEM

Oxidative stress is a key player in many neurodegenerative diseases. With age, oxidative stress in brain elevates due to imbalance of redox potential leading to generation of reactive oxygen species (ROS) (Andreyev et al., 2005; Wang and Michaelis, 2010). When the amount of ROS species produced is greater than scavenged by ROS defense mechanisms, it leads to oxidative stress leading to cell damage (Feng and Wang, 2012). Reports suggest that Aβ(1-42) accumulation is associated with oxidative stress in hippocampal neuron of *C. elegans* (Yatin et al., 1999). Phosphorylation of tau is also reported to be increased during oxidative stress via activation of glycogen synthase kinase 3-β (Lovell et al., 2004). Aberrant S-nitrosylation of proteins at cysteine residue of ApoE, Cdk5, and PDI leads to oxidative stress and neurodestruction (Zhao et al., 2014). In fact, oxidation of proteins in neurons that control Aβ solubilization and tau hyperphosphorylation severely affect progression of AD.

In GNEM, upregulation of cell stress molecules, such as Aβ oligomers, αβ-crystallin that signals to elevate APP protein was reported (Fischer et al., 2013). Upregulation of iNOS enzyme suggested that cell stress in GNE myopathy is mainly due to NO-related free radicals (Fischer et al., 2013). In GNEM patients and mouse model, proteins were found to be highly modified with S-nitrosylation (Cho et al., 2017). In AD, generation of NO correlates with the activation of iNOS in glial cells. Generation of NO by iNOS is robust and render neurotoxicity, contributing to neuronal death and injury (Zhao et al., 2014). Atrogenes and oxidative stress response proteins are highly upregulated in hyposialylated condition and supplementation with sialic acid restores ROS levels in muscle cells (Cho et al., 2017). Additionally, in HEK293 cell based model system for GNEM overexpressing pathologically relevant GNE mutation, PrdxIV, an ER resident Peroxiredoxin was found to be downregulated. The downregulation of Prdx IV may disturb the redox state of ER, affecting proper folding of proteins eventually leading to ER stress (Chanana et al., 2017). Also expression level of Prdx I and Prdx IV was substantially decreased in post-mortem brain of AD with higher level of protein oxidation (Majd and Power, 2018). These studies suggest that oxidative stress may be common to both the disorders. ER based peroxiredoxins may play an important role in the pathology of both the diseases.

Role of Endoplasmic Reticulum and Chaperones in Protein Aggregation

Endoplasmic reticulum is an important cellular organelle involved in proper folding and processing of proteins. Perturbation in functioning of ER leads to misfolding of proteins and eventually protein aggregation, which is the key feature in several neurodegenerative diseases. Accumulation of misfolded proteins in ER elicits ER stress and unfolded protein response (UPR) that triggers cell death by apoptosis to eliminate cell toxicity (Tabas and Ron, 2011). Misfolded proteins that are retained in ER undergo proteosomal degradation via ER-associated degradation or ERAD (Smith et al., 2011). Activation of UPR proteins such as IRE1 and chaperone, GRP78, have been reported in the cortex and hippocampal tissue of AD brain (Hoozemans et al., 2005; Lee et al., 2010a). Activation of UPR proteins such as IRE1α, PERK, and ATF6 have been reported in AD by Xiang et al. (2017). Even GNEM muscle biopsies revealed upregulation of different UPR proteins including GRP78/BiP, GRP94, calnexin, and calreticulin, which are ER resident chaperones. The same study showed localization of GRP78/BiP and GRP94 with Aβ in the ER (Li et al., 2013). Upregulation of chaperone GRP94 is reported in HEK cell based model of GNEM (Grover and Arya, 2014). Since upregulation of chaperones is also observed in GNEM, they may play an important role in protein aggregate and subsequently rimmed vacuole formation. Thus, small molecules affecting chaperone activity to enhance proper protein folding and inhibition of protein aggregation offer a promising therapeutic approach for GNEM.

Interestingly, calreticulin, molecular chaperone that modulates Ca^{2+} homeostasis, is downregulated in cortical neurons of AD patients and used as negative biomarker for AD progression (Lin et al., 2014). Another study reported that calreticulin co-localizes with both Aβ and APP and helps in proper folding of Aβ (Johnson et al., 2001). Stemmer et al have showed that calreticulin bound directly with Presenilin and Nicastrin molecular component of γ-secretase, along with Aβ (Stemmer et al., 2013). The binding of calreticulin with γ-secretase may direct the proper binding and cleavage of APP to Aβ. Due to the downregulation of calreticulin in neurons, serum γ-secretase losses its proper cleaving activity leading to misfolded Aβ and accumulation in neurons. Altered calreticulin levels could affect protein folding in GNEM as calreticulin interact with phosphodiisomerase (PDI) to serve chaperone function in ER. PDI interacts with peroxiredoxin IV, which is downregulated in GNE deficient cells (Chanana et al., 2017). Thus, calreticulin may need further investigation towards its role as molecular chaperones in GNEM.

Heat Shock Proteins (HSPs) present in the cytosol also help protein to achieve native structure and avoid aggregation (Franklin et al., 2005; Paul and Mahanta, 2014). Elevated levels of HSP70 and HSP27 were found in brain tissues of AD patients (Perez et al., 1991; Renkawek et al., 1993). HSP70 has been reported to interfere with the secretory pathway of APP by binding to APP and reducing Aβ production. Along with HSP70, HSP90 has been shown to degrade Aβ oligomers and tau via the proteasome degradation pathway (Lu et al., 2014). Overexpression of HSP70 and HSP90 helps to maintain tau homeostasis and increases its solubility, thereby preventing aggregation (Petrucelli et al., 2004). Overexpression of the chaperones also prevents the activation of Caspases, which may lead to neuronal death due to accumulation of aggregated proteins (Sabirzhanov et al., 2012). Proteomic study on GNEM patient biopsies also indicates an increase in HSP70, Crystallin and HSPB1 levels (Sela et al., 2011). Thus, more intensive research is demanded to explore chaperones as therapeutic drug targets for GNEM that can reduce protein aggregation and inhibit rimmed vacuole formation.

Autophagy in AD and GNEM

Autophagy is the major degradative pathway for recycling of various proteins and organelles inside the cell, as it is essential for maintaining a balance between protein synthesis and degradation (Yang et al., 2009). Autophagy has been reported to be elevated when cells sense any kind of stress (Kwang et al., 2008). In AD, number of autophagosomes increase indicative of impaired recycling of cellular constituents (Funderburk et al., 2010). Mutation in Presenilin-1 gene affects lysosome mediated autophagy, reduces p62 protein levels leading to imbalance in tau proteostasis (Chui et al., 1999; Lee et al., 2010b; Tung et al., 2014). Many genes common to autophagy and AD pathology have been identified such as autophagy-related 7 (ATG7), BCL2, Beclin 1 (BECN1/ATG6), cyclin dependent kinase 5 (CDK5), Cathepsin D (CTSD), microtubule associated protein tau (MAPT/TAU), Presenilin-1, α-Synuclein (SNCA/PARK1/NACP), Ubiquitin 1 etc., (Uddin et al., 2018). Aβ accumulated intracellularly also regulates autophagy (Son et al., 2012). Tau pro-aggregates act as targets for macrophagy and chaperone mediated autophagy (Zare-Shahabadi et al., 2015).

Rimmed vacuoles observed in GNEM pathology are also defined as clusters of autophagic vacuoles and multi-lamellar bodies, which contain congophilic amyloid proteins, ubiquitin and tau proteins (Nonaka et al., 2005). Higher expression of lysosomal-associated membrane proteins (LAMPs), LC3 and various other lysosomal proteins involved in autophagic pathway were observed in the skeletal muscle of the mice model for GNEM (Malicdan et al., 2007). Differential regulation of BCL2 in GNEM also supports that some common proteins of autophagy pathway in AD may play a role in GNEM autophagic vacuole formation. A comparison of the autophagic mechanisms in AD vs. GNEM is shown in **Figure 1**. Thus, it would be of interest to study and identify novel targets causing autophagy in GNEM and several autophagy stimulating drugs for AD may serve as therapeutic option for myopathy.

Cell Death and Apoptosis

Cell death is the most common feature of the neurodegenerative diseases and occurs massively. In AD, neuronal loss is mainly in cerebral cortex and limbic lobe (Alzheimer's Association, 2017). There are two major pathways for apoptosis, extrinsic pathway and intrinsic pathway. The extrinsic pathway involves

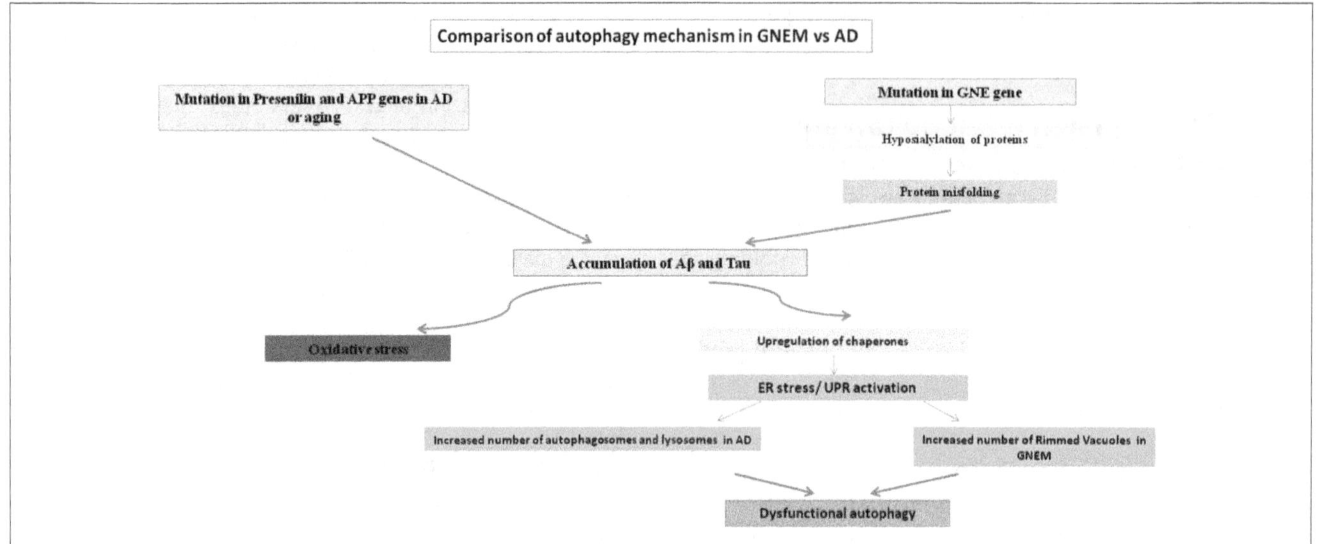

FIGURE 1 | Comparison of autophagy mechanism in AD and GNEM. Mutation in genes of Presenilin and APP for AD and GNE for GNEM leads to the accumulation of various proteins like Aβ and tau. This accumulation causes oxidative stress and ER stress/UPR activation due to upregulation of chaperones, ultimately leading to dysfunctional autophagy as the number of autophagosomes, lysosomes, and rimmed vacuoles increases.

cell surface receptors like TNF in which the binding of Aβ or Aβ oligomers to these receptors remains to be established but the pattern of activation of downstream Caspases (e.g., Caspases 2 and 8) involved in the extrinsic pathway is mediated by Aβ (Ghavami et al., 2014). In the intrinsic pathway, Aβ plays an important role as its intracellular accumulation in the ER cause ER stress and when it binding to a mitochondrial alcohol dehydrogenase leads to mitochondrial stress followed by activation of the downstream apoptotic markers (Lustbader et al., 2004). The upstream mediators of the apoptotic processes are yet to be determined, but the Caspases are activated in the process, which cleaves the tau protein leading to NFT formation (Dickson, 2004). Therefore, in AD, proteolysis of both APP and tau takes place leading to abnormal proteins, which aggregate and form lesions of fibrils extracellularly and intracellularly. Thus, direct involvement of Caspases in apoptosis of neurons is not yet established but many Caspases have been found to play a role in regulation of neuronal death upon Aβ accumulation (Behl, 2000; Dickson, 2004). Aβ(1-42) exposure leads to down regulation of anti-apoptotic proteins like Bcl-2 and upregulation of pro-apoptotic proteins like Bax, cytochrome-c and cleaved caspases in PC12 cells (Chen et al., 2018). Altered levels of various microRNAs that target neuropathological mechanisms have been reported in AD (Ma et al., 2017; Dehghani et al., 2018). Activation of programmed necrosis leading to cell death is reported in the brain of AD patients (Caccamo et al., 2017). The suppression of apoptotic cell signaling pathway proteins such as p38 MAPK can rescue tau pathology in AD (Maphis et al., 2016). These study suggest that various effector molecules targeting signaling proteins in the apoptotic pathway can play a role is preventing cell apoptosis caused due to Aβ accumulation or tau dysfunction and hence potential drug molecules for AD.

In GNEM, degeneration is seen in the myofibrils of the patient muscle biopsies, which might lead to rimmed vacuole formation (Yan et al., 2001). Similar to AD, activation of Caspases 3 and 9 was observed in the myoblast cells of the GNEM patient with M743T kinase mutation (Amsili et al., 2007). Along with this, increased pAKT levels was observed which suggests impairment in the apoptotic event (Amsili et al., 2007). Mitochondrial dependent apoptosis and disruption in both the structure and function of the mitochondria was observed in HEK cell based model system of GNEM over-expressing pathologically relevant GNE mutation (Singh and Arya, 2016). Also, activation of PTEN and PDK1 was observed in the myoblasts which might lead to muscle loss and on stimulation with insulin, activates PI3K and downstream signaling through AKT causing the activation of cell survival pathway (Harazi et al., 2014). Increased Anoikis, apoptosis due to loss of anchorage to extracellular matrix, was observed in pancreatic carcinoma cells when the GNE gene was silenced. Additionally, the level of CHOP has been reported to increase in GNE deficient cells indicative of apoptosis through ATF4-ATF3-CHOP pathway (Kemmner et al., 2012). Increased apoptosis due to internalization of Aβ peptides in hyposialylated C2C12 myotubes and skeletal muscles was observed in the patients of GNEM (Bosch-Morató et al., 2016). This suggests that sialylation has a role in Aβ uptake and cell apoptosis and molecules involved in apoptotic pathway can be therapeutic targets. Thus, molecular and cellular phenomenon for apoptosis in AD and GNEM seem to overlap despite difference in cell types, neuron vs. muscle cell, respectively.

A comparison of the apoptotic mechanisms in AD vs. GNEM has been described in **Figure 2**. Interestingly, treatment of GNE deficient cells with Insulin Growth Factor seems to rescue the apoptotic phenotype and hence could be a potential therapeutic target that counters apoptotic cell toward cell survival (Singh et al., 2018). In summary, proteins and drug molecules that rescue cell death phenomenon in AD by targeting common proteins, can be explored for GNEM therapy.

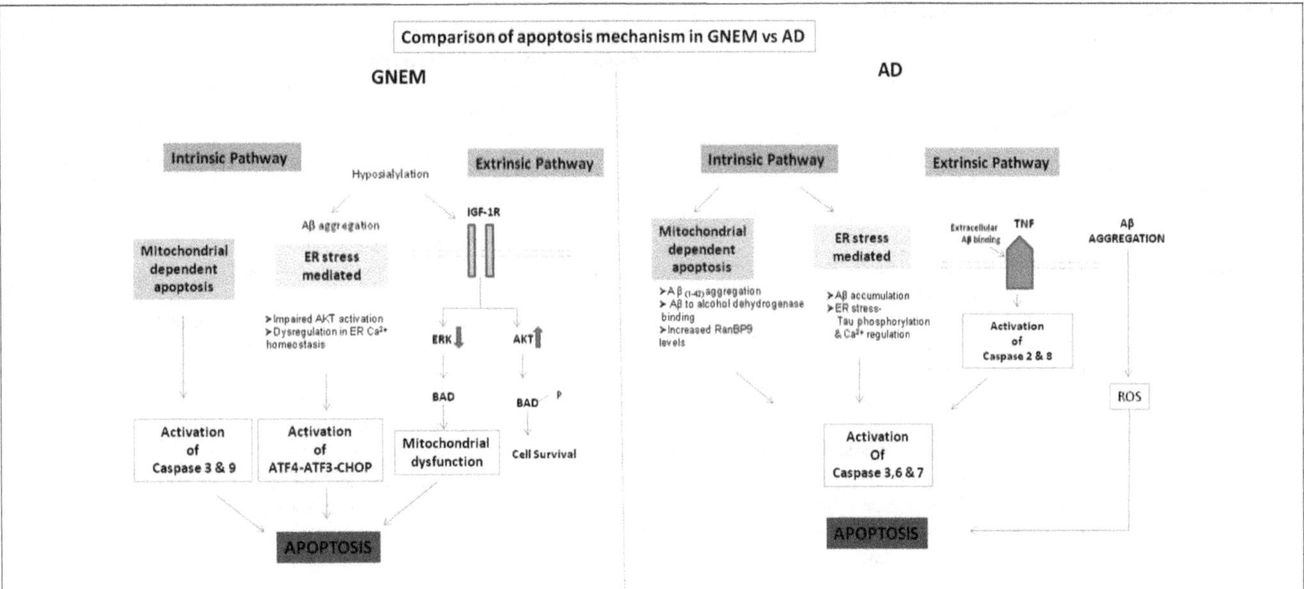

FIGURE 2 | Comparison of apoptosis mechanism in AD and GNEM. In GNEM, intrinsic pathway is mediated through mitochondria as a consequence of mitochondrial dysfunction and consequent release of cytochrome C and activation of executioner caspases-Caspase-3 and Caspase-9. Further, in the extrinsic pathway, mutation in GNE causes hyposialylation of Aβ leading to its aggregation progressing toward ER stress where AKT pathway is impaired and sarcoplasmic calcium is released into the cytoplasm, eventually leading to apoptosis. In the extrinsic pathway, hyposialylation of IGF1R receptor leads to impairment of ERK pathway and activation of BAD, inhibiting anti-apoptotic Bcl-2 and thus leading to apoptosis. Whereas in AD, in the intrinsic pathway, Aβ accumulation and tau phosphorylation in the ER leads to ER stress. In the mitochondria of AD patients, Aβ binds to Aβ binding-alcohol dehydrogenase (ABAD) leading to mitochondrial dysfunction. Both ER and mitochondrial stress lead to activation of effector caspases 3, 6, and 7, which might cleave tau leading to formation of NFTs. In the extrinsic pathway, accumulated Aβ binds to ligand TNF leading to activation of Caspase 2 and 8.

A complete comparison of molecular and cellular changes in AD and GNEM are listed in **Table 2**.

TREATMENT

There is no cure for AD till date as the medications available only help to control the symptoms of AD. The AD drug therapy includes drugs, which target neurotransmitter system of the brain such as Acetylcholinesterase (Ach esterase) inhibitors that increases neurotransmitter levels at synaptic junctions (Schenk et al., 2012). Three FDA approved acetylcholinesterase inhibitors are Rivastigmine, Galantamine (for mild AD), and Donepezil (for all stages of AD) are available (Schenk et al., 2012). Also Memantine, antagonist for *N*-methyl-D-aspartate (NMDA) receptor is used in combination with Ach esterase inhibitor. None of the pharmacological drugs are able to stop the damage and destruction of the neurons therefore, making the disease fatal.

Since, Aβ accumulation is one of the major causes leading to the disease; therefore drugs, which can lower the amount of Aβ accumulation in the brain are of prime importance. Secretase inhibitor drugs, inhibit the cleavage of APP into Aβ, therefore minimizing their accumulation (Imbimbo and Giardina, 2011). Another set of drugs used as a passive vaccination strategy in the form of antibodies, help in the clearance of Aβ species (Schenk et al., 2012). Several drugs were developed which completed Phase-III clinical trials but failed to demonstrate their efficacy in patients. The passive vaccination strategy in case of tau also proved to be ineffective (Wischik et al., 2014). A major limitation with respect to effectiveness of anti-amyloid drugs was thought to be late diagnosis of the disease. Thus, research focussing on the stage of initiation of amyloid formation could offer better drug targets. Indeed aducanumab, human monoclonal antibody, selective for aggregated form of Aβ showed reduced amyloid uptake and improved cognitive function in early AD patients (Scheltens et al., 2016).

In case of GNEM also, there is no treatment therapy available, which could reverse disease progression and stop muscle degeneration. Administration of *N*-acetylmannosamine, neuraminic acid, and sialyllactose in the mouse models of GNEM improved survival of the mouse by reduction in rimmed vacuole formation and β-amyloid deposition (Yonekawa et al., 2014). Gene therapy by administration of GNE gene lipoplex through intravenous infusion to the patients leads to an improvement in muscle strength and increased cell surface sialylation (Nemunaitis et al., 2010). An FDA approved molecular chaperone aiding in protein folding - 4-PBA (4-phenyl butyrate) has been proposed for GNEM (Krause, 2015). Anti-ActII activin antibody (bimagrumab or BYM338), an atrophic protein has been found to be helpful in preventing muscle atrophy in GNEM (Krause, 2015). Some of the compounds are under clinical trials such as sialic acid precursor, *N*-acetylmannosamine (ManNAc), and extended release sialic acid form, aceneuramic acid. However, due to lack of statistical significance in the cohort of patient study, the compound was discontinued by Ultragenyx (Mori-Yoshimura and Nishino, 2015; Argov et al., 2016).

TABLE 2 | Comparison of the molecular and cellular changes in AD and GNEM.

	Molecular and cellular changes in AD and GNEM	
	AD	**GNEM**
Glycosylation	• Impaired glucose metabolism • Glycosylation of proteins affected	• Glycosylation of NCAM, integrin, α-dystroglycan, IGF1R, neprilysin
Sialic acid involvement	Sialic acid dependent binding of Aβ to cells • Decrease Level sialyltransferases	Low Sialic acid production • Hyposialylation of glycoproteins.
Mitochondrial dysfunction	• Mitochondria number reduced • Aβ accumulation in mitochondria • Impaired TCA cycle • Mutation in mtDNA and cytochrome c oxidase • Impaired mitochondrial trafficking	• Vacuolar and swollen mitochondria • Increased branching of mitochondria • Upregulation of mitochondrial proteins like COX, Cytochrome C Oxidase, ATPases, NADH dehydrogenase
Oxidative stress	• Neurotoxicity and protein oxidation due to accumulated Aβ • Increased p-Tau • S-nitrosylation of different proteins like Cdk5, PDI, ApoE	• Upregulation of cell stress molecule • PrdxIV downregulated • Proteins found to be highly S-nitrosylated
ER stress	• XBP1 mRNA splicing leading to activation of IRE1α • GRP78/BiP, GRP94, calnexin and calreticulin upregulated • Co-localization of GRP78/BiP GRP94 and calreticulin with Aβ • Calreticulin binds with presenilin and neprisilin	• Upregulation of different UPR pathway proteins such as GRP78, GRP94, Calreticulin and Calnexin
Protein aggregation	• Aβ and p-tau proteins	• β-amyloid, phosphorylated Tau, TDP-43, α-synuclein
Chaperone involvement	• HSE (Heat Shock Element) associated with APP gene promoter • Elevated levels of HSP70 and HSP27 • HSP90 and HSP70 degrades Aβ oligomers and tau • Higher levels of HSP70 and HSP90 promotes the binding of tau to the microtubules	• Upregulation of various chaperones • The mutant protein preferentially retained in the ER
Apoptosis	• Activation of downstream caspases mediated by Aβ • Caspases cleaves the Tau protein • Nuclear chromatin clumping and apoptotic bodies	• Degeneration in myofibrils • Activation of Caspases 3 and 9 • Mitochondrial dependent apoptosis and disruption of mitochondria • Increased Anoikis • Increased levels of CHOP
Autophagy	• Failure of autophagy • Increased number of autophagosomes and lysosomes • Rab7 and LAMP proteins dysregulated	• Rimmed vacuoles-clusters of the autophagic vacuoles and multi-lamellar bodies • Higher expression of lysosomal-associated membrane proteins (LAMPs), LC3
Inflammation	**Occurs**	**Occurs rarely**
Cytoskeleton framework	• Aggregation of hyperphosphorylated tau • Inactivation of cofilin 1, SSH1 • Rac1 leads to APP accumulation • RhoA increases Aβ • Cofilin-actin rod results in synaptic loss	• GNE interact with Collapsin Response Mediator Protein-1 (CRMP-1), α-actinin-1 and α-actinin-2 • β-integrin mediated cell adhesion affected • Aβ induces FAK

Recent studies in GNEM indicate that sialic acid supplementation alone may not be sufficient to rescue disease phenotype. As discussed above several other cellular phenomena affect GNEM including accumulation of aggregated proteins such as β-amyloid and tau proteins. Sialic acid has been shown to affect β-amyloid uptake in C2C12 myoblast indicating role of sialic acid in β-amyloid uptake (Bosch-Morató et al., 2016). Thus, drug molecules affecting β-amyloid uptake and initiation of Aβ accumulation may serve as better therapeutic targets and offer common mechanism for AD as well as GNEM.

CONCLUSION

While much is known for AD, GNEM is poorly understood rare disease. Lack of number of patient samples for GNEM also limits the study. Also, absence of appropriate animal model system for GNEM, as $GNE^{-/-}$ mice are embryonically lethal at day E8.5, restricts the understanding for genotype to phenotype co-relation. There could be some interesting leads from AD studies that could help explore GNEM pathomechanism. While both diseases have lot of similarities at cellular level such as Aβ amyloid deposition, protein aggregation, autophagic vacuoles, major difference is that in AD, brain/neurons are affected while in GNEM, only muscles in particular anterior tibialis muscle cells are affected. No changes in the neurons of GNEM patients are reported. It would be of interest to study the stage of Aβ deposition in GNE deficient cells and whether protein aggregation could be prevented to slow the disease progression for GNEM. Also, whether there is any genetic predisposition of AD or GNEM in patient families would be important to understand epigenetics of these neurodegenerative disorders. Future studies could be planned toward deciphering common therapeutic targets for these disorders.

AUTHOR CONTRIBUTIONS

SD and RY have written the first draft of the manuscript. PC and RA revised and improved the first draft. RY prepared the tables and **Figure 2.** PC prepared **Figure 1.** RA edited and finalized the version. All authors have seen and agreed on the finally submitted version of the manuscript.

FUNDING

This work was supported by grants from the UPOE-II (Project ID:16), University Grants Commission, India, DST PURSE II (DST/SR/PURSE Phase II/11, Department of Science and Technology, Government of India and SERB (Science and Engineering Research Board) EMR/2015/001798, Government of India. We acknowledge Jawaharlal Nehru University, New Delhi for providing financial assistance towards publication and infrastructure.

ACKNOWLEDGMENTS

We thank Prof. M. A. Kamal, King Fahd Medical Research Center, King Abdulaziz University, Kingdom of Saudi Arabia for fruitful suggestions regarding conceptualizing the review. We also thank Dr. Kulvinder Singh Saini, Professor of Biotechnology, Department of Biology, King Abdulaziz University, Jeddah, Saudi Arabia for support and encouragement.

REFERENCES

Aisa, B., Gil-Bea, F. J., Solas, M., García-Alloza, M., Chen, C. P., Lai, M. K., et al. (2010). Altered NCAM expression associated with the cholinergic system in alzheimer's disease. *J. Alzheimers Dis.* 20, 659–668. doi: 10.3233/JAD-2010-1398

Alzheimer's Association (2017). Alzheimer's disease facts and figures. *Alzheimers Dement.* 13, 325–373. doi: 10.1016/j.jalz.2017.02.001

Amsili, S., Shlomai, Z., Levitzki, R., Krause, S., Lochmuller, H., Ben-Bassat, H., et al. (2007). Characterization of hereditary inclusion body myopathy myoblasts: possible primary impairment of apoptotic events. *Cell Death Differ.* 14, 1916–1924. doi: 10.1038/sj.cdd.4402208

Amsili, S., Zer, H., Hinderlich, S., Krause, S., Becker-Cohen, M., MacArthur, D. G., et al. (2008). UDP-N-acetylglucosamine-2-epimerase/N-acetylmannosamine kinase (GNE) binds to alpha-actinin 1: novel pathways in skeletal muscle? *PLoS One* 3:e2477. doi: 10.1371/journal.pone.0002477

Anada, R. P., Wong, K. T., Malicdan, M. C., Goh, K. J., Hayashi, Y., Nishino, I., et al. (2014). Absence of beta-amyloid deposition in the central nervous system of a transgenic mouse model of distal myopathy with rimmed vacuoles. *Amyloid* 21, 138–139. doi: 10.3109/13506129.2014.889675

Anderson, J. L., Head, S. I., Rae, C., and Morley, J. W. (2002). . Brain function in Duchenne muscular dystrophy. *Brain* 125(Pt 1), 4–13. doi: 10.1093/brain/awf012

Andreyev, A. Y., Kushnareva, Y. E., and Starkov, A. A. (2005). Mitochondrial metabolism of reactive oxygen species. *Biochemistry* 70, 200–214.

Ankarcrona, M., Mangialasche, F., and Winblad, B. (2010). Rethinking Alzheimer's disease therapy: Are mitochondria the key? *J. Alzheimers Dis.* 20, S579–S590. doi: 10.3233/JAD-2010-100327

Argov, Z., Caraco, Y., Lau, H., Pestronk, A., Shieh, P. B., Skrinar, A., et al. (2016). Aceneuramic acid extended release administration maintains upper limb muscle strength in a 48-week study of subjects with GNE myopathy: results from a phase 2, randomized, controlled study. *J. Neuromuscul. Dis.* 3, 49–66. doi: 10.3233/JND-159900

Argov, Z., and Yarom, R. (1984). "Rimmed vacuole myopathy" sparing the quadriceps. A unique disorder in iranian jews. *J. Neurol. Sci.* 64, 33–43. doi: 10.1016/0022-510X(84)90053-4

Ariga, T., Kobayashi, K., Hasegawa, A., Kiso, M., Ishida, H., and Miyatake, T. (2001). Characterization of high-affinity binding between gangliosides and amyloid beta-protein. *Arch Biochem. Biophys.* 388, 225–230. doi: 10.1006/abbi.2001.2304

Bamburg, J. R., Bernstein, B. W., Davis, R. C., Flynn, K. C., Goldsbury, C., Jensen, J. R., et al. (2010). ADF/Cofilin-actin rods in neurodegenerative diseases. *Curr. Alzheimers Res.* 7, 241–250. doi: 10.2174/156720510791050902

Barnes, D. E., and Yaffe, K. (2011). The projected effect of risk factor reduction on Alzheimer's disease prevalence. *Lancet Neurol.* 10, 819–828. doi: 10.1016/S1474-4422(11)70072-2

Barone, E., Mosser, S., and Fraering, P. C. (2014). Inactivation of brain Cofilin-1 by age, Alzheimer's disease and γ-secretase. *Biochim. Biophys. Acta* 1842(12 Pt A), 2500–2509. doi: 10.1016/j.bbadis.2014.10.004

Beach, T. G., Monsell, S. E., Phillips, L. E., and Kukull, W. (2012). Accuracy of the clinical diagnosis of Alzheimer disease at National Institute on Aging Alzheimer Disease Centers, 2005-2010. *J. Neuropathol. Exp. Neurol.* 71, 266–273. doi: 10.1097/NEN.0b013e31824b211b

Behl, C. (2000). Apoptosis and Alzheimer's disease. *J. Neural Transm.* 107, 1325–1344. doi: 10.1007/s007020070021

Bennmann, D., Weidemann, W., Thate, A., Kreuzmann, D., and Horstkorte, R. (2016). Aberrant O-GlcNAcylation disrupts GNE enzyme activity in GNE myopathy. *FEBS J.* 283, 2285–2294. doi: 10.1111/febs.13729

Bhattacharya, S., Khadilkar, S. V., Nalini, A., Ganapathy, A., Mannan, A. U., Majumder, P. P., et al. (2018). Mutation spectrum of GNE myopathy in the Indian sub-continent. *J Neuromuscul. Dis.* 5, 85–92. doi: 10.3233/JND-170270

Boo, J. H., Sohn, J. H., Kim, J. E., Song, H., and Mook-Jung, I. (2008). Rac1 changes the substrate specificity of gamma-secretase between amyloid precursor protein and Notch1. *Biochem. Biophys. Res. Commun.* 372, 913–917. doi: 10.1016/j.bbrc.2008.05.153

Bosch-Morató, M., Iriondo, C., Guivernau, B., Valls-Comamala, V., Vidal, N., Olivé, M., et al. (2016). Increased amyloid β-peptide uptake in skeletal muscle is induced by hyposialylation and may account for apoptosis in GNE myopathy. *Oncotarget* 7, 13354–13371. doi: 10.18632/oncotarget.7997

Broccolini, A., Gidaro, T., De Cristofaro, R., Morosetti, R., Gliubizzi, C., Ricci, E., et al. (2008). Hyposialylation of neprilysin possibly affects its expression and enzymatic activity in hereditary inclusion-body myopathy muscle. *J. Neurochem.* 105, 971–981. doi: 10.1111/j.1471-4159.2007.05208.x

Bubber, P., Haroutunian, V., Fisch, G., Blass, J. P., and Gibson, G. E. (2005). Mitochondrial abnormalities in Alzheimer brain: mechanistic implications. *Ann. Neurol.* 57, 695–703. doi: 10.1002/ana.20474

Caccamo, A., Branca, C., Piras, I. S., Ferreira, E., Huentelman, M. J., Liang, W. S., et al. (2017). Necroptosis activation in Alzheimer's disease. *Nat. Neurosci.* 20, 1236–1246. doi: 10.1038/nn.4608

Castellani, R., Hirai, K., Aliev, G., Drew, K. L., Nunomura, A., Takeda, A., et al. (2002). Role of mitochondrial dysfunction in Alzheimer's disease. *J. Neurosci. Res.* 70, 357–360. doi: 10.1002/jnr.10389

Cha, M. Y., Han, S. H., Son, S. M., Hong, H. S., Choi, Y. J., Byun, J., et al. (2012). Mitochondria-specific accumulation of amyloid β induces mitochondrial dysfunction leading to apoptotic cell death. *PLoS One* 7:e34929. doi: 10.1371/journal.pone.0034929

Chanana, P., Padhy, G., Bhargava, K., and Arya, R. (2017). Mutation in GNE downregulates peroxiredoxin IV altering ER redox homeostasis. *NeuroMolecular Med.* 19, 525–540. doi: 10.1007/s12017-017-8467-5

Chen, K., Lu, Y., Liu, C., Zhang, L., Fang, Z., and Yu, G. (2018). Morroniside prevents H2O2or Aβ1-42-induced apoptosis via attenuating JNK and p38 MAPK phosphorylation. *Eur. J. Pharmacol.* 834, 295–304. doi: 10.1016/j.ejphar.2018.07.047

Cho, A., Malicdan, M. C. V., Miyakawa, M., Nonaka, I., Nishino, I., and Noguchi, S. (2017). Sialic acid deficiency is associated with oxidative stress leading to muscle atrophy and weakness in the GNE myopathy. *Hum. Mol. Genet.* 274, 19792–19798. doi: 10.1093/hmg/ddx192

Chornenkyy, Y., Wang, W.-X., Wei, A., and Nelson, P. T. (2018). Alzheimer's disease and Type 2 Diabetes mellitus are distinct diseases with potential overlapping metabolic dysfunction upstream of observed cognitive decline. *Brain Pathol.* doi: 10.1111/bpa.12655 [Epub ahead of print].

Chui, D. H., Tanahashi, H., Ozawa, K., Ikeda, S., Checler, F., Ueda, O., et al. (1999). Transgenic mice with Alzheimer presenilin 1 mutations show accelerated neurodegeneration without amyloid plaque formation. *Nat. Med.* 5, 560–564. doi: 10.1038/8438

Chun, Y. S., Park, Y., Oh, H. G., Kim, T. W., Yang, H. O., Park, M. K., et al. (2015). O-GlcNAcylation promotes non-amyloidogenic processing of amyloid-β protein precursor via inhibition of endocytosis from the plasma membrane. *J. Alzheimers Dis.* 44, 261–275. doi: 10.3233/JAD-140096

DeHart, G. W., and Jones, J. C. R. (2004). Myosin-mediated cytoskeleton contraction and Rho GTPases regulate laminin-5 matrix assembly. *Cell Motil. Cytoskeleton* 57, 107–117. doi: 10.1002/cm.10161

Dehghani, R., Rahmani, F., and Rezaei, N. (2018). MicroRNA in Alzheimer's disease revisited: implications for major neuropathological mechanisms. *Rev. Neurosci.* 29, 161–182. doi: 10.1515/revneuro-2017-0042

Dickson, D. W. (2004). Apoptotic mechanisms in Alzheimer neurofibrillary degeneration: cause or effect? *J. Clin. Investigat.* 114, 23–27. doi: 10.1172/JCI22317

Eisenberg, I., Novershtern, N., Itzhaki, Z., Becker-Cohen, M., Sadeh, M., Willems, P. H., et al. (2008). Mitochondrial processes are impaired in hereditary inclusion body myopathy. *Hum. Mol. Genet.* 17, 3663–3674. doi: 10.1093/hmg/ddn261

Feng, Y., and Wang, X. (2012). Antioxidant therapies for Alzheimer's disease. *Oxid. Med. Cell. Longev.* 2012:472932. doi: 10.1155/2012/472932

Fischer, C., Kleinschnitz, K., Wrede, A., Muth, I., Kruse, N., Nishino, I., et al. (2013). Cell stress molecules in the skeletal muscle of GNE myopathy. *BMC Neurol.* 13:24. doi: 10.1186/1471-2377-13-24

Franklin, T. B., Krueger-Naug, A. M., Clarke, D. B., Arrigo, A. P., and Currie, R. W. (2005). The role of heat shock proteins Hsp70 and Hsp27 in cellular protection of the central nervous system. *Int. J. Hyperthermia* 21, 379–392. doi: 10.1080/02656730500069955

Fukui, H., Diaz, F., Garcia, S., and Moraes, C. T. (2007). Cytochrome c oxidase deficiency in neurons decreases both oxidative stress and amyloid formation in a mouse model of Alzheimer's disease. *Proc. Natl. Acad. Sci. U.S.A.* 104, 14163–14168. doi: 10.1073/pnas.0705738104

Funderburk, S. F., Marcellino, B. K., and Yue, Z. (2010). Cell "self-eating" (autophagy) mechanism in Alzheimer's disease. *Mt. Sinai J. Med.* 77, 59–68. doi: 10.1002/msj.20161

Garden, G. A., and La Spada, A. R. (2012). Intercellular (Mis)communication in neurodegenerative disease. *Neuron* 73, 886–901. doi: 10.1016/j.neuron.2012.02.017

Ghavami, S., Shojaei, S., Yeganeh, B., Ande, S. R., Jangamreddy, J. R., Mehrpour, M., et al. (2014). Autophagy and apoptosis dysfunction in neurodegenerative disorders. *Prog. Neurobiol.* 112, 24–49. doi: 10.1016/j.pneurobio.2013.10.004

Goate, A., Chartier-Harlin, M. C., Mullan, M., Brown, J., Crawford, F., Fidani, L., et al. (1991). Segregation of a missense mutation in the amyloid precursor protein gene with familial Alzheimer's disease. *Nature* 349, 704–706. doi: 10.1038/349704a0

Gong, C. X., Liu, F., Grundke-Iqbal, I., and Iqbal, K. (2005). Post-translational modifications of tau protein in Alzheimer's disease. *J. Neural Transm.* 112, 813–838. doi: 10.1007/s00702-004-0221-0

Grover, S., and Arya, R. (2014). Role of UDP-N-acetylglucosamine2-epimerase/N-acetylmannosamine kinase (GNE) in ??1-integrin-mediated cell adhesion. *Mol. Neurobiol.* 50, 257–273. doi: 10.1007/s12035-013-8604-6

Han, H. Y., Zhang, J. P., Ji, S. Q., Liang, Q. M., Kang, H. C., Tang, R. H., et al. (2013). αv and β1 integrins mediate Aβ-induced neurotoxicity in hippocampal neurons via the FAK signaling pathway. *PLoS One* 8:e64839. doi: 10.1371/journal.pone.0064839

Hanger, D. P., Byers, H. L., Wray, S., Leung, K. Y., Saxton, M. J., Seereeram, A., et al. (2007). Novel phosphorylation sites in Tau from Alzheimer brain support a role for casein kinase 1 in disease pathogenesis. *J. Biol. Chem.* 282, 23645–23654. doi: 10.1074/jbc.M703269200

Harazi, A., Becker-Cohen, M., Zer, H., Moshel, O., Hinderlich, S., and Mitrani-Rosenbaum, S. (2017). The interaction of UDP-N-acetylglucosamine 2-Epimerase/N-Acetylmannosamine Kinase (GNE) and Alpha-actinin 2 is altered in GNE Myopathy M743T mutant. *Mol. Neurobiol.* 54, 2928–2938. doi: 10.1007/s12035-016-9862-x

Harazi, A., Chaouat, M., Shlomai, Z., Levitzki, R., Becker-Cohen, M., Sadeh, M., et al. (2014). Survival-apoptosis associated signaling in GNE myopathy-cultured myoblasts. *J. Recept Signal Transduct. Res.* 35, 249–257. doi: 10.3109/10799893.2014.956755

Holtzman, D. M., Morris, J. C., and Goate, A. M. (2011)). Alzheimer's disease: the challenge of the second century. *Sci. Transl. Med.* 3:77sr1. doi: 10.1126/scitranslmed.3002369

Hoozemans, J. J. M., Veerhuis, R., Van Haastert, E. S., Rozemuller, J. M., Baas, F., Eikelenboom, P., et al. (2005). The unfolded protein response is activated in Alzheimer's disease. *Acta Neuropathol.* 110, 165–172. doi: 10.1007/s00401-005-1038-0

Huizing, M., and Krasnewich, D. M. (2009). Hereditary inclusion body myopathy: a decade of progress. *Biochim. Biophys. Acta* 1792, 881–887. doi: 10.1016/j.bbadis.2009.07.001

Huizing, M., Rakocevic, G., Sparks, S. E., Mamali, I., Shatunov, A., Goldfarb, L., et al. (2004). Hypoglycosylation of α-dystroglycan in patients with hereditary IBM due to GNE mutations. *Mol. Genet. Metab.* 81, 196–202. doi: 10.1016/j.ymgme.2003.11.012

Hutton, M., and Hardy, J. (1997). The presenilins and Alzheimer's disease. *Hum. Mol. Genet.* 6, 1639–1646. doi: 10.1093/hmg/6.10.1639

Imbimbo, B. P., and Giardina, G. A. (2011). γ-Secretase Inhibitors and Modulators for the treatment of Alzheimer's disease: disappointments and hopes. *Curr. Top. Med. Chem.* 11, 1555–1570. doi: 10.2174/156802611795860942

Iqbal, K., Alonso, A. D. C., and Grundke-Iqbal, I. (2008). Cytosolic abnormally hyperphosphorylated tau but not paired helical filaments sequester normal MAPs and inhibit microtubule assembly. *J. Alzheimers Dis.* 14, 365–370. doi: 10.3233/JAD-2008-14402

Jay, C. M., Levonyak, N., Nemunaitis, G., Maples, P. B., and Nemunaitis, J. (2009). Hereditary inclusion body myopathy (HIBM2). *Gene Regul. Syst. Biol.* 3, 181–190. doi: 10.4137/GRSB.S2594

Jiang, T., Yu, J. T., Hu, N., Tan, M. S., Zhu, X. C., and Tan, L. (2014). CD33 in Alzheimer's disease. *Mol. Neurobiol.* 49, 529–535. doi: 10.1007/s12035-013-8536-1

Johnson, R. J., Xiao, G., Shanmugaratnam, J., and Fine, R. E. (2001). Calreticulin functions as a molecular chaperone for the beta-amyloid precursor protein. *Neurobiol. Aging* 22, 387–395. doi: 10.1016/S0197-4580(00)00247-5

Kanekura, K., Suzuki, H., Aiso, S., and Matsuoka, M. (2009). ER stress and unfolded protein response in amyotrophic lateral sclerosis. *Mol. Neurobiol.* 39, 81–89. doi: 10.1007/s12035-009-8054-3

Kemmner, W., Kessel, P., Sanchez-Ruderisch, H., Moller, H., Hinderlich, S., Schlag, P. M., et al. (2012). Loss of UDP-N-acetylglucosamine 2-epimerase/N-acetylmannosamine kinase (GNE) induces apoptotic processes in pancreatic carcinoma cells. *FASEB J.* 26, 938–946. doi: 10.1096/fj.11-186700

Kizuka, Y., Kitazume, S., and Taniguchi, N. (2017). N-glycan and Alzheimer's disease. *Biochim. Biophys. Acta* 1861, 2447–2454. doi: 10.1016/j.bbagen.2017.04.012

Koistinen, H., Prinjha, R., Soden, P., Harper, A., Banner, S. J., Pradat, P.-F., et al. (2006). Elevated levels of amyloid precursor protein in muscle of patients with amyotrophic lateral sclerosis and a mouse model of the disease. *Muscle Nerve* 34, 444–450. doi: 10.1002/mus.20612

Köroğlu, Ç, Yılmaz, R., Sorgun, M. H., Solakoğlu, S., and Şener, Ö (2017). GNE missense mutation in recessive familial amyotrophic lateral sclerosis. *Neurogenetics* 18, 237–243. doi: 10.1007/s10048-017-0527-3

Krause, S. (2015). Insights into muscle degeneration from heritable inclusion body myopathies. *Front. Aging Neurosci.* 7:13. doi: 10.3389/fnagi.2015.00013

Kwang, W. K., Hwang, M., Moretti, L., Jaboin, J. J., Cha, Y. I., and Lu, B. (2008). Autophagy upregulation by inhibitors of caspase-3 and mTOR enhances radiotherapy in a mouse model of lung cancer. *Autophagy* 4, 659–668. doi: 10.4161/auto.6058

Lackner, L. L. (2013). Determining the shape and cellular distribution of mitochondria: The integration of multiple activities. *Curr. Opin. Cell Biol.* 25, 471–476. doi: 10.1016/j.ceb.2013.02.011

Lee, J. H., Won, S. M., Suh, J., Son, S. J., Moon, G. J., Park, U. J., et al. (2010a). Induction of the unfolded protein response and cell death pathway in Alzheimer's disease, but not in aged Tg2576 mice. *Exp. Mol. Med.* 42, 386–394. doi: 10.3858/emm.2010.42.5.040

Lee, J. H., Yu, W. H., Kumar, A., Lee, S., Mohan, P. S., Peterhoff, C. M., et al. (2010b). Lysosomal proteolysis and autophagy require presenilin 1 and are disrupted by Alzheimer-related PS1 mutations. *Cell* 141, 1146–1158. doi: 10. 1016/j.cell.2010.05.008

Letenneur, L., Launer, L. J., Andersen, K., Dewey, M. E., Ott, A., Copeland, J. R. M., et al. (2000). Education and the risk for Alzheimer's disease: sex makes a difference. EURODEM pooled analyses. *Am. J. Epidemiol.* 151, 1064–1071. doi: 10.1093/oxfordjournals.aje.a010149

Li, H., Chen, Q., Liu, F., Zhang, X., Li, W., Liu, S., et al. (2013). Unfolded Protein Response and activated degradative pathways regulation in GNE myopathy. *PLoS One* 8:e58116. doi: 10.1371/journal.pone.0058116

Lin, Q., Cao, Y., and Gao, J. (2014). Serum calreticulin is a negative biomarker in patients with Alzheimer's disease. *Int. J. Mol. Sci.* 15, 21740–21753. doi: 10.3390/ijms151221740

López-Otín, C., Blasco, M. A., Partridge, L., Serrano, M., and Kroemer, G. (2013). The hallmarks of aging. *Cell* 153, 1194–1217. doi: 10.1016/j.cell.2013.05.039

Lovell, M. A., Xiong, S., Xie, C., Davies, P., and Markesbery, W. R. (2004). Induction of hyperphosphorylated tau in primary rat cortical neuron cultures mediated by oxidative stress and glycogen synthase kinase-3. *J. Alzheimers Dis.* 6, 659–671. doi: 10.3233/JAD-2004-6610

Lu, R.-C., Tan, M.-S., Wang, H., Xie, A.-M., Yu, J.-T., and Tan, L. (2014). Heat shock protein 70 in Alzheimer's disease. *Biomed. Res. Int.* 2014, 1–8. doi: 10. 1155/2014/435203

Lustbader, J. W., Cirilli, M., Lin, C., Xu, H. W., Takuma, K., Wang, N., et al. (2004). ABAD directly links Abeta to mitochondrial toxicity in Alzheimer's disease. *Science.* 304, 448–452. doi: 10.1126/science.1091230

Ma, X., Liu, L., and Meng, J. (2017). MicroRNA-125b promotes neurons cell apoptosis and Tau phosphorylation in Alzheimer's disease. *Neurosci. Lett.* 661, 57–62. doi: 10.1016/j.neulet.2017.09.043

Maguire, T. M., and Breen, K. C. (1995). A decrease in neural sialyltransferase activity in Alzheimer's disease. *Dement Geriatr. Cogn. Disord.* 6, 185–190. doi: 10.1159/000106944

Maguire, T. M., Gillian, A. M., O'Mahony, D., Coughlan, C. M., and Breen, K. C. (1994). A decrease in serum sialyltransferase levels in Alzheimer's disease. *Neurobiol. Aging* 15, 99–102. doi: 10.1016/0197-4580(94)90149-X

Majd, S., and Power, J. H. (2018). Oxidative stress and decreased mitochondrial superoxide dismutase 2 and Peroxiredoxin 1 and 4 based mechanism of concurrent activation of AMPK and mTOR in Alzheimer's disease. *Curr. Alzheimer Res.* 15, 764–776. doi: 10.2174/1567205015666180223093020

Malicdan, M. C. V., Noguchi, S., Nonaka, I., Hayashi, Y. K., and Nishino, I. (2007). A Gne knockout mouse expressing human GNE D176V mutation develops features similar to distal myopathy with rimmed vacuoles or hereditary inclusion body myopathy. *Hum. Mol. Genet.* 16, 2669–2682. doi: 10.1093/hmg/ddm220

Maphis, N., Jiang, S., Xu, G., Kokiko-Cochran, O. N., Roy, S. M., Van Eldik, L. J., et al. (2016). Selective suppression of the α isoform of p38 MAPK rescues late-stage tau pathology. *Alzheimers Res. Ther.* 8:54. doi: 10.1186/s13195-016-0221-y

Mokhtar, S. H., Kim, M. J., Magee, K. A., Aui, P. M., Thomas, S., Bakhuraysah, M. M., et al. (2018). Amyloid-beta-dependent phosphorylation of collapsin response mediator protein-2 dissociates kinesin in Alzheimer's disease. *Neural Regen. Res.* 13, 1066–1080. doi: 10.4103/1673-5374.233451

Moniruzzaman, M., Ishihara, S., Nobuhara, M., Higashide, H., and Funamoto, S. (2018). Glycosylation status of nicastrin influences catalytic activity and substrate preference of γ-secretase. *Biochem. Biophys. Res. Commun.* 502, 98–103. doi: 10.1016/j.bbrc.2018.05.126

Montie, H. L., and Durcan, T. M. (2013). The cell and molecular biology of neurodegenerative diseases: an overview. *Front. Neurol.* 4:194. doi: 10.3389/fneur.2013.00194

Mori-Yoshimura, M., and Nishino, I. (2015). Sialic acid replacement therapy for distal myopathy with rimmed vacuoles. *Brain Nerve* 67, 1115–1123.

Mosconi, L. (2005). Brain glucose metabolism in the early and specific diagnosis of Alzheimer's disease: FDG-PET studies in MCI and AD. *Eur. J. Nucl. Med. Mol. Imaging* 32, 486–510. doi: 10.1007/s00259-005-1762-7

Murray, H. C., Low, V. F., Swanson, M. E. V., Dieriks, B. V., Turner, C., Faull, R. L. M., et al. (2016). Distribution of PSA-NCAM in normal, Alzheimer's and Parkinson's disease human brain. *Neuroscience* 330, 359–375. doi: 10.1016/j.neuroscience.2016.06.003

Nakagawa, K., Kitazume, S., Oka, R., Maruyama, K., Saido, T. C., Sato, Y., et al. (2006). Sialylation enhances the secretion of neurotoxic amyloid-β peptides. *J. Neurochem.* 96, 924–933. doi: 10.1111/j.1471-4159.2005.03595.x

Nalini, A., Gayathri, N., and Dawn, R. (2010). Distal myopathy with rimmed vacuoles: report on clinical characteristics in 23 cases. *Neurol. India* 58, 235–241. doi: 10.4103/0028-3886.63804

Nalini, A., Nishino, I., Gayathri, N., and Hayashi, Y. (2013). GNE myopathy in India. *Neurol. India* 61:371. doi: 10.4103/0028-3886.117609

Narici, M. V., and Maffulli, N. (2010). Sarcopenia: characteristics, mechanisms and functional significance. *Br. Med. Bull.* 95, 139–159. doi: 10.1093/bmb/ldq008

Nemunaitis, G., Maples, P. B., Jay, C., Gahl, W. A., Huizing, M., Poling, J., et al. (2010). Hereditary inclusion body myopathy: single patient response to GNE gene Lipoplex therapy. *J. Gene. Med.* 12, 403–412. doi: 10.1002/jgm.1450

Nogalska, A., D'Agostino, C., Engel, W. K., Cacciottolo, M., Asada, S., Mori, K., et al. (2015). Activation of the unfolded protein response in sporadic inclusion-body myositis but not in hereditary GNE inclusion-body myopathy. *J. Neuropathol. Exp. Neurol.* 74, 538–546. doi: 10.1097/NEN.0000000000000196

Noguchi, S., Keira, Y., Murayama, K., Ogawa, M., Fujita, M., Kawahara, G., et al. (2004). Reduction of UDP-N-acetylglucosamine 2-Epimerase/N-Acetylmannosamine kinase activity and sialylation in distal Myopathy with rimmed vacuoles. *J. Biol. Chem.* 279, 11402–11407. doi: 10.1074/jbc.M313171200

Nonaka, I., Noguchi, S., and Nishino, I. (2005). Distal myopathy with rimmed vacuoles and hereditary inclusion body myopathy. *Curr. Neurol. Neurosci. Rep.* 5, 61–65. doi: 10.1007/s11910-005-0025-0

Norfray, J. F., and Provenzale, J. M. (2004). Alzheimer's disease: neuropathologic findings and recent advances in imaging. *Am. J. Roentgenol.* 182, 3–13. doi: 10.2214/ajr.182.1.1820003

Ott, A., Stolk, R. P., van Harskamp, F., Pols, H. A., Hofman, A., and Breteler, M. M. (1999). Diabetes mellitus and the risk of dementia: the rotterdam study. *Neurology* 53, 1937–1942. doi: 10.1212/WNL.53.9.1937

Paul, S., and Mahanta, S. (2014). Association of heat-shock proteins in various neurodegenerative disorders: Is it a master key to open the therapeutic door? *Mol. Cell. Biochem.* 386, 45–61. doi: 10.1007/s11010-013-1844-y

Peila, R., Rodriguez, B. L., and Launer, L. J. (2002). Type 2 diabetes, APOE gene, and the risk for dementia and related pathologies. *Diabetes* 51, 1256–1262. doi: 10.2337/diabetes.51.4.1256

Penzes, P., and Rafalovich, I. (2012). Regulation of the actin cytoskeleton in dendritic spines. *Adv. Exp. Med. Biol.* 970, 81–95. doi: 10.1007/978-3-7091-0932-8_4

Perez, N., Sugar, J., Charya, S., Johnson, G., Merril, C., Bierer, L., et al. (1991). Increased synthesis and accumulation of heat shock 70 proteins in Alzheimer's disease. *Mol. Brain Res.* 11, 249–254. doi: 10.1016/0169-328X(91)90033-T

Petrucelli, L., Dickson, D., Kehoe, K., Taylor, J., Snyder, H., Grover, A., et al. (2004). CHIP and Hsp70 regulate tau ubiquitination, degradation and aggregation. *Hum. Mol. Genet.* 13, 703–714. doi: 10.1093/hmg/ddh083

Querfurth, H. W., and LaFerla, F. M. (2010). Alzheimer's disease. *N. Engl. J. Med.* 362, 329–344. doi: 10.1056/NEJMra0909142

Reilly, C. E. (2001). Neprilysin content is reduced in Alzheimer brain areas. *J. Neurol.* 248, 159–160. doi: 10.1007/s004150170259

Reiman, E. M., Chen, K., Alexander, G. E., Caselli, R. J., Bandy, D., Osborne, D., et al. (2005). Correlations between apolipoprotein E epsilon4 gene dose and brain-imaging measurements of regional hypometabolism. *Proc. Natl. Acad. Sci. U.S.A.* 102, 8299–8302. doi: 10.1073/pnas.0500579102

Renkawek, K., Bosman, G. J., and Gaestel, M. (1993). Increased expression of heat-shock protein 27 kDa in Alzheimer disease: a preliminary study. *Neuroreport* 5, 14–16. doi: 10.1097/00001756-199310000-00003

Ricci, E., Broccolini, A., Gidaro, T., Morosetti, R., Gliubizzi, C., Frusciante, R., et al. (2006). NCAM is hyposialylated in hereditary inclusion body myopathy due to GNE mutations. *Neurology* 66, 755–758. doi: 10.1212/01.wnl.0000200956.76449.3f

Ricotti, V., Roberts, R. G., and Muntoni, F. (2011). Dystrophin and the brain. *Dev. Med. Child Neurol.* 53, 12–12. doi: 10.1111/j.1469-8749.2010.03836.x

Roussel, B. D., Kruppa, A. J., Miranda, E., Crowther, D. C., Lomas, D. A., and Marciniak, S. J. (2013). Endoplasmic reticulum dysfunction in neurological disease. *Lancet Neurol.* 12, 105–118. doi: 10.1016/S1474-4422(12)70238-7

Rui, Y., Tiwari, P., Xie, Z., and Zheng, J. Q. (2006). Acute impairment of mitochondrial trafficking by beta-amyloid peptides in hippocampal neurons. *J. Neurosci.* 26, 10480–10487. doi: 10.1523/JNEUROSCI.3231-06.2006

Rust, M. B. (2015). ADF/cofilin: a crucial regulator of synapse physiology and behavior. *Cell. Mol. Life Sci.* 72, 3521–3529. doi: 10.1007/s00018-015-1941-z

Sabirzhanov, B., Stoica, B. A., Hanscom, M., Piao, C. S., and Faden, A. I. (2012). Over-expression of HSP70 attenuates caspase-dependent and caspase-independent pathways and inhibits neuronal apoptosis. *J. Neurochem.* 123, 542–554. doi: 10.1111/j.1471-4159.2012.07927.x

Salama, M., Shalash, A., Magdy, A., Makar, M., Roushdy, T., Elbalkimy, M., et al. (2018). Tubulin and tau: possible targets for diagnosis of Parkinson's and Alzheimer's diseases. *PLoS One* 13:e0196436. doi: 10.1371/journal.pone.0196436

Schedin-Weiss, S., Winblad, B., and Tjernberg, L. O. (2014). The role of protein glycosylation in Alzheimer disease. *FEBS J.* 281, 46–62. doi: 10.1111/febs.12590

Scheltens, P., Blennow, K., Breteler, M. M. B., de Strooper, B., Frisoni, G. B., Salloway, S., et al. (2016). Alzheimer's disease. *Lancet* 388, 505–517. doi: 10.1016/S0140-6736(15)01124-1

Schenk, D., Basi, G. S., and Pangalos, M. N. (2012). Treatment strategies targeting amyloid β-protein. *Cold Spring Harb. Perspect. Med.* 2:a006387. doi: 10.1101/cshperspect.a006387

Schnaar, R. L., Gerardy-Schahn, R., and Hildebrandt, H. (2014). Sialic acids in the brain: gangliosides and polysialic acid in nervous system development, stability, disease, and regeneration. *Physiol. Rev.* 94, 461–518. doi: 10.1152/physrev.00033.2013

Sela, I., Krentsis, I. M., Shlomai, Z., Sadeh, M., Dabby, R., Argov, Z., et al. (2011). The proteomic profile of hereditary inclusion body myopathy. *PLoS One* 6:e16334. doi: 10.1371/journal.pone.0016334

Serrano-Pozo, A., Frosch, M. P., Masliah, E., and Hyman, B. T. (2011). Neuropathological alterations in Alzheimer disease. *Cold Spring Harb. Perspect. Med.* 1:a006189. doi: 10.1101/cshperspect.a006189

Sibille, E. (2013). Molecular aging of the brain, neuroplasticity, and vulnerability to depression and other brain-related disorders. *Dialogues Clin. Neurosci.* 15, 53–65.

Siddiqui, S. S., Springer, S. A., Verhagen, A., Sundaramurthy, V., Alisson-Silva, F., Jiang, W., et al. (2017). The Alzheimer's Disease-protective CD33 splice variant mediates adaptive loss of function via diversion to an intracellular pool. *J. Biol. Chem.* 292, 15312–15320. doi: 10.1074/jbc.M117.799346

Singh, R., and Arya, R. (2016). GNE Myopathy and cell apoptosis: a comparative mutation analysis. *Mol. Neurobiol.* 53, 3088–3101. doi: 10.1007/s12035-015-9191-5

Singh, R., Chaudhary, P., and Arya, R. (2018). Role of IGF-1R in ameliorating apoptosis of GNE deficient cells. *Sci. Rep.* 8:7323. doi: 10.1038/s41598-018-25510-9

Siparsky, P. N., Kirkendall, D. T., and Garrett, W. E. (2014). Muscle changes in aging: understanding sarcopenia. *Sports Health* 6, 36–40. doi: 10.1177/1941738113502296

Smith, M. H., Ploegh, H. L., and Weissman, J. S. (2011). Road to ruin: targeting proteins for degradation in the endoplasmic reticulum. *Science* 334, 1086–1090. doi: 10.1126/science.1209235

Son, S. M., Jung, E. S., Shin, H. J., Byun, J., and Mook-Jung, I. (2012). Aβ-induced formation of autophagosomes is mediated by RAGE-CaMKKβ-AMPK signaling. *Neurobiol. Aging* 33:1006.e11-23. doi: 10.1016/j.neurobiolaging.2011.09.039

Souchay, C., and Moulin, C. (2009). Memory and consciousness in Alzheimers disease. *Curr. Alzheimer Res.* 6, 186–195. doi: 10.2174/156720509788486545

Spiro, R. G. (2002). Protein glycosylation: nature, distribution, enzymatic formation, and disease implications of glycopeptide bonds. *Glycobiology* 12, 43R–56R. doi: 10.1093/glycob/12.4.43R

Stemmer, N., Strekalova, E., Djogo, N., Plöger, F., Loers, G., Lutz, D., et al. (2013). Generation of amyloid-β is reduced by the interaction of calreticulin with amyloid precursor protein, presenilin and Nicastrin. *PLoS One* 8:e61299. doi: 10.1371/journal.pone.0061299

Stone, S., and Lin, W. (2015). The unfolded protein response in multiple sclerosis. *Front. Neurosci.* 9:264. doi: 10.3389/fnins.2015.00264

Supnet, C., and Bezprozvanny, I. (2010). Neuronal calcium signaling, mitochondrial dysfunction, and Alzheimer's disease. *J. Alzheimers Dis.* 20(Suppl. 2), S487–S498. doi: 10.3233/JAD-2010-100306

Swerdlow, R. H. (2018). Mitochondria and mitochondrial cascades in Alzheimer's disease. *J. Alzheimers Dis.* 62, 1403–1416. doi: 10.3233/JAD-170585

Tabas, I., and Ron, D. (2011). Integrating the mechanisms of apoptosis induced by endoplasmic reticulum stress. *Nat. Cell Biol.* 13, 184–190. doi: 10.1038/ncb0311-184

Taylor, J. P., Brown, R. H., and Cleveland, D. W. (2016). Decoding ALS: from genes to mechanism. *Nature* 539, 197–206. doi: 10.1038/nature20413

Thibault, O., Hadley, R., and Landfield, P. W. (2001). Elevated postsynaptic [Ca2 +]i and L-type calcium channel activity in aged hippocampal neurons: relationship to impaired synaptic plasticity. *J. Neurosci.* 21, 9744–9756. doi: 10.1523/JNEUROSCI.21-24-09744.2001

Thibault, O., Porter, N. M., Chen, K. C., Blalock, E. M., Kaminker, P. G., Clodfelter, G. V., et al. (1998). Calcium dysregulation in neuronal aging and Alzheimer's disease: History and new directions. *Cell Calcium* 24, 417–433. doi: 10.1016/S0143-4160(98)90064-1

Tung, Y. T., Wang, B. J., Hsu, W. M., Hu, M. K., Her, G. M., Huang, W. P., et al. (2014). Presenilin-1 regulates the expression of p62 to govern p62-dependent tau degradation. *Mol. Neurobiol.* 49, 10–27. doi: 10.1007/s12035-013-8482-y

Uddin, M. S., Stachowiak, A., Al Mamun, A., Tzvetkov, N. T., Takeda, S., Atanasov, A. G., et al. (2018). Autophagy and Alzheimer's disease: from molecular mechanisms to therapeutic implications. *Front. Aging Neurosci.* 10:04. doi: 10.3389/fnagi.2018.00004

Wang, B. (2009). Sialic Aacid is an essential nutrient for brain development and cognition. *Annu. Rev. Nutr.* 29, 177–222. doi: 10.1146/annurev.nutr.28.061807.155515

Wang, P.-L., Niidome, T., Akaike, A., Kihara, T., and Sugimoto, H. (2009). Rac1 inhibition negatively regulates transcriptional activity of the amyloid precursor protein gene. *J. Neurosci. Res.* 87, 2105–2114. doi: 10.1002/jnr.22039

Wang, X., and Michaelis, E. K. (2010). Selective neuronal vulnerability to oxidative stress in the brain. *Front. Aging Neurosci.* 2:12. doi: 10.3389/fnagi.2010.00012

Wang, Z., Sun, Z., Li, A. V., and Yarema, K. J. (2006). Roles for UDP-GlcNAc 2-epimerase/ManNAc 6-kinase outside of sialic acid biosynthesis: modulation of sialyltransferase and BiP expression, GM3 and GD3 biosynthesis, proliferation, and apoptosis, and ERK1/2 phosphorylation. *J. Biol. Chem.* 281, 27016–27028. doi: 10.1074/jbc.M604903200

Weidemann, W., Stelzl, U., Lisewski, U., Bork, K., Wanker, E. E., Hinderlich, S., et al. (2006). The collapsin response mediator protein 1 (CRMP-1) and the promyelocytic leukemia zinc finger protein (PLZF) bind to UDP-N-acetylglucosamine 2-epimerase/N-acetylmannosamine kinase (GNE), the key enzyme of sialic acid biosynthesis. *FEBS Lett.* 580, 6649–6654. doi: 10.1016/j.febslet.2006.11.015

Wischik, C. M., Harrington, C. R., and Storey, J. M. D. (2014). Tau-aggregation inhibitor therapy for Alzheimer's disease. *Biochem. Pharmacol.* 88, 529–539. doi: 10.1016/j.bcp.2013.12.008

Wiseman, F. K., Al-Janabi, T., Hardy, J., Karmiloff-Smith, A., Nizetic, D., Tybulewicz, V. L. J., et al. (2015). A genetic cause of Alzheimer disease: Mechanistic insights from Down syndrome. *Nat. Rev. Neurosci.* 16, 564–574. doi: 10.1038/nrn3983

Woodling, N. S., Colas, D., Wang, Q., Minhas, P., Panchal, M., Liang, X., et al. (2016). Cyclooxygenase inhibition targets neurons to prevent early behavioural decline in Alzheimer's disease model mice. *Brain* 139(Pt 7), 2063–2081. doi: 10.1093/brain/aww117

Xiang, C., Wang, Y., Zhang, H., and Han, F. (2017). The role of endoplasmic reticulum stress in neurodegenerative disease. *Apoptosis* 22, 1–26. doi: 10.1007/s10495-016-1296-4

Xie, T., Yan, C., Zhou, R., Zhao, Y., Sun, L., Yang, G., et al. (2014). Crystal structure of the γ-secretase component nicastrin. *Proc. Natl. Acad. Sci. U.S.A.* 111, 13349–13354. doi: 10.1073/pnas.1414837111

Yan, C., Ikezoe, K., and Nonaka, I. (2001). Apoptotic muscle fiber degeneration in distal myopathy with rimmed vacuoles. *Acta Neuropathol.* 101, 9–16.

Yang, D.-S., Lee, J.-H., and Nixon, R. A. (2009). Monitoring autophagy in Alzheimer's disease and related neurodegenerative diseases. *Methods Enzymol.* 453, 111–144. doi: 10.1016/S0076-6879(08)04006-8

Yang, D. S., Tandon, A., Chen, F., Yu, G., Yu, H., Arawaka, S., et al. (2002). Mature glycosylation and trafficking of nicastrin modulate its binding to presenilins. *J. Biol. Chem.* 277, 28135–28142. doi: 10.1074/jbc.M110871200

Yatin, S. M., Varadarajan, S., Link, C. D., and Butterfield, D. A. (1999). In vitro and in vivo oxidative stress associated with Alzheimer's amyloid beta-peptide (1-42). *Neurobiol. Aging* 20, 325–330.

Yonekawa, T., Malicdan, M. C. V., Cho, A., Hayashi, Y. K., Nonaka, I., Mine, T., et al. (2014). Sialyllactose ameliorates myopathic phenotypes in symptomatic GNE myopathy model mice. *Brain* 137, 2670–2679. doi: 10.1093/brain/awu210

Zare-Shahabadi, A., Masliah, E., Johnson, G. V. W., and Rezaei, N. (2015). Autophagy in Alzheimer's disease. *Rev. Neurosci.* 26, 385–395. doi: 10.1515/revneuro-2014-0076

Zhang, W., Huang, Y., and Gunst, S. J. (2012). The small GTPase RhoA regulates the contraction of smooth muscle tissues by catalyzing the assembly of cytoskeletal signaling complexes at membrane adhesion sites. *J. Biol. Chem.* 287, 33996–34008. doi: 10.1074/jbc.M112.369603

Zhang, Y., Thompson, R., Zhang, H., and Xu, H. (2011). APP processing in Alzheimer's disease. *Mol. Brain* 4:3. doi: 10.1186/1756-6606-4-3

Zhao, Q. F., Yu, J. T., and Tan, L. (2014). S-Nitrosylation in Alzheimer's disease. *Mol. Neurobiol.* 51, 268–280. doi: 10.1007/s12035-014-8672-2

6

Sex Differences in the Cognitive and Hippocampal Effects of Streptozotocin in an Animal Model of Sporadic AD

Jian Bao[1], Yacoubou A. R. Mahaman[1], Rong Liu[1], Jian-Zhi Wang[1,2], Zhiguo Zhang[3], Bin Zhang[4] and Xiaochuan Wang[1,2]*

[1] Key Laboratory of Ministry of Education of China for Neurological Disorders, Department of Pathophysiology, School of Basic Medicine and the Collaborative Innovation Center for Brain Science, Tongji Medical College, Huazhong University of Science and Technology, Wuhan, China, [2] Co-innovation Center of Neuroregeneration, Nantong University, Nantong, China, [3] School of Medicine and Health Management, Tongji Medical College, Huazhong University of Science and Technology, Wuhan, China, [4] Department of Genetics and Genomic Sciences, Icahn School of Medicine at Mount Sinai, New York, NY, United States

***Correspondence:**
Xiaochuan Wang
wxch@mails.tjmu.edu.cn

More than 95% of Alzheimer's disease (AD) belongs to sporadic AD (sAD), and related animal models are the important research tools for investigating the pathogenesis and developing new drugs for sAD. An intracerebroventricular infusion of streptozotocin (ICV-STZ) is commonly employed to generate sporadic AD animal model. Moreover, the potential impact of sex on brain function is now emphasized in the field of AD. However, whether sex differences exist in AD animal models remains unknown. Here we reported that ICV-STZ remarkably resulted in learning and memory impairment in the Sprague-Dawley male rats, but not in the female rats. We also found tau hyperphosphorylation, an increase of Aβ40/42 as well as increase in both GSK-3β and BACE1 activities, while a loss of dendritic and synaptic plasticity was observed in the male STZ rats. However, STZ did not induce above alterations in the female rats. Furthermore, estradiol levels of serum and hippocampus of female rats were much higher than that of male rats. In conclusion, sex differences exist in this sporadic AD animal model (Sprague-Dawley rats induced by STZ), and this should be considered in future AD research.

Keywords: Alzheimer's disease (AD), animal model, Streptozotocin (STZ), sex differences, learning and memory

INTRODUCTION

Alzheimer's disease (AD) is one of the most common neurodegenerative diseases, affecting about 35 million people all over the world. And its prevalence is expected to reach 115 million by 2050 due to aggravating trend of aging population, unless there are available treatments that can prevent or cure this disease (Mangialasche et al., 2010). Therefore, an appropriate animal model is an important research tool for finding valid AD treatments. Yet, over the last 20 years, many of the potential drugs that target tau and Aβ, the two hallmarks of AD, failed in clinical trials, though some of treatments were effective in AD animal models (Zahs and Ashe, 2010; Shineman et al., 2011; Hall and Roberson, 2012). Thus, it is crucial to re-evaluate the existing animal models of AD.

AD exists mainly in two forms: familial (fAD) and sporadic (sAD). More than 95% of cases belong to sAD, for which aging and metabolic disorders are the main non-genetic risk factors

(Kloppenborg et al., 2008). Intracerebroventricular streptozotocin (ICV-STZ) injection produces cognitive deficits in rats, as well as cholinergic dysfunction, tau hyperphosphorylation, insulin receptor dysfunction, impaired energy metabolism, and oxidative stress (Hong and Lee, 1997; Prickaerts et al., 1999; Salkovic-Petrisic and Hoyer, 2007; Deng et al., 2009). These changes are similar to those observed in the brain of patients with sporadic AD. Therefore, ICV-STZ treated rats have been proposed as a research model of sAD (Lannert and Hoyer, 1998; Mehla et al., 2013). Meanwhile, ICV-STZ animal model has been used to evaluate the therapeutic potential of numerous old and novel drugs and compounds, as well as other non-drug therapies (Jee et al., 2008; Rodrigues et al., 2010; Salkovic-Petrisic et al., 2013). Nevertheless, although effectiveness of the therapeutic strategies has been proved in ICV-STZ model, the therapies failed to achieve similar therapeutic effects on learning and memory deficits in sAD clinical trials, like those with NSAIDs and PPAR agonists or vitamin E and Ginkgo biloba (Woo, 2000; Salkovic-Petrisic et al., 2013; Dysken et al., 2014; Malkki, 2016; Prasad, 2017; Wightman, 2017). Thus, it is necessary to characterize and re-evaluate the ICV-STZ animal model.

Accumulating evidence indicates that there are some differences in structure, development, enzyme activity, and chemistry of the central nervous system (CNS) between female and male mammals (Becker et al., 2005; Cahill, 2006; McCarthy, 2009; Raznahan et al., 2010; Ruigrok et al., 2014; Forger et al., 2016). AD is one of major chronic neurodegenerative disorders that is histopathologically characterized by the intracellular neurofibrillary tangles (NFTs) that are composed of abnormally hyperphosphorylated tau and extracellular senile plaques that are accumulated of insoluble β-amyloid (Aβ), which result in a progressive cognitive impairment (Grundke-Iqbal et al., 1986; Alafuzoff et al., 1987). Although, it has been reported that ICV-STZ induces AD-like pathological changes, however, whether ICV STZ-induced sporadic AD in animal model is stable and universal in different sexes has not been reported. Here, we found that ICV-STZ remarkably induced AD-like pathological changes, including impaired learning and memory capacities; loss of dendritic and synaptic plasticity; tau hyperphosphorylation; increase in Aβ40/42 and increase in both GSK-3β and BACE1 activities in the male but not female STZ treated rats. Our study implies that sex difference should be taken into account during experiments design, results interpretation and drawing conclusions in AD research.

MATERIALS AND METHODS

Chemicals and Antibodies

STZ was from Sigma (Sigma, St. Louis, MO, USA). Antibodies employed in this study are listed in Supplementary Table 1.

Animal Experiments

Two-month-old male ($n = 24$) and female ($n = 24$) Sprague-Dawley (SD) rats were provided by the Experiment Animal Center of Tongji Medical College, Huazhong University of Science and Technology. All animal experiments were performed according to the "Policies on the Use of Animals and Humans in Neuroscience Research" approved by Society for Neuroscience in 1995 and approved by the Experiment Animal Center of Tongji Medical College, Huazhong University of Science and Technology. The animals were individually housed in cages (house temperature 24°C, controlled humidity 40% and 12/12 h inverted light cycle) with free access to water and food.

STZ, soluble in artificial cerebrospinal fluid (aCSF), was injected slowly (1 μl/min) into the ventriculus lateralis cerebri of rats (10 μl, 3 mg/kg). Control animals were identically treated with the same volume of aCSF. After 30 days, morris water maze was employed to train and test spatial learning and memory. After this procedure which lasted for 7 days, mice were sacrificed and other tests were proceeded (**Supplementary Figure 1**).

Morris Water Maze Assay

The water maze used was a circular, steel pool (1.6 m in diameter) that was filled with black water (temperature 25°C) that was non-toxic and contrast to rat. A black-colored, circular platform (12 cm in diameter) was placed below the water surface at a specific location. Distinctive visual cues were stuck to the wall. For spatial training, rats were subjected to 4 trials each day from 2:00 to 5:00 p.m. The training was lasted 6 days and 24 trials were given to every rat. For each trial, the rat was placed at different starting position spaced equally around the perimeter of the pool. Rats were allowed to find the submerged platform within 60 s. If the rat could not find the hidden platform, it was then gently guided to the platform and allowed to stay there for 30 s. The time that each rat took to reach the platform was recorded as the escape latency. For the probe trial test, rats were submitted to the same pool with the platform removed and a probe trial of 60 s was given. The number of crossings and the time in the target quadrant were recorded.

Western Blotting

The protocol was performed as previously described (Xu et al., 2014). Four left hippocampus per group for Western blotting. Hippocampi were rapidly dissected out and homogenized in a buffer containing NaF 50 mM, Tris-Cl (pH 7.6) 10 mM, 1 mM EDTA, 1 mM Na_3VO_4, 1 mM benzamidine, and 1 mM phenylmethylsulfonylfluoride (PMSF), 10 g/ml leupeptin, and 2 g/ml each of pepstatin A and aprotinin. The homogenates were added to one-third of sample buffer containing 200 mM Tris-HCl (pH 7.6), 8% sodium dodecyl sulfate, and 40% glycerol, boiled in a water bath for 10 min, and then centrifuged at 14,510 r for 10 min. Protein concentration of the supernatants were measured by the bicinchoninic acid Protein Assay Kit (Pierce, Rockford, IL, USA). Ten micrograms of protein for DMIA and pS396 antibodies, 20 μg protein for other antibodies, were loaded and separated by SDS-polyacrylamide gel electrophoresis (10% gel), and then transferred to a nitrocellulose membrane. After blocking in 3% non-fat milk for 1 h, the nitrocellulose membranes were incubated with primary antibodies at 4°C overnight. The membranes were then incubated with secondary antibodies conjugated to IRDye (800CW) for 1–2 h and visualized using the Odyssey Infrared Imaging System (LI-Cor Biosciences, Lincoln, NE, USA). Image J software was employed for the quantitative analysis of the western blots.

Golgi Staining

The Golgi staining protocol was performed as previously described (Morest, 1960). Three per group were used for Golgi Staining. The rats were anesthetized with 6% chloral hydrate and perfused with 300 ml of normal saline containing 0.5% sodium nitrite, followed by 400 ml of 4% formaldehyde solution and further by ~400 ml dying solution (4% formaldehyde, 5% potassium dichromate, and 5% chloral hydrate) for 5 h in the dark. The brains were removed and incubated in the same fixative in the dark. After 3 days, the brains were transferred to a solution containing 1% silver nitrate for 3 days in the dark. The silver solution was changed each day. Thirty-five micrometers of thick coronal brain sections were cut using a vibrating microtome (Leica, VT1000S, Germany).

Immunofluorescence

Three per group were used for Immunofluorescence Staining. The anesthetized rats were immediately perfused through the aorta with 300 ml normal saline, followed by a 300 ml solution containing 4% paraformaldehyde. The brains were dissected and post-fixed in 4% paraformaldehyde for another 48 h. Coronal sections (30 μm thick) were cut using a vibrating microtome. After incubation in 0.3% Triton-X100-PBS for 30 min at room temperature, free floating sections were blocked with 5% goat serum in PBS for 45 min at room temperature. Sections were then incubated overnight at 4°C with primary antibodies: polyclonal anti-MAP2 antibodies obtained from Abcam, (dilution 1:200, Cambridge, MA, USA). This was followed by incubation with secondary antibodies for 2 h at room temperature. The antibody staining was semi-quantitated by mean fluorescence intensities (MFIs) with Image J software.

BACE1 Enzymatic Assay

The protocol was performed as previously described (Qi et al., 2016). Five right hippocampus per group for the assay. Beta-secretase activity was monitored using a commercial kit, from Abnova (Neihu District, Taipei City 114 Taiwan) according to the manufacturer instructions and using a multi-well fluorescence plate reader capable of Ex = 335–355 nm and Em = 495–510 nm. In briefly, 50 μl of 4 μg/μl hippocampus lysate was added to a 96-well plate. Fifty microliters of 2× reaction buffer were added, followed by 2 μl of β-secretase substrate. The reaction mixtures were incubating for 1 h in the dark. Fluorescence was monitored at excitation wave (wavelength = 334–355 nm) and emission wave (emission wavelength = 490–510 nm). β-secretase activity can be expressed as the Relative Fluorescence Units (RFU) per μg of protein sample.

ELISA Quantification of Aβ

The protocol was performed as previously described (Zhang et al., 2015). Five right hippocampus per group for the Elisa assay. To detect the concentration of Aβ in hippocampi lysates, the rat hippocampi were homogenized in buffer (PBS with 5% BSA and 0.03% Tween-20, supplemented with protease inhibitor cocktail), and centrifuged at 16,000 g for 20 min. Aβ1-40 or Aβ1-42 was quantified using the rats Aβ1-40 or Aβ1-42 ELISA Kit (Elabscience, Wuhan, China) in accordance with the manufacturer's instructions. The Aβ concentrations were determined by comparison with the standard curve.

ELISA Quantification of Estradiol

Three right hippocampus per group for the assay. To measure the levels of estradiol in hippocampi lysates and serum, the rat hippocampi were homogenized in 1× PBS and blood is obtained from the orbital vessels, then centrifuged at 1,500 r for 20 min. Estradiol was quantified using the rat estradiol ELISA Kit (CZVV, Nanjing, China). The results were expressed in ng/L.

Statistical Analysis

Data are descriptively presented as means ± *SD* and analyzed by SPSS 17.0. Statistical analysis was performed using either Student's *t*-test (two-group comparison) for behavior test, dendritic plasticity, Western blot, enzymatic activity. For the levels of estradiol in serum and hippocampus, we firstly performed a descriptive analysis in Supplementary Tables 2, 3, and then a Shapiro–wilk test for a normal distribution of the samples from four group, finally a general linear model to be used for two-way ANOVA followed by *post-hoc* comparison, and differences with $P < 0.05$ were considered significant.

RESULTS

Sex Influences Spatial Learning and Memory Deficits in Sporadic AD Animal Model Induced by ICV-STZ

A study showed that a significant cognitive impairment was evoked at the 2nd week onwards, which persisted up to the 14th week with ICV-STZ (3 mg/kg) in rats (Mehla et al., 2013). To investigate whether sex differences exist in cognitive deficits induced by STZ, in the present study, we performed morris water maze to evaluate the memory and learning abilities of rats 30 days after ICV-STZ treatment. For male rats, we found that the escape latency to find a hidden platform dramatically increased while the traversing times and the time in the target quadrant were significantly decreased at the 7th day in ICV-STZ rats when compared to vehicle control (**Figures 1A–C**). This confirmed that ICV-STZ induced learning and memory deficits in male rats. For female rats, to our surprise, we failed to observe any learning and/or memory deficits. The latency to find the hidden platform, the crossing numbers and time spent in the target quadrant also did not change in female rats (**Figures 1E–G**). Both groups in male or female rats exhibited comparable swimming speed (**Figures 1D,H**), indicating that motor function was not affected. Altogether, the findings suggest that ICV-STZ injection induces cognitive impairments in male but not female rats.

Sex Influences Loss of Dendritic and Synaptic Plasticity in the Sporadic AD Animal Model Induced by ICV-STZ

Dendrite complexity (Li et al., 2008) and synaptic plasticity (Kasai et al., 2010) are neurobiological basis for learning and memory. We determined the effect of ICV-STZ on neuronal integrity, by examining levels of the dendritic marker MAP2. For male

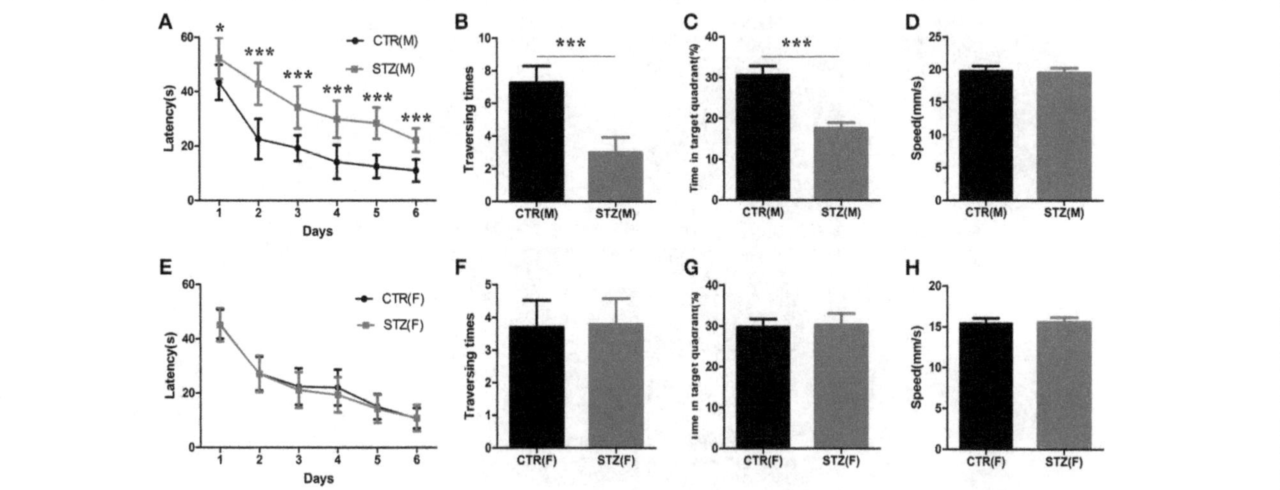

FIGURE 1 | Sex influences spatial learning and memory deficits in sporadic AD animal model induced by ICV-STZ. **(A,E)** Escape latencies to find the hidden platform for male or female rats. **(B,F)** The time spent in the target quadrant and **(C,G)** the crossed times after removing the platform. **(D,H)** The speed of male or female rats. Males are top figures **(A–D)**, females bottom figures **(E–H)**. The data were expressed as mean ± *SD* ($n = 12$). ***$P < 0.001$ vs. the vehicle control. Data were analyzed using *t*-test. *$P < 0.05$ vs. the vehicle control.

rats, the semi quantitative results showed a strongly reduced mean fluorescence intensities (MFIs) of MAP2 immunoreactivity in the pyramidal neurons of CA1 region of the hippocampus in ICV-STZ rats compared to vehicle control (**Figures 2A,B**). However, in female rats, MAP2 immunoreactivity showed that ICV-STZ had no effect on dendritic number compared to control (**Figures 2A,C**). We also examined alterations in dendritic spines using Golgi staining. Mushroom-type spines in the CA1 of ICV-STZ treated male rats decreased remarkably compared to control (**Figures 2D,E**), but the number of mushroom-type dendritic spines were not altered in the ICV-STZ treated female rats compared to control (**Figures 2D,F**).

Normal synaptic function is contingent upon the stable expression of synaptic proteins. Therefore, we evaluated several key synapse-associated proteins using Western blotting. ICV-STZ treatment remarkably suppressed the expressions of presynaptic synapsin I, synaptagmin and postsynaptic PSD95, PSD93, NR2A, and NR2B in male rats (**Figures 3A,B**). Nonetheless, there is no any significant difference between vehicle and ICV-STZ treated female rats (**Figures 3C,D**). These data demonstrate that ICV-STZ induces loss of dendritic and synaptic plasticity in male, but not in female rats.

Sex Influences Tau Hyperphosphorylation and GSK-3β Activity in the Sporadic AD Animal Model Induced by ICV-STZ

Abnormal hyperphosphorylation and accumulation of Tau play a key role in AD pathology (Wang and Liu, 2008), and hyperphosphorylated tau causes dendritic loss and neurodegeneration (Wang et al., 2010). In addition, ICV-STZ treatment induces tau hyperphosphorylation in rats (Zhou et al., 2013). In this study, we also explored whether ICV-STZ induces tau hyperphosphorylation in male or female rats, respectively. We detected a significantly increasing tau phosphorylation at the Ser199/202(AT8), Ser262, Ser396, and Ser404 sites in ICV-STZ treated male rats (**Figures 4A,B**). Conversely, in the female rats, ICV-STZ did not induce tau hyperphosphorylation (**Figures 4C,D**).

GSK-3β is the first identified and critical tau kinase (Singh et al., 1995), therefore we evaluated the total level and the activity-dependent phosphorylation of GSK-3β. In male rats, we found that the p-GSK-3β (Ser9) (the inactive form) level was remarkably decreased, while the level of total GSK-3β and p-GSK-3β (Tyr216) (the active form) didn't change (**Figures 5A,B**). In female rats, no significant difference was observed between ICV-STZ treated and vehicle control (**Figures 5C,D**). Taken together, these findings suggest that ICV-STZ activates GSK-3β and consequently leads to hyperphosphorylation of tau protein in male rats, but does not elicit these demonstrable pathological alterations in female rats.

Sex Influences the Activity of BACE1 and Aβ Production in the Sporadic AD Animal Model Induced by ICV-STZ

Another characterized histology of AD is extracellular senile plaques, which are composed of aggregated protein Aβ initiated by β-secretase (BACE1) (Alafuzoff et al., 1987; Vassar et al., 2009). We employed β-secretase Activity Assay Kit and Aβ40/42 Elisa Kit to detect BACE1 activity and Aβ levels of hippocampus. In ICV-STZ treated male rats, both BACE1 activity and Aβ40 level were significantly increased compared to control rats, while Aβ42 showed ascendant trend without significant difference (**Figures 6A,C,D**). However, in female rats, BACE1 activity and Aβ40/42 levels were not altered in both ICV-STZ and vehicle treated rats (**Figures 6B,E,F**). Thus, these data strongly support that ICV-STZ increases BACE1 activity and augments Aβ

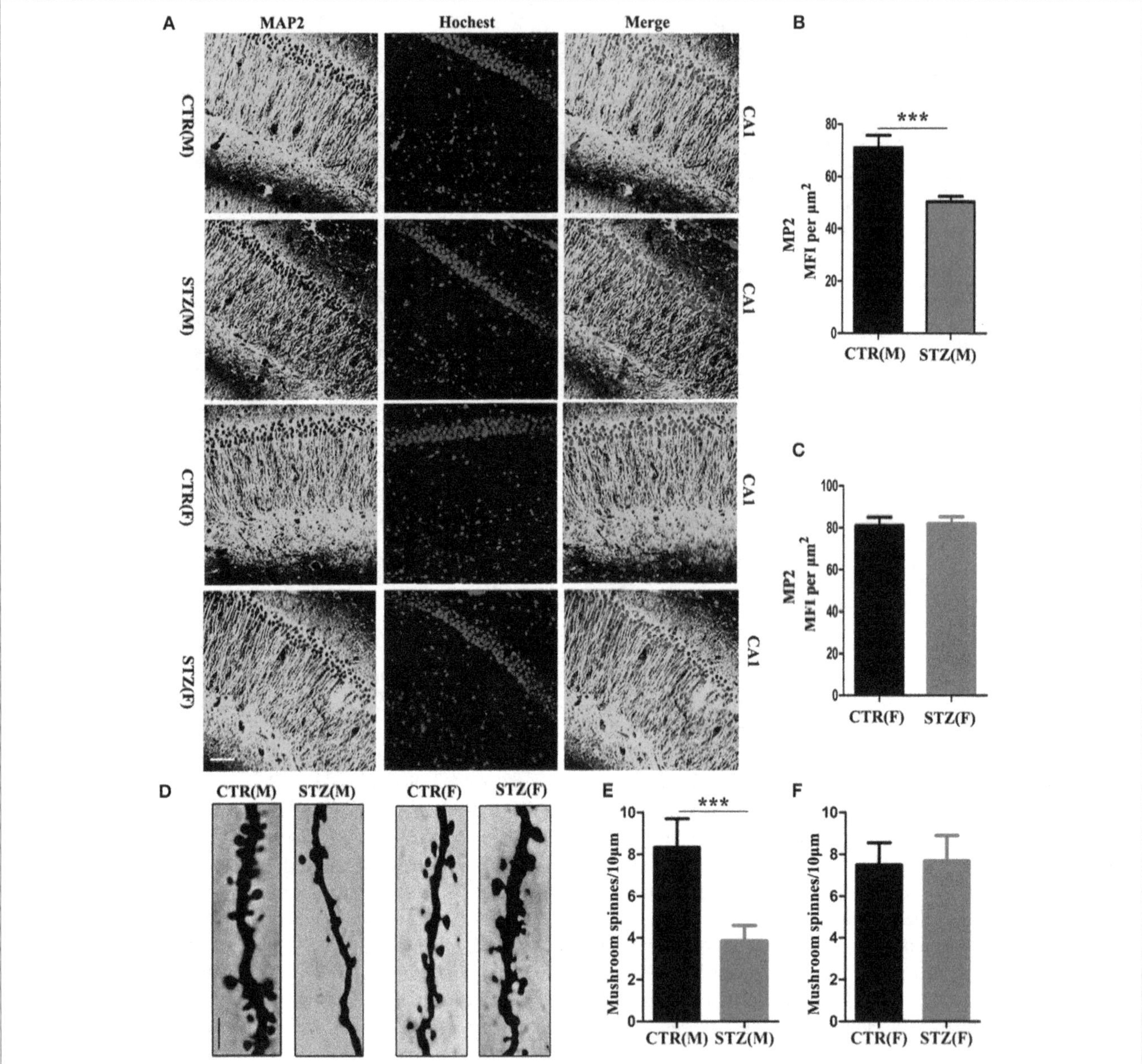

FIGURE 2 | Sex influences loss of dendritic plasticity in sporadic AD animal model. **(A)** MAP2 and DAPI co-staining in the hippocampal CA1 region for male or female rats. Scale bar = 100 μm. **(B,C)** Quantification of MAP2 immunofluorescence. The data were expressed as mean ± *SD* ($n = 3$). **(D)** Representative photomicrographs of dendritic spines in the hippocampal CA1 region. Scale bar = 5 μm. **(E,F)** Quantification of mushroom-type dendritic spines. The data were expressed as mean ± *SD* ($n = 3$). $^{***}P < 0.001$ vs. the vehicle control. Data were analyzed using *t*-test.

production in male rats, while did not exhibit these toxic effects in female rats.

Estradiol Levels in Serum and Hippocampus of ICV-STZ Treated Male and Female Rats

Previous studies have shown that estradiol reduces Aβ production via reducing total BACE1 activity, and decreases tau hyperphosphorylation by mediated GSK-3β activity (Singh et al., 1999; Zhang et al., 2008). To investigate whether estradiol influences the generation of the sporadic AD animal model induced by ICV-STZ, we measured estradiol levels in serum and hippocampus of ICV-STZ treated male and female rats. Shapiro–wilk test showed that all of the *p*-values were > 0.05, indicating estradiol levels in serum (Supplementary Table 4) and hippocampus (Supplementary Table 5) according with normal distribution from each group. And then, a general linear model was used for two-way ANOVA (Supplementary Tables 6, 7) followed by *post-hoc* comparison. We found that estradiol

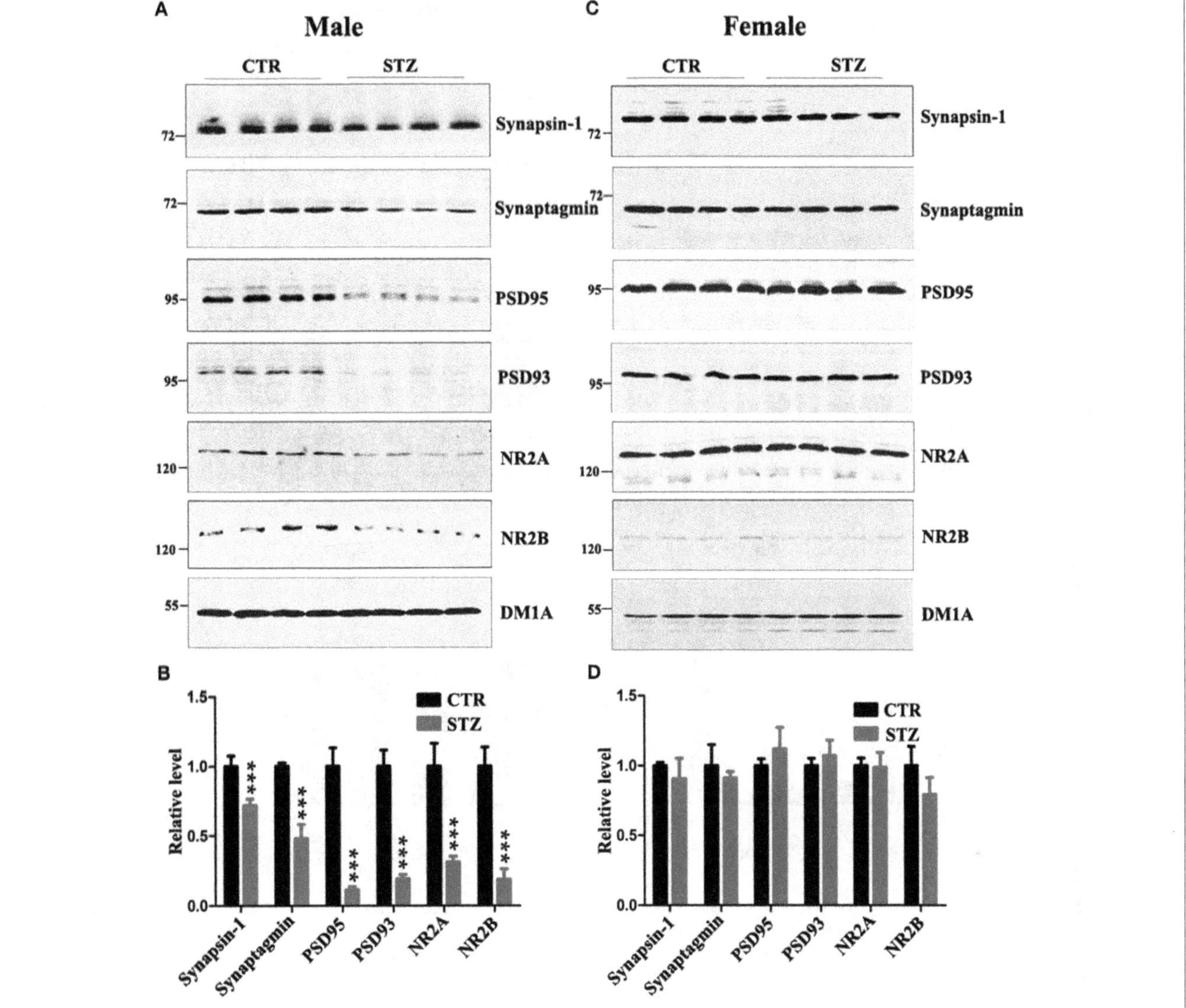

FIGURE 3 | Sex influences synaptic plasticity in the sporadic AD animal model. **(A,C)** Western blot analysis of the protein levels of synapsin-1, synaptagmin, psd95, psd93, NR2A, and NR2B and **(B,D)** their quantitative analysis for male or female rats. DM1A was used as a loading control. The data were expressed as mean ± *SD* ($n = 4$). $^{***}P < 0.001$ vs. the vehicle control. Data were analyzed using *t*-test.

levels of serum (**Figure 7A**) and hippocampus (**Figure 7B**) of female rats were much higher than that of male rats, while no difference was observed between the groups with same sex. The data suggest that high estradiol might protect from STZ induced neurotoxic effects in female rats.

DISCUSSION

Nowadays, AD is a major public health problem, which has been considered as a multifactorial disease associated with several etiopathogenic mechanisms (Iqbal and Grundke-Iqbal, 2010). The first step for a rational drug design is to study etiopathogenic mechanisms and to develop animal models based on these mechanisms. The late-onset sporadic form of AD, which mechanisms still remain unclear due to its multi-etiopathological factors, accounts for over 95% of all cases. However, few experimental animal model of sporadic AD badly limit the studies on its pathogenesis and drug development (Agrawal et al., 2011; Iqbal et al., 2013).

The majority of current animal models of AD are generated as familial one, which express human genes mutations, such as Aβ and tau related gene manipulation. However, animal model of familial AD cannot sufficiently exhibit all pathological alterations and processes (Chen et al., 2013). Therefore, experimental models that faithfully mimic the pathology of sAD are essential to study its mechanism and assess the effectiveness of the therapeutic strategies. Previous research has showed that sAD

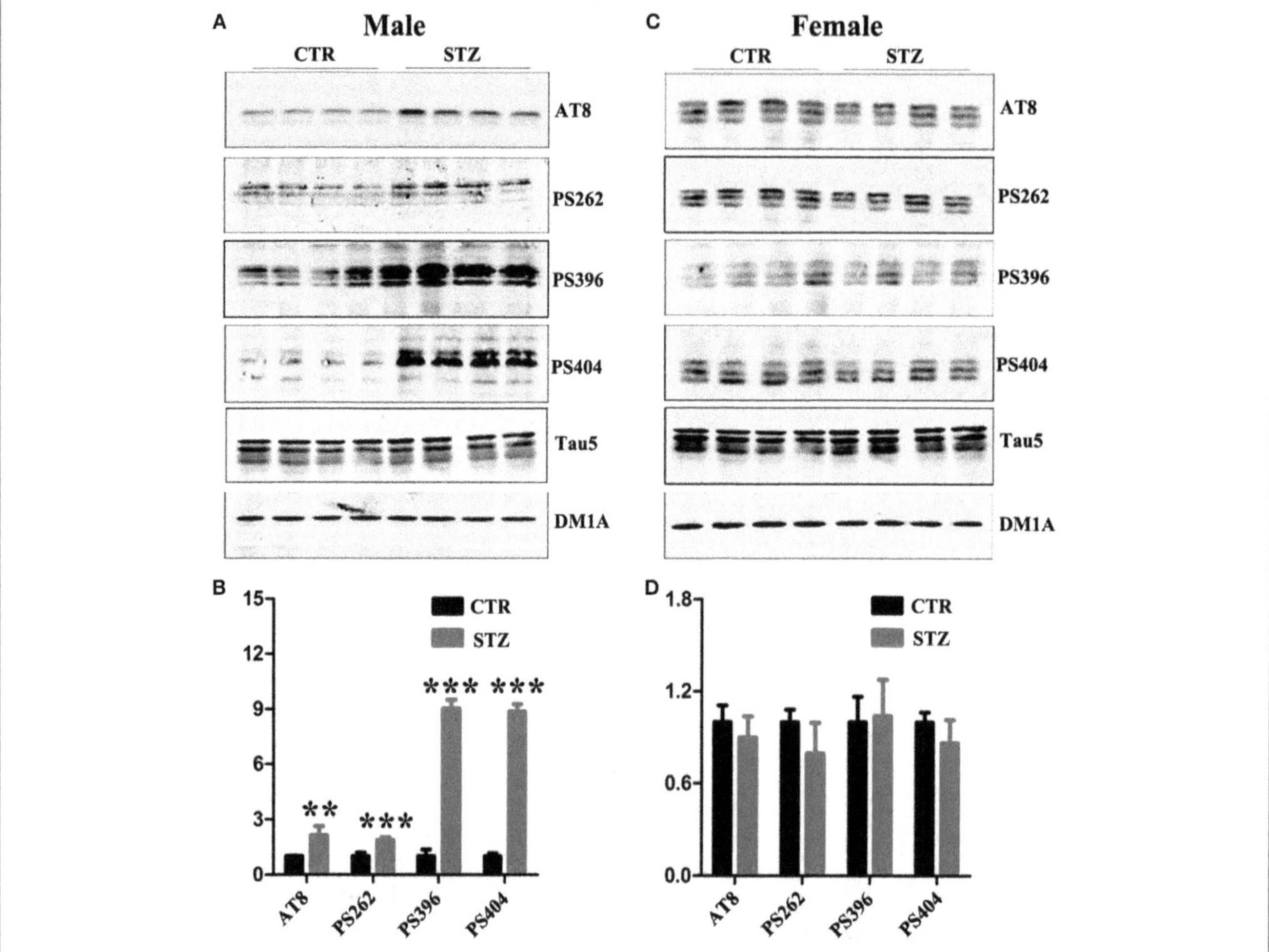

FIGURE 4 | Sex influences tau hyperphosphorylation in the sporadic AD animal model. **(A,C)** Western blot analysis of the protein levels of AT8, PS262, PS396, PS404, and Tau5 and **(B,D)** their quantitative analysis for male or female rats. The data were expressed as mean ± *SD* ($n = 4$). The phosphorylation level of tau was normalized to total tau level probed by tau5. The total level of tau was normalized DM1A. ****P* < 0.001 vs. the vehicle control. Data were analyzed using *t*-test. ***P* < 0.01 vs. the vehicle control.

is being recognized as an insulin resistant brains state (Valente et al., 2010; Bitel et al., 2012; Kamat et al., 2016). Therefore, a non-transgenic animal model generated by ICV-STZ has been proposed as a representative model of sAD. The ICV-STZ rats develop insulin resistant brains state associated with sAD like neuropathological changes and memory impairment (Carro and Torres-Aleman, 2004; Valente et al., 2010; Agrawal et al., 2011; Bitel et al., 2012; Chen et al., 2013; Iqbal et al., 2013; Kamat et al., 2016). Although, the mechanisms underlying ICV-STZ evoked AD pathology remain unknown, ICV-STZ rats have been used in many labs as an experimental model of sAD. For more than 20 years, although some of therapeutic strategies displayed very good effectiveness for AD in ICV-STZ animal models, the same therapies were hard to be reproduced on memory deficits in clinical trials with sAD patients (Salkovic-Petrisic et al., 2013). Thus, it is necessary to re-evaluate the ICV-STZ animal model once again.

Sex has a regulatory effect on brain functions (Brinton, 2009; Cui et al., 2013). We here investigated sex differences on cognitive deficits in the sporadic AD animal model induced by ICV-STZ. Similar to previous studies, the ICV administration of STZ induced cognitive deficits and loss of synaptic plasticity in male rats, but these neurotoxic effects were not observed in female rats. Thus, the ICV-STZ is only for generating animal model of sAD in male, but not in female rats. Consequently sex differences should be considered in AD researches in the future.

Estrogen reduces Aβ level by down-regulating total β secretase activity through MARK/ERK pathway, and modulates Aβ degradation (Pike, 1999; Singh et al., 1999; Vassar et al., 2009). In the present study, we found that ICV-STZ increased BACE1 activities and Aβ40/42 production in male rats, but these alterations were not observed in female rats. The studies have demonstrated that the number of NFTs consisting of hyperphosphorylated tau is positively correlated with the degree of clinical dementia (Iqbal and Grundke-Iqbal, 1991; Iqbal et al., 2008; Luo et al., 2014). Estrogens attenuate tau hperphosphorylation through kinases and phosphatases, such as the GSK-3β, Wnt, and PKA pathways (Zhang et al., 2008). The

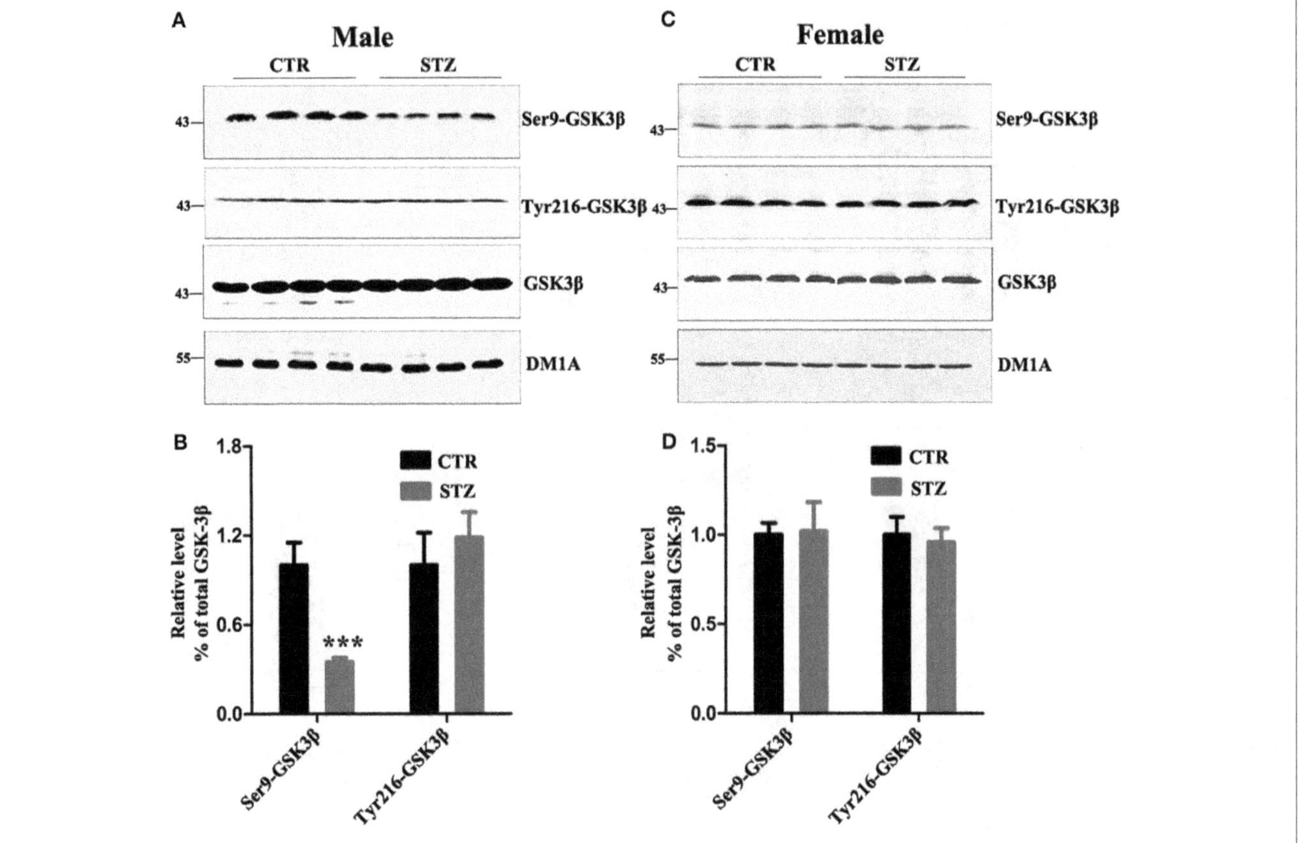

FIGURE 5 | Sex influences activity of GSK-3β in the sporadic AD animal model. **(A,C)** The total GSK-3β, GSK-3β (Ser9), GSK-3β (Tyr216) levels in whole hippocampus extracts were measured using Western blotting and **(B,D)** quantitative analysis. The phosphorylation level of GSK-3β was normalized to total GSK-3β level. The total level of GSK-3β was normalized DM1A. The data were expressed as mean ± *SD* ($n = 4$). $^{***}P < 0.001$ vs. the vehicle control. Data were analyzed using *t*-test.

ICV-STZ model in male rats shows hyperphosphorylation of tau and an increase of GSK-3β activity, but these tau pathologies are not observed in female rats. Together, sex hormones might account for functional discrepancy of ICV-STZ in the two sexes.

A large body of evidence shows that women have a higher incidence of AD than men happening after menopause, which suggest that estrogen might protect against AD pathology. Hormones have long been known to play key roles in regulating learning and memory and ample evidence has demonstrated that estradiol affects hippocampal morphology, plasticity, and memory (Packard, 1998; Brinton, 2009; Foster, 2012; Cui et al., 2013). Studies in the aromatase knock-out mouse suggest that estradiol induced spine and spine synapse formation in hippocampus, not in the cortex or the cerebellum (Zhou et al., 2014). Previous studies point to a role of hippocampus-derived estradiol in synaptic plasticity in cultured slices and *in vivo*, not just the role of gonads-derived estradiol (Zhou et al., 2010; Vierk et al., 2012). In addition, dendritic spines of CA1 pyramidal neurons vary during estrus cyclicity, which likely results from cycle of estradiol synthesis in the hippocampus, since gonadotropin releasing hormone regulates estradiol synthesis in the hippocampus in a dose-dependent manner (Woolley et al., 1990; Prange-Kiel et al., 2008, 2013). In the present study, 10 rats employed in each group is a small sample size. Therefore, we performed Shapiro–wilk test which showed that samples from each group was in accord with normal distribution. Relatively we found that hippocampal estradiol level of female rats is almost four times higher than that of male rats in both vehicle and ICV-STZ treated groups, which is in accordance with previous studies by using mass spectrometry (Fester et al., 2012). This implies that high estradiol levels in female rats might protect them from the ICV-STZ induced cognitive deficits and neurodegenerative pathologies, including synaptic damage, Aβ deposition, and tau hyperphosphorylation in hippocampus.

In reported literature, optimal female performance occurred during the phase of estrus on the spatial learning and memory, and the least efficient performance occurred during proestrus (Vina and Lloret, 2010). Since we did not determine the estrus stage of the control animals and cognitive ability and synaptic density are optimal during proestrus, the estradiol protective effects on hippocampal plasticity and memory would very likely have been greater if we had had exclusively taken proestrus female rats.

Although, the mouse- and monkey ICV-STZ models have also been developed, ICV-STZ rats are still widely used and employed to evaluate the therapeutic potential of drugs and

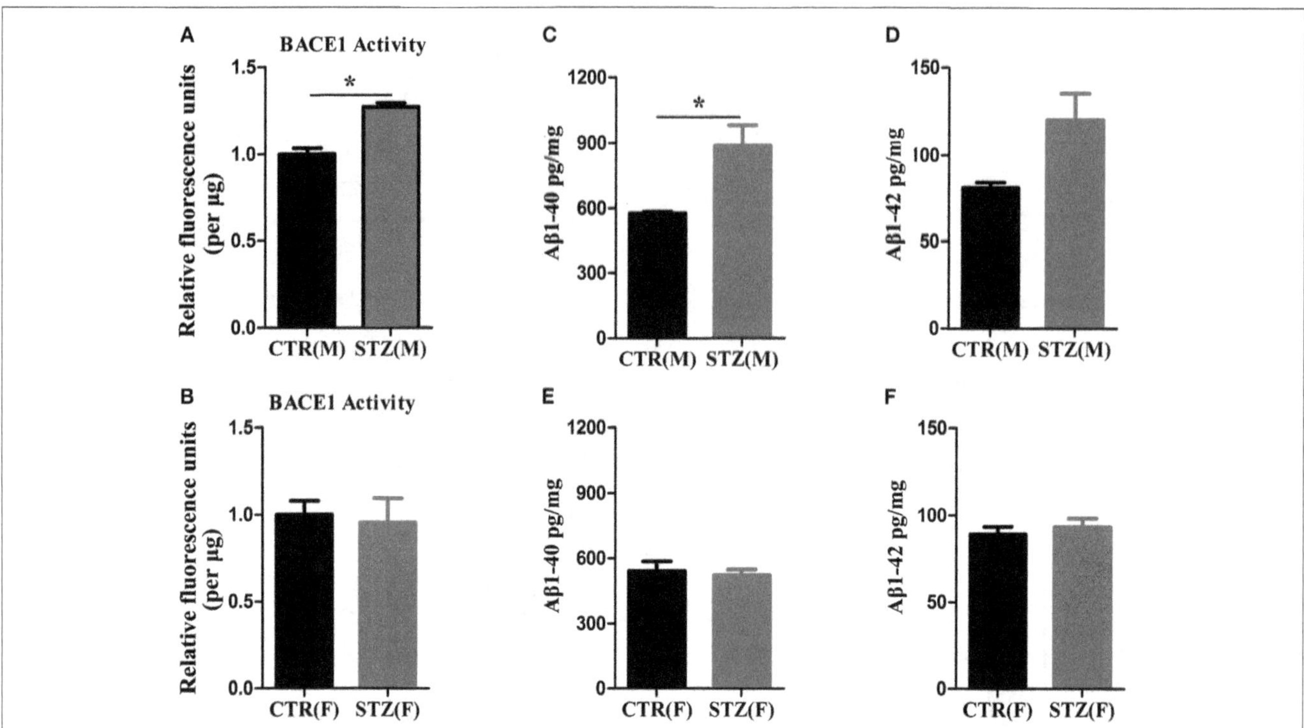

FIGURE 6 | Sex influences activity of BACE1 and Aβ production in the sporadic AD animal model. **(A,B)** BACE1 activity was determined using β-Secretase Activity Assay Kit. **(C–F)** Aβ40/42 levels were quantified through ELISA. The data were expressed as mean ± *SD* (*n* = 5). **P* < 0.05 vs. the vehicle group. Data were analyzed using *t*-test.

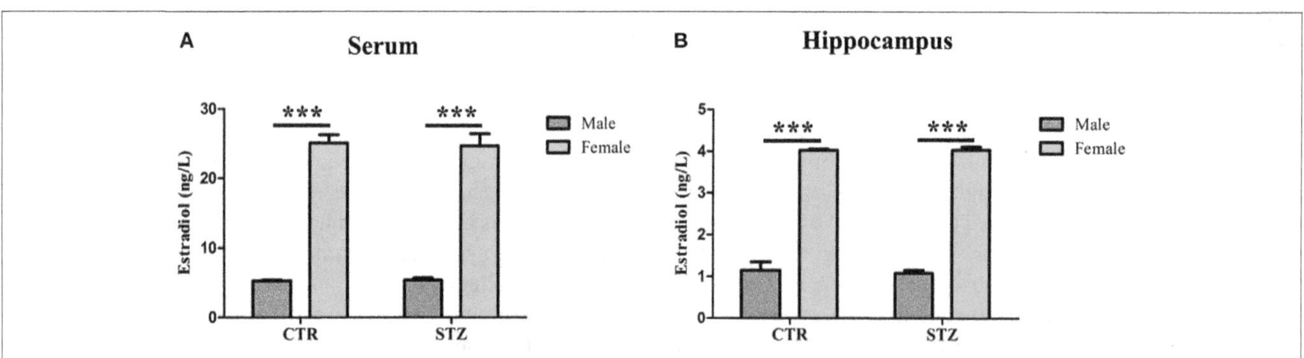

FIGURE 7 | Estradiol levels in serum and hippocampus. The Estradiol levels in the serum **(A)** and hippocampus **(B)** were measured. Estradiol levels of female rats were much higher than that of male rats, while no difference was observed between the groups with same sex. Data were presented as means ± *SD* (*n* = 3). ****P* < 0.001 vs. male rats. Data were analyzed using a general linear model was used for two-way ANOVA followed by *post-hoc* comparison.

non-drug therapies in numerous laboratories. Cognitive deficits and AD-like pathology, such as neuroinflammation, brain insulin resistance, tau hyperphosphorylation, Aβ overproduction, have been found both in female mice and monkeys (Chen et al., 2014; Park et al., 2015). Liu et al. have reported that STZ inhibits the Ras/ERK signaling cascade and decreased the phosphorylation of CREB, and induces cognitive impairment in rats (Liu et al., 2013). However, the study from Diao et al. shows the gender- and EC-dependent levels of proteins from the protein synthetic, chaperoning, and degradation machinery (Diao et al., 2007). Accordingly, it is necessary to re-evaluate the STZ-induced cognitive alterations between male and female rats. In the present study, we found that ICV-STZ remarkably results in cognitive impairments and AD like pathological alterations in the Sprague-Dawley male rats, but not in the female rats. It may conceivably be related with the gender- and EC-dependent levels of proteins from the protein synthetic, chaperoning, and degradation machinery, and consequently regulates tau related kinases and APP cleavage. Its molecular mechanism is worth further discussing. Our findings provide novel insights suggesting that sex differences exist in ICV-STZ rats which have been used as sporadic AD animal model for about 20 years. Therefore, our study encourages investigators to comply with National Institutes of Health policies to include females in biomedical research and to be aware that adding females to a study is not as simple as adding just another group.

AUTHOR CONTRIBUTIONS

XW and JW designed the experiments. JB performed the experiments and analyzed data. JB, YM, BZ, RL, ZZ, JW, and XW discussed and interpreted the results. JB, YM, and XW wrote the paper. All authors have approved the final version of the manuscript.

ACKNOWLEDGMENTS

This study was supported in parts by grants from Natural Science Foundation of China (81571255 and 31528010), the Hubei Province Key Technology R&D Program (2015BCE094) and the Academic Frontier Youth Team Project of HUST.

REFERENCES

Agrawal, R., Tyagi, E., Shukla, R., and Nath, C. (2011). Insulin receptor signaling in rat hippocampus: a study in STZ (ICV) induced memory deficit model. *Eur. Neuropsychopharmacol.* 21, 261–273. doi: 10.1016/j.euroneuro.2010.11.009

Alafuzoff, I., Iqbal, K., Friden, H., Adolfsson, R., and Winblad, B. (1987). Histopathological criteria for progressive dementia disorders: clinical-pathological correlation and classification by multivariate data analysis. *Acta Neuropathol.* 74, 209–225. doi: 10.1007/BF00688184

Becker, J. B., Arnold, A. P., Berkley, K. J., Blaustein, J. D., Eckel, L. A., and Hampson, E. (2005). Strategies and methods for research on sex differences in brain and behavior. *Endocrinology* 146, 1650–1673. doi: 10.1210/en.2004-1142

Bitel, C. L., Kasinathan, C., Kaswala, R. H., Klein, W. L., and Frederikse, P. H. (2012). Amyloid-βand tau pathology of Alzheimer's disease induced by diabetes in a rabbit animal model. *J. Alzheimers Dis.* 32, 291–305. doi: 10.3233/JAD-2012-120571

Brinton, R. D. (2009). Estrogen-induced plasticity from cells to circuits: predictions for cognitive function. *Trends Pharmacol. Sci.* 30, 212–222. doi: 10.1016/j.tips.2008.12.006

Cahill, L. (2006). Why sex matters for neuroscience. *Nat. Rev. Neurosci.* 7, 477–484. doi: 10.1038/nrn1909

Carro, E., and Torres-Aleman, I. (2004). The role of insulin and insulin-like growth factor I in the molecular and cellular mechanisms underlying the pathology of Alzheimer's disease. *Eur. J. Pharmacol.* 490, 127–133. doi: 10.1016/j.ejphar.2004.02.050

Chen, Y., Liang, Z., Blanchard, J., Dai, C. L., Sun, S., Lee, M. H., et al. (2013). A non-transgenic mouse model (icv-STZ mouse) of Alzheimer's disease: similarities to and differences from the transgenic model (3xTg-AD mouse). *Mol. Neurobiol.* 47, 711–725. doi: 10.1007/s12035-012-8375-5

Chen, Y., Liang, Z., Tian, Z., Blanchard, J., Dai, C. L., and Chalbot, S. (2014). Intracerebroventricular streptozotocin exacerbates Alzheimer-like changes of 3xTg-AD mice. *Mol. Neurobiol.* 49, 547–562. doi: 10.1007/s12035-013-8539-y

Cui, J., Shen, Y., and Li, R. (2013). Estrogen synthesis and signaling pathways during aging: from periphery to brain. *Trends Mol. Med.* 19, 197–209. doi: 10.1016/j.molmed.2012.12.007

Deng, Y., Li, B., Liu, Y., Iqbal, K., Grundke-Iqbal, I., and Gong, C. X. (2009). Dysregulation of insulin signaling, glucose transporters, O-GlcNAcylation, and phosphorylation of tau and neurofilaments in the brain: implication for Alzheimer's disease. *Am. J. Pathol.* 175, 2089–2098. doi: 10.2353/ajpath.2009.090157

Diao, W. F, Chen, W. Q., Höger, H., Shim, K. S., Pollak, A., and Lubec, G. (2007). The hippocampal protein machinery varies over the estrous cycle. *Proteomics Clin. Appl.* 1, 1462–1475. doi: 10.1002/prca.200700333

Dysken, M. W., Sano, M., Asthana, S., Vertrees, J. E., Pallaki, M., and Llorente, M. (2014). Effect of vitamin E and memantine on functional decline in Alzheimer disease: the TEAM-AD VA cooperative randomized trial. *JAMA* 311, 33–44. doi: 10.1001/jama.2013.282834

Fester, L., Prange-Kiel, J., Zhou, L., Blittersdorf, B.V., Bohm, J., Jarry, H., et al. (2012). Estrogen-regulated synaptogenesis in the hippocampus: sexual dimorphism *in vivo* but not *in vitro*. *J. Steroid Biochem. Mol. Biol.* 131, 24–29. doi: 10.1016/j.jsbmb.2011.11.010

Forger, N. G., Strahan, J. A., and Castillo-Ruiz, A. (2016). Cellular and molecular mechanisms of sexual differentiation in the mammalian nervous system. *Front. Neuroendocrinol.* 40, 67–86. doi: 10.1016/j.yfrne.2016.01.001

Foster, T. C. (2012). Role of estrogen receptor alpha and beta expression and signaling on cognitive function during aging. *Hippocampus* 22, 656–669. doi: 10.1002/hipo.20935

Grundke-Iqbal, I., Iqbal, K., Tung, Y. C., Quinlan, M., Wisniewski, H. M., and Binder, L. I. (1986). Abnormal phosphorylation of the microtubule-associated protein tau (tau) in Alzheimer cytoskeletal pathology. *Proc. Natl. Acad. Sci. U.S.A.* 83, 4913–4917. doi: 10.1073/pnas.83.13.4913

Hall, A. M., and Roberson, E. D. (2012). Mouse models of Alzheimer's disease. *Brain Res. Bull.* 88, 3–12. doi: 10.1016/j.brainresbull.2011.11.017

Hong, M., and Lee, V. M. (1997). Insulin and insulin-like growth factor-1 regulate tau phosphorylation in cultured human neurons. *J. Biol. Chem.* 272, 19547–19553. doi: 10.1074/jbc.272.31.19547

Iqbal, K., Bolognin, S., Wang, X., Basurto-Islas, G., Blanchard, J., Tung, Y. C., et al. (2013). Animal models of the sporadic form of Alzheimer's disease: focus on the disease and not just the lesions. *J. Alzheimers Dis.* 37, p469–p474. doi: 10.3233/JAD-130827

Iqbal, K., Alonso Adel, C, and Grundke-Iqbal, I. (2008). Cytosolic abnormally hyperphosphorylated tau but not paired helical filaments sequester normal MAPs and inhibit microtubule assembly. *J. Alzheimer's Dis.* 14, 365–370. doi: 10.3233/JAD-2008-14402

Iqbal, K., and Grundke-Iqbal, I. (1991). Ubiquitination and abnormal phosphorylation of paired helical filaments in Alzheimer's disease. *Mol. Neurobiol.* 5, 399–410.

Iqbal, K., and Grundke-Iqbal, I. (2010). Alzheimer disease, a multifactorial disorder seeking multi therapies. *Alzheimers Dement.* 6, 420–4. doi: 10.1016/j.jalz.2010.04.006

Jee, Y. S., Ko, I. G., Sung, Y. H., Lee, J. W., Kim, Y. S., and Kim, S. E. (2008). Effects of treadmill exercise on memory and c-Fos expression in the hippocampus of the rats with intracerebroventricular injection of streptozotocin. *Neurosci. Lett.* 443, 188–192. doi: 10.1016/j.neulet.2008.07.078

Kamat, P. K., Kalani, A., Rai, S., Tota, S. K., Kumar, A., and Ahmad, A. S. (2016). Streptozotocin intracerebro ventricular induced neurotoxicity and brain insulin resistance:a therapeutic intervention for treatment of Sporadic Alzheimer's Disease (sAD)-like pathology. *Mol. Neurobiol.* 53, 4548–4562. doi: 10.1007/s12035-015-9384-y

Kasai, H., Fukuda, M., Watanabe, S., Hayashi-Takagi, A., and Noguchi, J. (2010). Structural dynamics of dendritic spines in memory and cognition. *Trends Neurosci.* 33, 121–129. doi: 10.1016/j.tins.2010.01.001

Kloppenborg, R. P., van den Berg, E., Kappelle, L. J., and Biessels, G. J. (2008). Diabetes and other vascular risk factors for dementia: which factor matters most? A systematic review. *Eur. J. Pharmacol.* 585, 97–108. doi: 10.1016/j.ejphar.2008.02.049

Lannert, H., and Hoyer, S. (1998). Intracerebroventricular administration of streptozotocin causes long-term diminutions in learning and memory abilities and in cerebral energy metabolism in adult rats. *Behav. Neurosci.* 112, 1199–1208. doi: 10.1037/0735-7044.112.5.1199

Li, B., Yamamori, H., Tatebayashi, Y., Shafit-Zagardo, B., Tanimukai, H., and Chen, S. (2008). Failure of neuronal maturation in Alzheimer disease dentate gyrus. *J. Neuropathol. Exp. Neurol.* 67, 78–84. doi: 10.1097/nen.0b013e31816 0c5db

Liu, P., Zou, L., Jiao, Q., Chi, T., Ji, X., and Qi, Y. (2013). Xanthoceraside attenuates learning and memory deficits via improving insulin signaling in STZ-induced AD rats. *Neurosci. Lett.* 543, 115–120. doi: 10.1016/j.neulet.2013. 02.065

Luo, H. B., Xia, Y. Y., Shu, X. J., Liu, Z. C., Feng, Y., and Liu, X. H. (2014). SUMOylation at K340 inhibits tau degradation through deregulating its phosphorylation and ubiquitination. *Proc. Natl. Acad. Sci. U.S.A.* 111, 16586–16591. doi: 10.1073/pnas.1417548111

Malkki, H. (2016). Alzheimer disease: NSAIDs protect neurons and preserve memory in a mouse model of AD. *Nat. Rev. Neurol.* 12, 370–371. doi: 10.1038/nrneurol.2016.79

Mangialasche, F., Solomon, A., Winblad, B., Mecocci, P., and Kivipelto, M. (2010). Alzheimer's disease: clinical trials and drug development. *Lancet Neurol.* 9, 702–716. doi: 10.1016/S1474-4422(10)70119-8

McCarthy, M. M (2009). The two faces of estradiol: effects on the developing brain. *Neuroscientist* 15, 599–610. doi: 10.1177/10738584093 40924

Mehla, J., Pahuja, M., and Gupta, Y. K. (2013). Streptozotocin-induced sporadic Alzheimer's disease: selection of appropriate dose. *J. Alzheimers Dis.* 33, 17–21. doi: 10.3233/JAD-2012-120958

Morest, D. K (1960). A study of the structure of the area postrema with Golgi methods. *Am. J. Anat.* 107, 291–303. doi: 10.1002/aja.10010 70307

Packard, M. G. (1998). Posttraining estrogen and memory modulation. *Horm. Behav.* 34, 126–139. doi: 10.1006/hbeh.1998.1464

Park, S. J., Kim, Y. H., Nam, G. H., Choe, S. H., Lee, S. R., Kim, S. U., et al. (2015). Quantitative expression analysis of APP pathway and tau phosphorylation-related genes in the ICV STZ-induced non-human primate model of sporadic Alzheimer's disease. *Int. J. Mol. Sci.* 16, 2386–2402. doi: 10.3390/ijms160 22386

Pike, C. J. (1999). Estrogen modulates neuronal Bcl-xL expression and beta-amyloid-induced apoptosis: relevance to Alzheimer's disease. *J. Neurochem.* 72, 1552–1563. doi: 10.1046/j.1471-4159.1999.721552.x

Prange-Kiel, J., Jarry, H., Schoen, M., Kohlmann, P., Lohse, C., Zhou, L., et al. (2008). Gonadotropin-releasing hormone regulates spine density via its regulatory role in hippocampal estrogen synthesis. *Cell Biol. J.* 180, 417–426. doi: 10.1083/jcb.200707043

Prange-Kiel, J., Schmutterer, T., Fester, L., Zhou, L., Imholz, P., Brandt, N., et al. (2013). Endocrine regulation of estrogen synthesis in the hippocampus? *Prog. Histochem. Cytochem.* 48, 49–64. doi: 10.1016/j.proghi.2013. 07.002

Prasad, K. N (2017). Oxidative stress and pro-inflammatory cytokines may act as one of the signals for regulating microRNAs expression in Alzheimer's disease. *Mech. Ageing Dev.* 162, 63–71. doi: 10.1016/j.mad.2016. 12.003

Prickaerts, J., Fahrig, T., and Blokland, A. (1999). Cognitive performance and biochemical markers in septum, hippocampus and striatum of rats after an i.c.v. injection of streptozotocin: a correlation analysis. *Behav. Brain Res.* 102, 73–88. doi: 10.1016/S0166-4328(98)00158-2

Qi, C., Bao, J., Wang, J., Zhu, H., Xue, Y., Wang, X., et al. (2016). Asperterpenes, A., and B, two unprecedented meroterpenoids from *Aspergillus terreus* with BACE1 inhibitory activities. *Chem. Sci.* 7, 6563–6572. doi: 10.1039/C6SC02464E

Raznahan, A., Lee, Y., Stidd, R., Long, R., Greenstein, D., and Clasen, L. (2010). Longitudinally mapping the influence of sex and androgen signaling on the dynamics of human cortical maturation in adolescence. *Proc. Natl. Acad. Sci. U.S.A.* 107, 16988–16993. doi: 10.1073/pnas.1006025107

Rodrigues, L., Dutra, M. F, Ilha, J, Biasibetti, R., Quincozes-Santos, A., and Leite, M. C. (2010). Treadmill training restores spatial cognitive deficits and neurochemical alterations in the hippocampus of rats submitted to an intracerebroventricular administration of streptozotocin. *J. Neural Transm.* 117, 1295–1305. doi: 10.1007/s00702-010-0501-9

Ruigrok, A. N., Salimi-Khorshidi, G., Lai, M. C., Baron-Cohen, S., Lombardo, M. V., and Tait, R. J. (2014). A meta-analysis of sex differences in human brain structure. *Neurosci. Biobehav. Rev.* 39, 34–50. doi: 10.1016/j.neubiorev.2013.12.004

Salkovic-Petrisic, M., and Hoyer, S. (2007). Central insulin resistance as a trigger for sporadic Alzheimer-like pathology: an experimental approach. *J. Neural Transm. Suppl.* 72, 217–233. doi: 10.1007/978-3-211-73574-9_28

Salkovic-Petrisic, M., Knezovic, A., Hoyer, S., and Riederer, P. (2013). What have we learned from the streptozotocin-induced animal model of sporadic Alzheimer's disease, about the therapeutic strategies in Alzheimer's research. *J. Neural Transm.* 120, 233–252. doi: 10.1007/s00702-012-0877-9

Shineman, D. W., Basi, G. S., Bizon, J. L., Colton, C. A., Greenberg, B. D., and Hollister, B. A. (2011). Accelerating drug discovery for Alzheimer's disease: best practices for preclinical animal studies. *Alzheimers Res. Ther.* 3, 28. doi: 10.1186/alzrt90

Singh, M., Sétáló, G., Guan, X., Warren, M., and Toran-Allerand, C. D. (1999). Estrogen-induced activation of mitogen-activated protein kinase in cerebral cortical explants: convergence of estrogen and neurotrophin signaling pathways. *J. Neurosci.* 19, 1179–1188.

Singh, T. J., Zaidi, T., Grundke-Iqbal, I., and Iqbal, K. (1995). Modulation of GSK-3-catalyzed phosphorylation of microtubule-associated protein tau by non-proline-dependent protein kinases. *FEBS Lett.* 358, 4–8. doi: 10.1016/0014-5793(94)01383-C

Valente, T., Gella, A., Fernàndez-Busquets, X., Unzeta, M., and Durany, N. (2010). Immunohistochemical analysis of human brain suggests pathological synergism of Alzheimer's disease and diabetes mellitus. *Neurobiol. Dis.* 37, 67–76. doi: 10.1016/j.nbd.2009.09.008

Vassar, R., Kovacs, D. M., Yan, R., and Wong, P. C (2009). The beta-secretase enzyme BACE in health and Alzheimer's disease: regulation, cell biology, function, and therapeutic potential. *J. Neurosci.* 29, 12787–12794. doi: 10.1523/JNEUROSCI.3657-09.2009

Vierk, R., Glassmeier, G., Zhou, L., Brandt, N., Fester, L., Dudzinski, D., et al. (2012). Aromatase inhibition abolishes LTP generation in female but not in male mice. *Neurosci. J.* 32, 8116–8126. doi: 10.1523/JNEUROSCI.5319-11.2012

Vina, J., and Lloret, A. (2010). Why women have more Alzheimer's disease than men: gender and mitochondrial toxicity of amyloid-beta peptide. *J. Alzheimers Dis.* 20(Suppl. 2), S527–S533. doi: 10.3233/JAD-2010-100501

Wang, J. Z., and Liu, F. (2008). Microtubule-associated protein tau in development, degeneration and protection of neurons. *Prog. Neurobiol.* 85, 148–175. doi: 10.1016/j.pneurobio.2008.03.002

Wang, X., Blanchard, J., Kohlbrenner, E., Clement, N., Linden, R. M., and Radu, A. (2010). The carboxy-terminal fragment of inhibitor-2 of protein phosphatase-2A induces Alzheimer disease pathology and cognitive impairment. *FASEB J.* 24, 4420–4432. doi: 10.1096/fj.10-158477

Wightman, E. L. (2017). Potential benefits of phytochemicals against Alzheimer's disease. *Proc. Nutr. Soc.* 76, 106–112. doi: 10.1017/S0029665116002962

Woo, K. (2000). Is vitamin E the magic bullet for the treatment of Alzheimer's disease (AD)? *Perspectives* 24, 7–10.

Woolley, C. S., Gould, E., Frankfurt, M., and McEwen, B. S. (1990). Naturally-occurring fluctuation in dendritic spine density on adult hippocampal pyramidal neurons. *Neurosci. J.* 10, 4035–4039.

Xu, Z. P., Li, L., Bao, J., Wang, Z. H., Zeng, J., and Liu, E. J. (2014). Magnesium protects cognitive functions and synaptic plasticity in streptozotoc in-induced sporadic Alzheimer's model. *PLoS ONE* 9:e108645. doi: 10.1371/journal.pone.0108645

Zahs, K. R., and Ashe, K. H. (2010). 'Too much good news' - are Alzheimer mouse models trying to tell us how to prevent, not cure, Alzheimer's disease? *Trends Neurosci.* 33, 381–389. doi: 10.1016/j.tins.2010.05.004

Zhang, Q.G., Wang, R., Khan, M., Mahesh, V., and Brann, D. W. (2008). Role of Dickkopf-1, an antagonist of the Wnt/beta-catenin signaling pathway, in estrogen-induced neuroprotection and attenuation of tau phosphorylation. *J. Neurosci.* 28, 8430–8441. doi: 10.1523/JNEUROSCI.2752-08.2008

Zhang, Z., Song, M., Liu, X., Su Kang, S., Duong, D. M., and Seyfried, N. T. (2015). Delta-secretase cleaves amyloid precursor protein and regulates the pathogenesis in Alzheimer's disease. *Nat. Commun.* 9, 8762. doi: 10.1038/ncomms9762

Zhou, L., Fester, L., Haghshenas, S., de Vrese, X., von Hacht, R., Gloger, S., et al. (2014). Oestradiol-induced synapse formation in the female hippocampus:

7

Sleep Disorders Associated with Alzheimer's Disease

*Anna Brzecka[1], Jerzy Leszek[2], Ghulam Md Ashraf[3], Maria Ejma[4], Marco F. Ávila-Rodriguez[5], Nagendra S. Yarla[6], Vadim V. Tarasov[7], Vladimir N. Chubarev[7], Anna N. Samsonova[8], George E. Barreto[9,10] and Gjumrakch Aliev[8,11,12]**

[1] Department of Pulmonology and Lung Cancer, Wroclaw Medical University, Wroclaw, Poland, [2] Department of Psychiatry, Wroclaw Medical University, Wroclaw, Poland, [3] King Fahd Medical Research Center, King Abdulaziz University, Jeddah, Saudi Arabia, [4] Department of Neurology, Wroclaw Medical University, Wroclaw, Poland, [5] Facultad de Ciencias de la Salud, Universidad del Tolima, Ibagué, Colombia, [6] Department of Biochemistry and Bioinformatics, School of Life Sciences, Institute of Science, Gandhi Institute of Technology and Management University, Visakhapatnam, India, [7] Institute for Pharmaceutical Science and Translational Medicine, Sechenov First Moscow State Medical University, Moscow, Russia, [8] Institute of Physiologically Active Compounds of the Russian Academy of Sciences, Chernogolovka, Russia, [9] Departamento de Nutrición y Bioquímica, Facultad de Ciencias, Pontificia Universidad Javeriana, Bogotá, Colombia, [10] Instituto de Ciencias Biomédicas, Universidad Autónoma de Chile, Santiago, Chile, [11] GALLY International Biomedical Research and Consulting LLC, San Antonio, TX, United States, [12] School of Health Science and Healthcare Administration, University of Atlanta, Johns Creek, GA, United States

***Correspondence:**
Gjumrakch Aliev
aliev03@gmail.com;
cobalt55@gallyinternational.com

Sleep disturbances, as well as sleep-wake rhythm disturbances, are typical symptoms of Alzheimer's disease (AD) that may precede the other clinical signs of this neurodegenerative disease. Here, we describe clinical features of sleep disorders in AD and the relation between sleep disorders and both cognitive impairment and poor prognosis of the disease. There are difficulties of the diagnosis of sleep disorders based on sleep questionnaires, polysomnography or actigraphy in the AD patients. Typical disturbances of the neurophysiological sleep architecture in the course of the AD include deep sleep and paradoxical sleep deprivation. Among sleep disorders occurring in patients with AD, the most frequent disorders are sleep breathing disorders and restless legs syndrome. Sleep disorders may influence circadian fluctuations of the concentrations of amyloid-β in the interstitial brain fluid and in the cerebrovascular fluid related to the glymphatic brain system and production of the amyloid-β. There is accumulating evidence suggesting that disordered sleep contributes to cognitive decline and the development of AD pathology. In this mini-review, we highlight and discuss the association between sleep disorders and AD.

Keywords: AD, diagnosis, sleep disorders, disturbance, sleep-rhythm

INTRODUCTION

Alzheimer's disease (AD) is the most common cause of dementia, and its etiology is multifactorial (Chibber et al., 2016). The primary event in AD is the accumulation of amyloid-β (Aβ) in the brain (Karran et al., 2011). Abnormal deposition of Aβ triggers a cascade of events leading to neuroinflammation and neuronal cell death (Wyss-Coray and Mucke, 2002; Selkoe and Hardy, 2016). As a consequence, clinical manifestations of AD, mainly impaired cognitive function, develop progressively over 15 years since the beginning of accumulation of Aβ (Sen et al., 2017). Neuropathological modifications may develop progressively for several decades and during this preclinical period of AD, mild cognitive impairment (MCI) may occur (Drago et al., 2011; Bhat et al., 2017). In over 90% of cases, AD begins after the age of 65 as a sporadic form of dementia (Prince et al., 2013; Ashraf et al., 2016). Of late, AD has been found to coexist with other chronic diseases like cancer, diabetes, and cardiovascular diseases (Aliev et al., 2014; Jabir et al., 2015; Rizvi et al., 2015; Ashraf et al., 2016). This has opened up new dimensions of AD diagnosis and therapy based on proteomics (Ashraf et al., 2014, 2015) and nanotechnology (Soursou et al., 2015; Ansari et al., 2017).

In AD, and likely in other neurodegenerative diseases, sleep disorders appear early (Dos Santos et al., 2014, 2015). Although the time meant for sleeping extend during the day, sleeping and waking rhythms are disturbed (McCurry et al., 1999). Common symptoms include difficulties in falling asleep, arousal at night, repeated awakenings and waking up too early in the morning, and sleepiness and frequent naps during the day (McCurry and Ancoli-Israel, 2003; Most et al., 2012). Sleep disorders can be an important diagnostic indication that foreruns development of AD's pathological disorders in the form of Aβ deposition in the brain and during dementia onset (Lim et al., 2013; Spira et al., 2013). Sleep disorders worsen as the disease progresses (Bliwise et al., 1995), and their considerable intensification in the late stage of the disease is a strong predictive factor for mortality (Spalletta et al., 2015). In the present mini-review, we discuss the association of sleep disorders in AD (**Figure 1**).

Night-Time Sleep Duration and AD

Results of clinical and epidemiological studies regarding a connection between night-time sleep duration and risk of AD are not equivocal. Although a prospective, 2-years self-reporting study in 1,844 community-dwelling women in the age ≥70 has shown that women sleeping ≤5 h per night had poorer cognitive abilities than women sleeping longer, though the difference was small (Tworoger et al., 2006). Similar results were found in the Spanish study in 3,212 people at the age of ≥60, where no correlation was found between shortened (<7 h) sleep time (according to self reported data) and cognitive disorders, determined by Mini-Mental State Examination (MMSE) questionnaire (Faubel et al., 2009). However, among persons sleeping longer than 7 h, a statistically significant ($p < 0.001$) trend was proved, indicating that the longer the sleep (more than 7, 8, 9, 10, or 11 h), the worse the cognitive abilities are (Faubel et al., 2009). A progressive study based on the Pittsburgh Sleep Quality Index and encompassing 1,664 persons at the age of 65 years without cognitive disorders during a 1-year observation found that extended sleep time (>9 h) among women and shortened sleep time (<5 h) among men correlated with cognitive impairment (OR 3.70; 95% CI 1.49–9.17 and OR 4.95; 95% CI 1.72–14.27, respectively) (Potvin et al., 2012). Further, in a study in 298 women without dementia at the age of 82.3 ± 3.2 years, a total sleep time (TST) during polysomnography (PSG) did not show correlation with the degree of cognitive impairment (Yaffe et al., 2011).

Based on results obtained in empirical study conducted among healthy men in middle age, it has been hypothesized that $A\beta_{42}$ increases with chronic sleep deprivation (Ooms et al., 2014). In this study, encompassing men, aged 40–60 years, without cognitive impairments, 13 persons have not been allowed to fall asleep at night, while the other 13 persons were permitted to unlimitedly long sleep. In both groups, a concentration of $A\beta_{42}$ was measured in cerebrospinal fluid (CSF) collected in the evening and in the morning. In persons who slept at night, a 6% decrease of $A\beta_{42}$ level in the morning compared to evening hours had been observed (95% CI [0.94, 49.6], $p = 0.04$). However, among those who did not sleep, the physiological decrease of $A\beta_{42}$ level in the morning hours had not been noticed. Thus, observed increased levels of $A\beta_{42}$ in CSF after sleep deprivation might indicate a higher risk of development of AD. Moreover, there was a correlation between total sleep duration and maximal decrease of $A\beta_{42}$ ($r = -0.5, p = 0.04$).

Diagnostics of Sleep Disorders Based on Questionnaires in AD Patients

In patients with AD, the diagnostics of sleep disorders based on specific questionnaires is difficult due to cognitive impairment affecting reliability of self-report measures of sleep. It may happen that patients who suffer from severe difficulties in falling asleep and frequent awakenings at night do not complain of insomnia at all (Most et al., 2012). The study comparing results of sleep questionnaires, such as Pittsburgh Sleep Quality Index, the Sleep Disorders Questionnaire, and the Athens Insomnia Scale, with the results of actigraphy in 55 patients with AD and 26 controls revealed limited value of those sleep questionnaires in early and moderate AD stage (Most et al., 2012). Based on the results obtained in the questionnaires, it has been found that sleep disorders occurred in 24.5% of patients with mild to moderate form of AD (Moran et al., 2005). However, it appears that sleep disorders occur much more frequently in the course of this disease (Zhao et al., 2016).

PSG in the Diagnostics of Sleep Disorders in AD Patients

PSG is a basic and objective method of diagnosing sleep disorders. In the patients with AD, PSG usually shows prolonged sleep latency, i.e., time taken to fall asleep (McCurry and Ancoli-Israel, 2003). Indeed, increased number of awakenings and lengthened time of wakefulness after sleep onset causes reduced sleep efficiency (Bliwise, 1993; Rauchs et al., 2008).

The number of sleep cycles remains unchanged (Petit et al., 2004), but duration of both rapid eye movement (REM) sleep and deep sleep (N3) is usually shortened (Maestri et al., 2015). However, in AD, recognition of sleep stages—especially stage N3—is frequently difficult, because usually in electroencephalogram (EEG) recordings there are generalized slow waves (0.5–2 Hz) of low amplitude during both sleep and wakefulness (Petit et al., 2004; Peter-Derex et al., 2015). Also, during REM sleep, an increased amount of delta and theta waves and reduced number of faster α and β waves can be observed (Hassainia et al., 1997). Reduced activity of EEG is

Abbreviations: AD, Alzheimer's disease; CSF, Cerebrospinal fluid; EEG, Electroencephalogram; PSG, Polysomnography; MCI, Mild cognitive impairment; PLM, Periodic leg movements; REM, Rapid eye movement; RLS, Restless leg syndrome; TST, Total sleep time.

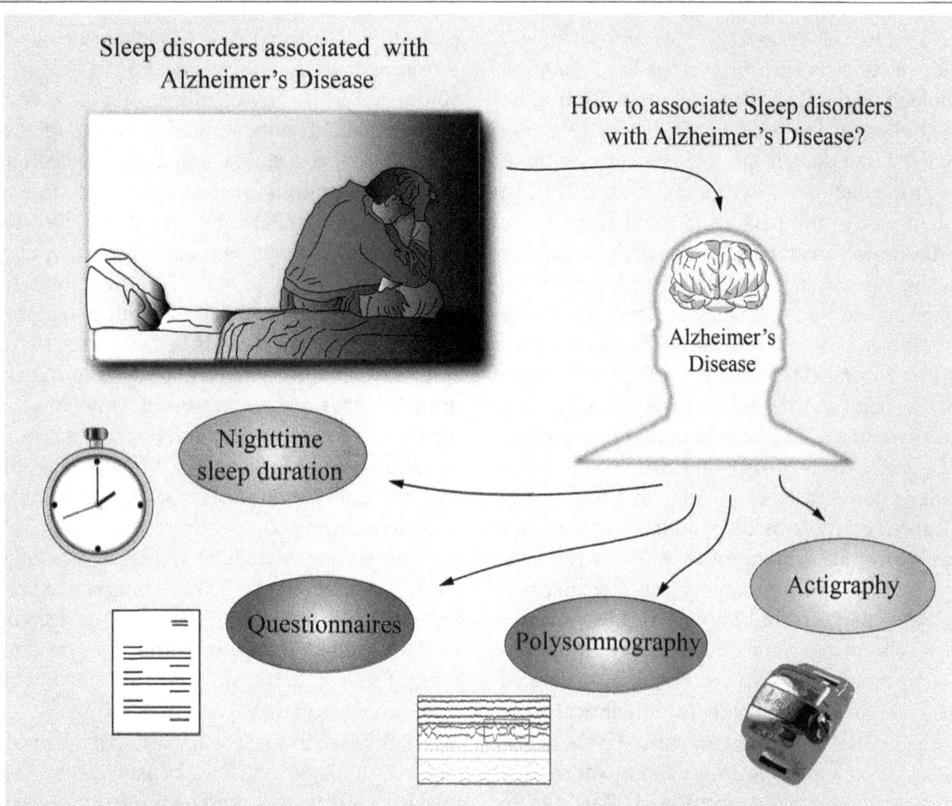

FIGURE 1 | Identification of sleep disorders and possible relationship with AD. Several sleep conditions may indicate the risk of undergo AD; for example, nighttime sleep (<5 h) is linked in many epidemiological studies as a risk factor for AD. Additionally, it is possible to qualitatively survey for sleep quality by means of questionnaires i.e., Athens Insomnia Scale or Pittsburg Sleep Quality Index. Polysomnography is a procedure to diagnose sleep disorders, and in AD patients, it is observed prolonged sleep latency and increased number of arousals. Finally, some portable equipment like Actigraph can provide key data of sleep quality by measuring the wakefulness and sleep activity in several days (10 days registration).

considered as a biological marker of AD (Prinz et al., 1982). Based on the measurements of the cyclic alternating pattern (CAP) in the PSG recordings, sleep instability was found both in the subjects with MCI (age 68.5 ± 7.0 years) and—to a greater extent—in patients with mild AD (age 72.7 ± 5.9 years) as compared to healthy persons without cognitive impairment (age 69.2 ± 12.6 years) (Maestri et al., 2015). In this study, encompassing 33 subjects in the three equally numerous groups, PSG revealed abnormalities in the microstructure of sleep, as indicated by decreased CAP rate and slow components of CAP. Thus, PSG abnormalities could serve as a potentially useful marker of neurodegeneration in subjects with cognitive impairments. Disordered sleep structure correlates with a degree of cognitive abilities impairment, including those assessed by MMSE. The correlations of cognitive impairments and sleep structure abnormalities in PSG recordings were found in a study of 48 patients with AD (21 patients with mild AD and 27 patients with moderate to severe AD) (Liguori et al., 2014). In this study, abnormalities of macrostructural sleep variables in PSG were more pronounced in patients with poorer cognitive function (MMSE score < 21).

Abnormalities in the PSG recordings were also noted in patients with preclinical AD. In a previous study of 25 subjects with MCI (age 70.5 ± 6.8 years, MMSE score 26.7 ± 2.4), higher density of arousals during slow wave sleep and decreased percentage of REM sleep during total sleep time as compared with healthy subjects in similar age were found (0.09 ± 0.11 vs. 0.19 ± 0.10; $p < 0.01$ and 14.7 ± 3.7 vs. 10.1 ± 5.4; $p < 0.007$, respectively) (Hita-Yañez et al., 2013).

In patients with amnestic MCI—who constitute a group of increased risk of progression to AD—abnormalities in the sleep structure were also observed. In a study of 8 amnestic MCI patients (age 72.1 ± 5.1), as compared with 16 age-matched healthy adults, there were fewer sleep spindles, shortened SWS and lower delta and theta power (Westerberg et al., 2012). However, PSG has limited usage for patients with AD. Its limitations rely in the fact that most patients with AD—especially in advanced stage—are not able to cooperate during the examination and do not tolerate any electrodes and sensors on the skin (Peter-Derex et al., 2015).

Actigraphy to Examine Sleep Disorders in Patients With AD

Actigraphy turned out to be appropriate method to examine sleep disorders in AD (Ancoli-Israel et al., 1997; Most et al., 2012). Prospective study based on actigraphy (10 days registration) conducted in 737 men and women at the age of 81.6 ± 7.2 has shown that after an average 3.3 years, risk of symptoms of AD was 1.5 times higher in subjects with high sleep fragmentation as compared to subjects with slight sleep fragmentation (Lim et al., 2013). Sleep studies on the basis of actigraphy (2 weeks registration) have been conducted in 142 persons without cognitive disorders at the age of ≥45 years (Ju et al., 2013). In this group, more than half of the persons (54.2%) were at the age >65 years, including 18 persons (12.7%) at the age over 75 years. TST (i.e., the amount of sleep) and the percentage of sleep in the time spent in bed (i.e., efficiency of sleep) have been determined. In this study, it has been arbitrarily stated that sleep efficiency <75% showed worse sleep quality, and correlation of quantity and quality of sleep and the level of $A\beta_{42}$ in CSF have been evaluated. No differences in TST have been found in persons with decreased and normal levels of $A\beta_{42}$ in CSF. In 32 persons (22.5%) on the basis of lowered level of $A\beta_{42}$ in CSF (≤ 500 pg/ml), pre-clinical form of AD was diagnosed. In this group, quality of sleep was worse than among other persons (80.4 vs. 83.7%, $p = 0.04$) (Ju et al., 2013). High proportions of the persons studied were at the age > 65 years, indicating possible influence of this factor on the obtained results. Additionally, it should be stated that $A\beta_{42}$ thresholds in CSF are not clearly defined in cognitively healthy persons. For persons in pre-clinical stage of AD, as defined on the basis of decreased $A\beta_{42}$ levels in the CSF, at least 3 naps in a week have been noted, i.e., more than for persons without signs of amyloid deposition (31.2 vs. 14.7%; $p = 0.03$). The results of the study have confirmed that the most important sleep disorder in AD is sleep fragmentation, causing worsening of the sleep quality (Ju et al., 2013). However, there might be bidirectional influence of amyloid deposition on sleep, and the authors indicate both the possibilities that $A\beta_{42}$ interferes with neuronal function related to sleep-wake cycle and that sleep disturbances contribute to amyloid deposition.

Breathing Disorders During Sleep in AD Patients

Sleep disorders in AD can be caused by breathing disorders during sleep and among them by repetitive obstructive sleep apnea (OSA). However, a correlation between breathing disorders during sleep and AD is not well explained. OSA syndrome occurs—similarly to AD—more often in older patients (Ancoli-Israel et al., 1991). The main risk factor of OSA syndrome is overweight or obesity. Obesity is diagnosed when body mass index (BMI) exceeds 30 kg/m^2. In the population of obese persons, with BMI >30 kg/m^2, OSA risk is about 20–40% (Saint Martin et al., 2015). A connection of AD with obesity is complex. High BMI in the middle of life relates with increased risk of AD in later life, while high BMI in later life is associated with lower risk (Whitmer et al., 2005; Emmerzaal et al., 2015). In a prospective study, where correlation between AD and body weight was analyzed, it has been stated that among patients who were obese at 50 years old, risk of AD was higher (HR 1.39; 95% CI 1.03–1.87) in comparison to patients with normal weight. A reversed correlation has been found by analyzing BMI in later life (i.e., in 65 years of age): among obese patients, the risk of AD was lower (HR 0.63, 95%CI 0.44–0.91) when compared to patients with normal BMI (Fitzpatrick et al., 2009). In the other prospective study comprising 1,394 persons, who at the age of 50 did not show any cognitive disorders, were followed-up for 14 years, and results showed that 142 of them had developed AD. It has been stated that among persons who were obese, upon the beginning of trial, AD developed, on the average, 6.7 months earlier (Chuang et al., 2016). Decrease of BMI before AD (about 0.21 kg/m^2 annually, otherwise about 0.6 kg annually for a person being 1.7 m tall) and stabilization or increase in BMI after the appearance of clinical symptoms of the disease were observed (Gu et al., 2014). Unfortunately, in the above cited studies on the link between obesity and AD risk, sleep breathing disorders have not been assessed. However, as there is increasing incidence of sleep apneas and hypopneas with increasing weight and sleep breathing disorders, and these variables should be taken into the consideration. According to some reports, breathing disorders during sleep occur more often in AD than among persons without dementia (Hoch et al., 1986; Gehrman et al., 2003; Janssens et al., 2009; Kinugawa et al., 2014). In other studies, differences in the frequency of sleep breathing disorders in PSG studies in AD, in comparison to control groups, were minor (Bliwise, 2002; Moraes et al., 2008); while in some studies these differences have not been noticed at all (Bliwise et al., 1989). A possibility of participation of breathing disorders during sleep in etiology of AD is considered by inflammation states, oxidative stress and hypoxemia being caused by them (Dyken et al., 2004; Daulatzai, 2012, 2013). Moreover, breathing disorders during sleep may contribute to progress of AD-related vascular changes. For example, in the study of Buratti et al. (2014) the intima-media thickness (IMT) and cerebrovascular reactivity to hypercapnia based on a breath-holding index (BHI) have been compared in groups of patients with and without OSA syndrome in the course of AD (Buratti et al., 2014). It has been stated that incorrect values of examined parameters (IMT > 1.0 mm, BHI < 0.69) occurred more often in patients with OSA syndrome than in patients without breathing disorders during sleep (HR respectively, 2.98; 95% CI: 1.37–6.46, $p < 0.05$ and 5.25; 95% CI: 2.35–11.74, $p < 0.05$). Indirectly, a correlation between sleep fragmentation and appearance of cognitive disorders was found in the observations conducted in 298 women at the age of 82.3 ± 3.2 years, who were diagnosed with OSA syndrome. Repeated breathing disorders in this syndrome caused sleep fragmentation, because arousals finish the periods of apneas and hypopneas. A prospective study revealed that after 5 years, the risk of mild cognitive disorders or dementi clearly grows (OR 2.04; 95% CI 1.10–3.78) together with increase of apneas and hypopneas frequency (Yaffe et al., 2011).

In a previous study encompassing 59 patients with dementia (MMSE 20.1 ± 6.6), who underwent PSG, OSA syndrome (moderate or severe form) was diagnosed in almost half of the patients (49%). It has been stated at the same time that risk of excitation at night was the smallest in the patients with high apnoe/hypopnoe index (AHI), i.e., with more severe OSA syndrome (Rose et al., 2011). It has been also proved that for some patients with mild or moderate form of AD, prevention of obstructive breathing disorders during sleep with continuous positive airway pressure (CPAP) can slow down development of dementia (Cooke et al., 2009). For instance, in the group of 23 patients with mild and moderate form of AD (MMSE > 15), as well as with severe form of OSA syndrome (AHI ≥ 30), cognitive disorders were compared after 3 years among patients who used or did not use CPAP and a reduction in the rate of cognitive disorders decline has been stated—measured in MMSE scale—in the group using CPAP [−0.7 (90% CI −1.7; +0.8 vs. −2.2 (90% CI 3.3–1.9); $p = 0.013$] (Troussière et al., 2014).

There is evidence indicating a link between OSA and AD (**Figure 2**). In a recently published study, it has been shown that OSA might induce early changes in CSF Aß 42 concentrations (Liguori et al., 2017). In this study, CSF $Aß_{42}$ concentrations were measured in 25 moderate or severe OSA patients with apnea and hypopnea index > 15/h, in 10 OSA patients treated with continuous positive airway pressure (CPAP, method of choice eliminating sleep apneas) and in 15 controls. In untreated OSA patients, CSF $Aß_{42}$ concentrations were lower than in controls and lower than in CPAP treated OSA patients. Additionally, in OSA patients, a correlation between CSF $Aß_{42}$ concentrations and arterial oxygen saturation during sleep was found, thus confirming the influence of the sleep disordered breathing on AD biomarkers. In another recent study, cognitively normal elderly persons (aged 55–90 years) were prospectively observed for 2 years (Sharma et al., 2017). After adjusting for age, sex and BMI, the association between severity of OSA, as indicated by apnea/hypopnea index, an annual rate change of CSF $Aß_{42}$ concentrations was found. These findings indicate that in cognitively normal older persons, OSA is associated with increased amyloid brain deposition. Repetitive arterial oxygen desaturations and/or sleep fragmentation, and known direct consequences of sleep apneas and hypopneas (Brzecka and Davies, 1993) are likely mechanisms linking OSA with MCI and AD. In a study of 38 cognitively normal persons −19 OSA patients (apnea/hypopnea index > 15/h, mean 21.2 ± 5.1/h, age 58.5 ± 4.1 years) and 19 controls of similar age—amyloid deposition in the brain was studied with Pittsburgh Compound B PET imaging (Yun et al., 2017). Higher amyloid deposition in the areas of right posterior cingulated gyrus and right temporal cortex was found in OSA patients as compared with controls, indicating the possibility of development or progression of AD as a consequence of sleep disordered breathing. Another confirmation of the link between OSA and AD was provided by a longitudinal 15-years long study of 1,667 participants (Lutsey et al., 2018). In the patients with severe OSA (with apnea/hypopnea index > 30/h)—but not in all OSA patients—there was higher risk ratio of AD dementia (1.66, 95% CI 1.06–5.18).

Periodic Limb Movements During Sleep and Restless Legs Syndrome

Periodic leg movements (PLM) can also lead to sleep fragmentation. In the study cited above (Rose et al., 2011), among 37% older people with dementia, PLM index (PLMI) was ≥15/h, indicating moderate to severe form of the disease. In comparison to results of the study conducted in 455 women at the age of 82.9 years, where PLMI ≥15/h has been found in 52% of patients (Claman et al., 2006), the percentage was smaller. In the other study, including 28 patients at the age of 67.8 ± 8.7 years with AD of moderate severity (MMSE 17.8 ± 6.8 points), not receiving any treatment possibly interfering with sleeps, and examined with PSG, more frequent occurrence of PLM was not observed in comparison to healthy people at similar age (Bliwise et al., 2012). PLM is usually accompanied by restless leg syndrome (RLS). This syndrome is diagnosed on the basis of medical history. However, it has been proved that patients with AD, even in the time of mild cognitive disorders, were not able to describe the symptoms of RLS properly (Tractenberg et al., 2005). On the other hand, based on the observations of the patients, it has been stated that symptoms indicating RLS (probable diagnosis of RLS) in the course of AD occur among about 4%–5.5% of patients (Ohayon and Roth, 2002; Talarico et al., 2013). In a study of 339 patients with AD, there were 14 patients meeting the criteria of RLS (Talarico et al., 2013). The patients with concomitant RLS were younger and more apathetic than AD patients without RLS ($p = 0.029$ and $p = 0.001$, respectively). This clinical observation suggested a dysfunction of dopaminergic system in the patients with RLS in the course of AD disease. The problem of RLS in AD may be important, as there are observations from other patients' groups that up to 90% of patients with RLS have sleep disruption caused by concomitant PLM syndrome (Skalski, 2017).

Sleep and Brain Glymphatic System in AD

Recent reports indicate an important relation between disrupted sleep, brain glymphatic system and AD (Mendelsohn and Larrick, 2013; Lee et al., 2015; O'Donnell et al., 2015; Krueger et al., 2016). For instance, glymphatic system consists of para-vascular channels located around blood vessels of the brain. CSF flows along para-arterial space, reaches the capillary bed and penetrates into the brain parenchyma, where it gets mixed with interstitial fluid and after collecting metabolic waste it is moved to para-venous space and then to cervical lymphatic vessels (Ratner et al., 2015). Thus, it can be stated that glymphatic system acts like the lymphatic system in the other body organs.

One of the glymphatic system functions is the removal of metabolites and neurotoxic compounds, including soluble Aβ from the CNS parenchyma (Kyrtsos and Baras, 2015; Bakker et al., 2016; Simon and Iliff, 2016). It has been demonstrated that more than half of Aβ could be removed from the brain through the glymphatic system (Iliff et al., 2012). It seems that sleep may influence glymphatic system function. During natural sleep, there is a marked increase of the brain's interstitial space as compared with wakefulness, possibly resulting from the shrinkage of astroglial cells (Mendelsohn and Larrick, 2013; Xie et al., 2013; Kress et al., 2014; O'Donnell et al., 2015). The enlargement of the extracellular space accelerates clearance processes. It has been found that in mice, the clearance of the Aβ during sleep was two-fold faster than during wakefulness (Xie et al., 2013). In the other animal study, it has been demonstrated that the speed of clearance through the glymphatic system depends also on the body posture (Lee et al., 2015). The glymphatic transport was the

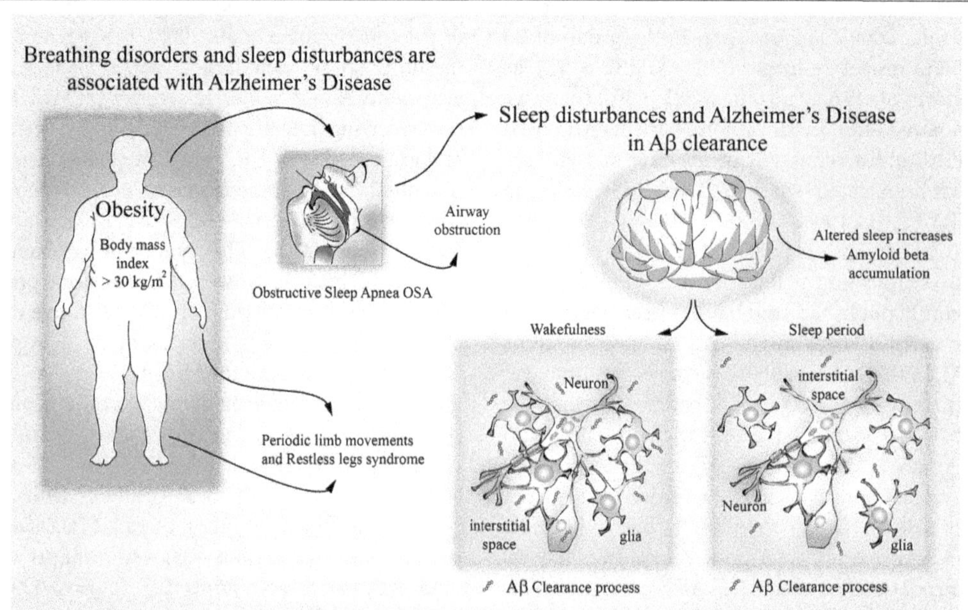

FIGURE 2 | Breathing disorders and amyloid beta clearance. It has been observed that sleep disorders in AD can be caused by obstructive sleep apnea (OSA). OSA is caused by an obstruction of respiratory airways, and its main risk overweight in obesity. Prospective studies have shown that patients with OSA may develop AD by several mechanisms such as neuroinflammation, oxidative stress and hypoxemia. Interestingly, clinical conditions like periodic limb movements and restless legs syndrome, which also lead to sleep disturbances, may be associated to AD. The removal of metabolites and neurotoxic compounds via glymphatic system is a function regulated by sleep and wakefulness activity. It is known that soluble amyloid beta can be cleared from the CNS parenchyma using the glymphatic system. Sleep may influence the clearance of amyloid beta due to the increased brain's interstitial space possibly by the shrinkage of astroglial cells.

most efficient in the lateral position, which is the most common during sleep.

As Aβ clearance is impaired in both early and late forms of AD (Tarasoff-Conway et al., 2015), it can be assumed that there is a link between impaired glymphatic system function and AD. Experiments in animal and humans revealed diurnal oscillation of the Aβ level in the brain interstitial fluid (Musiek, 2015). Indeed, as endogenous neuronal activity influences the regional concentration of the Aβ in the interstitial fluid (Bero et al., 2011), decreased neuronal activity in some stages of sleep may cause the oscillations of the Aβ concentrations. Slow wave sleep with periodic neuronal hyperpolarization and diminished neuronal firing in some brain regions can be associated with decreased Aβ production (Musiek, 2015). Thus, altered sleep quality might contribute to the onset and progression of the AD both through impaired glymphatic clearance and disturbances in the Aβ production in case of disordered slow wave sleep.

Although the presence of glymphatic system has been proved in animal studies, there is also evidence indicating its function in humans (Kiviniemi et al., 2016). The diffusion-based MR technique called diffusion tensor image analysis along the perivascular space has been used to reflect impairment of the glymphatic system in AD patients (Taoka et al., 2017). The usefulness of diffusion tensor imaging measurements has been also shown in distinguishing patients with early-stage AD from those with subcortical ischemic vascular disease (Tu et al., 2017).

Among sleep stages, specifically slow wave sleep, exert the influence on $A\beta_{42}$ level in the CSF. In a study encompassing 36 cognitively normal and elderly subjects, CSF $A\beta_{42}$ levels inversely correlated with slow wave sleep duration ($r = -0.35$, $p < 0.05$), slow wave sleep % of total sleep time ($r = -0.36$, $p < 0.05$) and slow wave activity in frontal EEG leads during sleep time ($r = -0.45$, $p < 0.01$) (Varga et al., 2016). Additionally, local Aβ accumulation was found to be associated specifically with diminished slow wave activity during sleep in the low frequency range (0.6–1 Hz) (Mander et al., 2015). These findings may indicate the association between decreased clearance and/or production of Aβ and slow wave sleep deficiency.

Final Remarks

The above listed clinical and experimental observations strongly suggest bidirectional relationship between sleep and AD. Sleep disorders, such as difficulties in falling asleep, sleep disruption and altered circadian sleep-wake cycle, are typical symptoms of AD and usually escalate with progression of the disease (Bliwise et al., 1995; McCurry et al., 1999; McCurry and Ancoli-Israel, 2003; Most et al., 2012; Lim et al., 2013; Spira et al., 2013; Dos Santos et al., 2014, 2015; Spalletta et al., 2015). PSG studies reveal macro- and micro-structure sleep abnormalities in both clinical and preclinical AD (Prinz et al., 1982; Bliwise, 1993; Rauchs et al., 2008; Westerberg et al., 2012; Hita-Yañez et al., 2013; Liguori et al., 2014; Maestri et al., 2015). There is a correlation between sleep-wake rhythm disturbance and signs of cerebral Aβ deposition (Lim et al., 2013). On the other hand, sleep abnormalities may increase the risk of AD development. There are empirical data showing increased levels of $A\beta_{42}$ in CSF after sleep deprivation (Ooms et al., 2014). There is also growing evidence showing that severe sleep disturbances caused by breathing disorders during sleep may influence AD development and progression (Dyken et al., 2004; Cooke et al., 2009; Rose et al., 2011; Daulatzai, 2013; Buratti et al., 2014; Troussière et al., 2014; Liguori et al., 2017; Sharma et al., 2017; Yun et al., 2017; Lutsey et al., 2018). In OSA patients the signs of increased amyloid deposition in the brain were observed (Sharma et al., 2017; Yun et al., 2017).

The key to understanding the link between sleep disturbances and AD development may be the function of glymphatic system. The activity of glymphatic system augments during sleep (Pistollato et al., 2016) and —to some extent —Aβ is cleared through the glymphatic system (Boespflug and Iliff, 2018). Thus, disrupted sleep may lead to glymphatic system function impairment and Aβ accumulation. Possible mechanisms of bidirectional relationship between sleep disturbances and Aβ clearance should be taken into consideration.

CONCLUSION

Clinical observations indicate the likelihood of a bidirectional relationship between abnormalities of sleep and AD. Changes in sleep structure, worse sleep quality in both preclinical and symptomatic AD, correlation of cognitive impairments with sleep structure abnormalities, changes in CSF Aß concentrations induced by sleep apneas and correlating with severity of sleep disordered breathing, the influence of physiological sleep on clearance of Aβ through the glymphatic system, possible influence of impaired glymphatic system on Aβ level, and observations with the use of the newest technical equipment reflecting impairment of the glymphatic system in AD patients allow to conclude that disordered sleep may contribute to the development of AD pathology.

Future Direction of the Research

1. Electrophysiologic sleep studies aimed to find early signs of risk of development of AD in target populations.
2. Development of specific procedures leading to improvement of sleep structure and quality.
3. The studies on glymphatic system in sleep breathing disorders in relation to the risk of $A\beta_{42}$ accumulation.
4. Testing possible relationship between worsening of cognitive abilities and inflammatory state, oxidative stress, hypoxemia or vascular pathology and other neuropathological signs in AD, and TAU protein production.
5. Based on the analysis of sleep and its disorders, identify new directions of AD therapy, especially at its pre-symptomatic stages.

AUTHOR CONTRIBUTIONS

All authors listed, have made substantial, direct and intellectual contribution to the work, and approved it for publication.

ACKNOWLEDGMENTS

This research was supported in part by RSF project #14-23-00160P and the scientific projects of IPAC (topics 48.8. and 48.9). Authors' also very grateful for the animal facilities were provided by Center for preclinical trials of IPAC RAS.

REFERENCES

Aliev, G., Priyadarshini, M., Reddy, V. P., Grieg, N. H., Kaminsky, Y., Cacabelos, R., et al. (2014). Oxidative stress mediated mitochondrial and vascular lesions as markers in the pathogenesis of Alzheimer disease. *Curr. Med. Chem.* 21, 2208–2217. doi: 10.2174/09298673216661312271613 03

Ancoli-Israel, S., Clopton, P., Klauber, M. R., Fell, R., and Mason, W. (1997). Use of wrist activity for monitoring sleep/wake in demented nursing-home patients. *Sleep* 20, 24–27. doi: 10.1093/sleep/20.1.24

Ancoli-Israel, S., Kripke, D. F., Klauber, M. R., Mason, W. J., Fell, R., and Kaplan, O., et al. (1991). Sleep-disordered breathing in community-dwelling elderly. *Sleep* 14, 486–495. doi: 10.1093/sleep/14.6.486

Ansari, S. A., Satar, R., Perveen, A., and Ashraf, G. M. (2017). Current opinion in Alzheimer's disease therapy by nanotechnology-based approaches. *Curr. Opin. Psychiatry* 30, 128–135. doi: 10.1097/YCO.0000000000000310

Ashraf, G. M., Chibber, S., Mohammad, Zaidi, S. K., Tabrez, S., Ahmad, A., et al. (2016). Recent updates on the association between Alzheimer's disease and vascular dementia. *Med. Chem.* 12, 226–237. doi: 10.2174/1573406411666151030111820

Ashraf, G. M., Greig, N. H., Khan, T. A., Hassan, I., Tabrez, S., and Shakil, S. (2014). Protein misfolding and aggregation in Alzheimer's disease and type 2 diabetes mellitus. *CNS Neurol. Disord. Drug Targets* 13, 1280–1293. doi: 10.2174/1871527313666140917095514

Ashraf, G. M., Tabrez, S., Jabir, N. R., Firoz, C. K., Ahmad, S., Hassan, I., et al. (2015). An overview on global trends in nanotechnological approaches for Alzheimer therapy. *Curr. Drug Metab.* 16, 719–727. doi: 10.2174/138920021608151107125757

Bakker, E. N., Bacska, B. J., Arbel-Ornath, M., Aldea, R., Bedussi, B., Morris, A. W., et al. (2016). Lymphatic clearance of the brain: perivascular, paravascular and significance for neurodegenerative diseases. *Cell Mol. Neurobiol.* 36, 181–194. doi: 10.1007/s10571-015-0273-8

Bero, A. W., Yan, P., Roh, J. H., Cirrito, J. R., Stewart, F. R., Raichle, M. E., et al. (2011). Neuronal activity regulates the regional vulnerability to amyloid-beta deposition. *Nat. Neurosci.* 14, 750–756. doi: 10.1038/nn .2801

Bhat, S. A., Kamal, M. A., Yarla, N. S., and Ashraf, G. M. (2017). Synopsis on managment strategies for neurodegenerative disorders: challenges from bench to bedside in successful drug discovery and development. *Curr. Top. Med. Chem.* 17, 1371–1378. doi: 10.2174/1568026616666161222121229

Bliwise, D. L. (1993). Sleep in normal aging and dementia. *Sleep* 16, 40–81. doi: 10.1093/sleep/16.1.40

Bliwise, D. L. (2002). Sleep apnea, APOE4 and Alzheimer's disease 20 years and counting? *J. Psychosom. Res.* 53, 539–546. doi: 10.1016/S0022-3999(02)00436-1

Bliwise, D. L., Hughes, M., McMahon, P. M., and Kutner, N. (1995). Observed sleep/wakefulness and severity of dementia in an Alzheimer's disease special care unit. *J. Gerontol. A Biol. Sci. Med. Sci.* 50, M303–M306. doi: 10.1093/gerona/50A.6.M303

Bliwise, D. L., Trotti, L. M., Yesavage, J. A., and Rye, D. B. (2012). Periodic leg movements in sleep in elderly patients with Parkinsonism and Alzheimer's disease. *Eur. J. Neurol.* 19, 918–923. doi: 10.1111/j.1468-1331.2012. 03673.x

Bliwise, D. L., Yesavage, J. A., Tinklenberg, J. R., and Dement, W. C. (1989). Sleep apnea in Alzheimer's disease. *Neurobiol. Aging* 10, 343–346. doi: 10.1016/0197-4580(89)90046-8

Boespflug, E. L., and Iliff, J. J. (2018). The emerging relationship between interstitial fluid-cerebrospinal fluid exchange, amyloid-β, and sleep. *Biol. Psychiatry* 83, 328–336. doi: 10.1016/j.biopsych.2017.11.031

Brzecka, A., and Davies, S. F. (1993). Profound sleep hypoxia in morbidly obese hypercapnic patients with obstructive sleep apnea. *Mater. Med. Pol.* 25, 63–71.

Buratti, L., Viticchi, G., Falsetti, L., Cagnetti, C., Luzzi, S., and Bartolini, M. (2014). Vascular impairment in Alzheimer's disease: the role of obstructive sleep apnea. *J. Alzheimers Dis.* 38, 445–453. doi: 10.3233/JAD-131046

Chibber, S., Alexiou, A., Alama, M. N., Barreto, G. E., Aliev, G., and Ashraf, G. M. (2016). A synopsis on the linkage between age-related dementias and vascular disorders. *CNS Neurol. Disord. Drug Targets.* 15, f250–f258. doi: 10.2174/1871527315666160202121809

Chuang, Y. F., An, Y., Bilgel, M., Wong, D. F., Troncoso, J. C., O'Brien, R. J., et al. (2016). Midlife adiposity predicts earlier onset of Alzheimer's dementia, neuropathology and presymptomatic cerebral amyloid accumulation. *Mol. Psychiatry* 21, 910–915. doi: 10.1038/mp.2015.129

Claman, D. M., Redline, S., Blackwell, T., Ancoli-Israel, S., Surovec, S., Scott, N., et al. (2006). Prevalence and correlates of periodic limb movements in older women. *J. Clin. Sleep Med.* 2, 438–445.

Cooke, J. R., Ayalon, L., Palmer, B. W., Loredo, J. S., Corey-Bloom, J., Natarajan, L., et al. (2009). Sustained use of CPAP slows deterioration of cognition, sleep, and mood in patients with Alzheimer's disease and obstructive sleep apnea: a preliminary study. *J. Clin. Sleep Med.* 5, 305–309. doi: 10.1016/j.sleep.2008.12.016

Daulatzai, M. A. (2012). Pathogenesis of cognitive dysfunction in patients with obstructive sleep apnea: a hypothesis with emphasis on the nucleus tractus solitarius. *Sleep Disord.* 2012:251096. doi: 10.1155/2012/251096

Daulatzai, M. A. (2013). Death by a thousand cuts in Alzheimer's disease: hypoxia–the prodrome. *Neurotox. Res.* 24, 216–243. doi: 10.1007/s12640-013-9379-2

Dos Santos, A. B., Barreto, G. E., and Kohlmeier, K. A. (2014). Treatment of sleeping disorders should be considered in clinical management of Parkinson's disease. *Front. Aging Neurosci.* 6:273. doi: 10.3389/fnagi.2014.00273

Dos Santos, A. B., Kohlmeier, K. A., and Barreto, G. E. (2015). Are sleep disturbances preclinical markers of Parkinson's disease? *Neurochem. Res.* 40, 421–427. doi: 10.1007/s11064-014-1488-7

Drago, V., Babiloni, C., Bartrés-Faz, D., Caroli, A., Bosch, B., Hensch, T., et al. (2011). Disease tracking markers for Alzheimer's disease at the prodromal (MCI) stage. *J. Alzheimers Dis.* 26, 159–199. doi: 10.3233/JAD-2011-0043

Dyken, M. E., Yamada, T., Glenn, C. L., and Berger, H. A. (2004). Obstructive sleep apnea associated with cerebral hypoxemia and death. *Neurology* 62, 491–493. doi: 10.1212/01.WNL.0000106952.84223.F3

Emmerzaal, T. L., Kiliaan, A. J., and Gustafson, D. R. (2015). 2003–2013: a decade of body mass index, Alzheimer's disease, and dementia. *J. Alzheimers Dis.* 43, 739–755. doi: 10.3233/JAD-141086

Faubel, R., López-García, E., Guallar-Castillón, P., Graciani, A., Banegas, J. R., and Rodríguez-Artalejo, F. (2009). Usual sleep duration and cognitive function in older adults in Spain. *J. Sleep Res.* 18, 427–435. doi: 10.1111/j.1365-2869.2009.00759.x

Fitzpatrick, A. L., Kuller, L. H., Lopez, O. L., Diehr, P., O'Meara, E. S., and Longstreth, W. T. Jr. (2009). Midlife and late-life obesity and the risk of dementia: cardiovascular health study. *Arch. Neurol.* 66, 336–342. doi: 10.1001/archneurol.2008.582

Gehrman, P. R., Martin, J. L., Shochat, T., Nolan, S., Corey-Bloom, J., and Ancoli-Israel, S. (2003). Sleep-disordered breathing and agitation in institutionalized adults with Alzheimer disease. *Am. J. Geriatr. Psychiatry* 11, 426–433. doi: 10.1097/00019442-200307000-00005

Gu, Y., Scarmeas, N., Cosentino, S., Brandt, J., Albert, M., Blacker, D., et al. (2014). Change in body mass index before and after Alzheimer's disease onset. *Curr. Alzheimer Res.* 11, 349–356. doi: 10.2174/15672050106661311201 10930

Hassainia, F., Petit, D., Nielsen, T., Gauthier, S., and Montplaisir, J. (1997). Quantitative EEG and statistical mapping of wakefulness and REM sleep in the evaluation of mild to moderate Alzheimer's disease. *Eur. Neurol.* 37, 219–224. doi: 10.1159/000117446

Hita-Yañez, E., Atienza, M., and Cantero, J. L. (2013). Polysomnographic and subjective sleep markers of mild cognitive impairment. *Sleep* 36, 1327–1334. doi: 10.5665/sleep.2956

Hoch, C. C., Reynolds, C. F. III., Kupfer, D. J., Houck, P. R., Berman, S. R., and Stack, J. A. (1986). Sleep-disordered breathing in normal and pathologic aging. *J. Clin. Psychiatry* 47, 499–503.

Iliff, J. J., Wang, M., Liao, Y., Plogg, B. A., Peng, W., Gundersen, G. A., et al. (2012). A paravascular pathway facilitates CSF flow through the brain parenchyma and the clearance of interstitial solutes, including amyloid β. *Sci. Transl. Med.* 4:147ra111. doi: 10.1126/scitranslmed.3003748

Jabir, N. R., Firoz, C. K., Baeesa, S. S., Ashraf, G. M., Akhtar, S., Kamal, W., et al. (2015). Synopsis on the linkage of Alzheimer's and Parkinson's disease with chronic diseases. *CNS Neurosci. Ther.* 21, 1–7. doi: 10.1111/cns.12344

Janssens, J. P., Metzger, M., and Sforza, E. (2009). Impact of volume targeting on efficacy of bi-level non-invasive ventilation and sleep in obesity-hypoventilation. *Respir. Med.* 103, 165–172. doi: 10.1016/j.rmed.2008.03.013

Ju, Y. E., McLeland, J. S., Toedebusch, C. D., Xiong, C., Fagan, A. M., Duntley, S. P., et al. (2013). Sleep quality and preclinical Alzheimer disease. *JAMA Neurol.* 70, 587–593. doi: 10.1001/jamaneurol.2013.2334

Karran, E., Mercken, M., and De Strooper, B. (2011). The amyloid cascade hypothesis for Alzheimer's disease: an appraisal for the development of therapeutics. *Nat. Rev. Drug Discov.* 10, f698–f712. doi: 10.1038/nrd3505

Kinugawa, K., Nguyen-Michel, V. H., and Mariani, J. (2014). [Obstructive sleep apnea syndrome: a cause of cognitive disorders in the elderly?]. *Rev. Med. Interne.* 35, 664–669. doi: 10.1016/j.revmed.2014.02.005

Kiviniemi, V., Wang, X., Korhonen, V., Keinänen, T., Tuovinen, T., Autio, J., et al. (2016). Ultra-fast magnetic resonance encephalography of physiological brain activity-Glymphatic pulsationmechanisms? *J. Cereb. Blood Flow Metab.* 36, 1033–1045. doi: 10.1177/0271678X15622047

Kress, B. T., Iliff, J. J., Xia, M., Wang, M., Wei, H. S., Zeppenfeld, D., et al. (2014). Impairment of paravascular clearance pathways in the aging brain. *Ann. Neurol.* 76, 845–861. doi: 10.1002/ana.24271

Krueger, J. M., Frank, M. G., Wisor, J. P., and Roy, S. (2016). Sleep function: toward elucidating an enigma. *Sleep Med. Rev.* 28, 46–54. doi: 10.1016/j.smrv.2015.08.005

Kyrtsos, C. R., and Baras, J. S. (2015). Modeling the role of the glymphatic pathway and cerebral blood vessel properties in Alzheimer's disease pathogenesis. *PLoS ONE* 10:e0139574. doi: 10.1371/journal.pone.0139574

Lee, H., Xie, L., Yu, M., Kang, H., Feng, T., Deane, R., et al. (2015). The effect of body posture on brain glymphatic transport. *J. Neurosci.* 35, 11034–11044. doi: 10.1523/JNEUROSCI.1625-15.2015

Liguori, C., Mercuri, N. B., Izzi, F., Romigi, A., Cordella, A., Sancesario, G., et al. (2017). Obstructive sleep apnea is associated with early but possibly modifiable Alzheimer's disease biomarkers changes. *Sleep* 40:zsx011. doi: 10.1093/sleep/zsx011

Liguori, C., Romigi, A., Nuccetelli, M., Zannino, S., Sancesario, G., Martorana, A., et al. (2014). Orexinergic system dysregulation, sleep impairment, and cognitive decline in Alzheimer disease. *JAMA Neurol.* 71, 1498–1505. doi: 10.1001/jamaneurol.2014.2510

Lim, A. S., Kowgier, M., Yu, L., Buchman, A. S., and Bennett, D. A. (2013). Sleep fragmentation and the risk of incident Alzheimer's disease and cognitive decline in older persons. *Sleep* 36, 1027–1032. doi: 10.5665/sleep.2802

Lutsey, P. L., Misialek, J. R., Mosley, T. H., Gottesman, R. F., Punjabi, N. M., Shahar, E., et al. (2018). Sleep characteristics and risk of dementia and Alzheimer's disease: the atherosclerosis risk in communities study. *Alzheimers Dement.* 14, 157–166. doi: 10.1016/j.jalz.2017.06.2269

Maestri, M., Carnicelli, L., Tognoni, G., Di Coscio, E., Giorgi, F. S., Volpi, L., et al. (2015). Non-rapid eye movement sleep instability in mild cognitive impairment: a pilot study. *Sleep Med.* 16, 1139–1145. doi: 10.1016/j.sleep.2015.04.027

Mander, B. A., Marks, S. M., Vogel, J. W., Rao, V., Lu, B., Saletin, J. M., et al. (2015). β-amyloid disrupts human NREM slow waves and related hippocampus-dependent memory consolidation. *Nat. Neurosci.* 18, 1051–1057. doi: 10.1038/nn.4035

McCurry, S. M., and Ancoli-Israel, S. (2003). Sleep dysfunction in Alzheimer's disease and other dementias. *Curr. Treat. Options Neurol.* 5, 261–272. doi: 10.1007/s11940-003-0017-9

McCurry, S. M., Logsdon, R. G., Teri, L., Gibbons, L. E., Kukull, W. A., Bowen, J. D., et al. (1999). Characteristics of sleep disturbance in community-dwelling Alzheimer's disease patients. *J. Geriatr. Psychiatry Neurol.* 12, 53–59. doi: 10.1177/089198879901200203

Mendelsohn, A. R., and Larrick, J. W. (2013). Sleep facilitates clearance of metabolites from the brain: glymphatic function in aging and neurodegenerative diseases. *Rejuvenation Res.* 16, 518–523. doi: 10.1089/rej.2013.1530

Moraes, W., Poyares, D., Sukys-Claudino, L., Guilleminault, C., and Tufik, S. (2008). Donepezil improves obstructive sleep apnea in Alzheimer disease: a double-blind, placebo-controlled study. *Chest* 133, 677–683. doi: 10.1378/chest.07-1446

Moran, M., Lynch, C. A., Walsh, C., Coen, R., Coakley, D., and Lawlor, B. A. (2005). Sleep disturbance in mild to moderate Alzheimer's disease. *Sleep Med.* 6, 347–352. doi: 10.1016/j.sleep.2004.12.005

Most, E. I., Aboudan, S., Scheltens, P., and Van Someren, E. J. (2012). Discrepancy between subjective and objective sleep disturbances in early- and moderate-stage Alzheimer disease. *Am. J. Geriatr. Psychiatry* 20, 460–467. doi: 10.1097/JGP.0b013e318252e3ff

Musiek, E. S. (2015). Circadian clock disruption in neurodegenerative diseases: cause and effect? *Front. Pharmacol.* 6:29. doi:10.3389/fphar.2015.00029

O'Donnell, J., Ding, F., and Nedergaard, M. (2015). Distinct functional states of astrocytes during sleep and wakefulness: is norepinephrine the master regulator? *Curr. Sleep Med. Rep.* 1, 1–8. doi: 10.1007/s40675-014-0004-6

Ohayon, M. M., and Roth, T. (2002). Prevalence of restless legs syndrome and periodic limb movement disorder in the general population. *J. Psychosom. Res.* 53, 547–554. doi: 10.1016/S0022-3999(02)00443-9

Ooms, S., Overeem, S., Besse, K., Rikkert, M. O., Verbeek, M., and Claassen, J. A. (2014). Effect of 1 night of total sleep deprivation on cerebrospinal fluid beta-amyloid 42 in healthy middle-aged men: a randomized clinical trial. *JAMA Neurol.* 71, 971–977. doi: 10.1001/jamaneurol.2014.1173

Peter-Derex, L., Yammine, P., Bastuji, H., and Croisile, B. (2015). Sleep and Alzheimer's disease. *Sleep Med. Rev.* 19, 29–38. doi: 10.1016/j.smrv.2014.03.007

Petit, D., Gagnon, J. F., Fantini, M. L., Ferini-Strambi, L., and Montplaisir, J. (2004). Sleep and quantitative EEG in neurodegenerative disorders. *J. Psychosom. Res.* 56, 487–496. doi: 10.1016/j.jpsychores.2004.02.001

Pistollato, F., Sumalla Cano, S., Elio, I., Masias Vergara, M., Giampieri, F., and Battino, M. (2016). Associations between sleep, cortisol regulation, and diet: possible implications for the risk of Alzheimer disease. *Adv. Nutr.* 7, 679–689. doi: 10.3945/an.115.011775

Potvin, O., Lorrain, D., Forget, H., Dubé, M., Grenier, S., Préville, M., et al. (2012). Sleep quality and 1-year incident cognitive impairment in community-dwelling older adults. *Sleep* 35, f491–f499. doi: 10.5665/sleep.1732

Prince, M., Bryce, R., Albanese, E., Wimo, A., Ribeiro, W., and Ferri, C. P. (2013). The global prevalence of dementia: a systematic review and metaanalysis. *Alzheimers. Dement.* 9, 63.e2–75.e2. doi: 10.1016/j.jalz.2012.11.007

Prinz, P. N., Peskind, E. R., Vitaliano, P. P., Raskind, M. A., Eisdorfer, C., Zemcuznikov, N., et al. (1982). Changes in the sleep and waking EEGs of nondemented and demented elderly subjects. *J. Am. Geriatr. Soc.* 30, 86–93. doi: 10.1111/j.1532-5415.1982.tb01279.x

Ratner, V., Zhu, L., Kolesov, I., Nedergaard, M., Benveniste, H., and Tannenbaum, A. (2015). Optimal-mass-transfer-based estimation of glymphatic transport in living brain. *Proc. SPIE Int. Soc. Opt. Eng.* 9413:94131J. doi: 10.1117/12.2076289

Rauchs, G., Schabus, M., Parapatics, S., Bertran, F., Clochon, P., Hot, P., et al. (2008). Is there a link between sleep changes and memory in Alzheimer's disease? *Neuroreport* 19, 1159–1162. doi: 10.1097/WNR.0b013e32830867c4

Rizvi, S. M., Shaikh, S., Waseem, S. M., Shakil, S., Abuzenadah, A. M., Biswas, D., et al. (2015). Role of anti-diabetic drugs as therapeutic agents in Alzheimer's disease. *EXCLI J.* 14, 684–696. doi: 10.17179/excli 2015-252

Rose, K. M., Beck, C., Tsai, P. F., Liem, P. H., Davila, D. G., Kleban, M., et al. (2011). Sleep disturbances and nocturnal agitation behaviors in older adults with dementia. *Sleep* 34, 779–786. doi: 10.5665/SLEEP.1048

Saint Martin, M., Roche, F., Thomas, T., Collet, P., Barthélémy, J. C., and Sforza, E. (2015). Association of body fat composition and obstructive sleep apnea in the elderly: a longitudinal study. *Obesity* 23, 1511–1516. doi: 10.1002/oby.21121

Selkoe, D., and Hardy, J. (2016). The amyloid hypothesis of Alzheimer's disease at 25 years. *EMBO Mol. Med.* 8, 595–608. doi: 10.15252/emmm.201606210

Sen, D., Majumder, A., Arora, V., Yadu, N., and Chakrabarti, R. (2017). Taming Alzheimer's disease: new perspectives, newer horizons. *Iran J. Neurol.* 16, 146–155.

Sharma, R. A., Varga, A. W., Bubu, O. M., Pirraglia, E., Kam, K., Parekh, A., et al. (2017). Obstructive sleep apnea severity affects amyloid burden in cognitively normal elderly: a longitudinal study. *Am. J. Respir. Crit. Care Med.* 197, 933–943. doi: 10.1164/rccm.201704-0704OC

Simon, M. J., and Iliff, J. J. (2016). Regulation of cerebrospinal fluid (CSF) flow in neurodegenerative, neurovascular and neuroinflammatory disease. *Biochim. Biophys. Acta.* 1862, 442–451. doi: 10.1016/j.bbadis.2015.10.014

Skalski, M. (2017). *[Sleep-Wake Disorders; DSM-5 Selections]*, Wroclaw: Edra, Urban and Partner.

Soursou, G., Alexiou, A., Ashraf, G. M., Siyal, A. A., Mushtaq, G., and Kamal, M. A. (2015). Applications of nanotechnology in diagnostics and therapeutics of Alzheimer's and Parkinson's disease. *Curr. Drug Metab.* 16, 705–712. doi: 10.2174/138920021608151107125049

Spalletta, G., Long, J. D., Robinson, R. G., Trequattrini, A., Pizzoli, S., Caltagirone, C., et al. (2015). Longitudinal neuropsychiatric predictors of death in Alzheimer's disease. *J. Alzheimers Dis.* 48, 627–636. doi: 10.3233/JAD-150391

Spira, A. P., Gamaldo, A. A., An, Y., Wu, M. N., Simonsick, E. M., and Bilgel, M. (2013). Self-reported sleep and beta-amyloid deposition in community-dwelling older adults. *JAMA Neurol.* 70, 1537–1543. doi: 10.1001/jamaneurol.2013.4258

Talarico, G., Canevelli, M., Tosto, G., Vanacore, N., Letteri, F., Prastaro, M., et al. (2013). Restless legs syndrome in a group of patients with Alzheimer's disease. *Am. J. Alzheimers Dis. Other Demen.* 28, 165–170. doi: 10.1177/1533317512470208

Taoka, T., Masutani, Y., Kawai, H., Nakane, T., Matsuoka, K., Yasuno, F., et al. (2017). Evaluation of glymphatic system activity with the diffusion MR technique: diffusion tensor image analysis along the perivascular space (DTI-ALPS) in Alzheimer's disease cases. *Jpn. J. Radiol.* 35, 172–178. doi: 10.1007/s11604-017-0617-z

Tarasoff-Conway, J. M., Carare, R. O., Osorio, R. S., Glodzik, L., Butler, T., Fieremans, E., et al. (2015). Clearance systems in the brain-implications for Alzheimer disease. *Nat. Rev. Neurol.* 11, 457–470. doi: 10.1038/nrneurol.2015.119

Tractenberg, R. E., Singer, C. M., and Kaye, J. A. (2005). Symptoms of sleep disturbance in persons with Alzheimer's disease and normal elderly. *J. Sleep Res.* 14, 177–185. doi: 10.1111/j.1365-2869.2005.00445.x

Troussière, A. C., Charley, C. M., Salleron, J., Richard, F., Delbeuck, X., Derambure, P., et al. (2014). Treatment of sleep apnoea syndrome decreases cognitive decline in patients with Alzheimer's disease. *J. Neurol. Neurosurg. Psychiatr.* 85, 1405–1408. doi: 10.1136/jnnp-2013-307544

Tu, M. C., Lo, C. P., Huang, C. F., Hsu, Y. H., Huang, W. H., Deng, J. F., et al. (2017). Effectiveness of diffusion tensor imaging in differentiating early-stage subcortical ischemic vascular disease, Alzheimer's disease and normal ageing. *PLoS ONE* 12:e0175143. doi: 10.1371/journal.pone.0175143

Tworoger, S. S., Lee, S., Schernhammer, E. S., and Grodstein, F. (2006). The association of self-reported sleep duration, difficulty sleeping, and snoring with cognitive function in older women. *Alzheimer Dis. Assoc. Disord.* 20, 41–48. doi: 10.1097/01.wad.0000201850.52707.80

Varga, A. W., Wohlleber, M. E., Giménez, S., Romero, S., Alonso, J. F., Ducca, E. L., et al. (2016). Reduced slow-wave sleep is associated with high cerebrospinal fluid Aβ42 levels in cognitively normal elderly. *Sleep* 39, 2041–2048. doi: 10.5665/sleep.6240

Westerberg, C. E., Mander, B. A., Florczak, S. M., Weintraub, S., Mesulam, M. M., Zee, P. C., et al. (2012). Concurrent impairments in sleep and memory in amnestic mild cognitive impairment. *J. Int. Neuropsychol. Soc.* 18, 490–500. doi: 10.1017/S135561771200001X

Whitmer, R. A., Gunderson, E. P., Barrett-Connor, E., Quesenberry, C. P. Jr, and Yaffe, K. (2005). Obesity in middle age and future risk of dementia: a 27 year longitudinal population based study. *BMJ* 330:1360. doi: 10.1136/bmj.38446.466238.E0

Wyss-Coray, T., and Mucke, L. (2002). Inflammation in neurodegenerative disease–a double-edged sword. *Neuron* 35, f419–f432. doi: 10.1016/S0896-6273(02)00794-8

Xie, L., Kang, H., Xu, Q., Chen, M. J., Liao, Y., Thiyagarajan, M., et al. (2013). Sleep drives metabolite clearance from the adult brain. *Science* 342, 373–377. doi: 10.1126/science.1241224

Yaffe, K., Laffan, A. M., Harrison, S. L., Redline, S., Spira, A. P., Ensrud, K. E., et al. (2011). Sleep-disordered breathing, hypoxia, and risk of mild cognitive impairment and dementia in older women. *JAMA* 306, 613–619. doi: 10.1001/jama.2011.1115

Yun, C. H., Lee, H. Y., Lee, S. K., Kim, H., Seo, H. S., Bang, S. A., et al. (2017). Amyloid burden in obstructive sleep apnea. *J. Alzheimers Dis.* 59, 21–29. doi: 10.3233/JAD-161047

Zhao, Q. F., Tan, L., Wang, H. F., Jiang, T., Tan, M. S., Tan, L., et al. (2016). The prevalence of neuropsychiatric symptoms in Alzheimer's disease: systematic review and meta-analysis. *J. Affect. Disord.* 190, 264–271. doi: 10.1016/j.jad.2015.09.069

8

Targeting Beta-Amyloid at the CSF: A New Therapeutic Strategy in Alzheimer's Disease

Manuel Menendez-Gonzalez[1,2,3*], *Huber S. Padilla-Zambrano*[4], *Gabriel Alvarez*[5], *Estibaliz Capetillo-Zarate*[6,7,8,9], *Cristina Tomas-Zapico*[3,10] *and Agustin Costa*[11]

[1] Servicio de Neurologia, Hospital Universitario Central de Asturias, Oviedo, Spain, [2] Department of Cellular Morphology and Biology, University of Oviedo, Oviedo, Spain, [3] Instituto de Investigacion Sanitaria del Principado de Asturias, Oviedo, Spain, [4] Centro de Investigaciones Biomedicas (CIB), University of Cartagena, Cartagena, Colombia, [5] HealthSens, S.L., Oviedo, Spain, [6] Departamento de Neurociencias, Universidad del Pais Vasco (UPV/EHU), Leioa, Spain, [7] El Centro de Investigación Biomédica en Red sobre Enfermedades Neurodegenerativas, Madrid, Spain, [8] Achucarro Basque Center for Neuroscience, Leioa, Spain, [9] Ikerbasque, Basque Foundation for Science, Bilbao, Spain, [10] Department of Functional Biology, University of Oviedo, Oviedo, Spain, [11] Department of Physical and Analytical Chemistry, University of Oviedo, Oviedo, Spain

***Correspondence:**
Manuel Menendez-Gonzalez
manuelmenendezgonzalez@gmail.com

Although immunotherapies against the amyloid-β (Aβ) peptide tried so date failed to prove sufficient clinical benefit, Aβ still remains the main target in Alzheimer's disease (AD). This article aims to show the rationale of a new therapeutic strategy: clearing Aβ from the CSF continuously (the "CSF-sink" therapeutic strategy). First, we describe the physiologic mechanisms of Aβ clearance and the resulting AD pathology when these mechanisms are altered. Then, we review the experiences with peripheral Aβ-immunotherapy and discuss the related hypothesis of the mechanism of action of "peripheral sink." We also present Aβ-immunotherapies acting on the CNS directly. Finally, we introduce alternative methods of removing Aβ including the "CSF-sink" therapeutic strategy. As soluble peptides are in constant equilibrium between the ISF and the CSF, altering the levels of Aβ oligomers in the CSF would also alter the levels of such proteins in the brain parenchyma. We conclude that interventions based in a "CSF-sink" of Aβ will probably produce a steady clearance of Aβ in the ISF and therefore it may represent a new therapeutic strategy in AD.

Keywords: Alzheimer disease, amyloid beta-peptides, cerebrospinal fluid, immunotherapy, "CSF sink hypothesis"

PHYSIOLOGICAL CLEARANCE OF Aβ

Amyloid beta (Aβ) denotes peptides of 36–43 amino acids that are intrinsically unstructured, meaning that in solution it does not acquire a unique tertiary fold but rather populates a set of structures. These peptides derive from the amyloid precursor protein (APP), which is cleaved by beta- (BACE) and gamma-secretases to yield Aβ (Menendez-Gonzalez et al., 2005; O'Nuallain et al., 2010).

Amyloid beta is cleared from the brain by several independent mechanisms (Malm et al., 2010; Diem et al., 2017; Zuroff et al., 2017), including drainage to the vascular and glymphatic systems (DeMattos et al., 2001; Iliff et al., 2012, 2013; Tarasoff-Conway et al., 2015; Bakker et al., 2016; Zuroff et al., 2017), and *in situ* degradation by glial cells (Ries and Sastre, 2016; Zuroff et al., 2017). Astrocytes and microglia can produce Aβ degrading proteases like neprilysin, as well as chaperones involved in the clearance of Aβ. There is also a receptor mediated endocytosis, where receptors located in the surface of glial cells are involved in the uptake and clearance of Aβ, like lipoprotein receptor-related protein 1 (LRP), receptor for advanced glycation end products (RAGE) and others (Ries and Sastre, 2016). In transcytosis, Aβ is removed from ISF across the blood brain barrier (BBB) by LRP (Yamada et al., 2009). LRP binds Aβ in the brain and then transports it across the BBB into the systemic blood. The LRP extracellular domain is cleaved allowing the LRP bound to Aβ. RAGE protein brings unbound Aβ back into the CNS. The whole process is regulated by PICALM (Zhao et al., 2015). A perivascular pathway facilitates CSF flow through the brain parenchyma and the clearance of interstitial solutes, including Aβ (Iliff et al., 2012, 2013). It was thought that changes in arterial pulsatility may contribute to accumulation and deposition of toxic solutes, including Aβ, in the aging brain (Iliff et al., 2012, 2013). However, mathematical simulation showed that arterial pulsations are not strong enough to produce drainage velocities comparable to experimental observations and that a valve mechanism such as directional permeability of the intramural periarterial drainage pathway is necessary to achieve a net reverse flow (Diem et al., 2017).

ALTERED CLEARANCE OF Aβ IN ALZHEIMER'S DISEASE

The pathophysiology of Alzheimer's disease (AD) is characterized by the accumulation of Aβ and phospho-tau protein in the form of neuritic plaques and neurofibrillary tangles, respectively (Braak and Braak, 1991; Atwood et al., 2002). Aβ molecules can aggregate to form flexible soluble oligomers, which exist in several forms and are toxic to neurons (Haass and Selkoe, 2007), and finally into diffuse and dense plaques. Moreover, variable amounts of misfolded oligomers (known as "seeds") are taken up by neurons then transmitted from neuron to neuron via the extracellular milieu and can propagate aggregates by a 'seeding' or "prion like" mechanism (Walker et al., 2016; Lei et al., 2017). Tau also forms such prion-like misfolded oligomers, and there is some evidence that misfolded Aβ can induce tau misfolding (Pulawski et al., 2012; Nussbaum et al., 2013).

Amyloid-β accumulation has been hypothesized to result from an imbalance between Aβ production and clearance. An overproduction is probably the main cause of the disease in the familial AD where a mutation in the *APP, PSEN1,* or *PSEN2* genes is present (presenilins are postulated to regulate APP processing through their effects on gamma-secretase) while altered clearance is probably the main cause of the disease in sporadic AD. A good amount of studies reporting altered clearance of Aβ in AD have been published in recent years (Atwood et al., 2002; Mawuenyega et al., 2010; Tarasoff-Conway et al., 2015; Ries and Sastre, 2016; de Leon et al., 2017; Zuroff et al., 2017), becoming one of the "hot-topics" in AD research today.

The different clearance systems probably contribute to varying extents on Aβ homeostasis. Any alteration to their function may trigger the progressive accumulation of Aβ (Morrone et al., 2015; Tarasoff-Conway et al., 2015; de Leon et al., 2017), which is the fundamental step in the hypothesis of the amyloid cascade (Lambert et al., 1998; Quan and Banks, 2007; Mawuenyega et al., 2010; Bateman et al., 2012; Fagan et al., 2014; Fleisher et al., 2015). There is a relationship between the decrease in the rate of turnover of amyloid peptides and the probability of aggregation due to incorrect protein misfolding (Patterson et al., 2015) resulting in its accumulation. As soluble molecules can move in constant equilibrium between the ISF and the CSF, Aβ monomers and oligomers can be detected in the CSF. The AP42, and Aβ oligomer/protofibril levels in cortical biopsy samples are higher in subjects with insoluble cortical Aβ aggregates than in subjects without aggregates, and brain tissue levels of AP42 are negatively correlated with CSF AP42 (Patel et al., 2012; Cesarini and Marklund, 2018). Indeed, measuring the levels of Aβ in the CSF is one of the main proposed biomarkers already accepted in the diagnostic criteria of AD (McKhann et al., 2011). It has been reported that levels of Aβ in the CSF vary with time. Results from cross-sectional analysis in familial AD demonstrate higher levels of Aβ in the CSF from mutation carriers compared to controls very early in the disease process (~20–30 years prior to estimated symptom onset), which then drop with disease progression, becoming significantly lower than controls ~10–20 years prior to symptom onset (Morrone et al., 2015; Tarasoff-Conway et al., 2015). These low levels then begin to plateau with the development of cognitive symptoms (Iliff et al., 2013). In sporadic AD at very early preclinical stage (transitional stage) there might be either elevations or reductions in CSF AP42 (Clark et al., 2018; de Leon et al., 2018).

THERAPEUTIC CLEARANCE OF Aβ

Different approaches have been investigated with the aim of removing brain Aβ. Decreasing Aβ production might be the first approach that one can think of to reduce ISF Aβ. For instance, the inhibition BACE is one of the first therapeutic strategies formulated after the amyloid cascade hypothesis, and it is still being explored today. Alternatively, increasing the elimination of Aβ by enzymatic degradation or by clearance enhancement may be able to slow down both the aggregation and the spread processes of the disease given the relevance of Aβ as a substrate in AD (Ryan et al., 2010). Among all strategies to enhance the clearance of Aβ, immunotherapy is the most explored approach so far.

Aβ Immunotherapy

Peripheral Aβ Immunotherapy and the Mechanism of Action of "Peripheral-Sink"

The Aβ immunotherapy consist on activating the immune system against Aβ through the induction (active immunotherapy) or administration (passive immunotherapy) of Aβ-antibodies (Menendez-Gonzalez et al., 2011). Passive immunotherapy can be either monoclonal (mAbs) or polyclonal (immunoglobulins). Active immunization activates the immune system to produce specific antigen antibodies. In AD, Aβ or fragments of Aβ can be used as an antigen, conjugated to a T-cell epitope-bearing protein, together with a booster of the immune system (adjuvant). Passive immunization avoids the need to activate and initiate an immune response to produce antigen-specific antibodies. In both active and passive immunization, Aβ-antibodies bind to Aβ, potentially promoting the clearance of the peptide (Georgievska et al., 2015).

Some interventions have been shown to produce some positive changes on brain Aβ, both in animal models and in human subjects. Unfortunately, these neuropathological benefits were not accompanied by sufficient clinical benefit; therefore, none of these therapies have been transferred to the clinic. One of the reasons may be that effective development of AD therapeutic strategies targeting Aβ require very early administration (before amyloid-plaques are in place) and consideration of the age- and ApoE-specific changes to endogenous Aβ clearance mechanisms in order to optimize efficacy (Morrone et al., 2015).

Understanding how Aβ-antibodies remove Aβ from the brain is a key in the design of Aβ immunotherapies for AD. Two distinct but not mutually exclusive mechanisms have been proposed: The "microglial phagocytosis" would require the antibodies to enter the brain, where they mediate the uptake of Aβ into local microglia. The "peripheral sink" mechanism of action relies only on peripheral antibodies to sequester Aβ in the systemic blood, lowering the level of free Aβ and inducing the brain to release its store of the peptide. This sequestration of circulating Aβ produces a shift in the concentration gradient of Aβ between the brain and the blood causing an efflux of Aβ out of the brain. Thus, it has been hypothesized that reducing Aβ peptides in the periphery would be a way to diminish Aβ levels and plaque load in the brain (Xiang et al., 2015). However, controversy still remains, with evidence both in favor and against the peripheral sink mechanism (Deane et al., 2009; Yamada et al., 2009). Studies with transgenic AD mice seem to validate the hypothesis of the peripheral sink as the main mechanism of Aβ removal after immunization. Some others showed that little or no antibody enters the brain (Vasilevko et al., 2007) and that peripheral anti-Aβ antibody alters CNS and plasma Aβ clearance decreasing brain Aβ burden (DeMattos et al., 2001). Additionally, mice with the Dutch and Iowa mutations have an Aβ peptide that is a poor substrate for the efflux transporter LRP, and so accumulates to high levels in the brain. Indeed, these mice have no peripheral sink effect, and despite a massive buildup of vascular amyloid and parenchymal plaque in brain, Aβ remains undetectable in their blood (Deane et al., 2004; Davis et al., 2006). Direct measurements of brain extracts revealed that little or no antibody was able to enter the brain from the periphery (Ryan et al., 2010). Sagare et al. (2007) showed that infusing in the blood a recombinant version of LRP (sLRP) binding Aβ lowers plaque burden in these mice, producing the peripheral sink effect. Authors also proved that Aβ shifted out of the CNS into the blood (Sagare et al., 2007).

On the other hand, sustained peripheral depletion of Aβ with a new form of neprilysin, which fuses with albumin to prolong plasma half-life, is designed to confer increased Aβ degradation activity and does not affect central Aβ levels in transgenic mice, rats and monkeys (Henderson et al., 2014). In other report (Deane et al., 2009), authors tested the peripheral sink hypothesis by investigating how selective inhibition of Aβ production in the periphery, using a BACE inhibitor or reducing BACE gene dosage, affects Aβ load in the brain. Selective inhibition of peripheral BACE activity in wildtype or transgenic mice reduced Aβ levels in the periphery but not in the brain, even after chronic treatment over several months. In contrast, a BACE inhibitor with improved brain disposition reduced Aβ levels in both brain and periphery already after acute dosing. BACE heterozygous mice displayed an important reduction in plasma Aβ, whereas Aβ reduction in the brain was much lower. These data suggest that reduction of Aβ in the periphery is not sufficient to reduce brain Aβ levels and that BACE is not the rate-limiting enzyme for Aβ processing in the brain (Georgievska et al., 2015). Recent research suggests that CSF naturally occurring antibodies against Aβ seem to have a protective effect for AD, while serum naturally occurring antibodies against Aβ do not seem to have any effect (Kimura et al., 2017; Menendez Gonzalez, 2017a). In line with this, Piazza et al. (2013) reported the first evidence about the participation of natural anti-Aβ autoantibodies in cerebral amyloid-related angiopathy (CAA) and the possible elimination mechanism of soluble Aβ in the CSF by antibodies. Today, CSF anti-Aβ autoantibodies are known to play a key role in the development of amyloid-related imaging abnormalities (ARIA) (DiFrancesco et al., 2015; Chen et al., 2016; Piazza and Winblad, 2016), which are MRI signal changes representing vasogenic edema (VE) and microhemorrhages (mH). VE and mH share some common underlying pathophysiological mechanisms, both in the natural history of AD and in immunotherapies (Sperling et al., 2011). Furthermore, this ARIA has been associated with a massive release of soluble Aβ, plaques and vascular deposits during the acute inflammatory phase (DiFrancesco et al., 2015; Chen et al., 2016; Piazza and Winblad, 2016).

Administered monoclonal antibodies also showed molecular effect, but clinical benefit in humans was not significant. For instance, Solanezumab increases the elimination of soluble Aβ and decreases the deposition of cerebral amyloid plaque in AD mice. In clinical trials, the administration of Solanezumab in patients with mild to moderate AD generated an increase of unbound Aβ in CSF, suggesting that the antibody has a direct peripheral effect with central indirect effect. However, clinical trials showed not improvement of the cognitive and functional capacities of patients (Doody et al., 2014; Chen et al., 2016; Siemers et al., 2016). Similarly, Bapineuzumab modifies Aβ accumulation and CSF biomarkers, but none of the trials showed a significant clinical benefit (Salloway et al., 2014).

Aβ-Immunotherapy Into the CNS

Many investigators have indicated that peripheral clearance through the BBB is not recommended in elderly people, in whom the normal transport of Aβ may present alterations. In addition, the risk of antibody-mediated hemorrhage in sites of cerebral amyloid angiopathy decreases the authors' interest in peripheral passive as well as in active reduction mediated by CNS Aβ antibodies. Due to this, it has been considered that the direct administration of immunotherapy to the CNS is more efficient than the peripheral one, but the intrinsic characteristics of the BBB make the pharmacological approach difficult. This has led to the search for strategies to overcome

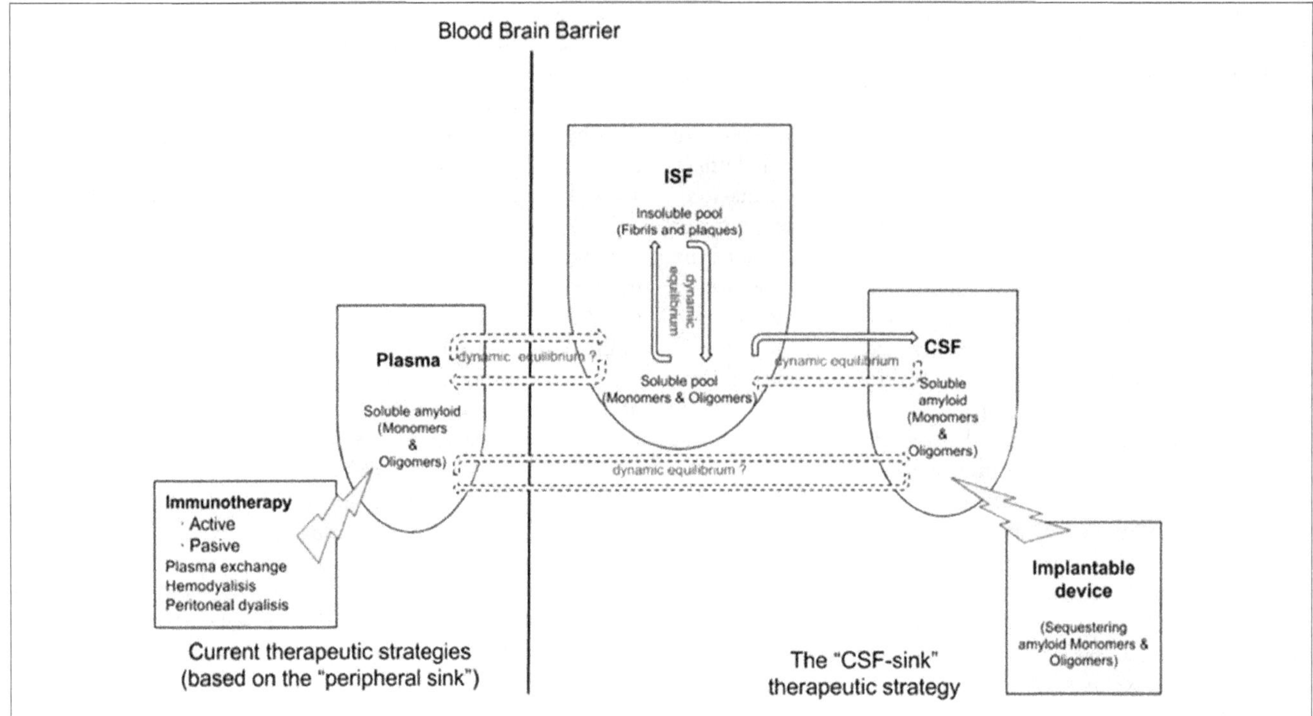

FIGURE 1 | Double dynamic equilibrium of Aβ: there is a bidirectional equilibrium between insoluble and soluble pools of Aβ in the ISF and there is a second equilibrium, also probably bidirectional, of soluble Aβ between the ISF and the CSF. The "CSF-sink therapeutic strategy" consists on sequestering target proteins from the CSF with implantable devices, thus inducing changes in the levels of these proteins in the ISF. Current therapeutic strategies rely on the "peripheral sink" hypothesis mostly. There is some controversy about the existence of a equilibrium of Aβ between plasma and the ISF/CSF.

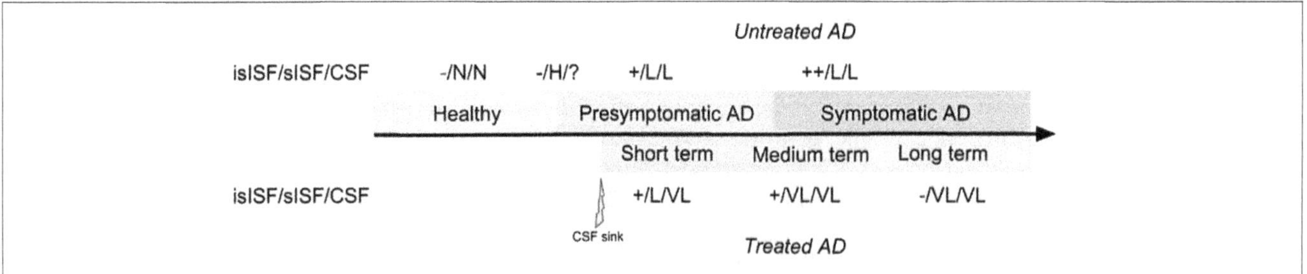

FIGURE 2 | Diagram representing the therapeutic effect of a "CSF-sink" intervention on the predicted levels of Aβ in the insoluble ISF (isISF), soluble ISF (sISF) and CSF pools in a patient with AD treated at presymptomatic stage. Legend: +, positive deposits; −, negative deposits; N, normal; H, high; VH, very high; L, low; VL, very low.

the BBB. These approaches were divided into two categories: the first comprises techniques that facilitate the passage of drugs through the BBB (for example, molecular "Trojan horses," oligopeptides transporters coupled to protons, exosomes, liposomes, nanoparticles, chimeric peptides, prodrugs); and the second consists on techniques that avoid BBB through direct delivery to the SNC. In this last category, the techniques have been investigated include the interruption of BBB (for example, with ultrasound and microbubbles) and intrathecal, intracerebroventricular and intranasal administration (Wilcock et al., 2003; Carty et al., 2006). Although much less explored, passive Aβ-immunotherapy into the CNS has been tested on animal models. Several groups have reported to have achieved clearance of brain Aβ after intracerebral or intraventricular injection of either Aβ antibodies (Wilcock et al., 2003, 2004; Oddo et al., 2004; Carty et al., 2006; Levites et al., 2006), antibodies to oligomeric assemblies of Aβ (Chauhan, 2007) or promoting cellular expression of Aβ-specific antibodies, delivered using viral vectors (Ryan et al., 2010). In most cases, the clearance was rapid (within a few days), but the benefits of the injections were transient because the decrease in amyloid plaques approached reversion at 30 days (Sevigny et al., 2016). Authors also observed a decrease in tau hyperphosphorylation, an increase in the number of microglia counts and an improved learning behavior (Doody et al., 2014). In different reports, the level of clearance achieved by this method varies significantly and ranges from what appears to be elimination throughout the CNS (Sakai et al., 2016) to the limited elimination of diffuse

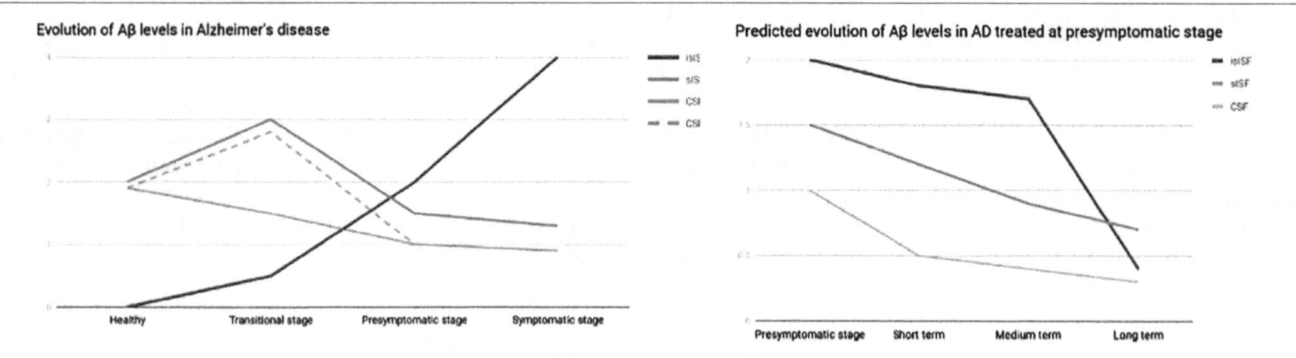

FIGURE 3 | Graph representing the evolution of Aβ in the different pools. On the left, evolution of Aβ levels across the different stages of a AD. On the right, predicted evolution of Aβ levels in a case of AD treated at presymptomatic stage. isISF, insoluble pool in the ISF; sISF, soluble pool in the ISF.

amyloid around the site of antibody injection (Ostrowitzki et al., 2012).

Some human monoclonal antibodies have been shown to enter the brain even when administered peripherally. In a transgenic mouse model of AD, Aducanumab is shown to enter the brain, bind parenchymal Aβ, and reduce soluble and insoluble Aβ in a dose-dependent manner. In patients with prodromal or mild AD, 1 year of monthly intravenous infusions of Aducanumab reduces brain Aβ in a dose- and time-dependent manner. This is accompanied by a slowing of clinical decline. The main safety issues are amyloid-related imaging abnormalities (Sevigny et al., 2016). Phase 3 clinical trials are ongoing. Gantenerumab preferentially interacts with aggregated brain Aβ, both parenchymal and vascular. This antibody acts centrally to disassemble and degrade amyloid plaques by recruiting microglia and activating phagocytosis (Ostrowitzki et al., 2012) but it does not alter plasma Aβ (Bohrmann et al., 2012). As with Adenacumab, trials showed positive trends in clinical scales, main safety worries are amyloid-related imaging abnormalities and clinical trials in different phases are ongoing.

In conclusion, no Aβ immunotherapy has demonstrated significant efficacy in humans to date. A meta-analysis of immunotherapies (Penninkilampi et al., 2017) found no significant treatment differences for typical primary outcome measures. Clinical benefits of peripheral immunotherapy in humans are limited, while the benefits of central immunotherapy in animal models are transient.

Alternative Therapeutic Strategies

Despite Aβ immunotherapy showed not conclusive results to date, Aβ remains the main target in AD. A study using an image biomarker determined that a 15% decrease in Aβ is related to a cognitive improvement of 15–20% (Liu et al., 2015). For all that, there is an urgent need to find alternative methods to achieve a depletion of Aβ in the brain.

A number of studies showed that blood dialysis and plasmapheresis reduces Aβ levels in plasma and CSF in humans and attenuates AD symptoms and pathology in AD mouse models (58,6165), suggesting that removing Aβ from the plasma seems to be an effective -albeit indirect- way of removing Aβ. Different methodologies, from peritoneal dialysis (Jin et al., 2017) to hemodialysis (Kitaguchi et al., 2015; Sakai et al., 2016; Tholen et al., 2016) and plasma exchange (Boada et al., 2009), reported some extent of success removing Aβ from the plasma, which in turn reduces Aβ in the CSF and in the ISF -this last compartment has been confirmed in animals only-. Again, the "peripheral-sink hypothesis" adds new sources of support from these alternative strategies (**Figure 1**).

However, there might be a much more direct way of removing Aβ from the ISF than clearing it from the plasma: clearing it from the CSF. A starting rationale is that there is an equilibrium of Aβ levels between the ISF and plasma in AD transgenic mice before developing Aβ deposits (DeMattos et al., 2002; Cirrito et al., 2003; Hong et al., 2011; Nag et al., 2011). However, this equilibrium is lost once Aβ deposits are in place while the equilibrium of Aβ between the ISF and the CSF still persists (DeMattos et al., 2002). Some studies also found a relationship between the load of cortical deposits and levels in the CSF in humans who underwent neurosurgery (ventriculo-peritoneal shunt) (Seppala et al., 2012; Pyykko et al., 2014; Herukka et al., 2015; Abu Hamdeh et al., 2018). At equilibrium, Aβ remains predominantly monomeric up to 3 pM, above which forms large aggregates (Nag et al., 2011). Once aggregated are in place, amyloid deposits can rapidly sequester soluble A from the ISF (Cirrito et al., 2003; Hong et al., 2011). Aβ in the ISF in plaque-rich mice is thought to be derived not from new A biosynthesis but rather from the large reservoir of less soluble Aβ in brain parenchyma (Cirrito et al., 2003). Moreover, a portion of the insoluble Amyloid pool is in dynamic equilibrium with ISF Amyloid. *In vitro* studies have shown that A aggregates contain a readily dissociable pool of Aβ, or "docked Aβ" as well as a long-lasting or stable "locked" pool of Aβ (Maggio et al., 1992; Esler et al., 2000). *In vitro*, as the concentration of Aβ in solution decreases, this docked pool can quickly dissociate from fibrils. *In vivo*, when Aβ production is inhibited and ISF Aβ levels begin to decrease, it is likely that this associated docked pool can return to solution over a finite period of time, as occurs *in vitro*, causing this pool of Aβ to dissociate from fibrils and become soluble. This results in a prolonged apparent half-life of ISF Aβ in animals with Aβ deposition (Cirrito et al., 2003).

We previously posed the hypothesis that soluble proteins can be cleared from the brain with interventions where soluble proteins are continuously removed from the CSF (Liu et al., 2015;

Menendez Gonzalez, 2017c). This is since soluble proteins are in constant equilibrium between the ISF and the CSF. Therefore, clearing Aβ from the CSF continuously will probably promote the efflux of Aβ from the ISF to the CSF (**Figure 2**).

The "CSF-sink" therapeutic strategy consists on sequestering Aβ from the CSF (**Figure 2**). Today, we can conceive several ways of accessing the CSF with implantable devices (Menendez Gonzalez, 2017b). These devices can be endowed with different technologies able to capture target molecules, such as Aβ, from the CSF. Thus, these interventions would work as a central sink of Aβ, reducing the levels of CSF Aβ, and by means of the CSF-ISF equilibrium would promote the efflux of Aβ from the ISF to the CSF (**Figure 2**).

A study on the Aβ clearance kinetics suggests that the speed and efficiency of Aβ clearance pathways may influence the effect on Aβ deposits (Yuede et al., 2016). A therapeutic strategy aimed at rapid clearance at only high concentrations may be different from a strategy that is designed for a sustained, possibly larger, suppression of Aβ. The "CSF-sink" therapeutic strategy is expected to provide an intense and sustained depletion of Aβ in the CSF and, in turn, a steady decrease Aβ in the ISF, preventing the formation of new aggregates and deposits in the short term and potentially reversing the already existing deposits in the medium and long terms (**Figure 3**).

Albeit AD is a complex disease, and targeting one single molecule might not be enough to hinder the whole neurodegenerative process, we consider this strategy is worth trying, since it is feasible and potentially efficient.

Finally, we would like to mention this strategy might also be valid for other neurodegenerative and neuroimmune diseases where target molecules are well identified and present in the CSF in equilibrium with the ISF. A series of studies in cellular and animal models are needed to prove this hypothesis.

CONCLUSION

We introduce the rationale basis for the "CSF-sink" hypothesis and conclude that continuous depletion of Aβ in the CSF will probably produce a steady clearance of Aβ in the ISF. Implantable devices aimed at sequestering Aβ from the CSF may represent a new therapeutic strategy in AD.

AUTHOR CONTRIBUTIONS

MM-G is the author of the hypothesis and wrote the whole manuscript. All the other authors revised the existing literature and critically reviewed the manuscript.

REFERENCES

Abu Hamdeh, S., Virhammar, J., Sehlin, D., Alafuzoff, I., Cesarini, K. G., and Marklund, N. (2018). Brain tissue Abeta42 levels are linked to shunt response in idiopathic normal pressure hydrocephalus. *J. Neurosurg.* doi: 10.3171/2017.7.JNS171005 [Epub ahead of print].

Atwood, C. S., Martins, R. N., Smith, M. A., and Perry, G. (2002). Senile plaque composition and posttranslational modification of amyloid-beta peptide and associated proteins. *Peptides* 23, 1343–1350. doi: 10.1016/S0196-9781(02)00070-0

Bakker, E. N., Bacskai, B. J., Arbel-Ornath, M., Aldea, R., Bedussi, B., Morris, A. W. J., et al. (2016). Lymphatic clearance of the brain: perivascular, paravascular and significance for neurodegenerative diseases. *Cell Mol. Neurobiol.* 36, 181–194. doi: 10.1007/s10571-015-0273-8

Bateman, R. J., Xiong, C., Benzinger, T. L. S., Fagan, A. M., Goate, A., Fox, N. C., et al. (2012). Clinical and biomarker changes in dominantly inherited Alzheimer's disease. *N. Engl. J. Med.* 367, 795–804. doi: 10.1056/NEJMoa1202753

Boada, M., Ortiz, P., Anaya, F., Hernandez, I., Munoz, J., Nunez, L., et al. (2009). Amyloid-targeted therapeutics in Alzheimer's disease: use of human albumin in plasma exchange as a novel approach for Abeta mobilization. *Drug News Perspect.* 22, 325–339. doi: 10.1358/dnp.2009.22.6.1395256

Bohrmann, B., Baumann, K., Benz, J., Gerber, F., Huber, W., Knoflach, F., et al. (2012). Gantenerumab: a novel human anti-Abeta antibody demonstrates sustained cerebral amyloid-beta binding and elicits cell-mediated removal of human amyloid-beta. *J. Alzheimers Dis.* 28, 49–69. doi: 10.3233/JAD-2011-110977

Braak, H., and Braak, E. (1991). Neuropathological stageing of Alzheimer-related changes. *Acta Neuropathol.* 82, 239–259. doi: 10.1007/BF00308809

Carty, N. C., Wilcock, D. M., Rosenthal, A., Grimm, J., Pons, J., Ronan, V., et al. (2006). Intracranial administration of deglycosylated C-terminal-specific anti-Aβ antibody efficiently clears amyloid plaques without activating microglia in amyloid-depositing transgenic mice. *J. Neuroinflammation* 3:11. doi: 10.1186/1742-2094-3-11

Cesarini, K. G., and Marklund, N. (2018). Brain tissue Aβ42 levels are linked to shunt response in idiopathic normal pressure hydrocephalus. *J. Neurosurg.* doi: 10.3171/2017.7.JNS171005 [Epub ahead of print].

Chauhan, N. B. (2007). Intracerebroventricular passive immunization with anti-oligoAbeta antibody in TgCRND8. *J. Neurosci. Res.* 85, 451–463. doi: 10.1002/jnr.21110

Chen, Y. F., Ma, X., Sundell, K., Alaka, K., Schuh, K., Raskin, J., et al. (2016). Quantile regression to characterize solanezumab effects in Alzheimer's disease trials. *Alzheimers Dement.* 2, 192–198. doi: 10.1016/j.trci.2016.07.005

Cirrito, J. R., May, P. C., O'Dell, M. A., Taylor, J. W., Parsadanian, M., Cramer, J. W., et al. (2003). In vivo assessment of brain interstitial fluid with microdialysis reveals plaque-associated changes in amyloid-beta metabolism and half-life. *J. Neurosci.* 23, 8844–8853.

Clark, L. R., Berman, S. E., Norton, D. L., Koscik, R., Jonaitis, E., Blennow, K., et al. (2018). Age-accelerated cognitive decline in asymptomatic adults with CSF β-amyloid. *Neurology*. doi: 10.1212/WNL.0000000000005291

Davis, J., Xu, F., Miao, J., Previti, M. L., Romanov, G., Ziegler, K., et al. (2006). Deficient cerebral clearance of vasculotropic mutant Dutch/Iowa Double A beta in human A betaPP transgenic mice. *Neurobiol. Aging* 27, 946–954. doi: 10.1016/j.neurobiolaging.2005.05.031

de Leon, M. J., Li, Y., Okamura, N., Tsui, W. H., Saint-Louis, L. A., Glodzik, L., et al. (2017). Cerebrospinal fluid clearance in Alzheimer disease measured with dynamic PET. *J. Nucl. Med.* 58, 1471–1476. doi: 10.2967/jnumed.116.187211

de Leon, M. J., Pirraglia, E., Osorio, R. S., Glodzik, L., Saint-Louis, L., Kim, H.-J., et al. (2018). The nonlinear relationship between cerebrospinal fluid Abeta42 and tau in preclinical Alzheimer's disease. *PLoS One* 13:e0191240. doi: 10.1371/journal.pone.0191240

Deane, R., Bell, R. D., Sagare, A., and Zlokovic, B. V. (2009). Clearance of amyloid-beta peptide across the blood-brain barrier: implication for therapies in Alzheimer's disease. *CNS Neurol. Disord. Drug Targets* 8, 16–30. doi: 10.2174/187152709787601867

Deane, R., Wu, Z., Sagare, A., Davis, J., Du Yan, S., Hamm, K., et al. (2004). LRP/amyloid beta-peptide interaction mediates differential brain efflux of Abeta isoforms. *Neuron* 43, 333–344. doi: 10.1016/j.neuron.2004.07.017

DeMattos, R. B., Bales, K. R., Cummins, D. J., Dodart, J. C., Paul, S. M., and Holtzman, D. M. (2001). Peripheral anti-A beta antibody alters CNS and plasma

A beta clearance and decreases brain A beta burden in a mouse model of Alzheimer's disease. *Proc. Natl. Acad. Sci. U.S.A.* 98, 8850–8855. doi: 10.1073/pnas.151261398

DeMattos, R. B., Bales, K. R., Parsadanian, M., O'Dell, M. A., Foss, E. M., Paul, S. M., et al. (2002). Plaque-associated disruption of CSF and plasma amyloid-beta (Abeta) equilibrium in a mouse model of Alzheimer's disease. *J. Neurochem.* 81, 229–236. doi: 10.1046/j.1471-4159.2002.00889.x

Diem, A. K., MacGregor Sharp, M., Gatherer, M., Bressloff, N. W., Carare, R. O., and Richardson, G. (2017). Arterial pulsations cannot drive intramural periarterial drainage: significance for Aβ drainage. *Front. Neurosci.* 11:475. doi: 10.3389/fnins.2017.00475

DiFrancesco, J. C., Longoni, M., and Piazza, F. (2015). Anti-Abeta autoantibodies in amyloid related imaging abnormalities (ARIA): candidate biomarker for immunotherapy in Alzheimer's disease and cerebral amyloid angiopathy. *Front. Neurol.* 6:207. doi: 10.3389/fneur.2015.00207

Doody, R. S., Thomas, R. G., Farlow, M., Iwatsubo, T., Vellas, B., Joffe, S., et al. (2014). Phase 3 trials of solanezumab for mild-to-moderate Alzheimer's disease. *N. Engl. J. Med.* 370, 311–321. doi: 10.1056/NEJMoa1312889

Esler, W. P., Stimson, E. R., Jennings, J. M., Vinters, H. V., Ghilardi, J. R., Lee, J. P., et al. (2000). Alzheimer's disease amyloid propagation by a template-dependent dock-lock mechanism. *Biochemistry* 39, 6288–6295. doi: 10.1021/bi992933h

Fagan, A. M., Xiong, C., Jasielec, M. S., Bateman, R. J., Goate, A. M., Benzinger, T. L. S., et al. (2014). Longitudinal change in CSF biomarkers in autosomal-dominant Alzheimer's disease. *Sci. Transl. Med.* 6:226ra30. doi: 10.1126/scitranslmed.3007901

Fleisher, A. S., Chen, K., Quiroz, Y. T., Jakimovich, L. J., Gutierrez Gomez, M., Langois, C. M., et al. (2015). Associations between biomarkers and age in the presenilin 1 E280A autosomal dominant Alzheimer disease kindred: a cross-sectional study. *JAMA Neurol.* 72, 316–324. doi: 10.1001/jamaneurol.2014.3314

Georgievska, B., Gustavsson, S., Lundkvist, J., Neelissen, J., Eketjall, S., Ramberg, V., et al. (2015). Revisiting the peripheral sink hypothesis: inhibiting BACE1 activity in the periphery does not alter beta-amyloid levels in the CNS. *J. Neurochem.* 132, 477–486. doi: 10.1111/jnc.12937

Haass, C., and Selkoe, D. J. (2007). Soluble protein oligomers in neurodegeneration: lessons from the Alzheimer's amyloid beta-peptide. *Nat. Rev. Mol. Cell Biol.* 8, 101–112. doi: 10.1038/nrm2101

Henderson, S. J., Andersson, C., Narwal, R., Janson, J., Goldschmidt, T. J., Appelkvist, P., et al. (2014). Sustained peripheral depletion of amyloid-β with a novel form of neprilysin does not affect central levels of amyloid-β. *Brain* 137, 553–564. doi: 10.1093/brain/awt308

Herukka, S.-K., Rummukainen, J., Ihalainen, J., von Und Zu Fraunberg, M., Koivisto, A. M., Nerg, O., et al. (2015). Amyloid-beta and tau dynamics in human brain interstitial fluid in patients with suspected normal pressure hydrocephalus. *J. Alzheimers Dis.* 46, 261–269. doi: 10.3233/JAD-142862

Hong, S., Quintero-Monzon, O., Ostaszewski, B. L., Podlisny, D. R., Cavanaugh, W. T., Yang, T., et al. (2011). Dynamic analysis of amyloid beta-protein in behaving mice reveals opposing changes in ISF versus parenchymal Abeta during age-related plaque formation. *J. Neurosci.* 31, 15861–15869. doi: 10.1523/JNEUROSCI.3272-11.2011

Iliff, J. J., Wang, M., Liao, Y., Plogg, B. A., Peng, W., Gundersen, G. A., et al. (2012). A paravascular pathway facilitates CSF flow through the brain parenchyma and the clearance of interstitial solutes, including amyloid beta. *Sci. Transl. Med.* 4:147ra111. doi: 10.1126/scitranslmed.3003748

Iliff, J. J., Wang, M., Zeppenfeld, D. M., Venkataraman, A., Plog, B. A., Liao, Y., et al. (2013). Cerebral arterial pulsation drives paravascular CSF-interstitial fluid exchange in the murine brain. *J. Neurosci.* 33, 18190–18199. doi: 10.1523/JNEUROSCI.1592-13.2013

Jin, W.-S., Shen, L.-L., Bu, X.-L., Zhang, W.-W., Chen, S.-H., Huang, Z.-L., et al. (2017). Peritoneal dialysis reduces amyloid-beta plasma levels in humans and attenuates Alzheimer-associated phenotypes in an APP/PS1 mouse model. *Acta Neuropathol.* 134, 207–220. doi: 10.1007/s00401-017-1721-y

Kimura, A., Takemura, M., Saito, K., Yoshikura, N., Hayashi, Y., and Inuzuka, T. (2017). Association between naturally occurring anti-amyloid β autoantibodies and medial temporal lobe atrophy in Alzheimer's disease. *J. Neurol. Neurosurg. Psychiatry* 88, 126L–131. doi: 10.1136/jnnp-2016-313476

Kitaguchi, N., Hasegawa, M., Ito, S., Kawaguchi, K., Hiki, Y., Nakai, S., et al. (2015). A prospective study on blood Abeta levels and the cognitive function of patients with hemodialysis: a potential therapeutic strategy for Alzheimer's disease. *J. Neural. Transm.* 122, 1593–1607. doi: 10.1007/s00702-015-1431-3

Lambert, M. P., Barlow, A. K., Chromy, B. A., Edwards, C., Freed, R., Liosatos, M., et al. (1998). Diffusible, nonfibrillar ligands derived from Abeta1-42 are potent central nervous system neurotoxins. *Proc. Natl. Acad. Sci. U.S.A.* 95, 6448–6453. doi: 10.1073/pnas.95.11.6448

Lei, Y., Han, H., Yuan, F., Javeed, A., and Zhao, Y. (2017). The brain interstitial system: anatomy, modeling, in vivo measurement, and applications. *Prog Neurobiol* 157, 230–246. doi: 10.1016/j.pneurobio.2015.12.007

Levites, Y., Das, P., Price, R. W., Rochette, M. J., Kostura, L. A., McGowan, E. M., et al. (2006). Anti-Abeta42- and anti-Abeta40-specific mAbs attenuate amyloid deposition in an Alzheimer disease mouse model. *J. Clin. Invest.* 116, 193–201. doi: 10.1172/JCI25410

Liu, Y.-H., Xiang, Y., Wang, Y.-R., Jiao, S.-S., Wang, Q.-H., Bu, X.-L., et al. (2015). Association between serum amyloid-beta and renal functions: implications for roles of kidney in amyloid-beta clearance. *Mol. Neurobiol.* 52, 115–119. doi: 10.1007/s12035-014-8854-y

Maggio, J. E., Stimson, E. R., Ghilardi, J. R., Allen, C. J., Dahl, C. E., Whitcomb, D. C., et al. (1992). Reversible in vitro growth of Alzheimer disease beta-amyloid plaques by deposition of labeled amyloid peptide. *Proc. Natl. Acad. Sci. U.S.A.* 89, 5462–5466. doi: 10.1073/pnas.89.12.5462

Malm, T., Koistinaho, M., Muona, A., Magga, J., and Koistinaho, J. (2010). The role and therapeutic potential of monocytic cells in Alzheimer's disease. *Glia* 58, 889–900. doi: 10.1002/glia.20973

Mawuenyega, K. G., Sigurdson, W., Ovod, V., Munsell, L., Kasten, T., Morris, J. C., et al. (2010). Decreased clearance of CNS beta-amyloid in Alzheimer's disease. *Science* 330:1774. doi: 10.1126/science.1197623

McKhann, G. M., Knopman, D. S., Chertkow, H., Hyman, B. T., Jack, C. R. J., Kawas, C. H., et al. (2011). The diagnosis of dementia due to Alzheimer's disease: recommendations from the National Institute on Aging-Alzheimer's Association workgroups on diagnostic guidelines for Alzheimer's disease. *Alzheimers Dement.* 7, 263–269. doi: 10.1016/j.jalz.2011.03.005

Menendez Gonzalez, M. (2017a). Association between naturally occurring antiamyloid β autoantibodies and medial temporal lobe atrophy in Alzheimer's disease. *J. Neurol. Neurosurg. Psychiatry* 88, 96–97. doi: 10.1136/jnnp-2016-314136

Menendez Gonzalez, M. (2017b). Implantable systems for continuous liquorpheresis and CSF replacement. *Cureus* 9:e1022. doi: 10.7759/cureus.1022

Menendez Gonzalez, M. (2017c). Mechanical dilution of beta-amyloid peptide and phosphorylated tau protein in Alzheimer's disease: too simple to be true? *Cureus* 9:e1062. doi: 10.7759/cureus.1062

Menendez-Gonzalez, M., Perez-Pinera, P., Martinez-Rivera, M., Calatayud, M. T., and Blazquez Menes, B. (2005). APP processing and the APP-KPI domain involvement in the amyloid cascade. *Neurodegener. Dis.* 2, 277–283. doi: 10.1159/000092315

Menendez-Gonzalez, M., Perez-Pinera, P., Martinez-Rivera, M., Muniz, A. L., and Vega, J. A. (2011). Immunotherapy for Alzheimer's disease: rational basis in ongoing clinical trials. *Curr. Pharm. Des.* 17, 508–520. doi: 10.2174/138161211795164112

Morrone, C. D., Liu, M., Black, S. E., and McLaurin, J. (2015). Interaction between therapeutic interventions for Alzheimer's disease and physiological Aβ clearance mechanisms. *Front. Aging Neurosci.* 7:64. doi: 10.3389/fnagi.2015.00064

Nag, S., Sarkar, B., Bandyopadhyay, A., Sahoo, B., Sreenivasan, V. K. A., Kombrabail, M., et al. (2011). Nature of the amyloid-beta monomer and the monomer-oligomer equilibrium. *J. Biol. Chem.* 286, 13827–13833. doi: 10.1074/jbc.M110.199885

Nussbaum, J. M., Seward, M. E., and Bloom, G. S. (2013). Alzheimer disease: a tale of two prions. *Prion* 7, 14–19. doi: 10.4161/pri.22118

Oddo, S., Billings, L., Kesslak, J. P., Cribbs, D. H., and LaFerla, F. M. (2004). Abeta immunotherapy leads to clearance of early, but not late, hyperphosphorylated tau aggregates via the proteasome. *Neuron* 43, 321–332. doi: 10.1016/j.neuron.2004.07.003

O'Nuallain, B., Freir, D. B., Nicoll, A. J., Risse, E., Ferguson, N., Herron, C. E., et al. (2010). Amyloid beta-protein dimers rapidly form stable synaptotoxic protofibrils. *J. Neurosci.* 30, 14411–14419. doi: 10.1523/JNEUROSCI.3537-10.2010

Ostrowitzki, S., Deptula, D., Thurfjell, L., Barkhof, F., Bohrmann, B., Brooks, D. J., et al. (2012). Mechanism of amyloid removal in patients with Alzheimer disease treated with gantenerumab. *Arch. Neurol.* 69, 198–207. doi: 10.1001/archneurol.2011.1538

Patel, S., Lee, E. B., Xie, S. X., Law, A., Jackson, E. M., Arnold, S. E., et al. (2012). Phosphorylated tau/amyloid beta 1-42 ratio in ventricular cerebrospinal fluid reflects outcome in idiopathic normal pressure hydrocephalus. *Fluids Barriers CNS* 9:7. doi: 10.1186/2045-8118-9-7

Patterson, B. W., Elbert, D. L., Mawuenyega, K. G., Kasten, T., Ovod, V., Ma, S., et al. (2015). Age and amyloid effects on human central nervous system amyloid-beta kinetics. *Ann. Neurol.* 78, 439–453. doi: 10.1002/ana.24454

Penninkilampi, R., Brothers, H. M., and Eslick, G. D. (2017). Safety and efficacy of anti-amyloid-beta immunotherapy in Alzheimer's disease: a systematic review and meta-analysis. *J. Neuroimmune Pharmacol.* 12, 194–203. doi: 10.1007/s11481-016-9722-5

Piazza, F., Greenberg, S. M., Savoiardo, M., Gardinetti, M., Chiapparini, L., Raicher, I., et al. (2013). Anti-amyloid β autoantibodies in cerebral amyloid angiopathy-related inflammation: implications for amyloid-modifying therapies. *Ann. Neurol.* 73, 449–458. doi: 10.1002/ana.23857

Piazza, F., and Winblad, B. (2016). Amyloid-related imaging abnormalities (ARIA) in immunotherapy trials for Alzheimer's disease: need for prognostic biomarkers? *J. Alzheimer's Dis.* 52, 417–420. doi: 10.3233/JAD-160122

Pulawski, W., Ghoshdastider, U., Andrisano, V., and Filipek, S. (2012). Ubiquitous amyloids. *Appl. Biochem. Biotechnol.* 166, 1626–1643. doi: 10.1007/s12010-012-9549-3

Pyykko, O. T., Lumela, M., Rummukainen, J., Nerg, O., Seppala, T. T., Herukka, S.-K., et al. (2014). Cerebrospinal fluid biomarker and brain biopsy findings in idiopathic normal pressure hydrocephalus. *PLoS One* 9:e91974. doi: 10.1371/journal.pone.0091974

Quan, N., and Banks, W. A. (2007). Brain-immune communication pathways. *Brain Behav. Immun.* 21, 727–735. doi: 10.1016/j.bbi.2007.05.005

Ries, M., and Sastre, M. (2016). Mechanisms of Aβ clearance and degradation by glial cells. *Front. Aging Neurosci.* 8:160. doi: 10.3389/fnagi.2016.00160

Ryan, D. A., Mastrangelo, M. A., Narrow, W. C., Sullivan, M. A., Federoff, H. J., and Bowers, W. J. (2010). Aβ-directed single-chain antibody delivery via a serotype-1 AAV vector improves learning behavior and pathology in Alzheimer's disease mice. *Mol. Ther.* 18, 1471–1481. doi: 10.1038/mt.2010.111

Sagare, A., Deane, R., Bell, R. D., Johnson, B., Hamm, K., Pendu, R., et al. (2007). Clearance of amyloid-beta by circulating lipoprotein receptors. *Nat. Med.* 13, 1029–1031. doi: 10.1038/nm1635

Sakai, K., Senda, T., Hata, R., Kuroda, M., Hasegawa, M., Kato, M., et al. (2016). Patients that have undergone hemodialysis exhibit lower amyloid deposition in the brain: evidence supporting a therapeutic strategy for Alzheimer's disease by removal of blood amyloid. *J. Alzheimers Dis.* 51, 997–1002. doi: 10.3233/JAD-151139

Salloway, S., Sperling, R., Fox, N. C., Blennow, K., Klunk, W., Raskind, M., et al. (2014). Two phase 3 trials of bapineuzumab in mild-to-moderate Alzheimer's disease. *N. Engl. J. Med.* 370, 322–333. doi: 10.1056/NEJMoa1304839

Seppala, T. T., Nerg, O., Koivisto, A. M., Rummukainen, J., Puli, L., Zetterberg, H., et al. (2012). CSF biomarkers for Alzheimer disease correlate with cortical brain biopsy findings. *Neurology* 78, 1568–1575. doi: 10.1212/WNL.0b013e3182563bd0

Sevigny, J., Chiao, P., Bussiere, T., Weinreb, P. H., Williams, L., Maier, M., et al. (2016). The antibody aducanumab reduces Aβ plaques in Alzheimer's disease. *Nature* 537, 50–56. doi: 10.1038/nature19323

Siemers, E. R., Sundell, K. L., Carlson, C., Case, M., Sethuraman, G., Liu-Seifert, H., et al. (2016). Phase 3 solanezumab trials: secondary outcomes in mild Alzheimer's disease patients. *Alzheimers Dement.* 12, 110–120. doi: 10.1016/j.jalz.2015.06.1893

Sperling, R. A., Jack, C. R. J., Black, S. E., Frosch, M. P., Greenberg, S. M., Hyman, B. T., et al. (2011). Amyloid-related imaging abnormalities in amyloid-modifying therapeutic trials: recommendations from the Alzheimer's association research roundtable workgroup. *Alzheimers Dement.* 7, 367–385. doi: 10.1016/j.jalz.2011.05.2351

Tarasoff-Conway, J. M., Carare, R. O., Osorio, R. S., Glodzik, L., Butler, T., Fieremans, E., et al. (2015). Clearance systems in the brain—implications for Alzheimer disease. *Nat. Rev. Neurol.* 11, 457–470. doi: 10.1038/nrneurol.2015.119

Tholen, S., Schmaderer, C., Chmielewski, S., Forstl, H., Heemann, U., Baumann, M., et al. (2016). Reduction of amyloid-beta plasma levels by hemodialysis: an anti-amyloid treatment strategy? *J. Alzheimers Dis.* 50, 791–796. doi: 10.3233/JAD-150662

Vasilevko, V., Xu, F., Previti, M. L., Van Nostrand, W. E., and Cribbs, D. H. (2007). Experimental investigation of antibody-mediated clearance mechanisms of amyloid-beta in CNS of Tg-SwDI transgenic mice. *J. Neurosci.* 27, 13376–13383. doi: 10.1523/JNEUROSCI.2788-07.2007

Walker, L. C., Schelle, J., and Jucker, M. (2016). The prion-like properties of amyloid-beta assemblies: implications for Alzheimer's disease. *Cold Spring Harb. Perspect. Med.* 6:a024398. doi: 10.1101/cshperspect.a024398

Wilcock, D. M., DiCarlo, G., Henderson, D., Jackson, J., Clarke, K., Ugen, K. E., et al. (2003). Intracranially administered anti-Abeta antibodies reduce beta-amyloid deposition by mechanisms both independent of and associated with microglial activation. *J. Neurosci.* 23, 3745–3751.

Wilcock, D. M., Munireddy, S. K., Rosenthal, A., Ugen, K. E., Gordon, M. N., and Morgan, D. (2004). Microglial activation facilitates Abeta plaque removal following intracranial anti-Abeta antibody administration. *Neurobiol. Dis.* 15, 11–20. doi: 10.1016/j.nbd.2003.09.015

Xiang, Y., Bu, X.-L., Liu, Y.-H., Zhu, C., Shen, L.-L., Jiao, S.-S., et al. (2015). Physiological amyloid-beta clearance in the periphery and its therapeutic potential for Alzheimer's disease. *Acta Neuropathol.* 130, 487–499. doi: 10.1007/s00401-015-1477-1

Yamada, K., Yabuki, C., Seubert, P., Schenk, D., Hori, Y., Ohtsuki, S., et al. (2009). Abeta immunotherapy: intracerebral sequestration of Abeta by an anti-Abeta monoclonal antibody 266 with high affinity to soluble Abeta. *J. Neurosci.* 29, 11393–11398. doi: 10.1523/JNEUROSCI.2021-09.2009

Yuede, C. M., Lee, H., Restivo, J. L., Davis, T. A., Hettinger, J. C., Wallace, C. E., et al. (2016). Rapid in vivo measurement of β-amyloid reveals biphasic clearance kinetics in an Alzheimer's mouse model. *J. Exp. Med.* 213, 677–685. doi: 10.1084/jem.20151428

Zhao, Z., Sagare, A. P., Ma, Q., Halliday, M. R., Kong, P., Kisler, K., et al. (2015). Central role for PICALM in amyloid-beta blood-brain barrier transcytosis and clearance. *Nat. Neurosci.* 18, 978–987. doi: 10.1038/nn.4025

Zuroff, L., Daley, D., Black, K. L., and Koronyo-Hamaoui, M. (2017). Clearance of cerebral Abeta in Alzheimer's disease: reassessing the role of microglia and monocytes. *Cell Mol. Life Sci.* 74, 2167–2201. doi: 10.1007/s00018-017-2463-7

9

Effects of Oligosaccharides from *Morinda officinalis* on Gut Microbiota and Metabolome of APP/PS1 Transgenic Mice

Yang Xin[1,2†], *Chen Diling*[3*†], *Yang Jian*[3], *Liu Ting*[2], *Hu Guoyan*[2], *Liang Hualun*[4], *Tang Xiaocui*[3], *Lai Guoxiao*[3,5], *Shuai Ou*[3], *Zheng Chaoqun*[3], *Zhao Jun*[6] *and Xie Yizhen*[3]

[1] Department of Pharmacy, The Fifth Affiliated Hospital of Guangzhou Medical University, Guangzhou, China, [2] The Fifth Clinical School of Guangzhou Medical University, Guangzhou, China, [3] State Key Laboratory of Applied Microbiology Southern China, Guangdong Provincial Key Laboratory of Microbial Culture Collection and Application, Guangdong Open Laboratory of Applied Microbiology, Guangdong Institute of Microbiology, Guangzhou, China, [4] Department of Pharmacy, The Second Clinical Medical College of Guangzhou University of Chinese Medicine, Guangzhou, China, [5] College of Pharmacy, Guangxi University of Traditional Chinese Medicine, Nanning, China, [6] Department of Obstetrics, Guangdong Women and Children Hospital, Guangzhou, China

***Correspondence:**
Chen Diling
diling1983@163.com

† These authors have contributed equally to this work.

Alzheimer's disease (AD), a progressive neurodegenerative disorder, lacks preclinical diagnostic biomarkers and therapeutic drugs. Thus, earlier intervention in AD is a top priority. Studies have shown that the gut microbiota influences central nervous system disorders and that prebiotics can improve the cognition of hosts with AD, but these effects are not well understood. Preliminary research has shown that oligosaccharides from *Morinda officinalis* (OMO) are a useful prebiotic and cause substantial memory improvements in animal models of AD; however, the mechanism is still unclear. Therefore, this study was conducted to investigate whether OMO are clinically effective in alleviating AD by improving gut microbiota. OMO were administered to APP/PS1 transgenic mice, and potential clinical biomarkers of AD were identified with metabolomics and bioinformatics. Behavioral experiments demonstrated that OMO significantly ameliorated the memory of the AD animal model. Histological changes indicated that OMO ameliorated brain tissue swelling and neuronal apoptosis and downregulated the expression of the intracellular AD marker $A\beta_{1-42}$. 16S rRNA sequencing analyses indicated that OMO maintained the diversity and stability of the microbial community. The data also indicated that OMO are an efficacious prebiotic in an animal model of AD, regulating the composition and metabolism of the gut microbiota. A serum metabolomics assay was performed using UHPLC-LTQ Orbitrap mass spectrometry to delineate the metabolic changes and potential early biomarkers in APP/PS1 transgenic mice. Multivariate statistical analysis showed that 14 metabolites were significantly upregulated, and 8 metabolites were downregulated in the model animals compared to the normal controls. Thus, key metabolites represent early indicators of the development of AD. Overall, we report a drug and signaling pathway with therapeutic potential, including proteins associated with cognitive deficits in normal mice or gene mutations that cause AD.

Keywords: oligosaccharides of *Morinda officinalis*, Alzheimer's disease, gut microbiota, metabolomics, APP/PS1 transgenic mice, metabolites

INTRODUCTION

As an irreversible neurodegenerative disease that causes cognitive deficits, Alzheimer's disease (AD) accounts for 60–80% of all types of dementia (1). The typical neuropathological features of AD include the extracellular aggregation of amyloid-β (Aβ) peptide, the formation of tau protein aggregates inside neurons and the malfunction and/or loss of synapses and axons (2–4). Since ~14 million people in the United States are predicted to be diagnosed with AD by 2050 (5), investigations of agents and reactions whose dysfunction causes AD are essential to provide insights into the etiology of the illness and to develop effective treatment strategies.

Some pathological features of AD, including cerebral atrophy, amyloid generation, altered gene expression, altered immune reactions, and cognitive deficits, have recently been linked to microbe infections (6–10). The brain and gut interact and modulate each other (11), and microbes in the gastrointestinal tract (GIT) are postulated to participate in AD development (12–14), although our understanding of the development and pathology of AD is insufficient and changing. Researchers have not determined how an imbalance in GIT microbes affects AD. The impact may be associated with the invasion of several pathogens, a decrease in the number of protective microbes, impaired immune tolerance, elevated membrane permeability and other defects in the immune system (15, 16). Probiotics have been shown to participate in the ability of the host to prevent and manage both chronic and acute conditions, such as AD (17). Alterations in the host physiology resulting from aging, genetics, diet, lifestyle and other factors might noticeably affect microbes (18–21). Metabolomics is a postgenomic field that offers new insights into the diagnostic and prognostic biomarkers of AD (22). Metabolomics has been used to identify metabolites and determine the expression of related genes in whole organisms, and it has recently been used in a wide range of applications in the clinic. Serum metabolites were discovered and considered potential biomarkers of AD (23), as retinoate has been used to help characterize and discriminate pathophysiological signatures of AD (24). According to recent reports, the gut microbiota and their metabolites influence the host metabolism (25). However, the roles of the gut microbiota and serum metabolites in AD are unclear.

Oligosaccharides from *Morinda officinalis* (OMO), a natural herbal extract used in traditional Chinese medicine, contain many active components. The saccharide content in the *M. officinalis* root is as high as 49.8–58.3%, mainly consisting of oligosaccharides with anti-dementia and memory-enhancing effects on many animal models (26–28). However, the mechanism underlying these beneficial effects has not been identified and will be elucidated in the present study. This study aims to provide a basis for the effective prediction and characterization of AD pathology by analyzing the gut microbiota and serum metabolite biomarkers.

Our research utilizes transgenic APPswe/PS1dE9 (APP/PS1) mouse models (29), which have been widely applied to investigations of the initial etiology of AD and evaluations of the efficacy of OMO treatments. Every specimen containing microbial 16S rRNA genes underwent concentration with the help of solid-phase reversible immobilization (SPRI) and subsequent quantification by electrophoresis utilizing an Agilent 2100 Bioanalyzer (Agilent, USA) prior to sequencing on an Illumina MiSeq sequencing system (30).

Whole-body blood specimens acquired from 8-month-old APP/PS1 and C57 mice were subjected to metabolomics evaluations using UHPLC-MS/MS. Subsequently, the entirety of the spectra were assessed using multivariate analysis to holistically investigate alterations in the levels of circulating metabolites. Fourteen metabolites were recognized that might contribute to the diagnosis and treatment of AD in the initial stage. Consequently, our research focused on assessing the therapeutic impact of OMO on AD by analyzing the diversity of microbes and performing metabolomics assays to provide insights into its etiology. Moreover, the results from this study will serve as the basis for the application of nutritional interventions and the AD-counteracting effects of OMO.

METHODS

Animal Model Preparation and Treatments

Adult male C57 mice and 2-month-old transgenic APP/PS1 mice weighing 18 to 22 grams were acquired from the Laboratory Animal Center of Guangdong Province (SCXK [Yue] 2008-0020, SYXK [Yue] 2008-0085) and were housed in pairs in the colony room on a 12/12-h light/dark cycle at 25°C in plastic cages and were allowed *ad libitum* access to food and water. Each procedure described in our study was approved by the Laboratory Animal Center of the Guangdong Institute of Microbiology. This study utilized as few mice as possible. 2-month-old APP/PS1 mice and age-matched C57 mice, which served as the control group ($n = 10$ animals), were utilized in the present study. Our research was approved by the Ethical Committee and complied with the Declaration of Helsinki.

Mice performed water maze tests (WMT) to identify adequate AD models before animals were randomized into the following 4 groups in this 6-month experiment: a C57 group (oral administration of distilled water), a transgenic APP/PS1 group [oral administration of distilled water], a high-dose transgenic APP/PS1 group [oral administration of 100 mg/(kg·d) OMO] and a low-dose transgenic APP/PS1 group (oral administration of 50 mg/(kg·d) OMO) ($n = 10$ animals per group).

WMTs

A Morris water maze (MWM, DMS-2, Chinese Academy of Medical Sciences Institute of Medicine) comprising a non-transparent circular fiberglass pool with a diameter of 20 cm that had been filled with water (25 ± 1°C) was used to examine murine spatial learning and memory. Wathet curtains tagged with three distal visual cues encircled the pool. Unified lighting of the examination room and pool was provided by four independent light sources of equivalent power. A CCD camera was placed over the center of the pool to record the swimming paths of each mouse. An EthoVision tracking system (Noldus, Leesburg, VA) was applied to digitize the video output. The

WMT consisted of three steps, as described in a previous study (31): primary spatial practice, reverse spatial practice and a probe examination.

Hematoxylin-Eosin (HE) and Immunohistochemical Staining

The look, activity and fur tint of each mouse were examined and recorded daily. The weight of each mouse was examined every 3 days when drugs were administered. Serum specimens were harvested, and murine cerebral samples were anatomically dissected after the WMT.

Three cerebral samples and three intestinum tenues were removed from randomly chosen mice in each experimental group, while the remaining tissues underwent fixation with four percent paraformaldehyde before processing into paraffin sections. Sections were stained with HE and immunohistochemistry before being examined under the light microscope (31, 32).

Microbiome Analysis

Fresh fecal specimens were acquired from murine nests and stored at −80°C. Microbe DNA specimens weighing from 1.2 to 20.0 ng were isolated from murine cecal specimens and stored at −20°C. The 16S rRNA genes of microbes were amplified with the following primers: forward 5′-ACTCCTACGGGAGGCAGCA-3′ and reverse 5′-GGACTACHVGGGTWTCTAAT-3′. Every amplified product was concentrated by SPRI and quantified by electrophoresis using an Agilent 2100 Bioanalyzer (Agilent). Every specimen was diluted to 1×10^9 molecules/μL in TE buffer and pooled into groups prior to the determination of DNA concentrations using a NanoDrop spectrophotometer. An Illumina MiSeq sequencing system was utilized to sequence 20 mL of the pooled admixture. The subsequent reads were analyzed as described in a previous study (30).

Serum Metabolomics Analysis

Eighty microliters of mouse serum was combined with 240 μL of a cold methanol-acetonitrile (2:1, v/v) mixture and 10 μL of an internal standard (0.3 mg/mL 2-chloro-L-phenylalanine in methanol). After vortexing for 2 min, the mixture was subjected to ultrasound disruption for 5 min, incubated in a −20°C freezer for 20 min, and centrifuged for 10 min at a low temperature (14,000 rpm at 4°C). Subsequently, 200 μL of the supernatant was loaded into the tube lining a sample vial and analyzed using LC-MS (33).

LC-MS Analysis Using an UHPLC-LTQ Orbitrap Spectrometer

An Ultimate 3000-Velos Pro system was utilized for LC-MS with the help of a binary solvent delivery manager and a specimen manager connected to an LTQ Orbitrap mass spectrometer equipped with an electrospray interface (Thermo Fisher Scientific, USA). LC settings are displayed below. The Acquity BEH C18 column (100 mm × 2.1 mm internal diameter, 1.7 μm; Waters, Milford, USA) was stored at 45°C. Isolation was performed with the following solvent gradient: 5% B−25% B from 0 to 1.5 min, 25% B−100% B from 1.5 to 10.0 min, 100% B−100% B from 10.0 to 13.0 min; 100% B−5% B from 13.0 to 13.5 min, and 13.5–14.5 min holding at 5% B at a flow rate of 0.40 mL/min. B represents acetonitrile (0.1% (v/v) acetonitrile), while A represents aqueous formic acid (0.1% (v/v) formic acid). The injection volume was 3 mL, and the column temperature was set to 45.0°C. Mass spectrometry data were recorded by the LTQ Orbitrap mass spectrometer in negative or positive electrospray ionization (ESI) mode. The capillary and source temperatures were 350°C, and the desolvation gas flow was maintained at 45 L/h. Centroid data were acquired from fifty to 1,000 m/z, with a 30,000 resolution.

Multivariate Statistical Analysis and Metabolite Identification

The XCMS program (https://xcmsonline.scripps.edu/landing_page.php?pgcontent=mainPage) was used for the non-linear alignment of data in the time domain and the spontaneous integration and isolation of peak intensities. The subsequent 3D matrix, including data such as retention time and m/z pairs (variable indices), specimen names (observations) and normalized ion intensities (variables), were integrated into the SIMCA program (version 14.0, Umetrics, Umeå, Sweden), in which a partial least squares discriminant analysis (PLS-DA), orthogonal partial least squares discriminant analysis (OPLS-DA) and principal component analysis (PCA) were conducted. Model quality was assessed using R^2X or R^2Y as well as Q^2-values. R^2X or R^2Y represent the percentage of variance in data interpreted using different models and suggested the goodness of fit, while Q^2 represented the prediction from the models detected using the cross-validation procedure. As a default, 7 rounds of cross-validation were conducted using SIMCA throughout the experiment to identify the most appropriate quantity of essential ingredients and prevent excessive model fitting. A permutation evaluation (200 times) was performed to confirm the OPLS-DA results.

Metabolomic Pathway Analysis

The web-based instrument Metabolomic Pathway Analysis (MetPA) (http://www.metaboanalyst.ca/faces/ModuleView.xhtml) was used to build and observe the metabolic pathways influenced by OMO by collecting information from databases such as the Kyoto Encyclopedia of Genes and Genomes (KEGG) and Human Metabolome Database (HMDB). The evaluation of KEGG pathways required Goatools (https://github.com/tanghaibao/Goatools) and KEGG (https://www.kegg.jp/) (34–37).

Statistical Analysis

The results are presented as the means ± SD from at least 3 independent experiments. ANOVA was employed to examine the significance of differences between groups using the Statistical Package for the Social Sciences software (SPSS, Abacus Concepts, Berkeley, CA) and Prism 5 (GraphPad Software, San Diego, USA) software. $P < 0.05$ indicated a significant difference.

RESULTS

OMO Administration Improved the AD Parameters in APP/PS1 Transgenic Mice

The average weight of the APP/PS1 group was increased compared with that of the control group ($p < 0.05$), and the former group exhibited abdominal swelling. The mice treated with OMO exhibited insignificant differences in weight compared with the control group ($p > 0.05$, **Figure 1A**).

The incubation time (IT) of every group treated with OMO was noticeably shorter than that of the APP/PS1 group. Mice that received a low dose of OMO displayed an IT of 86.49 ± 11.64 s, while mice receiving the high dose exhibited an IT of 82.06 ± 19.44 s on the 1st day; both values were noticeably different ($p < 0.01$) from the model group (113.75 ± 16.11). On the 4th day, the IT of mice treated with a low dose of OMO was reduced to 37.19 ± 5.36 s, while the IT of the high-dose group decreased to 28.27 ± 3.96 s, both of which differed remarkably from APP/PS1 mice (56.29 ± 9.69 s, $p < 0.01$, **Figure 1B**). Based on these findings, OMO reversed the learning and memory impairments observed in transgenic APP/PS1 mice.

According to the results of the probe trial, the differences in swimming distance and velocity were insignificant ($p > 0.05$). Mice in the control group swam for longer times in the northwest (target) quadrant (26.63 ± 3.83 s) than in the other quadrants ($p < 0.01$), while mice in the model group displayed a noticeably shorter swimming time (ST) of 20.77 ± 2.36 s ($p < 0.01$) in the aforementioned quadrant, indicating that mice in the control group recalled the position of the platform. The ST of mice receiving a low dose of OMO was 26.50 ± 3.59 s, while the ST of mice receiving the high dose was 27.36 ± 2.51 s, which was noticeably decreased compared with that of the control group. Mice receiving OMO exhibited noticeable differences in ST ($p < 0.01$) from mice in the control group, but the difference in swimming distance was not significant (**Figure 1C**).

HE staining did not reveal obvious alterations in hippocampal neurons in the control (**Figure 1D**). However, noticeable histopathological injury was observed in the hippocampus of APP/PS1 mice. Layered pyramidal neuron structure degeneration and neuronal loss (Nissl staining) were observed in the cortex and CA1 area. These alterations were ameliorated by the OMO supplement. Cells in mice receiving OMO displayed a better morphology, and the number of neurons was increased compared with that in mice that were not treated with OMO, particularly in mice receiving the high dose of OMO. The percentage of $A\beta_{1-42}$-positive cells exhibiting red IHC staining was substantially increased in the model group compared with that in the control group ($p < 0.05$). However, OMO administration decreased $A\beta_{1-42}$ expression (**Figure 1D**).

OMO Administration Improved the Gut Microbiota in APP/PS1 Transgenic Mice

The abundance of operational taxonomic units (OTUs) and the taxonomic profiles were evaluated (**Figure 2**).

Compared with the normal mice, the APP/PS1 transgenic mice exhibited a decrease in the microbial community diversity, as shown in **Figure 2A**, and all the APP/PS1 transgenic mice were clustered well using non-metric multidimensional scaling (NMDS) and PLS-DA (**Figures 2B,C**), indicating that the APP/PS1 transgenic mouse brain influenced the gut microbiota. After treatment with 50 mg/(kg·d) OMO, microbial diversity was improved to approximately the level of the normal control mice (**Figure 2B**).

Analysis revealed differences in the abundance of taxa between different groups, as displayed in **Figure 2D**. The abundance of some bacteria exhibited substantial changes at the genus and family levels in fecal samples from the APP/PS1 mice, while the OMO treatment changed those variations; in particular, obvious increases in the abundance of *Lactobacillus, Allobaculum, Lactobacillaceae,* and *Lachnospiraceae* were observed, indicating that OMO had a prebiotic role in protecting against intestinal dysbacteriosis in the AD model animals.

Moreover, at the genus level, the APP/PS1 transgenic mice exhibited an enrichment of some potential anti-AD microbes, such as *Lactobacillus, Akkermansia, Bacteroides, Adlercreutzia,* and *Desulfovibrio,* and reduced levels of other potential anti-AD microbes, such as *Ruminococcus, Bifidobacterium, Blautia, Oscillospira, Coprococcus, Sutterella,* and *Clostridium*, compared with the normal group (**Figure 4A**). At the family level, the APP/PS1 mice showed an enrichment of some potential anti-AD microbes, such as Lactobacillaceae, Lachnospiraceae, Bacteroidaceae, and Verrucomicrobiaceae, and reduced levels of other potential anti-AD microbes, such as S24-7, Ruminococcaceae, Coriobacteriaceae, Erysipelotrichaceae, and Bifidobacteriaceae, compared with the normal group (**Figure 4B**). Nevertheless, model mice treated with OMO displayed alterations in the quantity of microbes that counteracted AD. Based on these findings, OMO represents a promising treatment to modulate the community structure of GIT microbes.

GIT microbes have an obvious impact on the immune system of organisms. The differences in the gut microbiota among the APP/PS1 transgenic, OMO-treated and control mice are shown in **Figure 3**. A Venn diagram (**Figure 3A**) and a hierarchical tree (**Figure 3B**) revealed that Actinobacteria, Firmicutes, Coriobacterium, Lachnospiraceae, Bacilli, Clostridia, Bacteroidales, Clostridiales, Ruminococcaceae, Lactobacillales, Oscillospira, Bacteroidia, and Proteobacteria were the microbial types exhibiting increased levels after OMO administration and are thus promising candidates for future investigation. As shown in the heatmap (**Figure 3C**), OMO administration remarkably altered the composition of GIT microbes compared to the control group, as the relative abundance levels of the genera *Mucispirillum, Odoribacter, Rikenella, Faecalibacterium, Alistipes, Parabacteroides,* and *Anaerotruncus* were reduced, while the levels of *Arthrobacter, Phycicoccus, Streptococcus, Akkermansia, Blautia, Ruminococcus, Coprococcus, Allobaculum, Dehalobacterium, Methanolinea,* and *Candidatus Methanoregula* were increased. These findings indicate a relationship between the gut microbiota and AD.

According to the results of the KEGG pathway evaluation, categories of metabolic pathways such as the degeneration

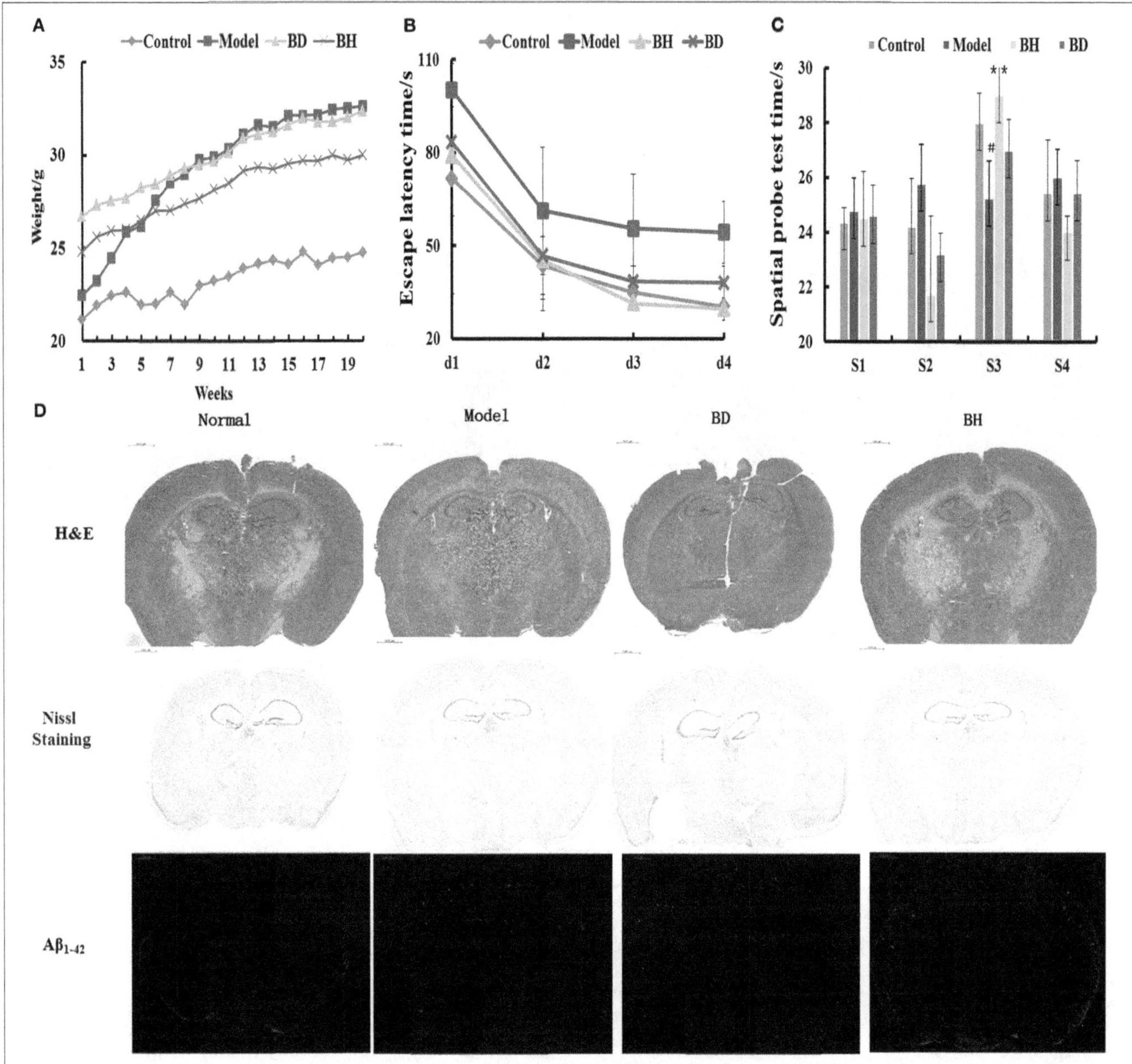

FIGURE 1 | Effect of OMO on APP/PS1 transgenic mice. Body weight changes were measured weekly **(A)**. Escape latencies in the H maze **(B)** and probe test results **(C)**, and histopathological changes in brain tissues **(D)** are shown. N represents the C57 group, M denotes the APP/PS1 transgenic group, BD indicates the group treated with 50 mg/kg OMO, and BH designates the group treated with 100 mg/kg OMO; the treatments were administered for 6 months ($n = 10$). Values are presented as the means ± SDs of six independent experiments. $^{\#}p < 0.05$ compared with the control group; $^{**}p < 0.01$ compared with the M group.

of xenobiotics, the generation and metabolism of glycan, the generation of secondary metabolic products, the enzyme families and metabolism of nucleotides, cofactors, terpenoids, amino acids, vitamins, polyketides, lipids, carbohydrate, and energy were altered in GIT microbes of APP/PS1 transgenic animals. Moreover, quite a few of these pathways were upregulated by the OMO supplement. Dynamic alterations in the 3 groups are displayed in **Figure 4C**, and the results suggested that OMO impacted the GIT microbial metabolism.

OMO Administration Changes On Metabolites in APP/PS1 Transgenic Mice

Multivariate Statistical Analysis

Typical negative and positive base peak APP/PS1 animals are displayed in **Figures 5A,B**, respectively. All the groups resembled one another in blood patterns of BPI chromatograms, with the exception of a few peaks. Multivariate statistical analysis was conducted with the aim of performing a more thorough investigation of the differences between complicated matrices.

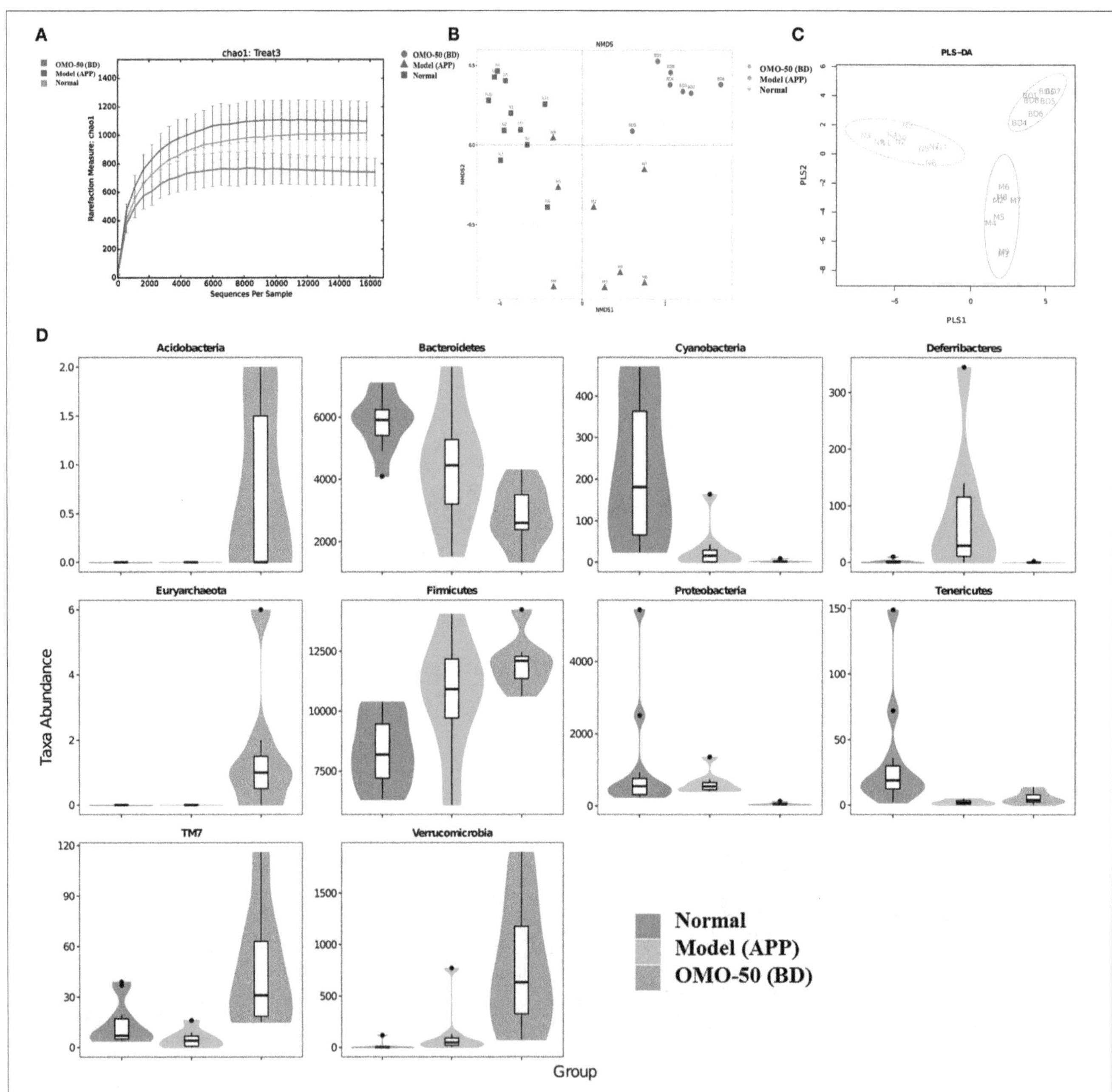

FIGURE 2 | Effects of OMO on the gut microbiota of the APP/PS1 transgenic mice, as determined from fecal samples. The rarefaction curve **(A)**, the results of the NMDS analysis **(B)**, PLS-DA results **(C)**, classification and abundance of fecal contents at the phylum level **(D)**, and the results of 16S rRNA sequencing of the gut microbiota using an Illumina MiSeq sequencing system are shown. N denotes the C57 group, M represents the APP/PS1 transgenic group, BD denotes the 50 mg/kg OMO-treated group, and BH indicates the 100 mg/kg OMO-treated group.

The loading plot showed a trend toward separation between any two groups (**Figure 6A**). Variables with higher loadings (positive and negative) exhibit greater contributions to the differences between the two groups of samples. The labeled metabolites may be relevant to the search for AD biomarkers. A supervised OPLS-DA was utilized to categorize the specimens into 2 blocks, aiming to differentiate between the two kinds of mice. Serum specimens from the two mouse strains were thoroughly isolated according to differences in metabolic patterns using the OPLS-DA loading plot assay. Furthermore, the categorized models were confirmed with the response permutation test (RPT) (38). A permutation plot assisted in the risk evaluation of obtaining a false result from the OPLS-DA. Every blue Q2 dot on the left side was elevated in comparison with primary dots on the right side, suggesting that the primary model was reliable and responsible for the differences observed between the two mouse strains (**Figure 6C**).

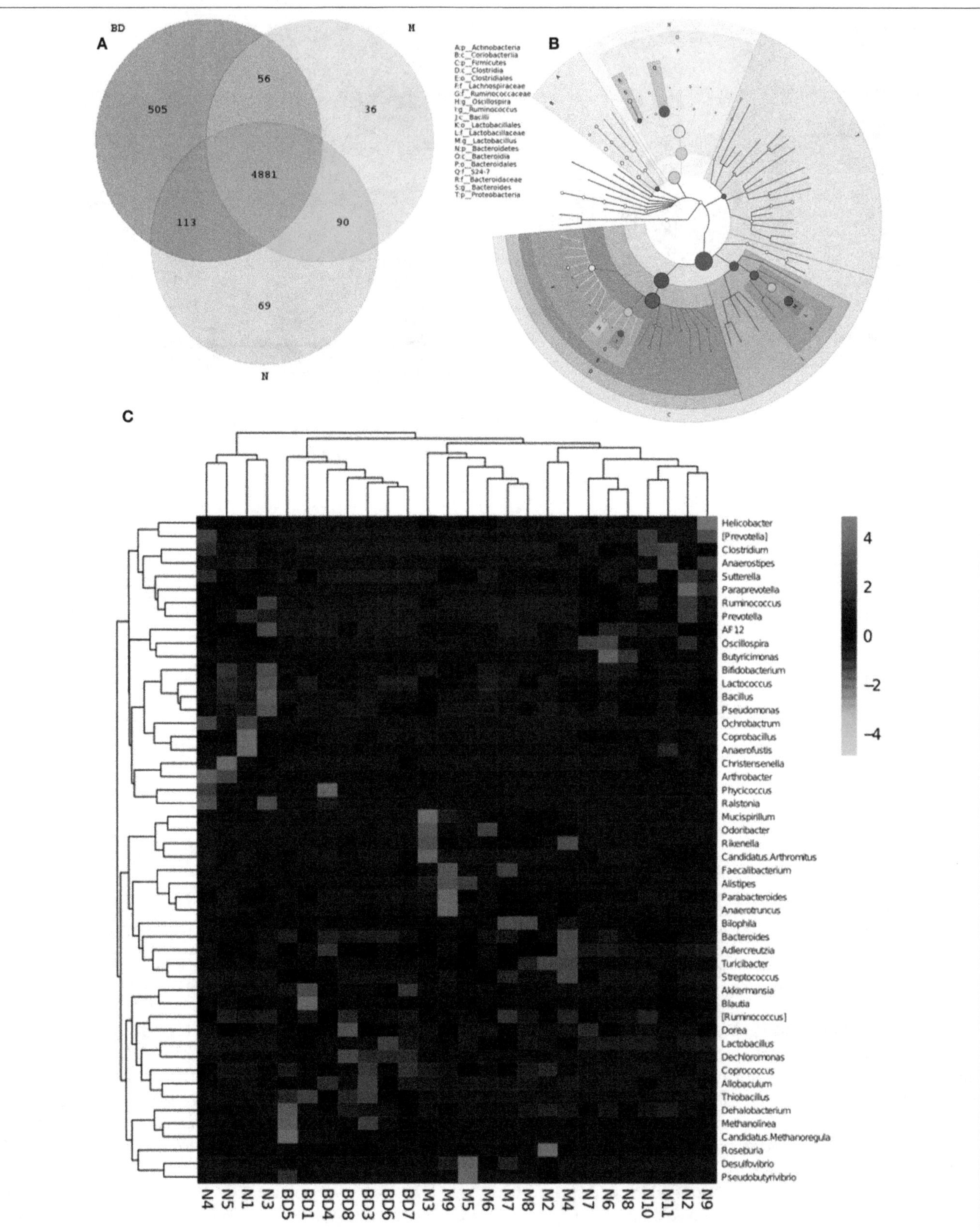

FIGURE 3 | Effects of OMO on the microbiota in fecal samples from the APP/PS1 transgenic mice. A Venn diagram of OTUs **(A)**, a sample species classification tree **(B)**, and the heatmap of 16S rRNA gene sequencing analysis of fecal contents at the genus level **(C)** are shown. N denotes the control group, M denotes the APP/PS1 transgenic group, and BD designates the 50 mg/kg OMO-treated group.

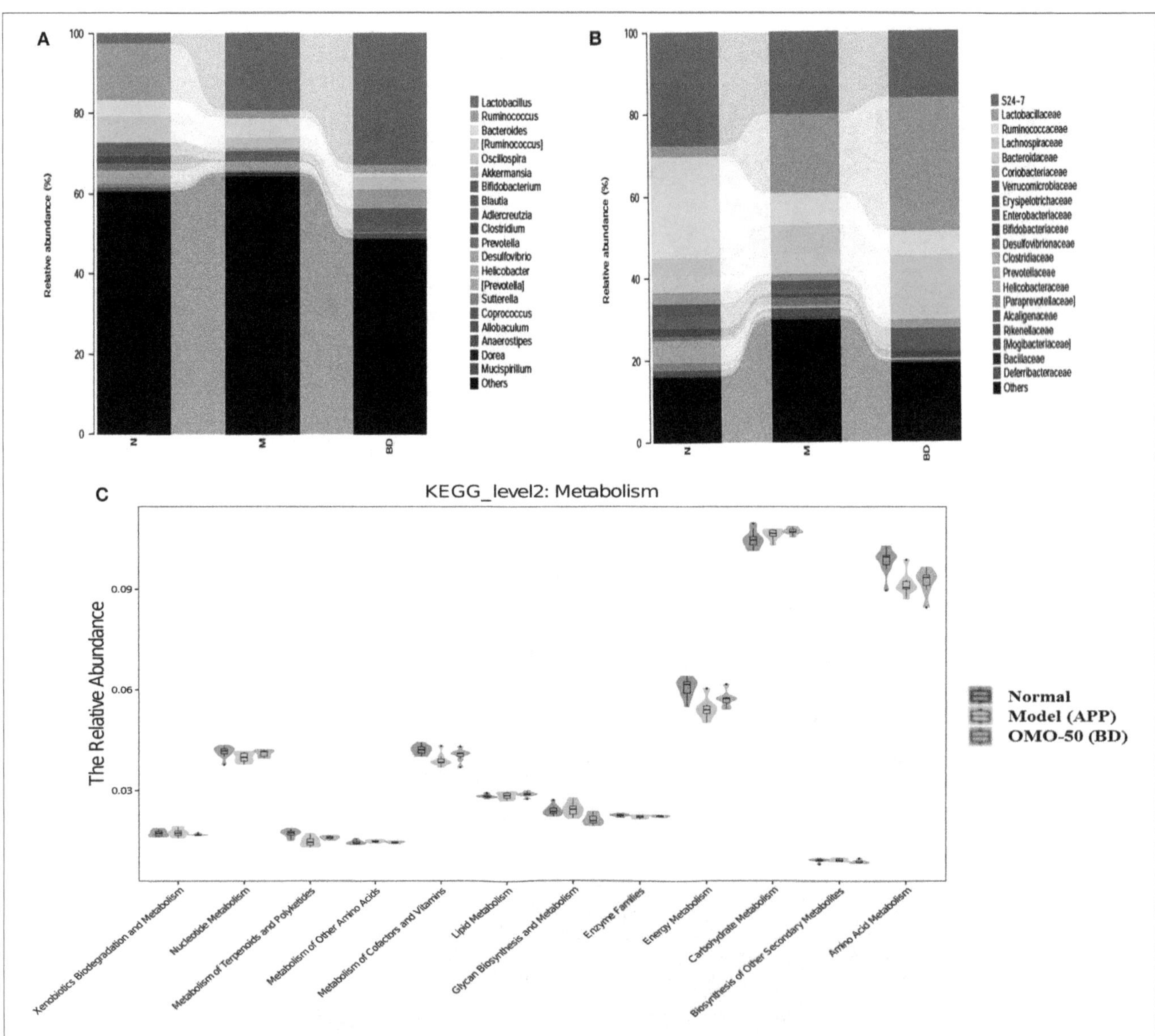

FIGURE 4 | Effects of OMO on the microbiota in fecal samples from the APP/PS1 transgenic mice. The graph in **(A)** shows the classification and abundance of fecal contents at the phylum level, **(B)** shows the classification and abundance of fecal contents at the family level, and **(C)** shows the results of the KEGG pathway enrichment analysis of the gut microbiota with respect to the metabolic systems. Values are presented as the means of six independent experiments. N denotes the control group, M represents the APP/PS1 transgenic group, and BD designates the 50 mg/kg OMO-treated group.

Identification of Candidate Metabolites

UHPLC-LTQ was used to evaluate metabolic pathways with the aim of investigating promising pathways that were influenced by APP/PS1 genes. The candidate metabolic products were identified from the MS/MS fragment data and subsequent searches of web-based databases, including KEGG, METLIN and HMDB. Twenty-two candidate markers were initially identified and featured in this way, a summary of which is displayed in **Figure 7A** (VIP > 1 and $p < 0.05$). We compared the relative intensity of the markers among the APP/PS1 mice, the C57 mice, and the low- and high-dose OMO-treated mice to determine the degree to which those candidate markers were altered. Fourteen metabolites were upregulated, including PI (22:3(10Z, 13Z, 16Z)/16:0), linolelaidic acid, PI (16:0/22:2(13Z, 16Z)), PE (22:1(13Z)/22:5(7Z, 10Z, 13Z, 16Z, 19Z)), PC (18:4(6Z, 9Z, 12Z, 15Z)/20:0), PE (22:1(13Z)/P-18:1(11Z)), 10-methyltridecanoic acid, LysoPC (22:5(7Z, 10Z, 13Z, 16Z, 19Z)), PC (22:6(4Z, 7Z, 10Z, 13Z, 16Z, 19Z)/18:1(9Z)), PE (22:0/P-18:1(9Z)), LysoPE (22:0/0:0), MG (22:5(7Z, 10Z, 13Z, 16Z, 19Z)/0:0/0:0), LysoPC (18:1(11Z)) and 11-β-hydroxyandrosterone-3-glucuronide. The levels of nine metabolites were significantly reduced: PC(20:0/18:3(6Z, 9Z, 12Z)), PC(20:3(5Z, 8Z, 11Z)/20:3(8Z, 11Z, 14Z)), 15(S)-hydroxyeicosatrienoic acid, PC(22:5(7Z, 10Z, 13Z, 16Z, 19Z)/18:0), LysoPC(20:3(8Z, 11Z, 14Z)), diethylphosphate, LysoPE(20:0/0:0) and 9,13-cis-retinoate. Moreover, a clustering analysis of the heatmap of all metabolites

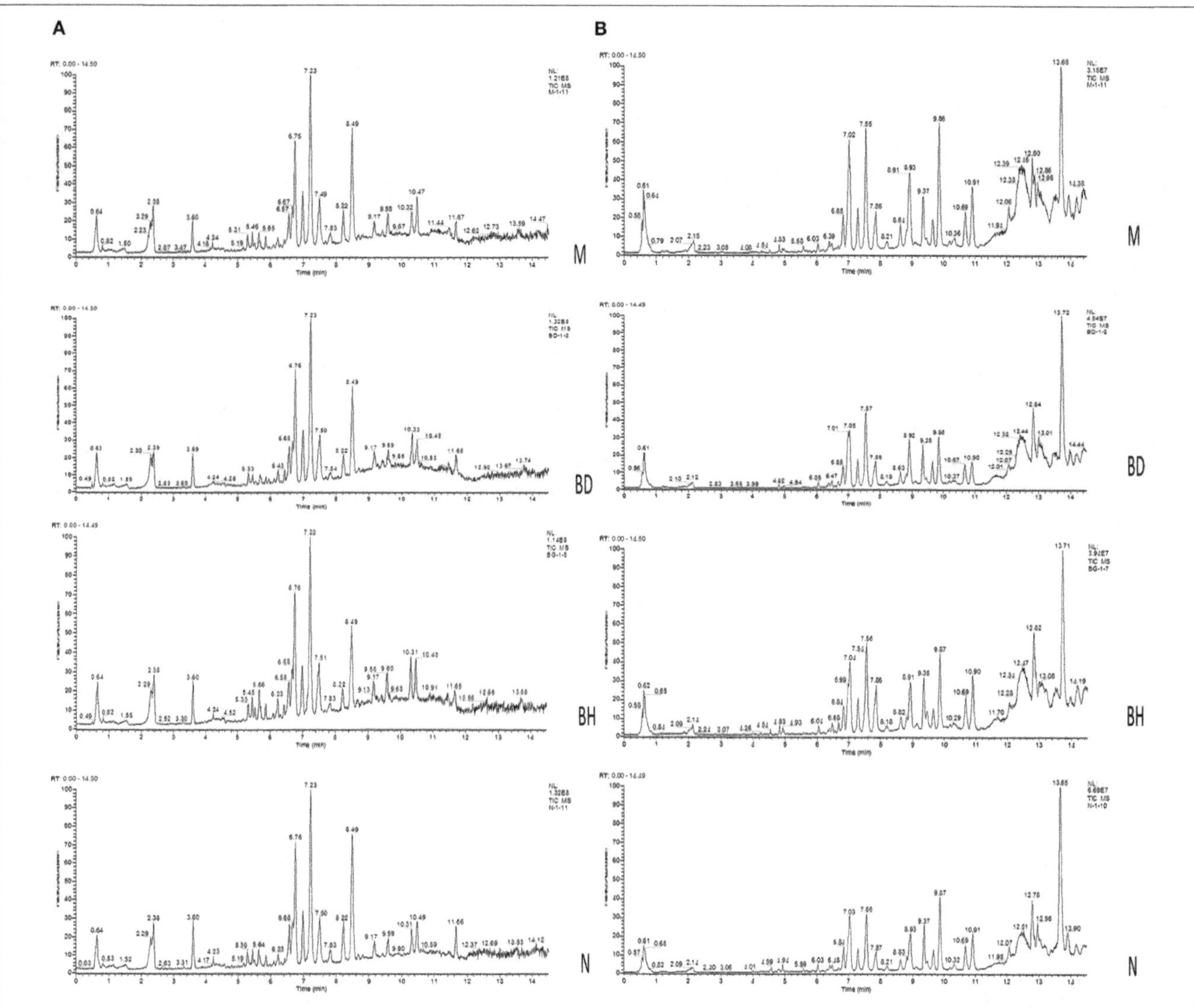

FIGURE 5 | Analysis of the metabolic profiles based on the UPLC/MS spectra of serum samples. Serum BPI chromatograms of APP/PS1 and wild-type mice collected in positive ion mode **(A)** and negative ion mode **(B)**. N denotes the control group, M represents the APP/PS1 transgenic group, BD denotes the 50 mg/kg OMO-treated group, and BH designates the 100 mg/kg OMO-treated group.

revealed the differences in relative levels between the four groups (**Figure 7B**). Furthermore, we obtained the KEGG pathway annotations of the metabolites (**Figure 7C**). In the figure, black indicates KEGG primary pathways, and colors represent KEGG secondary pathways; the number represents the counts of differentially produced metabolites in the metabolic pathway.

DISCUSSION

Pathological changes in AD are associated with microbial infections and gut microbes through four routes of interaction with the brain: direct effects on the vagus nerve, metabolites, direct production or alteration of neurotransmitters, and activation of immune signaling pathways (39). A study in *Nature* (14) also confirmed that the gut microbiota promotes neurodegenerative disease; the gut microbiota are closely associated with neurodegenerative disease in mouse models of Parkinson's disease, and the parkinsonian symptoms are relieved when the gut microbiota is altered. In the present study, OMO markedly modified behavior, regulated neurotransmitter secretion, and ameliorated brain tissue swelling. Moreover, OMO altered the diversity and steady-state composition of the microbial community, and the levels of metabolic products and AD biomarkers were altered. In addition, OMO was an efficacious prebiotic that regulated the composition and metabolism of the gut microbiota in an AD mouse model.

Mechanisms that regulate the GIT microbes have recently been shown to regulate cognition in the host, regardless of whether animals without germs, animals treated with antibiotics or probiotics administration or animals receiving a fecal microbial transplant (FMT) were used (40). The fecal microbial composition was noticeably altered by a 4-day treatment with

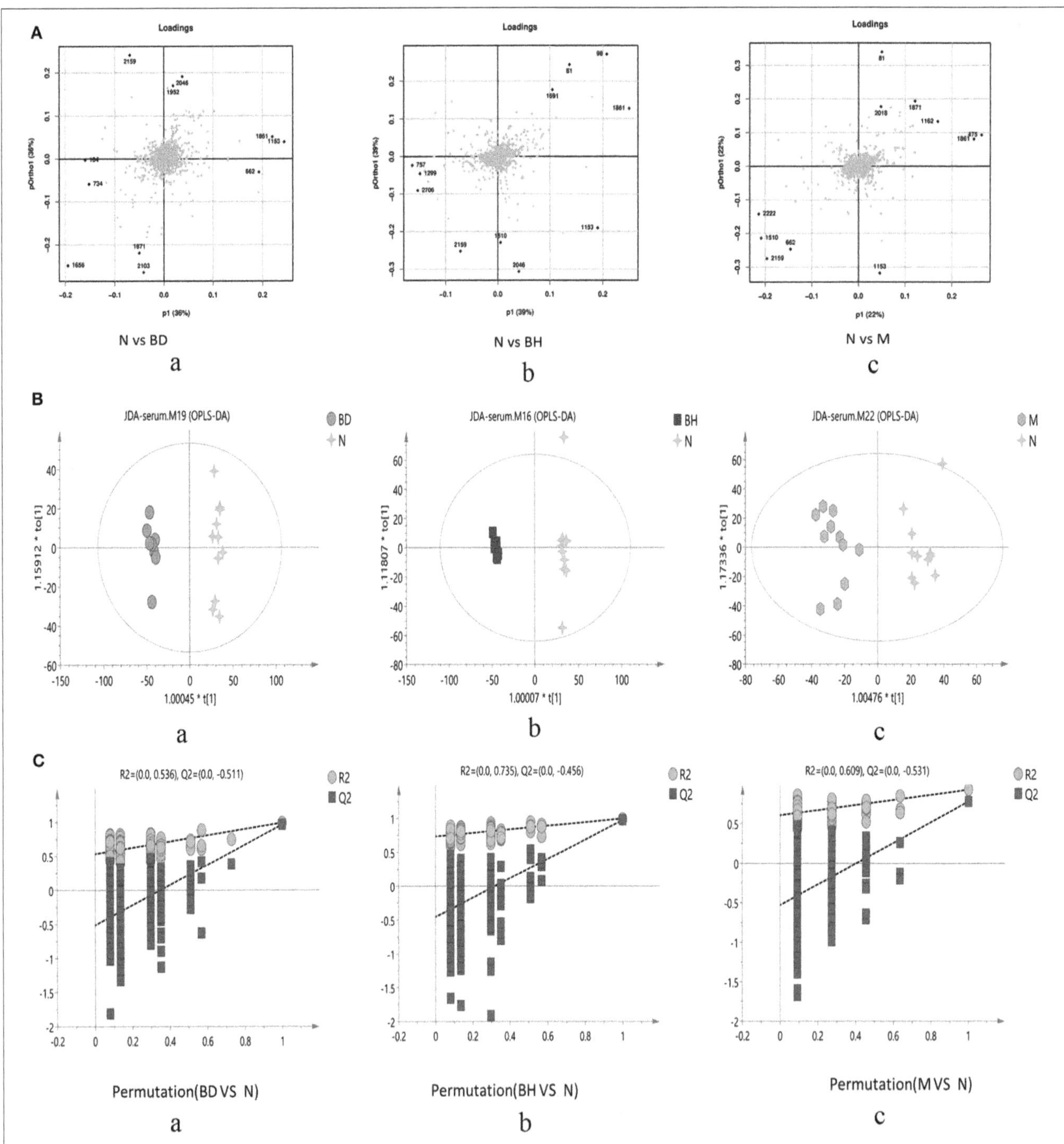

FIGURE 6 | Score plots of metabolite levels in a serum sample. OPLS-DA score plots of the serum metabolic profile **(A)**: (a) N vs. BD, (b) N vs. BH, and (c) N vs. M. Permutation score plots of serum metabolic profiles **(B)**: (a) N vs. BD, (b) N vs. BH, and (c) N vs. M. Loading score plot of the serum metabolic profile **(C)**: (a) N vs. BD, (b) N vs. BH, and (c) N vs. M. N denotes the control group, M represents the APP/PS1 transgenic group, BD denotes the 50 mg/kg OMO-treated group, and BH represents the 100 mg/kg OMO-treated group.

50 mg/(kg·day) OMO compared with that of the control group. Our data were consistent with findings from previous studies showing that alterations in the composition of the gut microbiota in APP/PS1 transgenic mice include a reduction in levels of *Bacteroidetes* and an increase in levels of *Firmicutes* ($p < 0.05$), while the OMO treatment reversed those changes ($p < 0.05$), as shown in **Figure 5** (Graphian), **Figure 6** (OUT and NMDS), indicating that GIT microbes are crucial contributors to host defense. Based on these findings, the gut microbiota acts as a barrier to protect the host from intestinal pathogen attacks (41).

Furthermore, through immunohistochemical staining of global brain tissues in the AD model mice, the present study

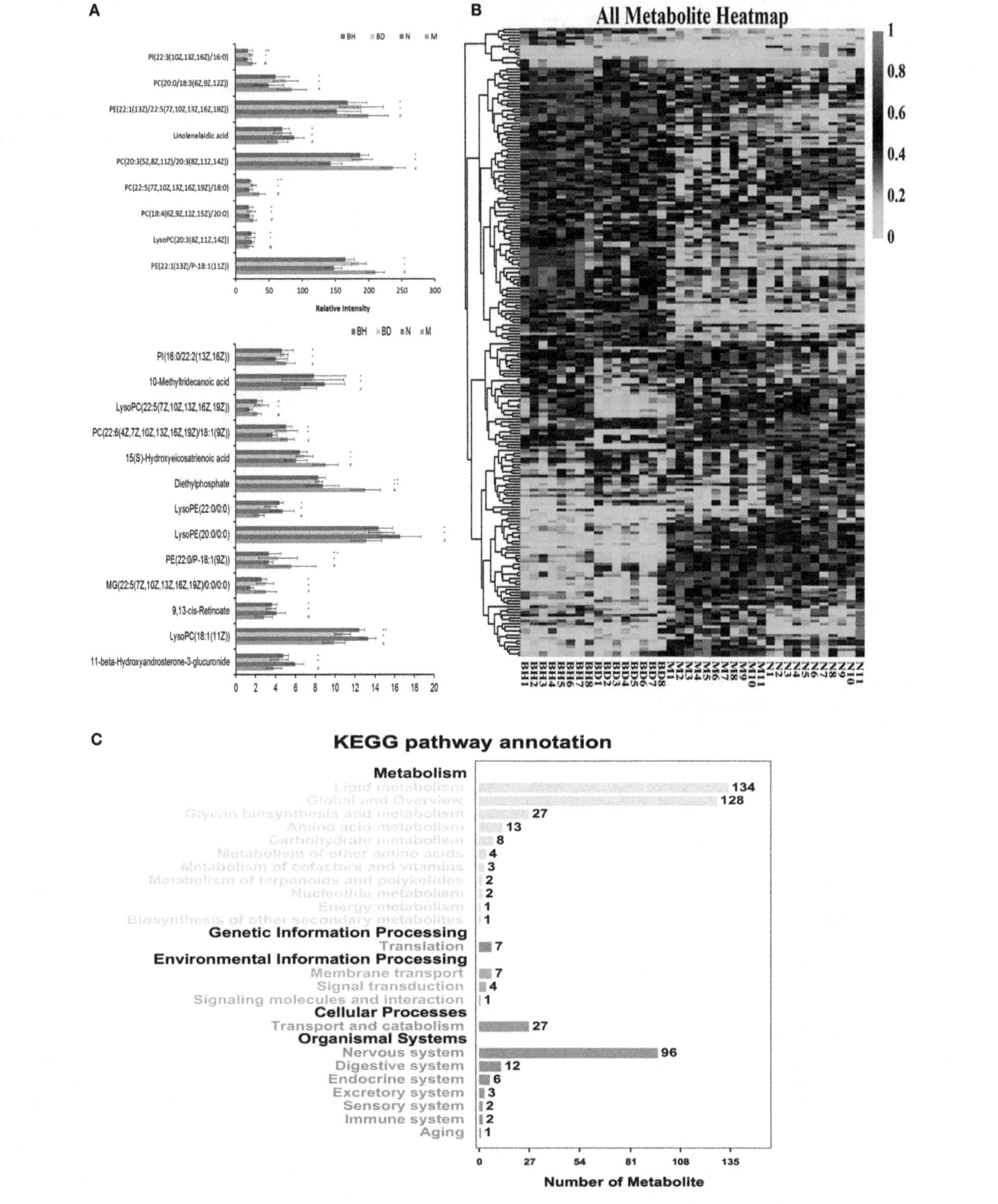

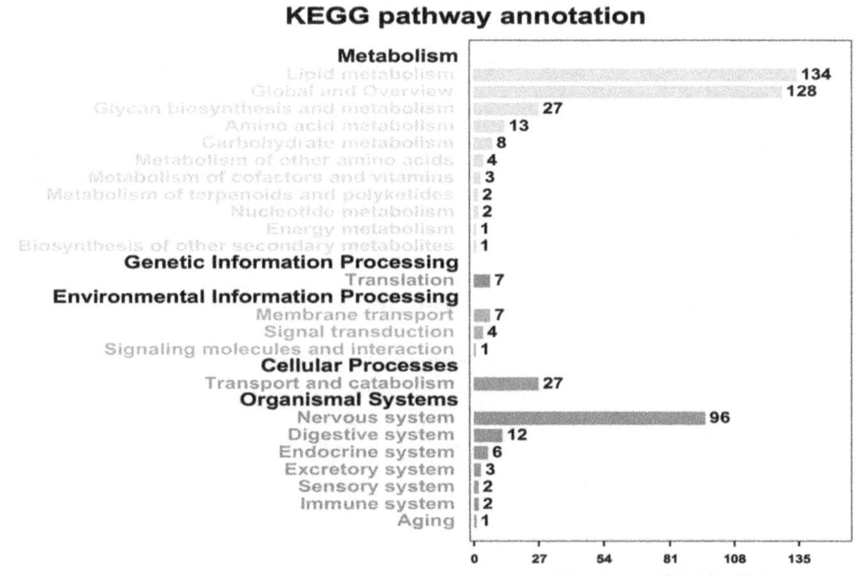

FIGURE 7 | Comparison of the relative intensities of the potential biomarkers **(A)**. KEGG pathway annotations of differentially expressed genes in serum samples **(B)**. Heatmap showing the levels of 24 different metabolites **(C)**. The degree of change is marked with different colors: red represents upregulation, and green indicates downregulation. Each row represents an individual sample, and each column represents a metabolite. N denotes the C57 mice, M represents the APP/PS1 transgenic mice, BD indicates the group treated with 50 mg/kg OMO, and BH denotes the group treated with 100 mg/kg OMO. Values are presented as the means ± SDs of six independent experiments. $^{\#}p < 0.05$ compared with the control group; $^{*}p < 0.05$ and $^{**}p < 0.01$ compared with the M group.

showed that weight, Aβ_{1-42} levels and staining improved to near normal levels (**Figure 1C**), indicating that OMO might regulate protein expression and signaling pathways in cells through the help of the gut microbiota. However, additional studies are required to extend the current findings on the effects of the microbiota on mice to humans to provide a basis for gut microbiota-based therapeutic applications of OMO.

In addition, the OMO treatment had an impact on the quantities of some typical GIT microbes, such as Lactobacillus, Bifidobacterium, Bacteroides, Lachnospiraceae, Akkermansia, Ruminococcus, Blautia, S24-7, Lachnospiraceae, Bacteroidaceae and Ruminococcaceae, in APP/PS1 transgenic animals (**Figures 4A,B**). OMO also affected the gut morphology, mucin production, and gut permeability and reduced dysbacteriosis. According to the results of the 16S metagenome analysis, OMO administration altered the balance of Bacteroidetes and Firmicutes and reduced the abundance of a few beneficial bacterial genera, namely, Akkermansia, Bacteroides, Roseburia, Bifidobacterium, Lactobacillus, and Desulfovibrio, which corroborated previous reports of their roles in metabolic deregulation (42–44).

Importantly, emerging studies have confirmed pathogenic links between GIT microbes and various disorders, particularly the noticeable alteration in quantities of typical microbes in these disorders (45–51). Thus, OMO influences several microbes that affect the generation and secretion of some neurotransmitters and neuromodulators. Murine models of chronic stress displayed similar effects, in which the examined activities, genetic, neuroendocrine and neurochemical alterations observed after the administration of a prebiotic supplement (oligosaccharides and galacto-oligosaccharides) seemed to be regulated in part by short-chain fatty acids (52). Consequently, the therapeutic effects of OMO may be partially attributed to modulatory effects on GIT microbes.

The changes in behavior and the gut microbiota after the administration of OMO coincided with changes in gene expression in blood samples collected from the whole body. A metabolomic analysis of whole-body blood revealed significant changes in the expression of some genes (**Figure 7**).

We have implemented a metabolomic approach using UHPLC-LTQ Orbitrap mass spectrometry to study the metabolites present in mouse serum, with a special emphasis on revealing whole-body metabolic alterations that might indicate early-stage AD and its progression. Based on the results of the enrichment analysis, lipid metabolites might be related to AD (53). In the category of lipid metabolism, *glycerophospholipid metabolism* and *α-linolenic acid metabolism pathway* were prominently altered in AD. Lipid metabolism is affected by levels of glycerol, propylene glycol, and fatty acid compounds in AD (54). These findings were supported by previous studies reporting elevated levels of polyunsaturated fatty acids in the brain (55, 56). Those fatty acids cause lipid peroxidation and promote the generation of toxic products in response to oxidative stress, resulting in neural damage and promoting AD development.

In the present study, levels of endogenous metabolic products in murine blood differed among the normal, model and OMO-treated groups. These alterations correlate with metabolic diseases, such as monoaminergic neurotransmitters in the nervous system (NS) (57). Thus, blood metabolites represent primary predictors of AD generation.

Pathway enrichment analyses in the metabolomics study indicated that the KEGG pathways *Glutamatergic synapse, Calcium signaling pathway, GnRH signaling pathway, Long-term potentiation, Circadian entrainment,* and *Oxytocin signaling pathway* displayed the greatest alterations during disease pathogenesis. These pathways share mutual hub metabolites, such as pyruvate and oxaloacetate, which are the main compounds required for the TCA cycle, gluconeogenesis, and glyoxylate and dicarboxylate metabolism (58). Pyruvate and pyruvate-oxaloacetate protect NS metabolism by promoting brain-to-blood glutamate efflux (59–61).

Although our understanding of the complicated relationship networks between GIT microbes and the brain is insufficient, prebiotics are known to forcefully regulate the microbial ecology. The influences of the microbial composition, abundance, diversity and functions of all GIT microbes must be examined since they are associated with brain function. Data from our study offer stronger proof of the defensive effect of OMO (which contains prebiotics) and help characterize its effects on the microbiota-brain-gut axis in AD. Using the promising natural chemical product OMO, we were able to identify new therapeutic targets for AD and provide a basis for the further study of AD pathogenesis.

AUTHOR CONTRIBUTIONS

YX, CD, YJ, LH, LG, SO, ZC, ZJ, and XY conceived and esigned the experiments. YX, CD, YJ, TX, and ZC performed the experiments. YX, CD, LT, HG, and ZJ analyzed the data. YX and CD wrote the paper and edited the manuscript. All the authors read and approved the final manuscript.

FUNDING

The present work received financial support from the Guangdong Science and Technology Plan Projects (2015A020211021; 2016A050502032), the Guangzhou Science and Technology Plan Projects (201504281708257; 201604020009), the High-level Leading Talent Introduction Program of GDAS (2016GDASRC-0102), Guangzhou Medical University Research Projects (2016C28), National Natural Science Foundation of China (81701086), and the Nanyue Microbial Talents Cultivation Fund of Guangdong Institute of Microbiology.

REFERENCES

Owen JB, Di DF, Sultana R, Perluigi M, Cini C, Pierce WM, et al. Proteomics-determined diffences in the concanavalin-A-fractionated proteome of hippocampus and inferior parietal lobule in subjects with Alzheimer's disease and mild cognitive impairment: implications for progression of AD. *J Proteome Res.* (2009) 8:471–82. doi: 10.1021/pr800667a

Arendt T, Bigl V, Arendt A, Tennstedt A. Loss of neurons in the nucleus basalis of Meynert in Alzheimer's disease, paralysis agitans and Korsakoff's Disease. *Acta Neuropathol.* (1983) 61:101–8. doi: 10.1007/BF00697388

Tu S, Okamoto S, Lipton SA, Xu H. Oligomeric Aβ-induced synaptic dysfunction in Alzheimer's disease. *Mol Neurodegener.* (2014) 9:48. doi: 10.1186/1750-1326-9-48

Adams IM. Structural plasticity of synapses in Alzheimer's disease. *Mol Neurobiol.* (1991) 5:411–9. doi: 10.1007/BF02935562

Hebert LE, Weuve J, Scherr PA, Evans DA. Alzheimer disease in the United States (2010-2050) estimated using the 2010 census. *Neurology* (2013) 80:1778–83. doi: 10.1212/WNL.0b013e31828726f5

Heintz C, Mair W. You are what you host: microbiome modulation of the aging process. *Cell* (2014) 156:408–11. doi: 10.1016/j.cell.2014.01.025

Miklossy J. Emerging roles of pathogens in Alzheimer disease. *Expert Rev Mol Med.* (2011) 13:e30. doi: 10.1017/S1462399411002006

Bhattacharjee S, Lukiw WJ. Alzheimer's disease and the microbiome. *Front Cell Neurosci.* (2013) 7:153. doi: 10.3389/fncel.2013.00153

Huang WS, Yang TY, Shen WC, Lin CL, Lin MC, Kao CH. Association between Helicobacter pylori infection and dementia. *J Clin Neurosci.* (2014) 21:1355–8. doi: 10.1016/j.jocn.2013.11.018

Mancuso R, Baglio F, Cabinio M, Calabrese E, Hernis A, Nemni R, et al. Titers of herpes simplex virus type 1 antibodies positively correlate with grey matter volumes in Alzheimer's disease. *J Alzheimers Dis.* (2014) 38:741–5. doi: 10.3233/JAD-130977

Mayer EA. Gut feelings:the emerging biology of gut-braincommunication. *Nat Rev Neurosci.* (2011) 12:453–66. doi: 10.1038/nrn3071

Pistollato F, Sumalla CS, Elio I, Masias VM, Giampieri F, Battino M. Role of gut microbiota and nutrients in amyloid formation and pathogenesis of Alzheimer disease. *Nutr Rev.* (2016) 74:624–34. doi: 10.1093/nutrit/nuw023

Zhao Y, Jaber V, Lukiw WJ. Secretory products of the human GI tract microbiome and their potential impact on Alzheimer's Disease (AD): detection of lipopolysaccharide (LPS) in AD. *Front Cell Infect Microbiol.* (2017) 7:318. doi: 10.3389/fcimb.2017.00318

Daniel E, Marco P. Microbiology: gut microbes augment neurodegeneration. Nature (2017) 544:304–5. doi: 10.1038/nature21910

Walker AW, Sanderson JD, Churcher C, Parkes GC, Hudspith BN, Rayment N, et al. High-throughput clone library analysis of the mucosa-associated microbiota reveals dysbiosis and differences between inflamed and non-inflamed regions of the intestine in inflammatory bowel disease. *BMC Microbiol.* (2011) 11:7. doi: 10.1186/1471-2180-11-7

Round JL, Mazmanian SK. The gut microbiota shapes intestinal immune responses during health and disease. *Nat Rev Immunol.* (2009) 9:313–23. doi: 10.1038/nri2515

Hsiao EY, McBride SW, Hsien S, Sharon G, Hyde ER, McCue T, et al. Microbiota modulate behavioral and physiological abnormalities associated with neurodevelopmental disorders. *Cell* (2013) 155:1451–63. doi: 10.1016/j.cell.2013.11.024

De Filippo C, Cavalieri D, Di Paola M, Ramazzotti M, Poullet JB, Massart S, et al. Impact of diet in shaping gut microbiota revealed by a comparative study in children from Europe and rural Africa. *Proc Natl Acad Sci USA.* (2010) 107:14691–6. doi: 10.1073/pnas.1005963107

Maslowski KM, Vieira AT, Ng A, Kranich J, Sierro F, Yu D, et al. Regulation of inflammatory responses by gut microbiota and chemoattractant receptor GPR43. *Nature* (2009) 461:1282–6. doi: 10.1038/nature 08530

Roca-Saavedra P, Mendez-Vilabrille V, Miranda JM, Nebot C, Cardelle- Cobas A, Franco CM, et al. Food additives contaminants and other minor components: effects on human gut microbiota-a review. *J Physiol Biochem.* (2017) 74:69–83. doi: 10.1007/s13105-017-0564-2

Neuman MG, Nanau RM. Inflammatory bowel disease: role of diet, microbiota, life style. *Transl Res.* (2012) 160:29–44. doi: 10.1016/j.trsl.2011.09.001

Kori M, Aydin B, Unal S, Arga KY, Kazan D. Metabolic biomarkers and neurodegeneration:a pathway enrichment analysis of Alzheimer's Disease, Parkinson's disease, and amyotrophic lateral sclerosis. *OMICS* (2016) 20:645–61. doi: 10.1089/omi.2016.0106

González-Domínguez R, Rupérez FJ, García-Barrera T, Barbas C, Gómez-Ariza JL. Metabolomic-driven elucidation of serum disturbances associated with Alzheimer's disease and mild cognitive impairment. *Curr Alzheimer Res.* (2016) 13:641–53. doi: 10.2174/1567205013666160129095138

Sahin M, Karauzum SB, Perry G, Smith MA, Aliciguzel Y. Retinoic acid isomers protect hippocampal neurons from amyloid-beta induced neurodegeneration. *Neurotox Res.* (2005) 7:243–50. doi: 10.1007/BF03036453

van de Wouw M, Schellekens H, Dinan TG, Cryan JF. Microbiota-gut-brain axis: modulator of host metabolism and appetite. *J Nutr.* (2017) 147:727–45. doi: 10.3945/jn.116.240481

Yang N, Wei Y, Xu Q, Tang B. Progress in epigenetic research on Alzheimer disease. *Chin J Med Genet.* (2016) 33:252–5. doi: 10.3760/cma.j.issn.1003-9406.2016.02.028

Chen DL, Zhang P, Lin L, Zhang HM, Liu SH. Protective effect of oligosaccharides from *Morinda officinalis* on β-amyloid-induced dementia rats. *China J Chin Mater Med.* (2013) 38:1306–9. doi: 10.4268/cjcmm20130908

Chen DL, Yang X, Yang J, Lai GX, Yong TQ, Tang XC, et al. Prebiotic effect of fructooligosaccharides from *Morinda officinalis* on Alzheimer's disease in rodent models by targeting the microbiota-gut-brain axis. *Front Aging Neurosci.* (2017) 9:403. doi: 10.3389/fnagi.2017.00403

Melnikova T, Savonenko A, Wang Q, Liang X, Hand T, Wu L, et al. Cycloxygenase-2 activity promotes cognitive deficits but not increased amyloid burden in a model of Alzheimer's disease in a sex-dimorphic pattern. *Neuroscience* (2006) 141:1149–62. doi: 10.1016/j.neuroscience.2006.05.001

Ling ZX, Xia L, Jia XY, Cheng YW, Luo YQ, Li Y, et al. Impacts of infection with different toxigenic Clostridium difficile strains on faecal microbiota in children. *Sci Rep.* (2014) 4:7485. doi: 10.1038/srep07485

Chen DL, Zhang P, Lin L, Zhang HM, Deng SD, Wu ZQ, et al. Protective effects of bajijiasu in a rat model of Aβ25–35 -induced neurotoxicity. *J Ethnopharmacol.* (2014) 154:206–17. doi: 10.1016/j.jep.2014.04.004

Zeng GF, Zhang ZY, Lu L, Xiao DQ, Zong SH, He JM. Protective effects of ginger root extract on Alzheimer disease-induced behavioral dysfunction in rats. *Rejuven Res.* (2013) 16:124–33. doi: 10.1089/rej.2012.1389

Tang Z, Liu LF, Li YL, Dong JY, Li M, Huang JD, et al. Urinary metabolomics reveals alterations of aromatic amino acid metabolism of Alzheimer's disease in the transgenic CRND8 mice. *Curr Alzheimer Res.* (2016) 13:764–76. doi: 10.2174/1567205013666160129095340

Wang L, Feng Z, Wang X, Wang X, Zhang X. DEGseq: an R package for identifying differentially expressed genes from RNA-seq data. *Bioinformatics* (2010) 26:136–8. doi: 10.1093/bioinformatics/btp612

Trapnell C, Hendrickson DG, Sauvageau M, Goff L, Rinn JL, Pachter L. Differential analysis of gene regulation at transcript resolution with RNA-seq. *Nat Biotech.* (2013) 31:46–53. doi: 10.1038/nbt.2450

Cabili MN, Trapnell C, Goff L, Koziol M, Tazon-Vega B, Regev A, et al. Integrative annotation of human large intergenic noncoding RNAs reveals global properties and specific subclasses. *Genes Dev.* (2011) 25:1915–27. doi: 10.1101/gad.17446611

Sun L, Luo H, Bu D, Zhao G, Yu K, Zhang C, et al. Utilizing sequence intrinsic composition to classify protein-coding and long non-coding transcripts. *Nucleic Acids Res.* (2013) 41:e166. doi: 10.1093/nar/gkt646

Golbraikh A, Tropsha A. Beware of q2!. *J Mol Graph Model.* (2002) 20:269–76. doi: 10.1016/S1093-3263(01)00123-1

Pochu H, David AR. More than a gut feeling: the implications of the gut microbiota in psychiatry. *Biol Psychiatry* (2017) 81:e35–7. doi: 10.1016/j.biopsych.2016.12.018

Hu X, Wang T, Jin F. Alzheimer's disease and gut microbiota. *Sci China Life Sci.* (2016) 59:1006–23. doi: 10.1007/s11427-016-5083-9

Vindigni SM, Zisman TL, Suskind DL, Damman CJ. The intestinal microbiome, barrier function, and immune system in inflammatory bowel disease: a tripartite pathophysiological circuit with implications for new therapeutic directions. *Ther Adv Gastroenterol.* (2016) 9:606–25. doi: 10.1177/1756283X16644242

Dao MC, Everard A, Aron-Wisnewsky J, Sokolovska N, Prifti E, Verger EO, et al. *Akkermansia muciniphila* and improved metabolic health during a dietary intervention in obesity: relationship with gut microbiome richness and ecology. *Gut* (2016) 65:426–36. doi: 10.1136/gutjnl-2014-308778

Neyrinck AM, Possemiers S, Druart C, Van de WT, De Backer F, Cani PD, et al. Prebiotic effects of wheat arabinoxylan related to the increase in bifidobacteria, Roseburia and Bacteroides/Prevotella in diet- induced obese mice. *PLoS ONE* (2011) 6:e20944. doi: 10.1371/journal.pone.0 020944

Wang J, Tang H, Zhang C, Zhao Y, Derrien M, Rocher E, et al. Modulation of gut microbiota during probiotic-mediated attenuation of metabolic syndrome in high fat diet-fed mice. *Isme J.* (2015) 9:1–15. doi: 10.1038/ismej.2014.99

Le CE, Nielsen T, Qin J, Prifti E, Hildebrand F, Falony G, et al. Richness of human gut microbiome correlates with metabolic markers. *Nature* (2013) 500:541–6. doi: 10.1038/nature12506

Cotillard A, Kennedy SP, Kong LC, Prifti E, Pons N, Le CE, et al. Dietary intervention impact on gut microbial gene richness. *Nature* (2013) 500:585–8. doi: 10.1038/nature12480

Arora T, Bäckhed F. The gut microbiota and metabolic disease: current understanding and future perspectives. *J Intern Med.* (2016) 280:339–49. doi: 10.1111/joim.12508

Ridaura VK, Faith JJ, Rey F, Cheng J, Duncan AE, Kau AL, et al. Gut microbiota from twins discordant for obesity modulate metabolism in mice. *Science* (2013) 341:1241214. doi: 10.1126/science.1241214

Turnbaugh PJ, Hamady M, Yatsunenko T. A core gut microbiome in obese and lean twins. *Nature* (2009) 457:480–4. doi: 10.1038/nature07540

Ott SJ, Musfeldt M, Wenderoth DF, Hampe J, Brant O, Fölsch UR, et al. Reduction in diversity of the colonic mucosa associated bacterial microflora in patients with active inflammatory bowel disease. *Gut* (2004) 53:685–93. doi: 10.1136/gut.2003.025403

Larsen N, Vogensen FK, van den Berg FW, Nielsen DS, Andreasen AS, Pedersen BK, et al. Gut microbiota in human adults with type 2 diabetes differsfrom non-diabetic adults. *PLoS ONE* (2010) 5:e9085. doi: 10.1371/journal.pone.0009085

Burokas A, Arboleya S, Moloney RD, Peterson VL, Murphy K, Clarke G, et al. Targeting the microbiota-gut-brain axis: prebiotics have anxiolytic and antidepressant-like effects and reverse the impact of chronic stress in mice. *Biol Psychiatry* (2017) 82:472–87. doi: 10.1016/j.biopsych.2016.12.031

González-Domínguez R, García-Barrera T, Vitorica J, Gómez-Ariza JL. Deciphering metabolic abnormalities associated with Alzheimer's disease in the APP/PS1 mouse model using integrated metabolomics approaches. *Biochimie* (2015) 110:119–28. doi: 10.1016/j.biochi.2015.01.005

Drolle E, Negoda A, Hammond K, Pavlov E, Leonenko Z. Changes in lipid membranes may trigger amyloid toxicity in Alzheimer's disease. *PLoS ONE* (2017) 12:e0182194. doi: 10.1371/journal.pone.0182194

Dias V, Junn E, Mouradian MM. The role of oxidative stress in Parkinson's disease. *J Parkinsons Dis.* (2013) 3:461–91. doi: 10.3233/JPD-130230

Liu X, Yamada N, Maruyama W, Osawa T. Formation of dopamine adducts derived from brain polyunsaturated fatty acids: mechanism for Parkinson disease. *J Biol Chem.* (2008) 283:34887–95. doi: 10.1074/jbc.M805682200

Yu J, Kong L, Zhang A, Han Y, Liu Z, Sun H, et al. High-throughput metabolomics for discovering potential metabolite biomarkers and metabolic mechanism from the APPswe/PS1dE9 transgenic model of Alzheimer's disease. *J Proteome Res.* (2017) 16:3219–28. doi: 10.1021/acs.jproteome.7b00206

Garrett RH, Grisham CM. *Principles of Biochemistry With a Human Focus.* Brooks/Cole; Thomson Learning (2002). p. 578–85.

Carvalho AS, Torres LB, Persike DS, Fernandes MJ, Amado D, Naffah-Mazzacoratti, MG, et al. Neuroprotective effect of pyruvate and oxaloacetate during pilocarpine induced status epilepticus in rats. *Neurochem Int.* (2011) 58:385–90. doi: 10.1016/j.neuint.2010.12.014

Zilberter Y, Gubkina O, Ivanov AI. A unique array of neuroprotective effects of pyruvate in neuropathology. *Front Neurosci.* (2015) 9:17. doi: 10.3389/fnins.2015.00017

Zlotnik A, Gurevich B, Tkachov S, Maoz I, Shapira Y, Teichberg VI. Brain neuroprotection by scavenging blood glutamate. *Exp Neurol.* (2007) 203:213–20. doi: 10.1016/j.expneurol.2006.08.021

10

Ethnopharmacological Approaches for Dementia Therapy and Significance of Natural Products and Herbal Drugs

Devesh Tewari[1†], Adrian M. Stankiewicz[2†], Andrei Mocan[3,4], Archana N. Sah[1], Nikolay T. Tzvetkov[5], Lukasz Huminiecki[2], Jarosław O. Horbańczuk[2] and Atanas G. Atanasov[2,6]*

[1] Department of Pharmaceutical Sciences, Faculty of Technology, Kumaun University, Nainital, India, [2] Institute of Genetics and Animal Breeding of the Polish Academy of Sciences, Jastrzebiec, Poland, [3] Department of Pharmaceutical Botany, Iuliu Haţieganu University of Medicine and Pharmacy, Cluj-Napoca, Romania, [4] ICHAT and Institute for Life Sciences, University of Agricultural Sciences and Veterinary Medicine, Cluj-Napoca, Romania, [5] Department of Molecular Biology and Biochemical Pharmacology, Institute of Molecular Biology Roumen Tsanev, Bulgarian Academy of Sciences, Sofia, Bulgaria, [6] Department of Pharmacognosy, University of Vienna, Vienna, Austria

***Correspondence:**
Atanas G. Atanasov
a.atanasov.mailbox@gmail.com

[†] These authors have contributed equally to this study.

Dementia is a clinical syndrome wherein gradual decline of mental and cognitive capabilities of an afflicted person takes place. Dementia is associated with various risk factors and conditions such as insufficient cerebral blood supply, toxin exposure, mitochondrial dysfunction, oxidative damage, and often coexisting with some neurodegenerative disorders such as Alzheimer's disease (AD), Huntington's disease (HD), and Parkinson's disease (PD). Although there are well-established (semi-)synthetic drugs currently used for the management of AD and AD-associated dementia, most of them have several adverse effects. Thus, traditional medicine provides various plant-derived lead molecules that may be useful for further medical research. Herein we review the worldwide use of ethnomedicinal plants in dementia treatment. We have explored a number of recognized databases by using keywords and phrases such as "dementia", "Alzheimer's," "traditional medicine," "ethnopharmacology," "ethnobotany," "herbs," "medicinal plants" or other relevant terms, and summarized 90 medicinal plants that are traditionally used to treat dementia. Moreover, we highlight five medicinal plants or plant genera of prime importance and discuss the physiological effects, as well as the mechanism of action of their major bioactive compounds. Furthermore, the link between mitochondrial dysfunction and dementia is also discussed. We conclude that several drugs of plant origin may serve as promising therapeutics for the treatment of dementia, however, pivotal evidence for their therapeutic efficacy in advanced clinical studies is still lacking.

Keywords: Alzheimer's disease, amyloid fibrils, β-amyloid, dementia, ethnopharmacology, herbal drugs

INTRODUCTION

Dementia is a clinical syndrome wherein gradual decline of mental and cognitive capabilities of an afflicted person takes place. As the disease progresses, the ability to function independently of an affected individual deteriorates due to memory loss (Burgess et al., 2002; Damasio and Gabrowski, 2004; Grand et al., 2011). The causes of dementia can be either reversible or irreversible. The reversible causes include, for example, substance abuse, subdural hematoma, removable tumors, and central nervous system (CNS) infections (Tripathi and Vibha, 2009). Some of the irreversible causes of dementia are neurodegenerative diseases such as Alzheimer's disease (AD), Parkinson's disease (PD), and Huntington's disease (HD) (Mehan et al., 2012).

Thus, dementia is associated with multiple predisposing conditions and risk factors, among which aging is the greatest and most obvious one (Blennow et al., 2006; Corrada et al., 2010). The most widespread group of dementias is related to neurodegenerative disorders, including AD, PD, and HD, or amyotrophic lateral sclerosis (ALS). Another important group of dementias are vascular cognitive impairments. These pathologies often coexist with neurodegenerative dementias (Iadecola, 2013). Vascular cognitive impairments arise due to various cerebrovascular pathologies, such as hypoperfusions or hemorrhages causing disruption of the blood-brain barrier (BBB) and neurovascular units, usually in hemispheric white matter (Iadecola, 2013). Other diseases may also contribute to development of dementia. Such diseases include metabolic disorders, which participate in the pathology via dysregulation of energy management (Cai et al., 2012), AIDS, which causes indirect damage to the brain through immune activated macrophages (Navia and Rostasy, 2005), or even systemic infections (Lim et al., 2015). Various environmental factors also increase the risk of developing dementia. For example toxins contained in abused substances (Ridley et al., 2013), pesticides (Yan et al., 2016), or air pollution (Rivas-Arancibia et al., 2013; Power et al., 2016) may cause oxidative stress and subsequent neuronal cell death. In addition to the above factors, the etiology of dementia includes a genetic component. The occurrence of dementia is connected with numerous gene polymorphisms and other mutations (Weksler et al., 2013). For example, mutations in three deterministic autosomal dominant genes, i.e., presenilin 1 (PSEN1) on chromosome 14q, presenilin 2 (PSEN2) on 1q, and amyloid precursor protein (APP) on 21q, are associated with early-onset AD (EOAD) (Giri et al., 2016). The apolipoprotein E (APOE) gene, located at locus 19q13.2, is the strongest genetic risk factor for sporadic lead-onset AD (LOAD) (Corder et al., 1993; Giri et al., 2016; Swerdlow et al., 2017). There are three common APOE alleles, namely APOE ε2, ε3, and ε4 alleles, among which the APOE ε4 genotype is mainly associated with the higher risk of AD development (Mahley and Rall, 2000; Giri et al., 2016; Swerdlow et al., 2017). The link between the APOE ε4 genotype and development of AD pathology is complex (Giri et al., 2016). Studies suggest that APOE ε4 is associated with 3- up to 12-fold increased risk of LOAD and earlier onset of dementia in individuals with PSEN1 mutation, whereas APOE ε2 decreases the risk of LOAD (Pastor et al., 2003; Giri et al., 2016). In addition, APOE ε4 contributes to AD pathogenesis by Aβ-independent mechanisms involving neurovascular functions, synaptic plasticity, cholesterol homeostasis, and neuroinflammation (Giri et al., 2016). Thus, the presence of APOE4 ε4 allele is considered one of the risk factors for AD; more specifically, it is associated with increased risk of cerebral amyloid angiopathy and age-related cognitive decline during aging (Liu et al., 2013).

Dementia is a highly prevalent syndrome. Despite its prevalence, some evidence suggest that only 10% (low-middle-income countries) to 50% (high-income countries) of all dementia cases are diagnosed (Prince et al., 2016). In addition, the number of dementia cases will grow in consecutive years, as dementia mostly affects the elderly, and the number of people with advanced age is rising rapidly due to the global increase in life expectancy. Quaglio et al. (2016) approximate, that 1.5–2% of the Europeans are currently affected by dementia. On a similar note, Prince et al. (2016) estimated that in 2015 around 47 million people globally suffered from dementia. This number may reach roughly 131 million in 2050 (Prince et al., 2016). In the year 2021, one million people will be affected by dementia in the UK alone (Knapp et al., 2007). The importance of developing novel dementia treatments was recognized by the G7 summit in December 2014. The forum participants recommended that dementia should be treated as a global priority with the main objective to introduce effective therapy by 2025 (Cummings et al., 2016).

Dementia is a significant burden on society both by eliciting human suffering and financially. Dementia is the fifth most frequent cause of death in high-income countries (Dolgin, 2016). Their caregivers were also negatively affected by the health conditions of the patients and showed moderately high levels of depressive symptoms (Schulz et al., 2008). According to the World Alzheimer Report 2016 (Prince et al., 2016), not only in the low-income countries, but also in the high-income countries people with dementia have poor access to healthcare due to its high cost and ineffective diagnostic systems. Dementia management is very expensive due to long-lasting and costly care that the patients receive (Hurd et al., 2013). Various costs related to dementia, including health services, social services, unpaid careers, and others reach around €23 billion per year alone in the UK (Luengo-Fernandez et al., 2010). This economic burden can be further illustrated by the fact that, in the UK, the current annual cost of dementia is higher than current annual costs of heart disease and cancer combined (Luengo-Fernandez et al., 2010). Another prediction suggests that by 2050 dementia and Alzheimer's disease may cost the United States alone around USD 1 trillion (Dolgin, 2016).

In this review, we present a global overview on the worldwide use of ethnomedicine for the management of dementia. Moreover, we also focus on five prominent plants traditionally used for dementia treatment and highlight the constituents, which may be responsible for plant's bioactivity.

Currently, there is no highly effective medicine that stops the progressive course of dementia (Abbott, 2011). We propose that learning about the active substances produced by some plants and

TABLE 1 | Most common forms of dementia (according to Abbott, 2011).

Dementia form	Neuropathology	Symptoms	Dementia cases (%)
AD-related dementia	Aβ plaques, neurofibrillary tangles	Memory deficits, depression, poor judgment or evidence of mental confusion	50–80
Vascular dementia	Decreased or interrupted blood flow to the brain, hypoperfusion, oxidative stress	Similar to AD, but less affected memory	20–30
Dementia with Lewy bodies	α-Synuclein aggregates in neurons and glial cells (cortical Lewy bodies)	Similar to AD and less to PD, hallucinations, tremors, impaired attention	<5
Frontotemporal dementia	Accumulation of MAP tau, atrophy of frontal and temporal lobes	Changes in social behavior, difficulties with language	5–10

their mechanism of action may lead to the development of novel therapies for dementia. The natural products pool represents a continuous major source for drug discovery (Atanasov et al., 2015). In this context, the present review could serve as a useful resource for the development of ethnomedicine-derived pharmaceuticals for the dementia therapy.

FREQUENT FORMS OF DEMENTIA

The most common types of dementia are AD-related dementia (approximately 50–80% of all dementia cases) (Qiu et al., 2009; Abbott, 2011), vascular dementia (approximately 20–30%) (Abbott, 2011; Iadecola, 2013), dementia with Lewy bodies (between 15 and 35% according to Zupancic et al., 2011, or less than 5% according to Abbott, 2011) and the frontotemporal dementia (FTD), which is the fourth most frequent form of presenile dementia (between 5 and 10%) (Abbott, 2011; **Table 1**).

Common to these dysfunctions is a presence of abnormal accumulated proteins in the brains of patients. For example, in AD amyloid beta (Aβ) peptides aggregate into amyloid plaques (Hardy and Higgins, 1992), while TDP-43 protein accumulates in the human brain during the course of FTD (Baloh, 2011). Brains of FTD patients show gross atrophy of frontal and anterior temporal lobes (Brun, 1987; McKhann et al., 2001), and their histopathology reveals microvacuolar degeneration and loss of pyramidal neurons in the frontal and temporal cortex (Rabinovici and Miller, 2010). Furthermore, pathologic accumulation of microtubule-associated protein (MAP) tau is a process also common for AD and FTD (Iqbal et al., 2016). Abnormal hyperphosphorylation of tau protein leads to its aggregation into intraneuronal neurofibrillary tangles (Iqbal et al., 2010). Vascular dementia is a heterogeneous group of brain disorders associated with a cognitive impairment that is attributed to multifactorial cerebrovascular pathologies, such as hypoperfusion, oxidative stress, and inflammation (Iadecola, 2013). Dementia with Lewy bodies is characterized by the presence of α-synuclein aggregates in neurons and glial cells (Zupancic et al., 2011), and also associated with cholinergic as well as glutamate transmission deficiencies (Zupancic et al., 2011). It may also be concluded, that there is a great deal of overlap between the symptoms of different types of dementia (Abbott, 2011).

Naturally, the pathology of these diseases is more complicated (Blennow et al., 2006). Various markers of AD can be found in the brains of afflicted patients (Blennow et al., 2006). These markers include, e.g., dysregulation of signaling of memory-related neurotransmitter acetylcholine (ACh) (Kihara and Shimohama, 2004), vascular damage (Franzblau et al., 2013), loss of neurons (Niikura et al., 2006) and synapses (Shankar and Walsh, 2009). Mitochondrial dysfunction is another pathology, which was recognized as an important early event in the AD progression and, therefore, may be considered as promising target for the treatment of AD and AD-related dementia (Kumar and Singh, 2015). We briefly describe the mitochondrial dysfunction in the context of dementia in section Mitochondrial Dysfunction and Neurodegeneration.

MITOCHONDRIAL DYSFUNCTION AND NEURODEGENERATION

Mitochondria are double membrane-enclosed organelles that are responsible to exert a broad range of cellular functions that include the most important adenosine triphosphate (ATP) production (energy conversion), but also involvement in several homeostatic processes, such as regulation of cell cycle and cell growth, calcium handling, and apoptosis-programmed cell death (van Horssen et al., 2017). Moreover, mitochondria play a crucial role in many other essential metabolic processes (van Horssen et al., 2017). Thus, mitochondrial diseases often have an associated metabolic component and, therefore, mitochondrial defects are predictable in energy-dependent disturbances, inflammation, and aging (Chan, 2006; Banasch et al., 2011). Hence, mitochondrial dysfunction is one of the key pathological features in various age-related neurodegenerative diseases including AD-associated dementia due to the pivotal role of mitochondria in neuronal cell survival or death (Moreira et al., 2010). For example, it has been proposed that mitochondrial network remodeling plays a prominent role in neurodegeneration (Zhu et al., 2013; Burte et al., 2015). The mitochondrial cascade hypothesis proposed the mitochondrial dysfunction as a principal episode in AD pathology (Moreira et al., 2010; Swerdlow et al., 2010). Moreover, mitochondrial dysfunction, which is also described as an impairment of electron transport chain, is responsible to increase the production of reactive oxagen species (ROS) and change mitochondrial dynamics (Beal, 2005; Lin and Beal, 2006; Hung et al., 2018). A recent study has shown the reciprocal relationship between ROS and mitochondrial dynamics during early stages

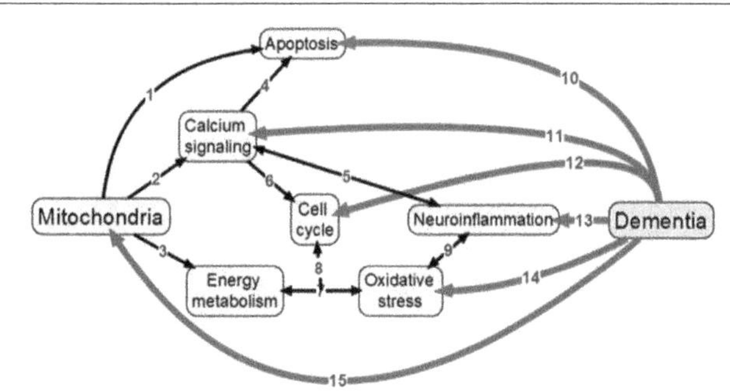

FIGURE 1 | Overview of mechanisms linking mitochondrial activity with dementia: (1) Mitochondria are crucially important for activating apoptosis (Wang and Youle, 2009); (2) Mitochondria regulate calcium signaling pathway (Walsh et al., 2009); (3) Oxidative phosphorylation occurs in electron transport chain of mitochondria; (4) Calcium signaling induces apoptosis (Hajnoczky et al., 2003); (5) Calcium and neuroinflammatory signaling pathways interact with each other (Sama and Norris, 2013); (6) Cell cycle requires calcium signaling (Berridge, 1995); (7) Mitochondrial oxidative phosphorylation is one of the main sources of reactive oxygen species (Dai et al., 2014); (8) Oxidative phosphorylation and reactive oxygen species regulate cell cycle (Antico Arciuch et al., 2012); (9) Oxidative stress and neuroinflammation are highly interconnected processes (Gao et al., 2014); (10) Neuronal apoptosis (LeBlanc, 2005; Favaloro et al., 2012); (11) Impaired calcium signaling (Berridge, 2011; Nimmrich and Eckert, 2013); (12) Changes in cell cycle (Raina et al., 2000; Katsel et al., 2013); (13) Presence of neuroinflammation (Pasqualetti et al., 2015); (14) Increased oxidative stress (Bennett et al., 2009; Kumar and Singh, 2015); (15) Changes in mitochondrial morphology and functions (Spano et al., 2015; Hung et al., 2018).

of neurodegeneration (Hung et al., 2018). It has also been found that the cause for mitochondria-mediated toxicity is the progressive accumulation of Aβ in mitochondria (Chen and Yan, 2010). Recent studies provided the crucial role of mitochondrial dysfunction in regulating the ROS and intracellular calcium levels in neuronal cells (Aminzadeh et al., 2018). In addition, Lee et al. investigated the relationship between the NAD-dependent deacetylase sirtuin-3 (SIRT3) protein and mitochondrial function using AD human brain samples, demonstrating that dysfunction of SIRT3 leads to mitochondrial and neuronal damage, and may improve the mitochondrial pathology and neurodegeneration in AD (Lee et al., 2017). Therefore, mitochondrial dysfunction is considered as a cardinal pathological hallmark for neurodegenerative diseases including AD and AD-related dementia (Lin and Beal, 2006; van Horssen et al., 2017). Detailed information of mitochondrial activities that may be associated with dementia is presented in **Figure 1**.

Summarizing the above, the oxidative stress and mitochondrial dysfunction are of high importance in the pathology and pathogenesis of AD and dementia. Therefore, natural antioxidants and mitochondria targeting molecules can be important strategies to treat elderly individuals with AD (Reddy and Reddy, 2017). Several naturally occurring antioxidants, such as *Ginkgo biloba* (Gb) and curcumin, showed blocking effect on the age-dependent spatial cognitive behavior and also increased the Aβ-degrading enzymes in transgenic mouse models (Stackman et al., 2003; Wang et al., 2014). Moreover, several other antioxidants, including ferulic acid, α-lipoic acid, R-lipoic acid, vitamin E, vitamin C, melatonin, CoQ10, *N*-acetyl-L-cysteine, pyrrolyl-alpha-nitronyl nitroxide, and zeolite supplementation, also showed beneficial effects on AD in different transgenic mouse models (Reddy and Reddy, 2017). Most of these naturally occurring compounds revealed reduction in Aβ levels, mitochondrial dysfunction, phosphorylated tau, and microglial activation, and also increased the synaptic activity (Reddy and Reddy, 2017). Therefore, many of them are available as supplements or can be used as alternative treatment strategies that may help certain neurological conditions, such as PD, AD, some dementia types, and other clinical conditions.

CURRENT PHARMACEUTICAL TREATMENTS OF DEMENTIA

Approved (Semi-)Synthetic Drugs

Several (semi-)synthetic drugs are available worldwide for the treatment of AD and some dementia types. The selective, reversible acetylcholinesterase (AChE) inhibitor donepezil, the non-selective butyrylcholinetserase (BuChE) and AChE inhibitor rivastigmine, as well as the *N*-methyl-D-aspartate (NMDA) receptor antagonist memantine are some of the most widely used therapeutics for AD-associated dementia (Blennow et al., 2006; Winblad et al., 2016). Some of these drugs, like the (semi-)synthetic drug rivastigmine, are also approved for treating other dementia types like PD-related dementia (Winblad et al., 2016). Most prominent drugs approved for clinical use in AD and different forms of dementia are present in **Table 2**. A combined donepezil–memantine drug with the brand name Namzaric® was approved by the FDA in 2014 for the treatment of moderate-to-severe AD in people who are taking donepezil hydrochloride at the recommended clinically efficient dose of 10 mg/day (http://www.alz.org AD report). However, this combinative medicine may cause various side effects, including muscle problems, slow heartbeat and fainting, increased stomach acid levels, nausea, vomiting, and seizures. In addition, some findings suggest that abovementioned drugs do not provide therapeutic benefits for agitation present in patients with severe behavioral symptoms (Howard et al., 2007; Fox et al., 2012). Some neuroleptic/antipsychotic drugs, such as haloperidol, risperidone, and olanzapine, are currently being used to treat behavioral and psychological symptoms of dementia (BPSD), however, their use is controversial (Ballard and Howard, 2006). Therefore, such drugs are not approved by FDA for the treatment of BPSD. Nevertheless, they are still often prescribed off-label as no better treatment for BPSD exists currently (Ibrahim et al., 2012).

The (semi-)synthetic drugs that are currently used for the treatment of dementia have an impact on several symptoms in different disease stages, but do not stop the progressive course of the disease (Tzvetkov and Antonov, 2017). Therefore, the investigation of naturally occurring compounds with potential therapeutic properties for the treatment of different dementia forms is of great medical and socioeconomic importance.

TABLE 2 | Approved (semi-)synthetic drugs used for the treatment of dementia.

	Memantine	Rivastigmine	Donepezil
Brand name	Namenda® (USA) Axura® (Europe) Ebixa® (Europe) Memando® (Ger)	Exelon® (USA, Europe)	Aricept® (USA, Europe)
Chemical structure	Chem. formula: $C_{12}H_{21}N$ Mol. wt.: 179.3 g/mol	Chem. formula: $C_{14}H_{22}N_2O_2$ Mol. wt.: 250.3	Chem. formula: $C_{24}H_{29}NO_3$ Mol. wt.: 379.5 g/mol
Indications	Moderate-to-severe AD, AD-related dementia	Mild-to-moderate AD, AD-related dementia	Mild-to-moderate AD, early-to-mid AD dementia
Mode of action	Non-competitive NMDA-receptor antagonist	Slowly reversible, non-selective AChE and BuChE inhibitor	Reversible, selective AChE inhibitor
Side effects (http://www.alz.org)	Confusion, dizziness, constipation, and headache	Nausea, vomiting, loss of appetite, increased frequency of bowel movements	Nausea, vomiting, loss of appetite, increased frequency of bowel movements
Half-life (Blennow et al., 2006)	60–100 h (long)	1 h (very short)	70 h (long)
Doses per day (Blennow et al., 2006)	One (first week)	Two	One
Initial dose (Blennow et al., 2006)	5 mg/day	3 mg/day (2 × 1.5 mg)	5 mg/day
Recommended clinically efficient dose (Blennow et al., 2006)	20 mg/day	6–12 mg/day	10 mg/day

Galantamine—the Only Current Drug of Plant Origin against Dementia

Galantamine is an important drug of plant origin that is widely prescribed for the treatment of mild-to-moderate AD and AD-related dementia (Lilienfeld, 2002). Efficacy of galantamine has been confirmed in several clinical trials (Olin and Schneider, 2002). Galantamine, also known as galanthamine (for structure, see **Figure 2**), is an isoquinoline alkaloid produced by plants from *Amaryllidaceae* family. It was first discovered and isolated from bulbs of *Galanthus nivalis* (common snowdrop) by the Bulgarian chemist D. Paskov and his team in 1956 (Paskov, 1958). The original industrial phytopreparation of the pure galantamine extract (named Nivalin®) was prepared in late 1950s by the same research group (Chrusciel and Varagić, 1966). Galantamine was first applied to treat poliomyelitis and later, for the treatment of neuropathic pain and as an anesthetic (Ng et al., 2015). Today, galantamine is mainly obtained from *Galanthus woronowi* Losinsk and *Galanthus alpines* Sosn. (Caucasian snowdrop) daffodil bulbs and also synthesized artificially (Loy and Schneider, 2006).

Galantamine has a unique dual mode of action affecting the brain's cholinergic system (**Figure 2**). It is a reversible, competitive inhibitor of the AChE enzyme and an allosteric enhancer of the nicotinic acetylcholine receptor (nAChR) (Albuquerque et al., 2001).

Galantamine also prevents mitochondrial dysfunction, as shown by its capability to rescue changes in mitochondrial membrane potential (MMP) and morphology induced by Aβ25/35 or hydrogen peroxide treatment (Ezoulin et al., 2008; Liu et al., 2010). Oxidative stress is caused by toxic reactive oxygen species (ROS), which are generated mainly during the electron transport in mitochondria. By protecting the mitochondria and inhibiting AChE activity galantamine decreases oxidative damage to cells and thus mediates neuroprotection (Tsvetkova et al., 2013).

Furthermore, galantamine may interact with other brain-targeted drugs by decreasing activity of P-glycoprotein, a multi-drug resistance transporter present in brain's vascular endothelium (Namanja et al., 2009). It is responsible for actively effluxing drugs back into the bloodstream, thus preventing them from crossing into the brain (Namanja et al., 2009). Hence, galantamine may allow drugs that were co-administered with it to reach the brain more easily. Galantamine also enhances the protective effect of rofecoxib (an anti-inflammatory COX-2 inhibitor) and caffeic acid (a plant-derived phenol) against neurotoxicity-induced mitochondrial dysfunction, oxidative damage, and cognitive impairment in rats (Kumar et al., 2011). Similarly, galantamine potentiates antioxidative activity of melatonin, a brain sleep hormone (Romero et al., 2010). Combined galantamine and memantine treatment is also hypothesized to be a potential novel therapy for schizophrenia (Koola et al., 2014).

Treatment with galantamine has shown to consistently delay the onset of different behavioral symptoms of dementia, such as anxiety, euphoria, depression, irritability, delusions, and unusual motor behavior (Monsch and Giannakopoulos, 2004). A review by Loy and Schneider (2006) described in detail 10 clinical trials comprising the total of 6,805 demented patients, who were submitted to galantamine treatment. The results revealed that the galantamine is well-tolerated by the majority of patients. Some

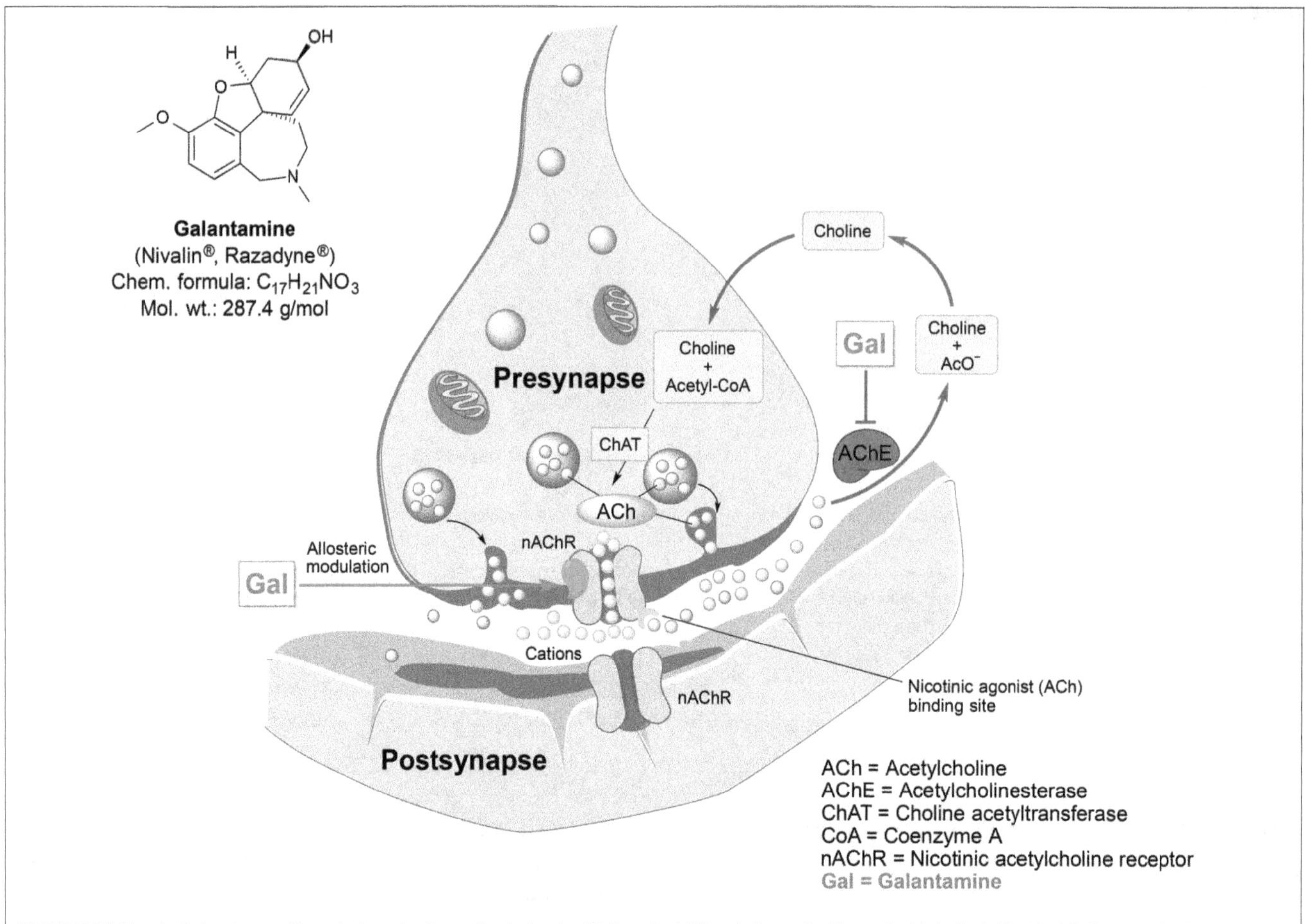

FIGURE 2 | Chemical structure and targeted mechanisms of galantamine (Gal) against AD and dementia. The major biological effects of Gal lead to significant neuroprotection via dual AChE inhibition and allosteric stimulation of nAChRs.

common side effects were observed in the treatment groups in a dose-dependent manner (Loy and Schneider, 2006).

Because of its efficacy, the drug is recommended by Alzheimer's disease/dementia treatment guidelines of the USA and Europe (Doody et al., 2001; Waldemar et al., 2007). The drug is also approved for use in roughly 29 countries including Canada, in the European Union (except for The Netherlands, under the name Nivalin® in 2000), Japan, Korea, Mexico, Singapore, South Africa, Thailand, etc. The FDA approved galantamine in the United States under the brand name Razadyne® in 2001 for the treatment of AD and AD-related dementia. In summary, the plant-derived galantamine is a well-established medicine for dementia treatment, which acts via modulation of acetylcholine signaling and inhibition of oxidative damage.

GENERAL OVERVIEW OF THE DIVERSITY OF PLANTS USED IN DEMENTIA TREATMENT

Modern research on dementias showed that they are complex diseases with multiple molecular mechanisms involved in their pathogenesis. With this realization emerged the new paradigm for treating these pathologies: therapies for dementia should target multiple underling molecular targets, instead of concentrating on any single one. Correspondingly, plant and plant extracts are composed of many substances that are hypothesized to act on multiple molecular targets in an additive or even synergistic manner (Long et al., 2015). Many herbal medicines are already being used for dementia treatment. Unfortunately, active ingredients of these herbs are poorly described. Similarly, we still know very little on how this myriad of substances interact with each other and with prescription medications (Zhou et al., 2016b). The research on these topics will be essential for developing therapeutics, comprised of substances that amplify each other activity and which are devoid of harmful side effects.

In this work, we attempted to collect and document scattered information from various ethnopharmacological reports. We searched several web databases namely, ScienceDirect, Pubmed, Scopus, and Google Scholar using keywords such as "dementia," "Alzheimer's," "traditional medicine," "ethnopharmacology," and "ethnobotany." Web hits from Google scholar were gathered through Boolean information retrieval method using plant name with "AND" operator (Pohl et al., 2010) followed by "dementia" or "Alzheimer's." An overview of the identified medicinal plants used for treating dementia or AD is presented in **Table 3.**

SELECTED PROMINENT MEDICINAL PLANTS AND PLANT GENERA USED FOR THE TREATMENT OF DEMENTIA

After the extensive web-search for medicinal plants used for dementia treatment in various regions worldwide, the following five plants or plant genera described below were selected for detailed discussion according to the highest observed number of web hits.

Ginkgo biloba L.

Ginkgo is among the most unique plants on earth and belongs to world's oldest tree species (IARC Working Group, 2016). It is a living fossil which gross morphology did not change for around 200 million years (Guan et al., 2016). Gingko is the last living member of the *Ginkgoaceae* family, which appeared during the Mesozoic era. Gb was cultivated in ancient China due to its diverse medicinal properties. Extracts from this plant were utilized for the treatment of various ailments and symptoms viz. poor circulation, fatigue, vertigo, and tinnitus (Sun et al., 2013). Gingko extract is available on market in some countries (e.g., China) as a herbal supplement named Gingium. It is intended for use in certain age-related cognitive disorders including memory impairment and it alleviates the symptoms of dementias and AD (Zhou et al., 2016a). There are two main categories of chemical phytoconstituents likely responsible for the neuro-therapeutic potential of Gingko: terpene lactones (ginkgolides and bilobalide) and flavonoids (flavonols and flavone glycosides) (**Figure 3**; Solfrizzi and Panza, 2015; IARC Working Group, 2016).

The triterpene ginkgolides A, B, and C are unique to Gb (Solfrizzi and Panza, 2015). However, there are some other constituents such as the ginkgotoxin (found in Gb seeds) and the phenolic type lipid bilobol (found in Gb fruits) that possess some specific biological effects (IARC Working Group, 2016). For example, ginkgotoxin exhibit neurotoxic activity (induce the epileptic seizures) (IARC Working Group, 2016), whereas bilobol and its derivatives show cytotoxic and antibacterial activity (Tanaka et al., 2011).

Ginkgo leaf extract was first developed for therapeutic purposes in Germany in 1965 (Isah, 2015). The first commercially available extract was registered in France in 1974 under the name EGb761; it contains about 24% flavonoids and 6% terpene lactones (Isah, 2015). The standardized Gb extract (EGb761) belongs to the most widely tested in clinical trials herbal medications worldwide for cognitive impairment, AD, and AD-related dementia (Solfrizzi and Panza, 2015). EGb761 affects a multitude of mechanisms associated with proper brain functions (Zhou et al., 2016a; **Figure 4**).

It was reported to mediate neuroprotection by modulating circulating glucocorticoid levels, as well as Aβ aggregation, ion homeostasis and growth factors synthesis (Amri et al., 1996; Ahlemeyer and Krieglstein, 2003). These processes are likely involved in regulation of oxidative stress (Butterfield et al., 2013; Ruttkay-Nedecky et al., 2013; Dávila et al., 2016; Alam et al., 2017; Gómez-Sámano et al., 2017) which is in agreement with various reports showing antioxidative activity of Gb extract (Bridi et al., 2001; Chandrasekaran et al., 2003). Moreover, the influence of Ginkgo constituents on mitochondrial function is well recognized. Multiple *in vitro* studies show that Ginkgo constituents protect MMP from various toxicants and oxidative stress (Eckert et al., 2005; Abdel-Kader et al., 2007; Wang and Wang, 2016). Gingko extract affects many aspects of mitochondrial morphology such as fission (Zhou et al., 2017), swelling (Schwarzkopf et al., 2013), and coupling (Rhein et al., 2010). Gingko extract also interacts with mitochondrial electron transport chain (Abdel-Kader et al., 2007). Interestingly, it was found that improvement of the oxidative phosphorylation efficiency was more pronounced in cells overexpressing APP than in control cells (Rhein et al., 2010). This suggests that Ginkgo extract may be effective specifically in AD therapy. The extract also protected rodent neurons and glial cells against cerebral ischemia/reperfusion or scopolamine-induced toxicity (Chandrasekaran et al., 2003; Domoráková et al., 2006; Paganelli et al., 2006; Jahanshahi et al., 2012, 2013). Moreover, EGb761 enhanced the functional integrity and protected cerebral microvascular endothelial cells cultured *in vitro* from damage (Yan et al., 2008; Wan et al., 2014). These effects may be related to a known antiplatelet activity of Gingko extract (Kim et al., 2011). Antiplatelet agents are proposed as a possible therapeutics for vascular syndromes (Geeganage et al., 2010; Heim et al., 2017). Thus, EGb761 may counteract dysfunction of neurovascular unit, which is one of the pathologies associated with AD (Farkas and Luiten, 2001; Zlokovic, 2011).

The use of Ginkgo for the treatment of several cerebral dysfunctions connected to neurodegenerative dementia and brain aging has a long history (Abdou et al., 2016). Studies performed on several animal models suggest that Gingko extract may enhance the cognitive and behavioral functions in aged individuals and Parkinson's disease patients (Kim et al., 2004; Takuma et al., 2007; Ribeiro et al., 2016). Apart from the animal studies, several clinical trials also reported the lack of significant adverse effects and effectiveness of EGb 761 in the therapy of AD and vascular dementia (Kanowski et al., 1996; Napryeyenko et al., 2009; Ihl et al., 2012). Although the gingko extract seems to be beneficial for the treatment of cognitive impairments, further studies are required to assess its possible interaction with other drugs. Such studies may translate to better efficacy and safety of gingko extract therapy. Few important interactions between Ginkgo constituents and drugs are currently known (Izzo, 2012). Nevertheless, there are reports of single patients, which suffered serious neurological side effects after administering Ginkgo herb along with risperidone, valproic acid/phenytoin or trazodone (Izzo, 2012). In summary, Ginkgo extract shows neuroprotective effect, which may be underlined by its antioxidative and/or antiplatelet activities. Clinical studies confirm the effectiveness of Ginkgo extract for dementia treatment. Thus, we speculate that some Ginkgo-based drugs may reach the market in near future.

TABLE 3 | Overview of medicinal plants used to treat dementia worldwide.

Plant (Plant family)	References for the use of the plants for dementia treatment in ethnomedicine	Number of google scholar hits for keyword "dementia"	Number of google scholar hits for keyword "Alzheimer's"
Acorus calamus L. (Acoraceae)	Howes and Houghton, 2003	492	730
Aframomum melegueta (Roskoe) K. Schum. (Zingiberaceae)	Fatumbi, 1995	46	104
Agapanthus africanus (Agapanthaceae)	Stafford et al., 2008	06	06
Ammocharis coranica (Ker-Gawl.) Herb. (Amaryllidaceae)	Stafford et al., 2008	13	26
Ananas comosus (Bromeliaceae)	Wolters, 1994; Adams et al., 2007	129	414
Angelica sinensis (Oliv.) Diels (Apiaceae)	Mantle et al., 2000	1,010	1,660
Angelica archangelica (Apiaceae)	Ross, 2001; Howes and Houghton, 2003	196	318
Angelica species (Apiaceae)	Perry and Howes, 2011	4,670	3,140
Annona senegalensis Pers. (Annonaceae)	Stafford et al., 2008	139	80
Artemisia absinthium L. (Asteraceae)	Howes and Houghton, 2003; Adams et al., 2007	242	439
Asparagus africanus Lam. (Asparagaceae)	Stafford et al., 2008	26	34
Asparagus concinnus (Baker) Kies (Asparagaceae)	Stafford et al., 2008	01	01
Bacopa monnieri (L.) Wettst. (Plantaginaceae)	Manyam, 1999	1,370	1,990
Barbieria pinnata (Pers.) Baill. (Fabacea)	Schultes, 1993, 1994; Adams et al., 2007	04	06
Platycladus orientalis (L.) Franco (Syn. *Biota orientalis* (L.)Endl.) (Cupressaceae)	Nishiyama et al., 1995; Howes et al., 2003	150	236
Boophone disticha (L.f.) Herb. (Amaryllidaceae)	Stafford et al., 2008	39	78
Brugmansia ×*candida* Pers. (Solanaceae)	González Ayala, 1994; Adams et al., 2007	12	55
Bupleurum species (Apiaceae)	Perry and Howes, 2011	518	717
Camellia sinensis Kuntze (Theaceae)	Perry and Howes, 2011	1,420	3,910
Cannabis sativa L. (Cannabaceae)	Perry and Howes, 2011	1,740	3,260
Carum carvi L. (Apiaceae)	Adsersen et al., 2006	163	340
Caryophyllus spp. (Caryophyllaceae)	Tabernaemontanus, 1987; Adams et al., 2007	161	292
Cassia lucens Vog. (Fabaceae)	Schultes, 1993, 1994; Adams et al., 2007	28	93
Celastrus paniculatus Willd. (Celastraceae)	Howes and Houghton, 2003	189	274
Centella asiatica (L.) Urb (Apiaceae)	Stafford et al., 2008	1,060	1,970
Dysphania ambrosioides (L.) Mosyakin&Clemants (Amaranthaceae) {Syn. *Chenopodium ambrosioides* L.(Chenopodiaceae)}	de Barradas, 1957; CESA, 1992, 1993; Adams et al., 2007	94	154
Clitoria ternatea L. (Fabaceae)	Howes and Houghton, 2003	185	294
Codonopsis pilulosa (Franch.) Nannf. (Campanulaceae)	Howes and Houghton, 2003	198	245
Coffea arabica L. (Rubiaceae)	Perry and Howes, 2011	484	1,180
Convallaria majalis L. (Convallariaceae)	Tabernaemontanus, 1987; Adams et al., 2007	82	95
Coriandrum sativum L. (Apiaceae)	Tabernaemontanus, 1987; Adams et al., 2007	310	765
Corydalis cava (L.) Schw. et K. (Papaveraceae)	Adsersen et al., 2006; Adams et al., 2007	65	86
Corydalis intermedia (L.) M'erat (Papaveraceae)	Adsersen et al., 2006; Adams et al., 2007	71	141
Corydalis solida (L.) Swartz ssp. *laxa* (Papaveraceae)	Adsersen et al., 2006; Adams et al., 2007	21	30
Corydalis solida (L.) Swartz ssp. *slivenensis* (Papaveraceae)	Adsersen et al., 2006; Adams et al., 2007	04	04
Crinum bulbispermum (Burm.f.) Milne-Redh. & Schweick. (Amaryllidaceae)	Stafford et al., 2008	47	97
Crinum moorei Hook.f (Syn.*Crinum imbricatum* Baker) (Amaryllidaceae)	Stafford et al., 2008	20	54
Crinum macowanii Baker (Amaryllidaceae)	Stafford et al., 2008	41	93
Crocus sativus L. (Iridaceae)	Perry and Howes, 2011	678	1,310
Curcuma longa L. (Zingiberaceae)	Howes and Houghton, 2003; Perry and Howes, 2011	2,130	6,270
Euphrasia nemorosa (Pers.) Wallr. (Scrophulariaceae)	Adsersen et al., 2006	09	16

(Continued)

TABLE 3 | Continued

Plant (Plant family)	References for the use of the plants for dementia treatment in ethnomedicine	Number of google scholar hits for keyword "dementia"	Number of google scholar hits for keyword "Alzheimer's"
Tetradium ruticarpum (A.Juss.) T.G.Hartley (Syn. *Evodia rutaecarpa* Hook.f.&Thoms.) (Rutaceae)	Mantle et al., 2000; Howes and Perry, 2011	366	367
Ferula gummosa Boiss. (Apiaceae)	Tabernaemontanus, 1987; Adams et al., 2007	22	32
Galanthus woronowii Losinsk. (Amaryllidaceae)	Perry and Howes, 2011	155	286
Galanthus alpinus Sosn. (Syn. *Galanthus caucasicus*) (Amaryllidaceae)	Perry and Howes, 2011	27	55
Ginkgo biloba L. (Ginkgoaceae)	Gurib-Fakim, 2006; Perry and Howes, 2011	14,000	17,300
Glycyrrhiza species (Leguminosae)	Perry and Howes, 2011	2,410	4,050
Huperzia serrate (Thunb.) Trevis. (Lycopodiaceae)	Howes et al., 2003; Adams et al., 2007; Perry and Howes, 2011	1,130	1,710
Hydrolea glabra Schum. and Thonn. (Hydrophilaceae)	Fatumbi, 1995; Adams et al., 2007	01	03
Hypericum perforatum L. (Clusiaceae)	Perry and Howes, 2011	2,500	3,180
Lactuca sativa L. (Asteraceae)	Schweitzer de Palacios, 1994; Adams et al., 2007	287	895
Lannea schweinfurthii Engl. (Anacardiaceae)	Stafford et al., 2008	12	22
Lantana camara L. (Verbenaceae)	Müller-Ebeling and Rätsch, 1989; Adams et al., 2007	97	262
Lavandula angustifolia Miller (Lamiaceae)	Adsersen et al., 2006; Perry and Howes, 2011	800	981
Leucojum aestivum L. (Amaryllidaceae)	Perry and Howes, 2011	133	447
Lycoris radiata Herb. (Amaryllidaceae)	Howes and Houghton, 2003	227	273
Magnolia officinalis Rehder and Wilson (Magnoliaceae)	Howes and Houghton, 2003	389	715
Matricaria recutita L. (Asteraceae)	Tabernaemontanus, 1987; Adams et al., 2007	575	1,150
Medicago sativa L. (Fabaceae)	Finkler, 1985; Adams et al., 2007	390	1,180
Melissa officinalis L. (Lamiaceae)	Lonicerus, 1679; Mills, 1991; Perry et al., 1998; Mantle et al., 2000; Adsersen et al., 2006; Adams et al., 2007; Perry and Howes, 2011	1,140	1,920
Mentha spicata L. (Lamiaceae)	Adsersen et al., 2006	223	537
Narcissus spp. (Amaryllidaceae)	Perry and Howes, 2011	1,480	745
Nicotiana species (Solanaceae)	Perry and Howes, 2011	900	3,060
Ocimum basilicum L. (Lamiaceae)	Fuchs, 1543; Sfikas, 1980; Adams et al., 2007	407	997
Origanum majorana Moench (Lamiaceae)	Fuchs, 1543; Adams et al., 2007	675	1,550
Origanum vulgare L. (Lamiaceae)	Adsersen et al., 2006	358	978
Paeonia ×suffruticosa Andrews (Paeoniaceae)	Mantle et al., 2000	189	345
Panax ginseng C.A.Mey. (Araliaceae)	Perry and Howes, 2011	4,790	6,950
Paullinia cupana Kunth ex. H. B. K (Sapindaceae)	Taylor, 1998; Adams et al., 2007	248	515
Petroselinum crispum (Mil.) Nym.exA.W.Hill. (Apiaceae)	Adsersen et al., 2006	308	562
Physostigma venenosa Balf.f. (Leguminosae)	Mantle et al., 2000	08	11
Pimpinella anisum L. (Apiaceae)	Adsersen et al., 2006	214	493
Piper methysticum G.Forst. (Piperaceae)	Perry and Howes, 2011	768	953
Polygala tenuifolia Willd. (Polygalaceae)	Duke and Ayensu, 1985; Chang et al., 1986; Howes and Houghton, 2003	549	679
Pteroselinum vulgare (Mill.) Nym. and A.W. Hill (Apiaceae)	Adams et al., 2007	82	221
Rosmarinus officinalis L. (Lamiaceae)	Price and Price, 1995; Chevallier, 1996; Perry et al., 1998; Mantle et al., 2000; Adams et al., 2007	1,140	2,440
Rosmarinus officinalis L. (Lamiaceae)	Adsersen et al., 2006	1,140	2,440
Ruta graveolens L. (Rutaceae)	Adsersen et al., 2006	351	420
Salvia lavandulifolia Vahl. (Lamiaceae)	Perry and Howes, 2011	103	190
Salvia miltiorrhiza Bung. (Lamiaceae)	Howes and Houghton, 2003	1,430	2,090

(Continued)

TABLE 3 | Continued

Plant (Plant family)	References for the use of the plants for dementia treatment in ethnomedicine	Number of google scholar hits for keyword "dementia"	Number of google scholar hits for keyword "Alzheimer's"
Salvia officinalis L. (Lamiaceae)	Sfikas 1980; Tabernaemontanus, 1987; Akhondzadeh et al., 2003; Howes et al., 2003; Savelev et al., 2004; Adams et al., 2007	1,610	2,960
Scadoxus multiflorus (Martyn) Raf. (Amaryllidaceae)	Stafford et al., 2008	06	31
Syzygium aromaticum (L.) Merrill and Perry (Myrtaceae)	Tabernaemontanus, 1987; Adams et al., 2007	248	647
Tagetes lucida Cav. (Asteraceae)	Ortiz de Montellano, 1990; Adams et al., 2007	25	54
Terminalia chebula Retz. (Combretaceae)	Misra, 1998; Manyam, 1999; Howes and Houghton, 2003	545	938
Theobroma cacao L. (Sterculiaceae)	Roeder, 1988; Adams et al., 2007	535	1,400
Thymus vulgaris L. (Lamiaceae)	Adsersen et al., 2006	1,440	2,760
Valeriana officinalis L. (Valerianaceae)	Perry and Howes, 2011	973	1,340
Vinca minor L. (Apocynaceae)	Perry and Howes, 2011	1,520	2,070
Vitis vinifera L. (Vitaceae)	Perry and Howes, 2011	994	3,010

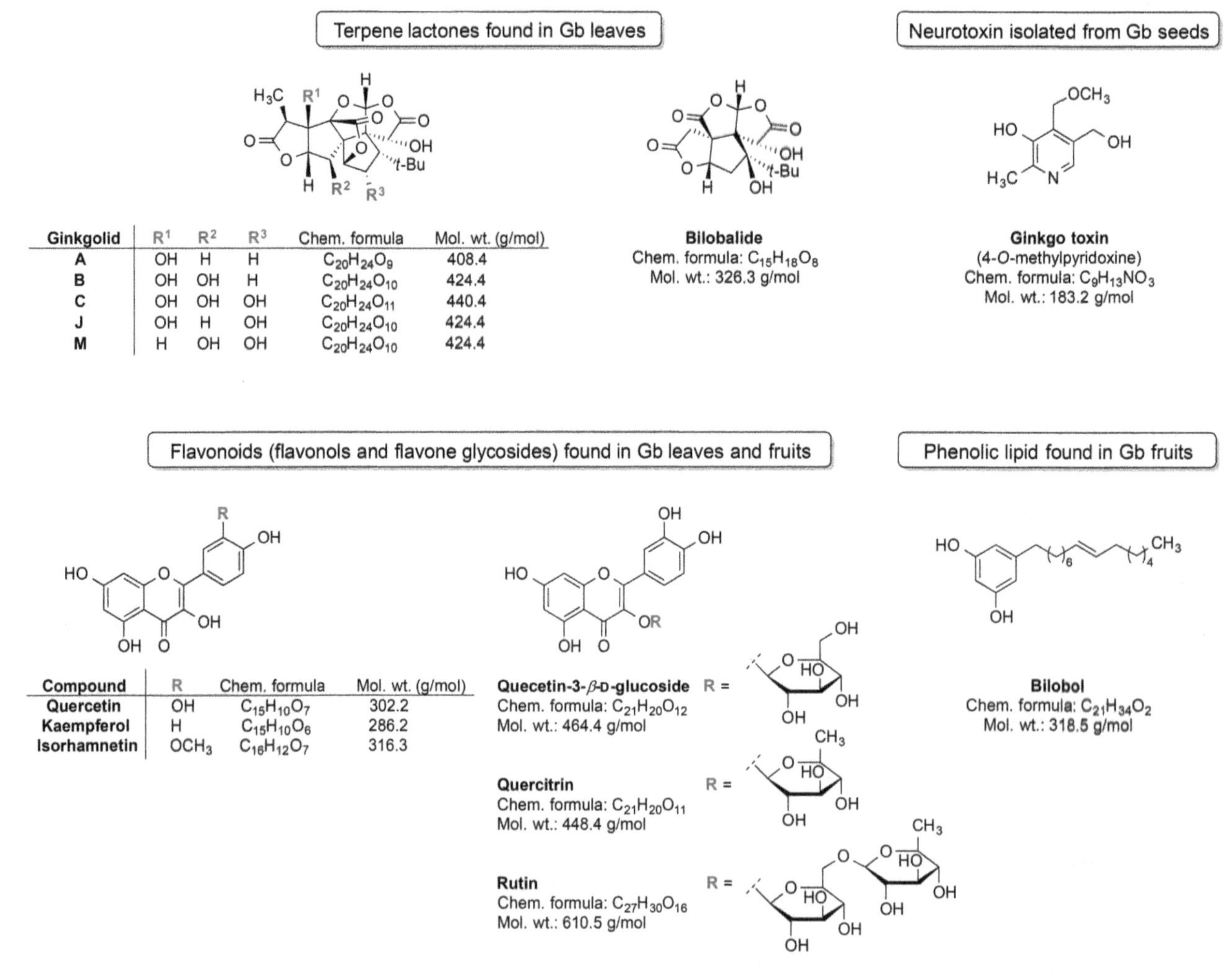

Terpene lactones found in Gb leaves

Ginkgolid	R^1	R^2	R^3	Chem. formula	Mol. wt. (g/mol)
A	OH	H	H	$C_{20}H_{24}O_9$	408.4
B	OH	OH	H	$C_{20}H_{24}O_{10}$	424.4
C	OH	OH	OH	$C_{20}H_{24}O_{11}$	440.4
J	OH	H	OH	$C_{20}H_{24}O_{10}$	424.4
M	H	OH	OH	$C_{20}H_{24}O_{10}$	424.4

Bilobalide
Chem. formula: $C_{15}H_{18}O_8$
Mol. wt.: 326.3 g/mol

Neurotoxin isolated from Gb seeds

Ginkgo toxin
(4-*O*-methylpyridoxine)
Chem. formula: $C_9H_{13}NO_3$
Mol. wt.: 183.2 g/mol

Flavonoids (flavonols and flavone glycosides) found in Gb leaves and fruits

Compound	R	Chem. formula	Mol. wt. (g/mol)
Quercetin	OH	$C_{15}H_{10}O_7$	302.2
Kaempferol	H	$C_{15}H_{10}O_6$	286.2
Isorhamnetin	OCH_3	$C_{16}H_{12}O_7$	316.3

Quecetin-3-β-D-glucoside R =
Chem. formula: $C_{21}H_{20}O_{12}$
Mol. wt.: 464.4 g/mol

Quercitrin R =
Chem. formula: $C_{21}H_{20}O_{11}$
Mol. wt.: 448.4 g/mol

Rutin R =
Chem. formula: $C_{27}H_{30}O_{16}$
Mol. wt.: 610.5 g/mol

Phenolic lipid found in Gb fruits

Bilobol
Chem. formula: $C_{21}H_{34}O_2$
Mol. wt.: 318.5 g/mol

FIGURE 3 | Most prominent phytochemical constituents found in *Gingko biloba* (Gb).

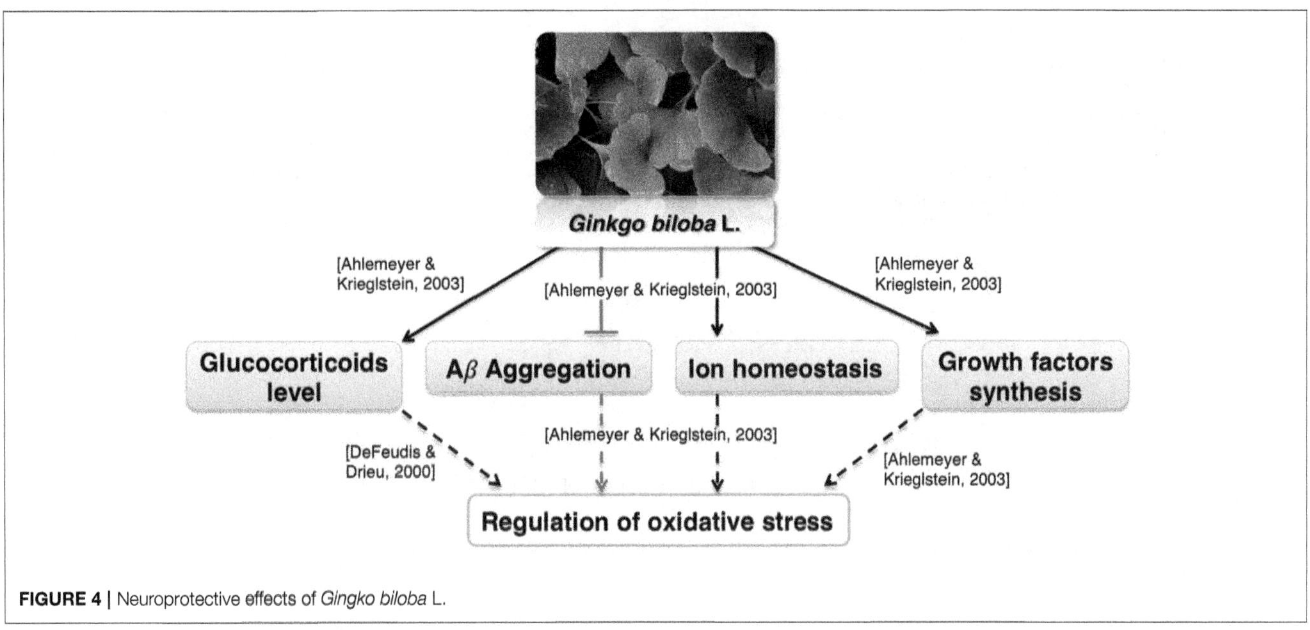

FIGURE 4 | Neuroprotective effects of *Gingko biloba* L.

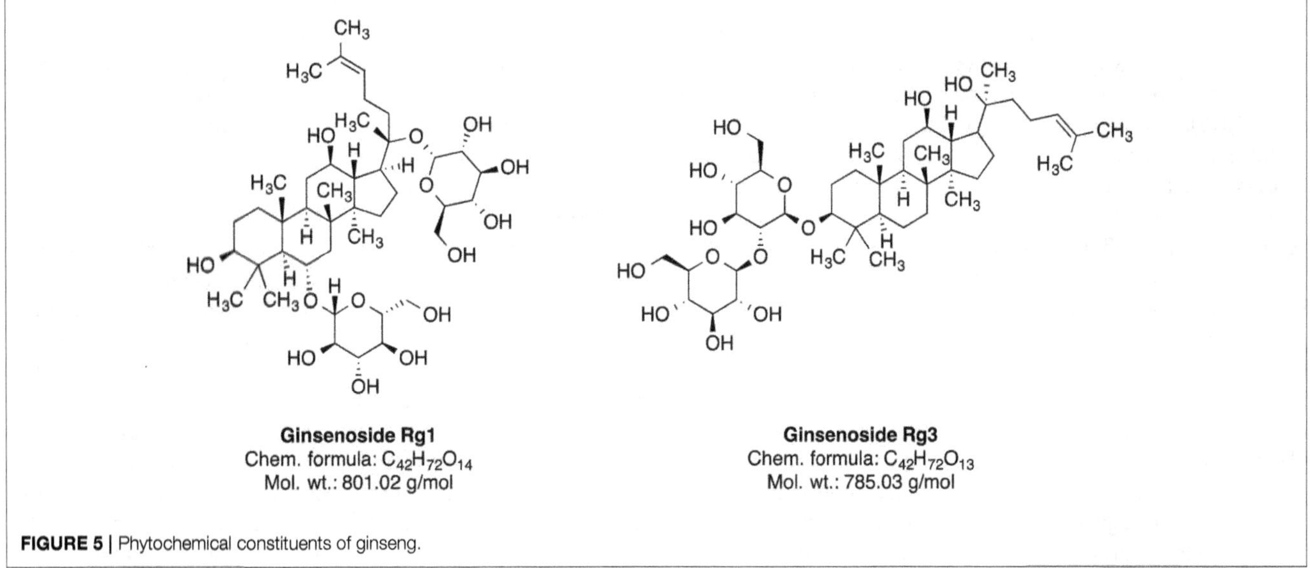

FIGURE 5 | Phytochemical constituents of ginseng.

Panax ginseng C.A. Meyer (Ginseng)

Ginseng is broadly used as an additive for dietary supplements or medicines. It serves as an adaptogen, which is a substance promoting homeostasis and protecting against various biological stressors. The dried root of this plant was used in the traditional medicine mainly in China and Korea (Yun, 2001).There are several species of *Panax* including *P. ginseng* (Oriental ginseng), *P. japonicus* (Japanese ginseng), *P. quinquefolius* (American ginseng), *P. trifolius*, *P. notoginseng* (Burkill), and *P. major* (Ngan et al., 1999). *Panax ginseng* CA Meyer is the most frequently used and extensively researched species of ginseng (Lee et al., 2005). The species is widely distributed in the northeastern part of China. The plant has been used in traditional Chinese medicine for a more than 2000 years as a tonic for fatigue, weakness and aging (Wang et al., 2010). Some constituents of this plant, such as ginsenosides Rgl and Rg3 (**Figure 5**) and ginseng polysaccharides, have been investigated for their therapeutic potential (Yin et al., 2013; Song et al., 2017; Sun et al., 2017). The neuroprotective effect of ginseng is mainly attributed to the 20(*S*)-ginsenoside Rg3 (**Figure 5**), which has a steroidal backbone structure with carbohydrate part and aliphatic side chain (Yang et al., 2009). Rg3 is generated by heating the roots at high temperature (Popovich and Kitts, 2004; Sun et al., 2010).

A significant reduction of the amyloid-β40 and amyloid-β42 levels was reported after the ginsenoside Rg3 treatment in the brains of transgenic mice (Tg2576 line), as well as in

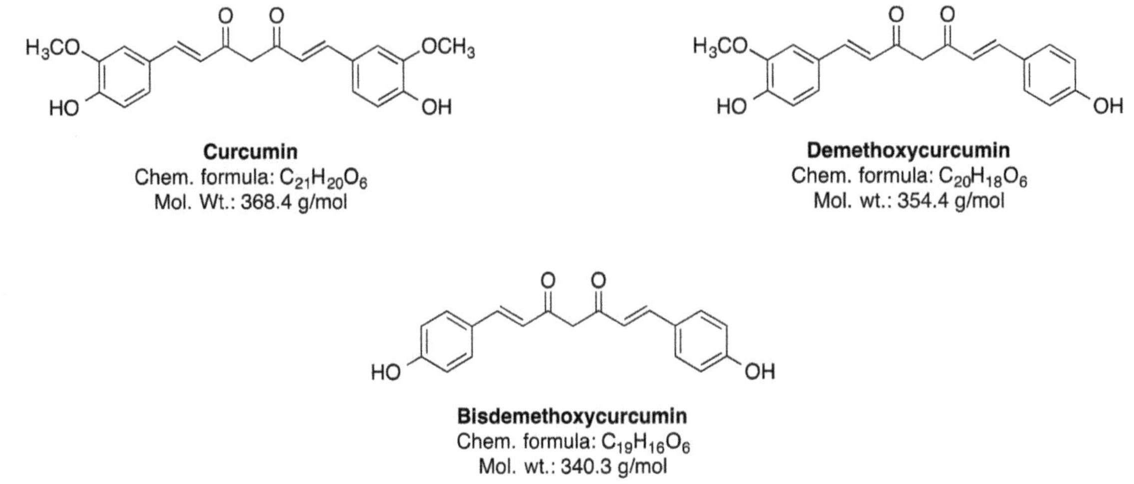

Curcumin
Chem. formula: $C_{21}H_{20}O_6$
Mol. Wt.: 368.4 g/mol

Demethoxycurcumin
Chem. formula: $C_{20}H_{18}O_6$
Mol. wt.: 354.4 g/mol

Bisdemethoxycurcumin
Chem. formula: $C_{19}H_{16}O_6$
Mol. wt.: 340.3 g/mol

FIGURE 6 | Chemical structures of curcuminoids.

cultured cells (Chen et al., 2006). Ginsenoside Rg3 also protects against glutamate-induced neurotoxicity in cultured cortical neurons (Kim et al., 1998). Similarly, another ginseng constituent ginsenoside Rg1 (GRg1) suppressed Aβ-induced neurotoxicity, likely through p38 pathway activation in neuroblastoma cells (Li et al., 2012). Ginsenosides also regulate nicotinic acetylcholine receptor channel activity (Nah, 2014). As acetylcholine signaling mediates learning and memory, modulation of acetylcholine receptor activity may be involved in the compound effectiveness against dementia (Bartus et al., 1982; Giacobini, 2004). The ginseng extract specifically enriched with ginsenoside Rg3 rescues scopolamine-induced memory impairment possibly through modulation of the AChE activity and the NF-κB signaling pathway in the hippocampus of mice (Kim et al., 2016). NF-κB is a protein complex, which regulates neuroinflammation and is activated by ROS (Kaur et al., 2015). On a similar note, GRg1 reduces the Aβ-associated generation of ROS and cell death (Wang and Du, 2009). Correspondingly, many publications show protective effect of ginseng constituents on brain mitochondrial activity under multiple toxic conditions, including ischemia (Ye et al., 2011), calcium treatment (Tian et al., 2009; Zhou et al., 2014), hydrogen peroxide treatment (Tian et al., 2009), and even incubation of cells with Aβ *in vitro* (Ma et al., 2014).

A recent meta-analysis of randomized clinical trials showed inconsistent effect of ginseng on AD (Wang et al., 2016). Generally, the trials suffered from small sample size and poor design, including lack of placebo groups (Wang et al., 2016). Thus, there is a need of larger trials to determine the efficacy of ginseng in AD.

In summary, ginseng constituents are suggested to modulate a number of dementia-related mechanisms, such as amyloid-β metabolism, oxidative stress, neuroinflammation, and acetylcholine signaling. Unfortunately, the effect of gingseng on dementia patients remains poorly understood despite some efforts.

Curcuminoids from Genus Curcuma

The genus Curcuma (commonly termed as Turmeric) comprises around 80 species and is considered as one of the biggest genera of the *Zingiberaceae* family (Sirirugsa et al., 2007). Curcumin and its curcuminoid analogs, demethoxycurcumin and bisdemethoxycurcumin, are responsible for the typically yellow color of turmeric (Chin et al., 2013). However, the main bioactive phytoconstituent of Curcuma genus is curcumin (**Figure 6**).

It is an approved natural food colorant (E100) and can be easily obtained from turmeric through solvent extraction and crystallization (Chin et al., 2013). Furthermore, curcumin is widely used in traditional Indian medicine for the treatment of anorexia, hepatic diseases, cold, cough, and other disorders (Chin et al., 2013; Huminiecki et al., 2017). Nowadays, *in vivo* studies suggest that curcumin has potential neuroprotective properties including antioxidant, anti-neuroinflammatory, antiproliferative, anti-amyloidogenic, and neuro-regulative effects (Chin et al., 2013). A large epidemiological Indo-US Cross National Dementia study showed that the peasant Indian population has a low prevalence of AD and AD-associated dementia compared to the US population, and that may be linked to the high curcumin consumption in the Indian population (Chin et al., 2013), although such correlation does not necessarily imply causative connection.

Curcumin is comprised of two feruloyl moieties with 3-methoxy-4-hydroxy substituents (**Figure 7A**; Sahne et al., 2017). Both side units are linked together by an unsaturated seven-carbon spacer that includes a β-diketo function so that the molecule of curcumin is almost symmetric. Depending on pH of the environment, curcumin can exist in two possible tautomeric forms: enol and diketo (Sahne et al., 2017). The keto form is predominant in acidic and neutral media ($pH \leq 7.4$) as well as in solid state, while in non-polar and basic milieu ($pH \geq 8.0$) the enol form is occurring (Sahne et al., 2017). Moreover, the enol form co-exists in two equivalent tautomers that undergo

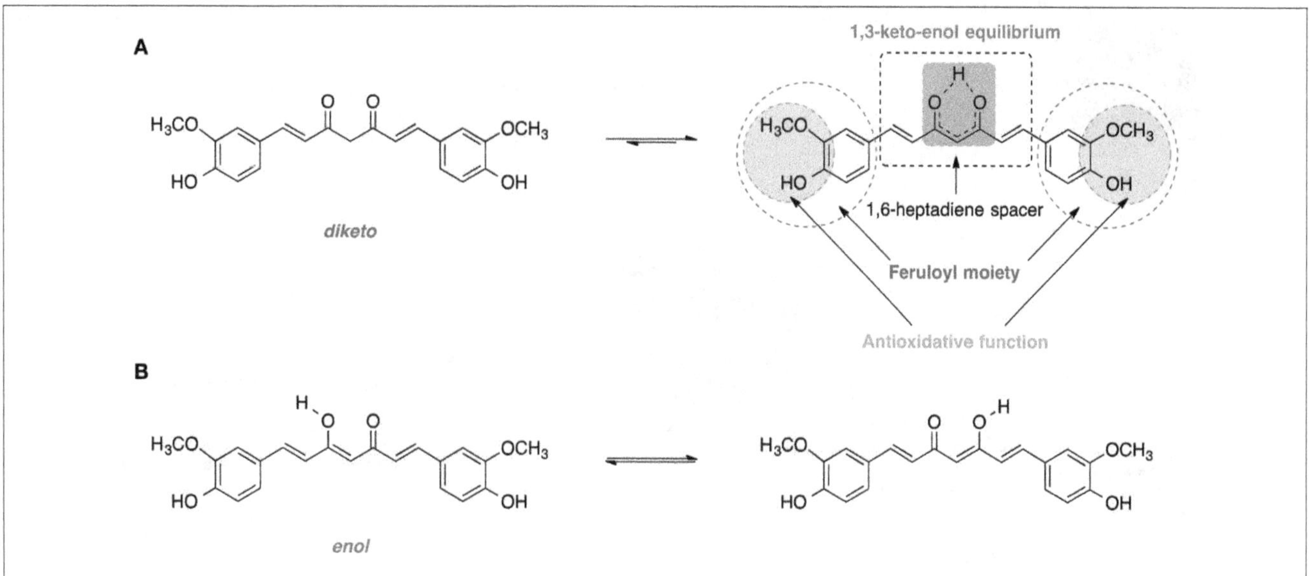

FIGURE 7 | Tautomerism of curcumin: **(A)** Diketo and 1,3-keto-enol equilibrium form of curcumin with its biologically relevant structural units. **(B)** Hydrogen transfer in the most stable enol form.

intramolecular hydrogen transfer (**Figure 7B**; Anjomshoa et al., 2016). Under physiological conditions (pH ~7.4) curcumin can reach its 1,3-keto-enol equilibrium state. Some of the most important antioxidant properties of curcumin and its ability to scavenge ROS are associated with the stability and the antioxidative capability of the methoxy phenolic type groups that are present. The structural features of curcumin including its tautomeric forms and pharmacophores are present in **Figure 7**.

Curcumin suppresses tumor necrosis factor (TNF) activity, formation of Aβ plaques and protects brain cells from noxious agents (Belkacemi et al., 2011). In recent years, the natural polyphenols are being implemented in the treatment of different neurological disorders (Pathak et al., 2013; Hügel and Jackson, 2015).

Curcumin-enriched diet enhances memory and hippocampal neurogenesis in aged rats (Dong et al., 2012). This effect may be mediated by curcumin-induced modulation of expression of genes involved in cell growth and synaptic plasticity (Dong et al., 2012). Neuroprotective properties of curcumin are often attributed to its anti-inflammatory, antioxidant and lipophilic potential (Mishra and Palanivelu, 2008). For example, enhanced hippocampal expression of pro-inflammatory proteins TNF-α and IL-1 beta, which was caused by intracerebroventricular infusion of Aβ42 peptide solution, was at least partially normalized by infusion with curcumin-loaded lipid-core nanocapsules (but not free curcumin) (Hoppe et al., 2013a). Similarly, in neuroblastoma cells, curcumin suppressed the radiation-induced increase in activity of the pro-neuroinflammatory complex NF-κB (Aravindan et al., 2008). Activity of the neuroinflammation- and oxidative damage-related proteins NF-κB, Nrf2, and Sirtl was also regulated in presence of curcumin in human neuroblastoma cells (Doggui et al., 2013). Curcumin treatment reduces ROS level in neuroblastoma cell lines treated with the noxious agent acrolein and in rat primary neurons with induced Ab42 hyper-expression (Ye and Zhang, 2012; Doggui et al., 2013). Curcumin protects mitochondria from noxious factors such as oxidative stress and rotenone (inhibitor of electron transport chain) *in vitro* (Daverey and Agrawal, 2016; Ramkumar et al., 2017). It also alleviates the age-associated loss of mitochondrial and oxidative activity in rodent brains (Dkhar and Sharma, 2010; Eckert et al., 2013; Rastogi et al., 2014). Curcumin also was shown to stimulate Sirtl and Bcl-2 expression and to decrease brain cell death in experimental stroke (Miao et al., 2016). Reports also show that curcumin increases cell viability at low dosages (Ye and Zhang, 2012) and binds Aβ peptides, thus preventing them from aggregation into Aβ plaques (Yanagisawa et al., 2011). Due to its lipophillic properties, the curcumin can cross the BBB, bind to the plaques and decrease the β-amyloid plaques in AD by inducing phagocytosis of Aβ (Mishra and Palanivelu, 2008). Some of the curcumin derived pyrazoles and isoxazoles also bind to Aβ42 (**Figure 8**; Narlawar et al., 2008).

Curcumin treatment decreases Aβ40/42 and PSEN1 protein and mRNA levels in APP-overexpressing neuroblastoma cells (Xiong et al., 2011). Curcumin derivatives also increased the uptake of Aβ by macrophages, which were isolated from blood of AD patients and cultivated *in vitro* (Zhang et al., 2006). This is a relevant information, because peripheral macrophages are known to infiltrate brains of AD patients and participate in clearance of amyloid plaques (Gate et al., 2010). Moreover, in human neuroblastoma cells curcumin inhibits Aβ-induced tau phosphorylation likely via PTEN/Akt/GSK-3β pathway (Huang et al., 2014). Other researchers report, that Akt/GSK-3β and ERK pathways mediate the protective effect of curcumin on Aβ induced memory impairments (Hoppe et al., 2013b; Zhang et al., 2015). Curcumin treatment also improved hippocampal-dependent memory of Aβ-infused rats (Hoppe et al., 2013b).

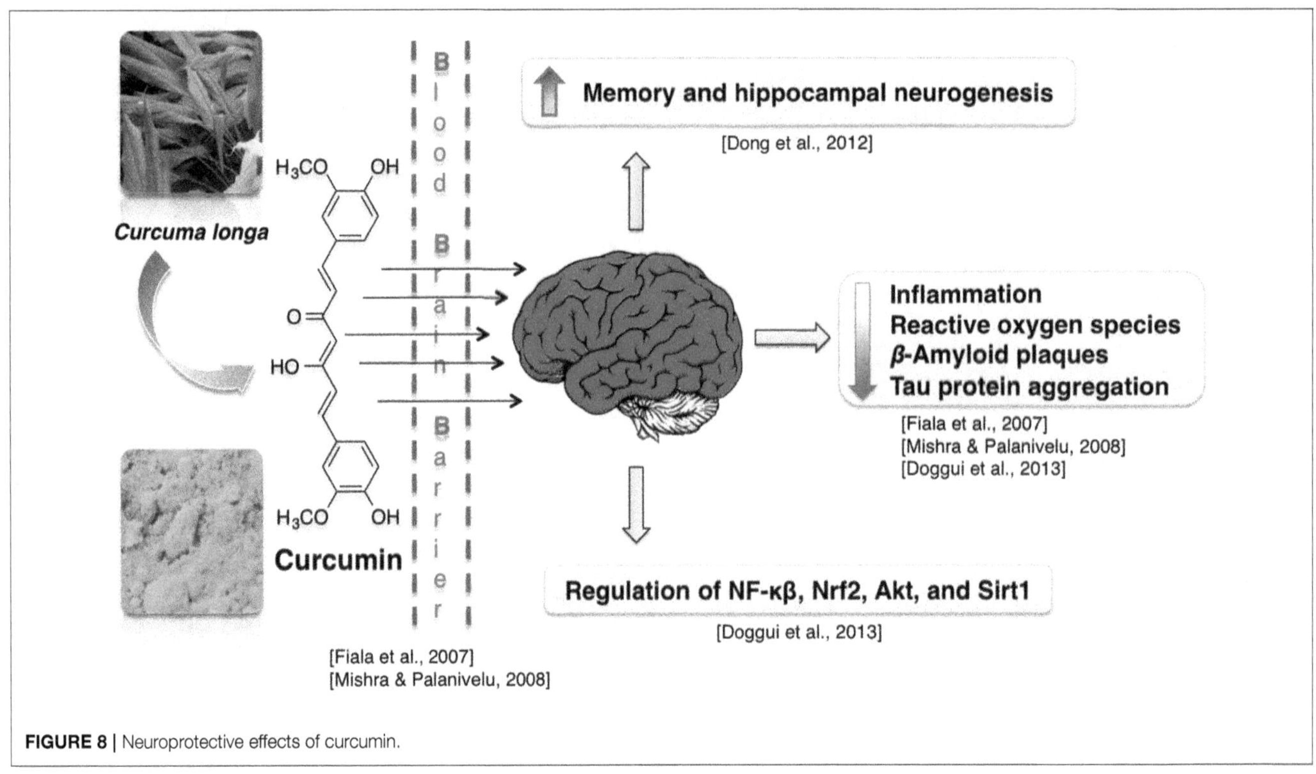

FIGURE 8 | Neuroprotective effects of curcumin.

A systematic review by Brondino et al. showed, that the few clinical trials studying the effect of curcumin on AD yielded inconclusive results (Brondino et al., 2014). Although curcumin was found to be safe during short-term use, future clinical studies need to determine its long-term safety and efficacy on human subjects (Brondino et al., 2014). Since the systematic review arrival, another clinical study was published on the topic, showing improvement of working memory and mood after curcumin treatment in a fairly small group of elderly participants (Cox et al., 2015). There is also a study showing correlation between consumption of curcumin-containing spice—curry—with cognitive performance in elderly (Ng et al., 2006). This finding should be taken with a grain of salt in context of curcumin-dementia research, as curcumin concentration in curry is fairly low (Tayyem et al., 2006) and the extent of biologically available curcumin ingested with curry is disputed. Co-administration of curcumin and donepezil (reversible cholinesterase inhibitor) had synergistic effect on cognition and oxidative stress (Akinyemi et al., 2017). Combined donepezil/curcumin therapeutic also showed good BBB permeability (Yan et al., 2017). Concluding, curcumin protects brain cells against damage induced by oxidative stress and Aβ pathology. These properties may underlie beneficial effects of curcumin for treatment of dementia symptoms, as seen in animal model studies. The data suggest, that curcumin may be a promising candidate for novel dementia medication, but conclusive clinical research that could verify this hypothesis is still lacking. Moreover, to date, researchers analyzed the efficacy of curcumin exclusively against AD-associated dementia, leaving out other dementias.

Glycyrrhiza Genus

Genus *Glycyrrhiza*, also known as licorice (liquorice), is a member of Fabaceae family and consists of about 30 species. Most of the plants of this genus are perennial herbs native to Mediterranean region, Asia, Southern Russia, and Iran (Asl and Hosseinzadeh, 2008). The *Glycyrrhiza* species are cultivated all throughout Europe and Asia (Blumenthal et al., 2000; Asl and Hosseinzadeh, 2008). The licorice roots and rhizomes are used worldwide as natural sweetener and a herbal medicine mainly for the therapy of autoimmune hepatitis C, jaundice, peptic ulcer, and skin diseases such as atopic dermatitis and inflammation-induced hyperpigmentation (Asl and Hosseinzadeh, 2008; Callender et al., 2011; Tewari et al., 2017); further studies suggest that licorice roots may also have pharmacologically useful properties such as anticancer, antioxidative, anti-inflammatory, antiviral, antimicrobial, hepato- and cardioprotectitve effects (Asl and Hosseinzadeh, 2008; Waltenberger et al., 2016). The main bioactive phytoconstituents of *Glycyrrhiza glabra* (liquorice) root are the sweet-tasting triterpene saponin glycyrrhizin (glycyrrhizic acid) and the phenolic type compound isoliquiritigenin (**Figure 9**). Other important constituents also include several isoflavonoid derivatives such as shinpterocarpin, glabrone, glabridin, galbrene, lico-isoflavones A and B (Asl and Hosseinzadeh, 2008).

Due to their antioxidative properties, several species of *Glycyrrhiza* were investigated for possible therapeutic effects as neuroprotectants against neurodegenerative disorders such as PD, AD, and dementia. For example, extract from *Glycyrrhiza inflata* prevents tau misfolding *in vitro* (Chang et al., 2016). Thus, the extract of this plant may be effective against various

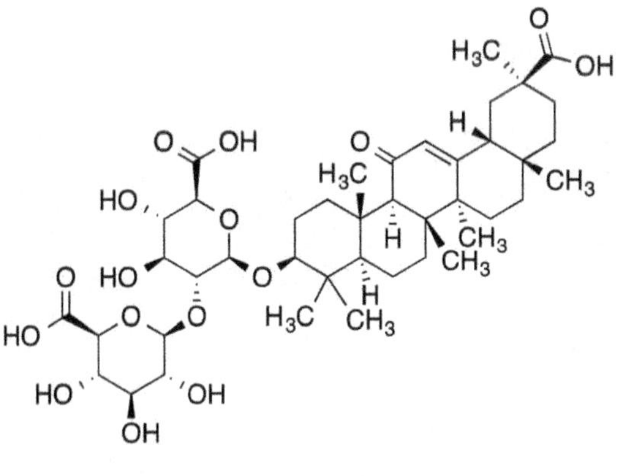

Glycyrrhizin (Epigen™, Glycyron™)
(glycyrrhizic acid or glycyrrhizinic acid)
Chem. formula: $C_{42}H_{62}O_{16}$
Mol. wt.: 822.9 g/mol

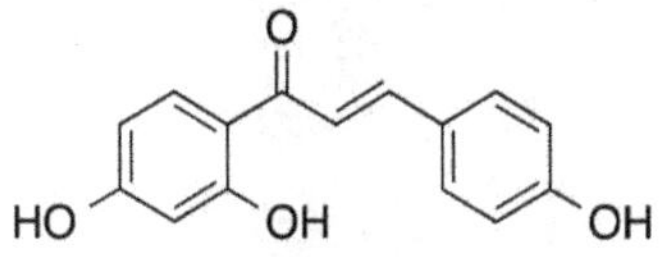

Isoliquiritigenin
Chem. formula: $C_{15}H_{12}O_4$
Mol. wt.: 256.3

FIGURE 9 | Chemical structures of the major phytoconstituents of *Glycyrrhiza glabra*.

taupathies and AD. *G. inflata* extract decreased oxidative stress in cell models of spinocerebellar ataxia type 3 (SCA3), also known as Machado-Joseph disease (MJD), by upregulating the activity of PPARGC1A and the NFE2L2-ARE pathway (Chen et al., 2014). Glycyrrhizin prevents cytotoxicity, ROS generation and downregulation of glutathione (GSH), which are elicited by 1-methyl-4-phenylpyridinium (MPP^+) (Yim et al., 2007). MPP+ is a neurotoxic substance acting via interference with the mitochondrial oxidative phosphorylation (Yim et al., 2007). The GSH downregulation is noteworthy, because it is a crucial element of the antioxidative system of the brain (Dringen, 2000). Increased oxidative stress in dementia is attributed to dwindled levels of GSH (Yim et al., 2007; Saharan and Mandal, 2014). Similarly, *G. inflata* extract was shown to inhibit oxidative stress *in vitro* (Chang et al., 2016). The brain cells are susceptible to the oxidative stress. The effect of licorice extract on the oxidative stress may be connected to the beneficial effect of isoliquiritigenin on mitochondrial function (Yang et al., 2012). Licorice may reduce the damage to the brain cells, improve the neuronal function and prevent the memory impairment by diminishing oxidative stress associated with several dementia types (Ju et al., 1989; Dhingra et al., 2004).

Figure 10 summarizes the valuable effects of licorice root extract that may be useful for the treatment of dementia and/or AD-related dementia. Some authors suggest that memory-enhancing activity of the licorice root extract may be connected to its anti-inflammatory effect (Yokota et al., 1998; Dhingra et al., 2004). This data is in agreement with the known tight relationship between inflammation and oxidative stress (Dandekar et al., 2015). *Glycyrrhiza* is used in various polyherbal formulations. One of such formulations used in traditional Japanese Kampo medicine is yokukansan, which is composed of seven different plants including *Glycyrrhiza uralensis* Fisher. *Glycyrrhiza* extract antagonizes α2A adrenoceptors (Ikarashi and Mizoguchi, 2016). Several phytoconstituents of *Glycyrrhiza*: glycyrrhizin, glycycoumarin, liquiritin and isoliquiritigenin show neuroprotective effects when applied as a component of the yokukansan (Ikarashi and Mizoguchi, 2016). Isoliquiritigenin inhibited the activity of the NMDA receptors (Ikarashi and Mizoguchi, 2016). Noteworthy, memantine, an important synthetic drug against dementia, also shows antagonism for NMDA receptors (Danysz and Parsons, 2003). Moreover, the neuroprotective effect of glycycoumarin may be due to its ability to suppress the pro-apoptotic activity of caspase-3 (Kanno et al., 2015; Ikarashi and Mizoguchi, 2016).

Extract from another *Glycyrrhiza* species—*Glycyrrhiza glabra*—improved the learning ability of mice after 7 days of oral administration (Parle et al., 2004). However, another study reported the paradoxical sedative properties of the extract (Hikino, 1985). This shows that the *G. glabra* extract is useful for the improvement of the learning ability but its dose should be established carefully to prevent the sedative effects. A glycyrrhizin salt, diammonium-glycyrrhizinate, prevented the mitochondrial and cognitive dysfunctions induced by Aβ42 in mice (Zhu et al., 2012). Although not yet proven in context of brain function, licorice constituents have a potential to interact with other drugs because of its modulating activity of P450 proteins, which belong to the main regulators of xenobiotic metabolism (Qiao et al., 2014). In summary, glycyrrhiza extracts show anti-inflammatory and antioxidative properties and modulate glutamate signaling and apoptosis. Similarly to above described herbal medicines curcumin and ginseng, despite animal model-based evidence for glycyrrhiza effectiveness in regulating cognitive deficits, there are currently no studies on effectiveness of this plant for dementia therapy in patients.

Camellia sinensis Kuntze

Camellia sinensis Kuntze (green tea) brew is one of the most extensively consumed beverages in the world (Goenka et al., 2013). Several beneficial effects of green tea consumption

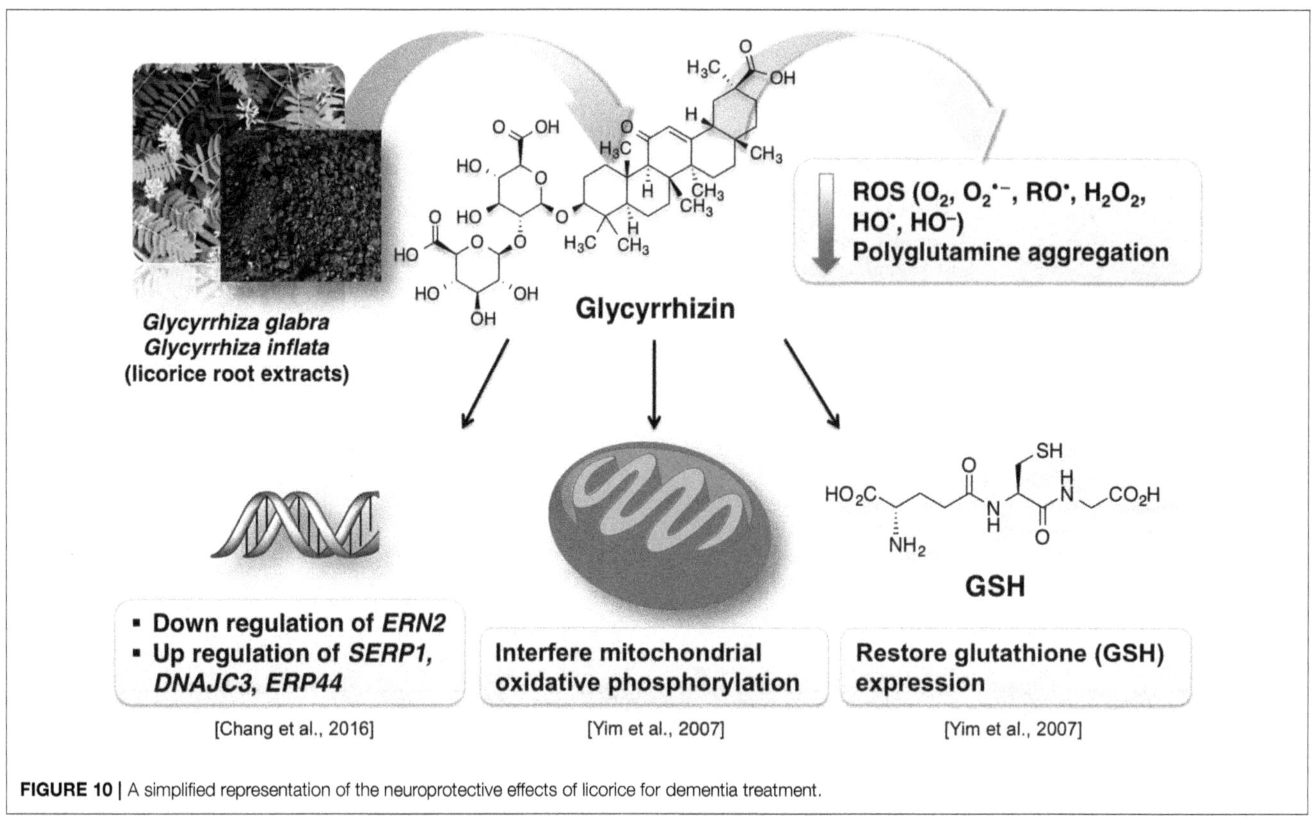

FIGURE 10 | A simplified representation of the neuroprotective effects of licorice for dementia treatment.

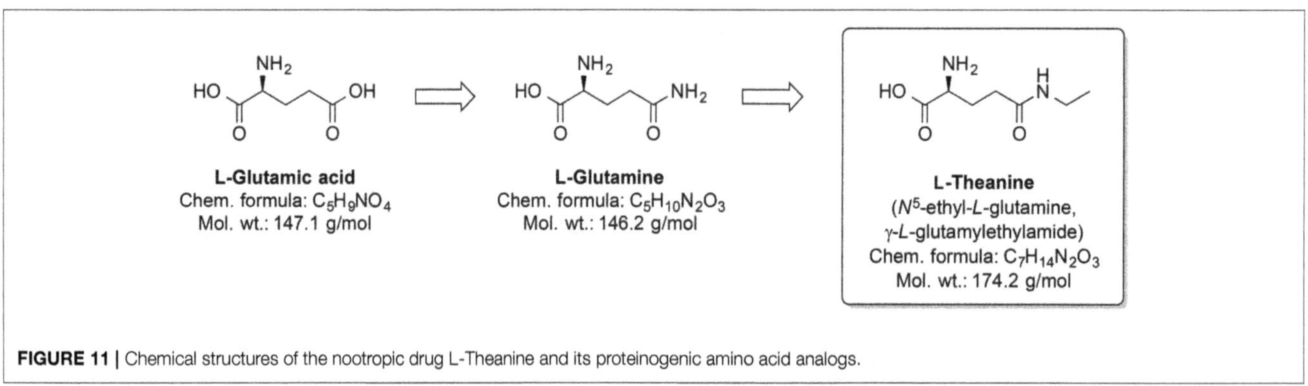

FIGURE 11 | Chemical structures of the nootropic drug L-Theanine and its proteinogenic amino acid analogs.

are reported for various conditions like obesity, diabetes, inflammation, coronary artery disease, stroke and some malignancies (de Mejia et al., 2009; Chacko et al., 2010). Consumption of green tea-related compounds [e.g., (-)-epigallocatechin-3-gallate] improves cognitive functions and prevents memory impairment in animals and humans (Rezai-Zadeh et al., 2008; de Mejia et al., 2009; Mandel et al., 2011).

Around one-third out of 4,000 bioactive compounds of *C. sinensis* are polyphenols (Mahmood et al., 2010). The gene expression and activity of the membrane metalloendopeptidase (MME) were enhanced by green tea extract. Several MME are capable of degrading Aβ peptides (Wang et al., 2006). Pretreatment by infusion with extract of green tea leaves into the left hippocampus of a rat prevented cognitive impairments and superoxide dismutase activity changes, and corrected deregulated activity of pro-inflammatory enzyme COX and AChE, which were induced by injecting $AlCl_3$ into the same brain area (Jelenkovic et al., 2014). When injected i.p. L-theanine, one of the amino acid components of *C. sinensis,* protects against memory impairment and cell death caused by ischemia (Egashira et al., 2007, 2008). Interestingly, chronic ingestion of L-theanine in rats also caused improvement in cognitive functions (Yamada et al., 2008) and decreased oxidation levels in the brain of the rats (Nishida et al., 2008). Similarly, in transgenic mouse AD model, the green tea constituent epigallocatechin-3-gallate normalized the dysregulated ROS production, as well as mitochondrial respiration and MMP (Dragicevic et al., 2011). Generally,

L-theanine is an *N*-amino-ethylated analog of the proteinogenic neurotransmitter L-glutamic acid and its precursor L-glutamine (**Figure 11**). L-theanine protects against Aβ42-induced memory deficits and death of cortical and hippocampal cells, possibly by suppressing the ERK/p38 and NF-κB signaling pathways and reducing the oxidative damage (Kim et al., 2009).

Daily consumption of green tea is hypothesized to reduce the risk of AD and age-related dementia (Ayoub and Melzig, 2006). In some clinical studies, L-theanine improved the cognitive functions and mood in combination with caffeine in healthy human subjects (Haskell et al., 2008; Owen et al., 2008). On the other hand, the results of studies on the effects of L-theanine alone on mood are inconclusive (Kimura et al., 2007; Haskell et al., 2008). Green tea catechins can regulate activity of P-glycoprotein (Zhou et al., 2004), which may influence brain availability of co-administered substances. Summarizing, green tea extract shows antiapoptotic and antioxidative activities and may even directly inhibit Aβ plaque formation. Moreover, several human studies provide credibility to the hypothesis that green tea constituents may be effective for modulation of human cognition and perhaps in dementia treatment.

CONCLUSIONS

In this work, we discuss that a large number of plants have been used for dementia treatment worldwide. The mechanisms of action of the reviewed five prominent representative plants generally involve anti-inflammatory, antioxidative, and antiapoptotic activity that are mainly associated with the neuroprotective effects of these plants or their bioactive constituents. Some of such naturally occurring compounds exhibit promising potential as alternative therapeutic strategies. For example, curcumin showed remarkable synergetic effects on cognition and oxidative stress, as well as good BBB permeability, when co-administrated with the approved reversible ChE inhibitor donepezil. Moreover, such combined donepezil/curcumin application may be useful for treatment of dementia symptoms, as seen in animal model studies. Furthermore, combined supplement treatment with some mitochondrial antioxidants, such as α-lipoic acid and acetyl-L-carnitine has been shown to reduce both physical and mental weariness or even to restore memory function in age-related diseases, including AD and different types of dementia, as provided in transgenic mouse model of AD. However, there are still many unknowns in this research area that need to be clarified by planning future studies. The scientific community needs more comprehensive research focused on identifying active ingredients of plants and investigating their mechanism of action. Such research will facilitate clinical studies evaluating the potential of the featured herbal products in dementia treatment. We conclude that further research on plants used in different ethnomedicinal practices and the traditional medicine could lead to the development of novel therapeutics for dementia and, therefore, is of a very high interest.

AUTHOR CONTRIBUTIONS

DT, AMS, and AA have written the first draft of the manuscript. AM, ANS, LH, JH, and NT revised and improved the first draft. All authors have seen and agreed on the finally submitted version of the manuscript.

ACKNOWLEDGMENTS

The authors acknowledge the support by the Polish KNOW (Leading National Research Centre) Scientific Consortium "Healthy Animal—Safe Food," decision of Ministry of Science and Higher Education No. 05-1/KNOW2/2015.

REFERENCES

Abbott, A. (2011). Dementia: a problem for our age. *Nature* 475, S2–S4. doi: 10.1038/475S2a

Abdel-Kader, R., Hauptmann, S., Keil, U., Scherping, I., Leuner, K., Eckert, A., et al. (2007). Stabilization of mitochondrial function by *Ginkgo biloba* extract (EGb 761). *Pharmacol. Res.* 56, 493–502. doi: 10.1016/j.phrs.2007.09.011

Abdou, H. M., Yousef, M. I., El Mekkawy, D. A., and Al-Shami, A. S. (2016). Prophylactic neuroprotective efficiency of co-administration of *Ginkgo biloba* and Trifolium pretense against sodium arsenite-induced neurotoxicity and dementia in different regions of brain and spinal cord of rats. *Food Chem. Toxicol.* 94, 112–127. doi: 10.1016/j.fct.2016.05.015

Adams, M., Gmünder, F., and Hamburger, M. (2007). Plants traditionally used in age related brain disorders—a survey of ethnobotanical literature. *J. Ethnopharmacol.* 113, 363–381. doi: 10.1016/j.jep.2007.07.016

Adsersen, A., Gauguin, B., Gudiksen, L., and Jäger, A. K. (2006). Screening of plants used in Danish folk medicine to treat memory dysfunction for acetylcholinesterase inhibitory activity. *J. Ethnopharmacol.* 104, 418–422. doi: 10.1016/j.jep.2005.09.032

Ahlemeyer, B., and Krieglstein, J. (2003). Neuroprotective effects of *Ginkgo biloba* extract. *Cell. Mol. Life Sci. C.* 60, 1779–1792. doi: 10.1007/s00018-003-3080-1

Akhondzadeh, S., Noroozian, M., Mohammadi, M., Ohadinia, S., Jamshidi, A. H., and Khani, M. (2003). Salvia officinalis extract in the treatment of patients with mild to moderate Alzheimer's disease: a double blind, randomized and placebo-controlled trial. *J. Clin. Pharm. Ther.* 28, 53–59. doi: 10.1046/j.1365-2710.2003.00463.x

Akinyemi, A. J., Oboh, G., Oyeleye, S. I., and Ogunsuyi, O. (2017). Anti-amnestic effect of curcumin in combination with donepezil, an anticholinesterase drug: involvement of cholinergic system. *Neurotox. Res.* 31, 560–569. doi: 10.1007/s12640-017-9701-5

Alam, M. M., Okazaki, K., Nguyen, L. T. T., Ota, N., Kitamura, H., Murakami, S., et al. (2017). Glucocorticoid receptor signaling represses the antioxidant response by inhibiting histone acetylation mediated by the transcriptional activator NRF2. *J. Biol. Chem.* 292, 7519–7530. doi: 10.1074/jbc.M116.773960

Albuquerque, E. X., Santos, M. D., Alkondon, M., Pereira, E. F., and Maelicke, A. (2001). Modulation of nicotinic receptor activity in the central nervous system: a novel approach to the treatment of Alzheimer disease. *Alzheimer Dis. Assoc. Disord.* 15(Suppl. 1), S19–25. doi: 10.1097/00002093-200108001-00004

Aminzadeh, M., Roghani, M., Sarfallah, A., and Riazi, G. H. (2018). TRPM2 dependence of ROS-induced NLRP3 activation in Alzheimer's disease. *Int. Immunopharmacol.* 54, 78–85. doi: 10.1016/j.intimp.2017.10.024

Amri, H., Ogwuegbu, S. O., Boujrad, N., Drieu, K., and Papadopoulos, V. (1996). *In vivo* regulation of peripheral-type benzodiazepine receptor and glucocorticoid synthesis by *Ginkgo biloba* extract EGb 761 and isolated ginkgolides. *Endocrinology* 137, 5707–5718. doi: 10.1210/endo.137.12.8940403

Anjomshoa, S., Namazian, M., and Noorbala, M. R. (2016). The effect of solvent on tautomerism, acidity and radical stability of curcumin and its derivatives based on thermodynamic quantities. *J. Solution Chem.* 45, 1021–1030. doi: 10.1007/s10953-016-0481-y

Antico Arciuch, V. G., Elguero, M. E., Poderoso, J. J., and Carreras, M. C. (2012). Mitochondrial regulation of cell cycle and proliferation. *Antioxid. Redox Signal.* 16, 1150–1180. doi: 10.1089/ars.2011.4085

Aravindan, N., Madhusoodhanan, R., Ahmad, S., Johnson, D., and Herman, T. S. (2008). Curcumin inhibits NFκB mediated radioprotection and modulate apoptosis related genes in human neuroblastoma cells. *Cancer Biol. Ther.* 7, 569–576. doi: 10.4161/cbt.7.4.5534

Asl, M. N., and Hosseinzadeh, H. (2008). Review of pharmacological effects of *Glycyrrhiza* sp. and its bioactive compounds. *Phyther. Res.* 22, 709–724. doi: 10.1002/ptr.2362

Atanasov, A. G., Waltenberger, B., Pferschy-Wenzig, E.-M., Linder, T., Wawrosch, C., Uhrin, P., et al. (2015). Discovery and resupply of pharmacologically active plant-derived natural products: a review. *Biotechnol. Adv.* 33, 1582–1614. doi: 10.1016/j.biotechadv.2015.08.001

Ayoub, S., and Melzig, M. F. (2006). Induction of neutral endopeptidase (NEP) activity of SK-N-SH cells by natural compounds from green tea. *J. Pharm. Pharmacol.* 58, 495–501. doi: 10.1211/jpp.58.4.0009

Ballard, C., and Howard, R. (2006). Neuroleptic drugs in dementia: benefits and harm. *Nat. Rev. Neurosci.* 7, 492–500. doi: 10.1038/nrn1926

Baloh, R. H. (2011). TDP-43: the relationship between protein aggregation and neurodegeneration in amyotrophic lateral sclerosis and frontotemporal lobar degeneration. *FEBS J.* 278, 3539–3549. doi: 10.1111/j.1742-4658.2011.08256.x

Banasch, M., Ellrichmann, M., Tannapfel, A., Schmidt, W. E., and Goetze, O. (2011). The non-invasive (13)C-methionine breath test detects hepatic mitochondrial dysfunction as a marker of disease activity in non-alcoholic steatohepatitis. *Eur. J. Med. Res.* 16:258. doi: 10.1186/2047-783X-16-6-258

Bartus, R. T., Dean, R. L. III., Beer, B., and Lippa, A. S. (1982). The cholinergic hypothesis of geriatric memory dysfunction. *Science* 217, 408–414. doi: 10.1126/science.7046051

Beal, M. F. (2005). Mitochondria take center stage in aging and neurodegeneration. *Ann. Neurol.* 58, 495–505. doi: 10.1002/ana.20624

Belkacemi, A., Doggui, S., Dao, L., and Ramassamy, C. (2011). Challenges associated with curcumin therapy in Alzheimer disease. *Expert Rev. Mol. Med.* 13, e34. doi: 10.1017/S1462399411002055

Bennett, S., Grant, M. M., and Aldred, S. (2009). Oxidative stress in vascular dementia and Alzheimer's disease: a common pathology. *J. Alzheimers. Dis.* 17, 245–257. doi: 10.3233/JAD-2009-1041

Berridge, M. J. (1995). Calcium signalling and cell proliferation. *Bioessays* 17, 491–500. doi: 10.1002/bies.950170605

Berridge, M. J. (2011). Calcium signalling and Alzheimer's disease. *Neurochem. Res.* 36, 1149–1156. doi: 10.1007/s11064-010-0371-4

Blennow, K., de Leon, M. J., and Zetterberg, H. (2006). Alzheimer's disease. *Lancet (London, England)* 368, 387–403. doi: 10.1016/S0140-6736(06)69113-7

Blumenthal, M., Goldberg, A., and Brinkmann, J. (2000). *Herbal Medicine, Expanded Commission E Monographs Cd-Rom.* Austin, TX: American Botanical Council/Integrative Medical.

Bridi, R., Crossetti, F. P., Steffen, V. M., and Henriques, A. T. (2001). The antioxidant activity of standardized extract of *Ginkgo biloba* (EGb 761) in rats. *Phytother. Res.* 15, 449–451. doi: 10.1002/ptr.814

Brondino, N., Re, S., Boldrini, A., Cuccomarino, A., Lanati, N., Barale, F., et al. (2014). Curcumin as a therapeutic agent in dementia: a mini systematic review of human studies. *Sci. World J.* 2014:174282. doi: 10.1155/2014/174282

Brun, A. (1987). Frontal lobe degeneration of non-Alzheimer type. *I. Neuropathology. Arch. Gerontol. Geriatr.* 6, 193–208. doi: 10.1016/0167-4943(87)90021-5

Burgess, L., Page, S., and Hardman, P. (2002). Changing attitudes in dementia care and the role of nurses. *Nurs. Times* 99, 18–19.

Burte, F., Carelli, V., Chinnery, P. F., and Yu-Wai-Man, P. (2015). Disturbed mitochondrial dynamics and neurodegenerative disorders. *Nat. Rev. Neurol.* 11, 11–24. doi: 10.1038/nrneurol.2014.228

Butterfield, D. A., Swomley, A. M., and Sultana, R. (2013). Amyloid beta-peptide (1-42)-induced oxidative stress in Alzheimer disease: importance in disease pathogenesis and progression. *Antioxid. Redox Signal.* 19, 823–835. doi: 10.1089/ars.2012.5027

Cai, H., Cong, W., Ji, S., Rothman, S., Maudsley, S., and Martin, B. (2012). Metabolic dysfunction in Alzheimer's disease and related neurodegenerative disorders. *Curr. Alzheimer Res.* 9, 5–17. doi: 10.2174/1567205127990 15064

Callender, V. D., St Surin-Lord, S., Davis, E. C., and Maclin, M. (2011). Postinflammatory hyperpigmentation: etiologic and therapeutic considerations. *Am. J. Clin. Dermatol.* 12, 87–99. doi: 10.2165/11536930-000000000-00000

CESA (1992). *Usos Tradicionales de las Especies Forestales Nativas en el Ecuador.* Tomo II. CESA: Central Ecuatoriana de Servicios Agrícolas.

CESA (1993). *Usos Tradicionales de las Especies Forestales Nativas en el Ecuador.* Tomo III. CESA: Central Ecuatoriana de Servicios Agrícolas.

Chacko, S. M., Thambi, P. T., Kuttan, R., and Nishigaki, I. (2010). Beneficial effects of green tea: a literature review. *Chin. Med.* 5:13. doi: 10.1186/1749-8546-5-13

Chan, D. C. (2006). Mitochondria: dynamic organelles in disease, aging, and development. *Cell* 125, 1241–1252. doi: 10.1016/j.cell.2006.06.010

Chandrasekaran, K., Mehrabian, Z., Spinnewyn, B., Chinopoulos, C., Drieu, K., and Fiskum, G. (2003). Neuroprotective effects of bilobalide, a component of *Ginkgo biloba* extract (EGb 761®) in global brain ischemia and in excitotoxicity-induced neuronal death. *Pharmacopsychiatry* 36, 89–94. doi: 10.1055/s-2003-40447

Chang, H.-M., But, P. P. H., and Yao, S.-C. (1986). *Pharmacology and Applications of Chinese Materia Medica.* Singapore: World Scientific.

Chang, K.-H., Chen, I.-C., Lin, H.-Y., Chen, H.-C., Lin, C.-H., Lin, T.-H., et al. (2016). The aqueous extract of Glycyrrhiza inflata can upregulate unfolded protein response-mediated chaperones to reduce tau misfolding in cell models of Alzheimer's disease. *Drug Des. Devel. Ther.* 10, 885–896. doi: 10.2147/DDDT.S96454

Chen, C.-M., Weng, Y.-T., Chen, W.-L., Lin, T.-H., Chao, C.-Y., Lin, C.-H., et al. (2014). Aqueous extract of Glycyrrhiza inflata inhibits aggregation by upregulating PPARGC1A and NFE2L2-ARE pathways in cell models of spinocerebellar ataxia 3. *Free Radic. Biol. Med.* 71, 339–350. doi: 10.1016/j.freeradbiomed.2014.03.023

Chen, F., Eckman, E. A., and Eckman, C. B. (2006). Reductions in levels of the Alzheimer's amyloid beta peptide after oral administration of ginsenosides. *FASEB J. Off. Publ. Fed. Am. Soc. Exp. Biol.* 20, 1269–1271. doi: 10.1096/fj.05-5530fje

Chen, J. X., and Yan, S. S. (2010). Role of mitochondrial amyloid-beta in Alzheimer's disease. *J. Alzheimers. Dis.* 20(Suppl. 2), S569–S578. doi: 10.3233/JAD-2010-100357

Chevallier, A. (1996). *The Encyclopedia of Medicinal Plants.* London: Dorling Kindersley publishers.

Chin, D., Huebbe, P., Pallauf, K., and Rimbach, G. (2013). Neuroprotective properties of curcumin in Alzheimer's disease–merits and limitations. *Curr. Med. Chem.* 20, 3955–3985. doi: 10.2174/09298673113209990210

Chrusciel, M., and Varagić, V. (1966). The effect of galantamine on the blood pressure of the rat. *Br. J. Pharmacol.* 26, 295–301. doi: 10.1111/j.1476-5381.1966.tb01908.x

Corder, E. H., Saunders, A. M., Strittmatter, W. J., Schmechel, D. E., Gaskell, P. C., Small, G. W., et al. (1993). Gene dose of apolipoprotein E type 4 allele and the risk of Alzheimer's disease in late onset families. *Science* 261, 921–923.

Corrada, M. M., Brookmeyer, R., Paganini-Hill, A., Berlau, D., and Kawas, C. H. (2010). Dementia incidence continues to increase with age in the oldest old: the 90+ study. *Ann. Neurol.* 67, 114–121. doi: 10.1002/ana.21915

Cox, K. H. M., Pipingas, A., and Scholey, A. B. (2015). Investigation of the effects of solid lipid curcumin on cognition and mood in a healthy older population. *J. Psychopharmacol.* 29, 642–651. doi: 10.1177/0269881114552744

Cummings, J., Aisen, P. S., DuBois, B., Frölich, L., Jack, C. R., Jones, R. W., et al. (2016). Drug development in Alzheimer's disease: the path to 2025. *Alzheimer's Res. Ther.* 8:39. doi: 10.1186/s13195-016-0207-9

Dai, D.-F., Chiao, Y. A., Marcinek, D. J., Szeto, H. H., and Rabinovitch, P. S. (2014). Mitochondrial oxidative stress in aging and healthspan. *Longev. Heal.* 3:6. doi: 10.1186/2046-2395-3-6

Damasio, A. R., and Gabrowski, T. J. (2004). "Definition, clinical features and neuroanatomical basis of dementia," in *The Neuropathology of Dementia*, eds M. M. Esiri, V. M.-Y. Lee, and J. Q. Trojanowski (Cambridge: Cambridge University Press), 1–34.

Dandekar, A., Mendez, R., and Zhang, K. (2015). Cross talk between ER stress, oxidative stress, and inflammation in health and disease. *Methods Mol. Biol.* 1292, 205–214. doi: 10.1007/978-1-4939-2522-3_15

Danysz, W., and Parsons, C. G. (2003). The NMDA receptor antagonist memantine as a symptomatological and neuroprotective treatment for Alzheimer's disease: preclinical evidence. *Int. J. Geriatr. Psychiatry* 18, S23–S32. doi: 10.1002/gps.938

Daverey, A., and Agrawal, S. K. (2016). Curcumin alleviates oxidative stress and mitochondrial dysfunction in astrocytes. *Neuroscience* 333, 92–103. doi: 10.1016/j.neuroscience.2016.07.012

Dávila, D., Fernández, S., and Torres-Alemán, I. (2016). Astrocyte resilience to oxidative stress induced by insulin-like growth factor I (IGF-I) involves preserved AKT (protein kinase B) activity. *J. Biol. Chem.* 291, 12039. doi: 10.1074/jbc.A115.695478

de Barradas, J. P. (1957). *Plantas Mágicas Americanas*. Consejo Superior de Investigaciones Científicas, Instituto "Bernardino de Sahagún."

de Mejia, E. G., Ramirez-Mares, M. V., and Puangpraphant, S. (2009). Bioactive components of tea: cancer, inflammation and behavior. *Brain. Behav. Immun.* 23, 721–731. doi: 10.1016/j.bbi.2009.02.013

Dhingra, D., Parle, M., and Kulkarni, S. K. (2004). Memory enhancing activity of Glycyrrhiza glabra in mice. *J. Ethnopharmacol.* 91, 361–365. doi: 10.1016/j.jep.2004.01.016

Dkhar, P., and Sharma, R. (2010). Effect of dimethylsulphoxide and curcumin on protein carbonyls and reactive oxygen species of cerebral hemispheres of mice as a function of age. *Int. J. Dev. Neurosci.* 28, 351–357. doi: 10.1016/j.ijdevneu.2010.04.005

Doggui, S., Belkacemi, A., Paka, G. D., Perrotte, M., Pi, R., and Ramassamy, C. (2013). Curcumin protects neuronal-like cells against acrolein by restoring Akt and redox signaling pathways. *Mol. Nutr. Food Res.* 57, 1660–1670. doi: 10.1002/mnfr.201300130

Dolgin, E. (2016). How to defeat dementia. *Nature* 539, 156–158. doi: 10.1038/539156a

Domoráková, I., Burda, J., Mechírová, E., and Feriková, M. (2006). Mapping of rat hippocampal neurons with NeuN after ischemia/reperfusion and *Ginkgo biloba* extract (EGb 761) pretreatment. *Cell. Mol. Neurobiol.* 26, 1191–1202. doi: 10.1007/s10571-006-9080-6

Dong, S., Zeng, Q., Mitchell, E. S., Xiu, J., Duan, Y., Li, C., et al. (2012). Curcumin enhances neurogenesis and cognition in aged rats: implications for transcriptional interactions related to growth and synaptic plasticity. *PLoS ONE* 7:e31211. doi: 10.1371/journal.pone.0031211

Doody, R. S., Stevens, J. C., Beck, C., Dubinsky, R. M., Kaye, J. A., Gwyther, L., et al. (2001). Practice parameter: management of dementia (an evidence-based review) Report of the Quality Standards Subcommittee of the American Academy of Neurology. *Neurology* 56, 1154–1166. doi: 10.1212/WNL.56.9.1154

Dragicevic, N., Smith, A., Lin, X., Yuan, F., Copes, N., Delic, V., et al. (2011). Green tea epigallocatechin-3-gallate (EGCG) and other flavonoids reduce Alzheimer's amyloid-induced mitochondrial dysfunction. *J. Alzheimers. Dis.* 26, 507–521. doi: 10.3233/JAD-2011-101629

Dringen, R. (2000). Metabolism and functions of glutathione in brain. *Prog. Neurobiol.* 62, 649–671. doi: 10.1016/S0301-0082(99)00060-X

Duke, J. A., and Ayensu, E. S. (1985). *Medicinal Plants of China*. Algonac: Reference Publications.

Eckert, A., Keil, U., Scherping, I., Hauptmann, S., and Muller, W. E. (2005). Stabilization of mitochondrial membrane potential and improvement of neuronal energy metabolism by *Ginkgo biloba* extract EGb 761. *Ann. N. Y. Acad. Sci.* 1056, 474–485. doi: 10.1196/annals.1352.023

Eckert, G. P., Schiborr, C., Hagl, S., Abdel-Kader, R., Muller, W. E., Rimbach, G., et al. (2013). Curcumin prevents mitochondrial dysfunction in the brain of the senescence-accelerated mouse-prone 8. *Neurochem. Int.* 62, 595–602. doi: 10.1016/j.neuint.2013.02.014

Egashira, N., Hayakawa, K., Osajima, M., Mishima, K., Iwasaki, K., Oishi, R., et al. (2007). Involvement of GABA(A) receptors in the neuroprotective effect of theanine on focal cerebral ischemia in mice. *J. Pharmacol. Sci.* 105, 211–214. doi: 10.1254/jphs.SCZ070901

Egashira, N., Ishigami, N., Pu, F., Mishima, K., Iwasaki, K., Orito, K., et al. (2008). Theanine prevents memory impairment induced by repeated cerebral ischemia in rats. *Phytother. Res.* 22, 65–68. doi: 10.1002/ptr.2261

Ezoulin, M. J. M., Ombetta, J.-E., Dutertre-Catella, H., Warnet, J.-M., and Massicot, F. (2008). Antioxidative properties of galantamine on neuronal damage induced by hydrogen peroxide in SK-N-SH cells. *Neurotoxicology* 29, 270–277. doi: 10.1016/j.neuro.2007.11.004

Farkas, E., and Luiten, P. G. (2001). Cerebral microvascular pathology in aging and Alzheimer's disease. *Prog. Neurobiol.* 64, 575–611. doi: 10.1016/S0301-0082(00)00068-X

Fatumbi, P. V. P. (1995). *Ewé: The Use of Plants in Yoruba Society*. Salvador: Oderbrecht.

Favaloro, B., Allocati, N., Graziano, V., Di Ilio, C., and De Laurenzi, V. (2012). Role of Apoptosis in disease. *Aging (Albany NY)* 4, 330–349. doi: 10.18632/aging.100459

Finkler, K. (1985). *Spiritualist Healers in Mexico: Successes and Failures of Alternative Therapeutics*. Salem, WI: Praeger Publishers.

Fox, C., Crugel, M., Maidment, I., Auestad, B. H., Coulton, S., Treloar, A., et al. (2012). Efficacy of memantine for agitation in Alzheimer's dementia: a randomised double-blind placebo controlled trial. *PLoS ONE* 7:e35185. doi: 10.1371/journal.pone.0035185

Franzblau, M., Gonzales-Portillo, C., Gonzales-Portillo, G. S., Diamandis, T., Borlongan, M. C., Tajiri, N., et al. (2013). Vascular damage: a persisting pathology common to Alzheimer's disease and traumatic brain injury. *Med. Hypotheses* 81, 842–845. doi: 10.1016/j.mehy.2013.09.012

Fuchs, L. (1543). *Kräuterbuch. Michael Isingrin*. Basel.

Gao, H.-M., Zhou, H., and Hong, J.-S. (2014). "Oxidative stress, neuroinflammation, and neurodegeneration," in *Neuroinflammation, and Neurodegeneration*, eds P. K. Peterson and M. Toborek (New York, NY: Springer New York), 81–104.

Gate, D., Rezai-Zadeh, K., Jodry, D., Rentsendorj, A., and Town, T. (2010). Macrophages in Alzheimer's disease: the blood-borne identity. *J. Neural Transm.* 117, 961–970. doi: 10.1007/s00702-010-0422-7

Geeganage, C., Wilcox, R., and Bath, P. M. W. (2010). Triple antiplatelet therapy for preventing vascular events: a systematic review and meta-analysis. *BMC Med.* 8:36. doi: 10.1186/1741-7015-8-36

Giacobini, E. (2004). Cholinesterase inhibitors: new roles and therapeutic alternatives. *Pharmacol. Res.* 50, 433–440. doi: 10.1016/j.phrs.2003.11.017

Giri, M., Zhang, M., and Lu, Y. (2016). Genes associated with Alzheimer's disease: an overview and current status. *Clin. Interv. Aging* 11, 665–681. doi: 10.2147/CIA.S105769

Goenka, P., Sarawgi, A., Karun, V., Nigam, A. G., Dutta, S., and Marwah, N. (2013). Camellia sinensis (Tea): implications and role in preventing dental decay. *Pharmacogn. Rev.* 7, 152–156. doi: 10.4103/0973-7847.120515

Gómez-Sámano, M. Á., Grajales-Gómez, M., Zuarth-Vázquez, J. M., Navarro-Flores, M. F., Martínez-Saavedra, M., Juárez-León, Ó. A., et al. (2017). Fibroblast growth factor 21 and its novel association with oxidative stress. *Redox Biol.* 11, 335–341. doi: 10.1016/j.redox.2016.12.024

González Ayala, J. C. (1994). *Botánica Medicinal Popular: Etnobotánica Medicinal de El Salvador*. Jardín Botànico La Laguna.

Grand, J. H., Caspar, S., and Macdonald, S. W. (2011). Clinical features and multidisciplinary approaches to dementia care. *J Multidiscip Heal.* 2011, 125–147. doi: 10.2147/JMDH.S17773

Guan, R., Zhao, Y., Zhang, H., Fan, G., Liu, X., Zhou, W., et al. (2016). Draft genome of the living fossil *Ginkgo biloba*. *Gigascience* 5, 49. doi: 10.1186/s13742-016-0154-1

Gurib-Fakim, A. (2006). Medicinal plants: traditions of yesterday and drugs of tomorrow. *Mol. Aspects Med.* 27, 1–93. doi: 10.1016/j.mam.2005.07.008

Hajnoczky, G., Davies, E., and Madesh, M. (2003). Calcium signaling and apoptosis. *Biochem. Biophys. Res. Commun.* 304, 445–454. doi: 10.1016/S0006-291X(03)00616-8

Hardy, J. A., and Higgins, G. A. (1992). Alzheimer's disease: the amyloid cascade hypothesis. *Science (*256, 184.

Haskell, C. F., Kennedy, D. O., Milne, A. L., Wesnes, K. A., and Scholey, A. B. (2008). The effects of L-theanine, caffeine and their combination on cognition and mood. *Biol. Psychol.* 77, 113–122. doi: 10.1016/j.biopsycho.2007.09.008

Heim, C., Khan, M. A., Motsch, B., Gocht, A., Ramsperger-Gleixner, M., Stamminger, T., et al. (2017). microvascular integrity can be preserved by anti-platelet therapy and in combination with mTOR inhibitor. *J. Hear. Lung Transplant.* 36, S376. doi: 10.1016/j.healun.2017.01.1069

Hikino, H. (1985). Recent research on oriental medicinal plants. *Econ. Med. Plant. Res.* 1, 53–85.

Hoppe, J. B., Coradini, K., Frozza, R. L., Oliveira, C. M., Meneghetti, A. B., Bernardi, A., et al. (2013a). Free and nanoencapsulated curcumin suppress beta-amyloid-induced cognitive impairments in rats: involvement of BDNF and Akt/GSK-3beta signaling pathway. *Neurobiol. Learn. Mem.* 106, 134–144. doi: 10.1016/j.nlm.2013.08.001

Hoppe, J. B., Haag, M., Whalley, B. J., Salbego, C. G., and Cimarosti, H. (2013b). Curcumin protects organotypic hippocampal slice cultures from Abeta1-42-induced synaptic toxicity. *Toxicol. In Vitro* 27, 2325–2330. doi: 10.1016/j.tiv.2013.10.002

Howard, R. J., Juszczak, E., Ballard, C. G., Bentham, P., Brown, R. G., Bullock, R., et al. (2007). Donepezil for the treatment of agitation in Alzheimer's disease. *N. Engl. J. Med.* 357, 1382–1392. doi: 10.1056/NEJMoa066583

Howes, M.-J. R., and Houghton, P. J. (2003). Plants used in Chinese and Indian traditional medicine for improvement of memory and cognitive function. *Pharmacol. Biochem. Behav.* 75, 513–527. doi: 10.1016/S0091-3057(03)00128-X

Howes, M.-J. R., and Perry, E. (2011). The role of phytochemicals in the treatment and prevention of dementia. *Drugs Aging* 28, 439–468. doi: 10.2165/11591310-000000000-00000

Howes, M. R., Perry, N. S. L., and Houghton, P. J. (2003). Plants with traditional uses and activities, relevant to the management of Alzheimer's disease and other cognitive disorders. *Phyther. Res.* 17, 1–18. doi: 10.1002/ptr.1280

Huang, H.-C., Tang, D., Xu, K., and Jiang, Z.-F. (2014). Curcumin attenuates amyloid-beta-induced tau hyperphosphorylation in human neuroblastoma SH-SY5Y cells involving PTEN/Akt/GSK-3beta signaling pathway. *J. Recept. Signal Transduct. Res.* 34, 26–37. doi: 10.3109/10799893.2013.848891

Hügel, H. M., and Jackson, N. (2015). Polyphenols for the prevention and treatment of dementia diseases. *Neural Regen. Res.* 10, 1756–1758. doi: 10.4103/1673-5374.169609

Huminiecki, L., Horbanczuk, J., and Atanasov, A. G. (2017). The functional genomic studies of curcumin. *Semin. Cancer Biol.* 46, 107–118. doi: 10.1016/j.semcancer.2017.04.002

Hung, C. H.-L., Cheng, S. S.-Y., Cheung, Y.-T., Wuwongse, S., Zhang, N. Q., Ho, Y.-S., et al. (2018). A reciprocal relationship between reactive oxygen species and mitochondrial dynamics in neurodegeneration. *Redox Biol.* 14, 7–19. doi: 10.1016/j.redox.2017.08.010

Hurd, M. D., Martorell, P., and Langa, K. M. (2013). Monetary costs of dementia in the United States. *N. Engl. J. Med.* 369, 489–490. doi: 10.1056/NEJMc1305541

Iadecola, C. (2013). The pathobiology of vascular dementia. *Neuron* 80, 844–866. doi: 10.1016/j.neuron.2013.10.008

IARC Working Group (2016). *Some Drugs and Herbal Products.* Lyon: Ginkgo Biloba. International Agency for Research and Cancer (IARC) Monographs, WHO.

Ibrahim, F., Knight, S. R., and Cramer, R. L. (2012). Addressing the controversial use of antipsychotic drugs for behavioral and psychological symptoms of dementia. *J. Pharm. Technol.* 28, 3–9. doi: 10.1177/875512251202800102

Ihl, R., Tribanek, M., and Bachinskaya, N. (2012). Efficacy and tolerability of a once daily formulation of *Ginkgo biloba* extract EGb 761(R) in Alzheimer's disease and vascular dementia: results from a randomised controlled trial. *Pharmacopsychiatry* 45, 41–46. doi: 10.1055/s-0031-1291217

Ikarashi, Y., and Mizoguchi, K. (2016). Neuropharmacological efficacy of the traditional Japanese Kampo medicine yokukansan and its active ingredients. *Pharmacol. Ther.* 166, 84–95. doi: 10.1016/j.pharmthera.2016.06.018

Iqbal, K., Liu, F., and Gong, C.-X. (2016). Tau and neurodegenerative disease: the story so far. *Nat. Rev. Neurol.* 12, 15–27. doi: 10.1038/nrneurol.2015.225

Iqbal, K., Liu, F., Gong, C.-X., and Grundke-Iqbal, I. (2010). Tau in Alzheimer disease and related tauopathies. *Curr. Alzheimer Res.* 7, 656–664. doi: 10.2174/156720510793611592

Isah, T. (2015). Rethinking *Ginkgo biloba* L.: medicinal uses and conservation. *Pharmacogn. Rev.* 9, 140–148. doi: 10.4103/0973-7847.162137

Izzo, A. A. (2012). Interactions between herbs and conventional drugs: overview of the clinical data. *Med. Princ. Pract.* 21, 404–428. doi: 10.1159/000334488

Jahanshahi, M., Nickmahzar, E. G., and Babakordi, F. (2013). Effect of Gingko biloba extract on scopolamine-induced apoptosis in the hippocampus of rats. *Anat. Sci. Int.* 88, 217–222. doi: 10.1007/s12565-013-0188-8

Jahanshahi, M., Nikmahzar, E., Yadollahi, N., and Ramazani, K. (2012). Protective effects of *Ginkgo biloba* extract (EGB 761) on astrocytes of rat hippocampus after exposure with scopolamine. *Anat. Cell Biol.* 45, 92–96. doi: 10.5115/acb.2012.45.2.92

Jelenkovic, A., Jovanovic, M. D., Stevanovic, I., Petronijevic, N., Bokonjic, D., Zivkovic, J., et al. (2014). Influence of the green tea leaf extract on neurotoxicity of aluminium chloride in rats. *Phytother. Res.* 28, 82–87. doi: 10.1002/ptr.4962

Ju, H. S., Li, X. J., Zhao, B. L., Han, Z. W., and Xin, W. J. (1989). Effects of glycyrrhiza flavonoid on lipid peroxidation and active oxygen radicals. *Yao Xue Xue Bao* 24, 807–812.

Kanno, H., Kawakami, Z., Tabuchi, M., Mizoguchi, K., Ikarashi, Y., and Kase, Y. (2015). Protective effects of glycycoumarin and procyanidin B1, active components of traditional Japanese medicine yokukansan, on amyloid beta oligomer-induced neuronal death. *J. Ethnopharmacol.* 159, 122–128. doi: 10.1016/j.jep.2014.10.058

Kanowski, S., Herrmann, W. M., Stephan, K., Wierich, W., and Horr, R. (1996). Proof of efficacy of the *Ginkgo biloba* special extract EGb 761 in outpatients suffering from mild to moderate primary degenerative dementia of the Alzheimer type or multi-infarct dementia. *Pharmacopsychiatry* 29, 47–56. doi: 10.1055/s-2007-979544

Katsel, P., Tan, W., Fam, P., Purohit, D. P., and Haroutunian, V. (2013). Cell cycle checkpoint abnormalities during dementia: a plausible association with the loss of protection against oxidative stress in Alzheimer's disease [corrected]. *PLoS ONE* 8:e68361. doi: 10.1371/journal.pone.0068361

Kaur, U., Banerjee, P., Bir, A., Sinha, M., Biswas, A., and Chakrabarti, S. (2015). Reactive oxygen species, redox signaling and neuroinflammation in Alzheimer's disease: the NF-kappaB connection. *Curr. Top. Med. Chem.* 15, 446–457. doi: 10.2174/1568026615666150114160543

Kihara, T., and Shimohama, S. (2004). Alzheimer's disease and acetylcholine receptors. *Acta Neurobiol. Exp. (Wars).* 64, 99–105.

Kim, J. M., Ryou, S. H., Kang, Y. H., and Kang, J. S. (2011). Effect of *Ginkgo biloba* leaf powder and extract on plasma and liver lipids, platelet aggregation and erythrocyte Na+ efflux in rats fed hypercholesterolemic diet. *FASEB J.* 25, 980–988.

Kim, J., Shim, J., Lee, S., Cho, W.-H., Hong, E., Lee, J. H., et al. (2016). Rg3-enriched ginseng extract ameliorates scopolamine-induced learning deficits in mice. *BMC Complement. Altern. Med.* 16:66. doi: 10.1186/s12906-016-1050-z

Kim, M.-S., Lee, J.-I., Lee, W.-Y., and Kim, S.-E. (2004). Neuroprotective effect of *Ginkgo biloba* L. extract in a rat model of Parkinson's disease. *Phytother. Res.* 18, 663–666. doi: 10.1002/ptr.1486

Kim, T. I., Lee, Y. K., Park, S. G., Choi, I. S., Ban, J. O., Park, H. K., et al. (2009). l-Theanine, an amino acid in green tea, attenuates beta-amyloid-induced cognitive dysfunction and neurotoxicity: reduction in oxidative damage and inactivation of ERK/p38 kinase and NF-kappaB pathways. *Free Radic. Biol. Med.* 47, 1601–1610. doi: 10.1016/j.freeradbiomed.2009.09.008

Kim, Y. C., Kim, S. R., Markelonis, G. J., and Oh, T. H. (1998). Ginsenosides Rb1 and Rg3 protect cultured rat cortical cells from glutamate-induced neurodegeneration. *J. Neurosci. Res.* 53, 426–432.

Kimura, K., Ozeki, M., Juneja, L. R., and Ohira, H. (2007). L-Theanine reduces psychological and physiological stress responses. *Biol. Psychol.* 74, 39–45. doi: 10.1016/j.biopsycho.2006.06.006

Knapp, M., Prince, M., Albanese, E., Banerjee, S., Dhanasiri, S., and Fernandez, J. L. (2007). *Dementia UK: The Full Report.* London: Alzheimer's Society.

Koola, M. M., Buchanan, R. W., Pillai, A., Aitchison, K. J., Weinberger, D. R., Aaronson, S. T., et al. (2014). Potential role of the combination of galantamine and memantine to improve cognition in schizophrenia. *Schizophr. Res.* 157, 84–89. doi: 10.1016/j.schres.2014.04.037

Kumar, A., Prakash, A., and Pahwa, D. (2011). Galantamine potentiates the protective effect of rofecoxib and caffeic acid against intrahippocampal Kainic acid-induced cognitive dysfunction in rat. *Brain Res. Bull.* 85, 158–168. doi: 10.1016/j.brainresbull.2011.03.010

Kumar, A., and Singh, A. (2015). A review on mitochondrial restorative mechanism of antioxidants in Alzheimer's disease and other neurological conditions. *Front. Pharmacol.* 6:206. doi: 10.3389/fphar.2015.00206

LeBlanc, A. C. (2005). The role of apoptotic pathways in Alzheimer's disease neurodegeneration and cell death. *Curr. Alzheimer Res.* 2, 389–402. doi: 10.2174/156720505774330573

Lee, J., Kim, Y., Liu, T., Hwang, Y. J., Hyeon, S. J., Im, H., et al. (2017). SIRT3 deregulation is linked to mitochondrial dysfunction in Alzheimer's disease. *Aging Cell.* doi: 10.1111/acel.12679. [Epub ahead of print].

Lee, T.-K., Johnke, R. M., Allison, R. R., O'Brien, K. F., and Dobbs, L. J. J. (2005). Radioprotective potential of ginseng. *Mutagenesis* 20, 237–243. doi: 10.1093/mutage/gei041

Li, W., Chu, Y., Zhang, L., Yin, L., and Li, L. (2012). Ginsenoside Rg1 attenuates tau phosphorylation in SK-N-SH induced by Abeta-stimulated THP-1 supernatant and the involvement of p38 pathway activation. *Life Sci.* 91, 809–815. doi: 10.1016/j.lfs.2012.08.028

Lilienfeld, S. (2002). Galantamine–a novel cholinergic drug with a unique dual mode of action for the treatment of patients with Alzheimer's disease. *CNS Drug Rev.* 8, 159–176. doi: 10.1111/j.1527-3458.2002.tb00221.x

Lim, S. L., Rodriguez-Ortiz, C. J., and Kitazawa, M. (2015). Infection, systemic inflammation, and Alzheimer's disease. *Microbes Infect.* 17, 549–556. doi: 10.1016/j.micinf.2015.04.004

Lin, M. T., and Beal, M. F. (2006). Mitochondrial dysfunction and oxidative stress in neurodegenerative diseases. *Nature* 443, 787–795. doi: 10.1038/nature05292

Liu, C.-C., Liu, C.-C., Kanekiyo, T., Xu, H., and Bu, G. (2013). Apolipoprotein E and Alzheimer disease: risk, mechanisms and therapy. *Nat. Rev. Neurol.* 9, 106–118. doi: 10.1038/nrneurol.2012.263

Liu, X., Xu, K., Yan, M., Wang, Y., and Zheng, X. (2010). Protective effects of galantamine against Aβ-induced PC12 cell apoptosis by preventing mitochondrial dysfunction and endoplasmic reticulum stress. *Neurochem. Int.* 57, 588–599. doi: 10.1016/j.neuint.2010.07.007

Long, F., Yang, H., Xu, Y., Hao, H., and Li, P. (2015). A strategy for the identification of combinatorial bioactive compounds contributing to the holistic effect of herbal medicines. *Sci. Rep.* 5:12361. doi: 10.1038/srep12361

Lonicerus, A. (1679). *Kräuterbuch, Matthias Wagner*. Ulm.

Loy, C., and Schneider, L. (2006). Galantamine for Alzheimer's disease and mild cognitive impairment. *Cochrane database Syst. Rev.* 25:CD001747. doi: 10.1002/14651858.CD001747.pub3

Luengo-Fernandez, R., Leal, J., and Gray, A. (2010). *Dementia 2010: The Economic Burden of Dementia and Associated Research Funding in the United Kingdom*. Oxford: Cambridge Alzheimer's Research Trust.

Ma, B., Meng, X., Wang, J., Sun, J., Ren, X., Qin, M., et al. (2014). Notoginsenoside R1 attenuates amyloid-beta-induced damage in neurons by inhibiting reactive oxygen species and modulating MAPK activation. *Int. Immunopharmacol.* 22, 151–159. doi: 10.1016/j.intimp.2014.06.018

Mahley, R. W., and Rall, S. C. Jr. (2000). Apolipoprotein E: far more than a lipid transport protein. *Annu. Rev. Genomics Hum. Genet.* 1, 507–537. doi: 10.1146/annurev.genom.1.1.507

Mahmood, T., Akhtar, N., and Khan, B. A. (2010). The morphology, characteristics, and medicinal properties of Camellia sinensis tea. *J. Med. Plants Res.* 4, 2028–2033. doi: 10.5897/JMPR10.010

Mandel, S. A., Amit, T., Weinreb, O., and Youdim, M. B. H. (2011). Understanding the broad-spectrum neuroprotective action profile of green tea polyphenols in aging and neurodegenerative diseases. *J. Alzheimers. Dis.* 25, 187–208. doi: 10.3233/JAD-2011-101803

Mantle, D., Pickering, A. T., and Perry, E. K. (2000). Medicinal plant extracts for the treatment of dementia. *CNS Drugs* 13, 201–213. doi: 10.2165/00023210-200013030-00006

Manyam, B., V (1999). Dementia in ayurveda. *J. Altern. Complement. Med.* 5, 81–88. doi: 10.1089/acm.1999.5.81

McKhann, G. M., Albert, M. S., Grossman, M., Miller, B., Dickson, D., and Trojanowski, J. Q. (2001). Clinical and pathological diagnosis of frontotemporal dementia: report of the Work Group on Frontotemporal Dementia and Pick's Disease. *Arch. Neurol.* 58, 1803–1809. doi: 10.1001/archneur.58.11.1803

Mehan, S., Sharma, D., Sharma, G., Arora, R., and Sehgal, V. (2012). *Dementia-A Complete Literature Review on Various Mechanisms Involves in Pathogenesis and an Intracerebroventricular Streptozotocin Induced Alzheimer's Disease*. INTECH Open Access Publisher. Available online at: http://www.intechopen.com/books/inflammatory-diseases-immunopathology-clinical-and-pharmacologicalbases/alzheimer-s-disease-an-updated-review-on-pathogenesis-and-intracerebroventricular-streptozotocin-ind

Miao, Y., Zhao, S., Gao, Y., Wang, R., Wu, Q., Wu, H., et al. (2016). Curcumin pretreatment attenuates inflammation and mitochondrial dysfunction in experimental stroke: the possible role of Sirt1 signaling. *Brain Res. Bull.* 121, 9–15. doi: 10.1016/j.brainresbull.2015.11.019

Mills, S. Y. (1991). *Out of the Earth: The Essential Book of Herbal Medicine*. London: Viking.

Mishra, S., and Palanivelu, K. (2008). The effect of curcumin (turmeric) on Alzheimer's disease: an overview. *Ann. Indian Acad. Neurol.* 11, 13–19. doi: 10.4103/0972-2327.40220

Misra, R. (1998). Modern drug development from traditional medicinal plants using radioligand receptor-binding assays. *Med. Res. Rev.* 18, 383–402.

Monsch, A. U., and Giannakopoulos, P. (2004). Effects of galantamine on behavioural and psychological disturbances and caregiver burden in patients with Alzheimer's disease. *Curr. Med. Res. Opin.* 20, 931–938. doi: 10.1185/030079904125003890

Moreira, P. I., Carvalho, C., Zhu, X., Smith, M. A., and Perry, G. (2010). Mitochondrial dysfunction is a trigger of Alzheimer's disease pathophysiology. *Biochim. Biophys. Acta* 1802, 2–10. doi: 10.1016/j.bbadis.2009.10.006

Müller-Ebeling, C., and Rätsch, C. (1989). *Heilpflanzen der Seychellen. VWB-Verlag für Wissenschaft und Bildung*. Berlin.

Nah, S.-Y. (2014). Ginseng ginsenoside pharmacology in the nervous system: involvement in the regulation of ion channels and receptors. *Front. Physiol.* 5:98. doi: 10.3389/fphys.2014.00098

Namanja, H. A., Emmert, D., Pires, M. M., Hrycyna, C. A., and Chmielewski, J. (2009). Inhibition of human P-glycoprotein transport and substrate binding using a galantamine dimer. *Biochem. Biophys. Res. Commun.* 388, 672–676. doi: 10.1016/j.bbrc.2009.08.056

Napryeyenko, O., Sonnik, G., and Tartakovsky, I. (2009). Efficacy and tolerability of *Ginkgo biloba* extract EGb 761 by type of dementia: analyses of a randomised controlled trial. *J. Neurol. Sci.* 283, 224–229. doi: 10.1016/j.jns.2009.02.353

Narlawar, R., Pickhardt, M., Leuchtenberger, S., Baumann, K., Krause, S., Dyrks, T., et al. (2008). Curcumin-derived pyrazoles and isoxazoles: swiss army knives or blunt tools for Alzheimer's disease? *ChemMedChem* 3, 165–172. doi: 10.1002/cmdc.200700218

Navia, B. A., and Rostasy, K. (2005). The AIDS dementia complex: clinical and basic neuroscience with implications for novel molecular therapies. *Neurotox. Res.* 8, 3–24. doi: 10.1007/BF03033817

Ng, T.-P., Chiam, P.-C., Lee, T., Chua, H.-C., Lim, L., and Kua, E.-H. (2006). Curry consumption and cognitive function in the elderly. *Am. J. Epidemiol.* 164, 898–906. doi: 10.1093/aje/kwj267

Ng, Y. P., Or, T. C. T., and Ip, N. Y. (2015). Plant alkaloids as drug leads for Alzheimer's disease. *Neurochem. Int.* 89, 260–270. doi: 10.1016/j.neuint.2015.07.018

Ngan, F., Shaw, P., But, P., and Wang, J. (1999). Molecular authentication of Panax species. *Phytochemistry* 50, 787–791. doi: 10.1016/S0031-9422(98)00606-2

Niikura, T., Tajima, H., and Kita, Y. (2006). Neuronal cell death in Alzheimer's disease and a neuroprotective factor, humanin. *Curr. Neuropharmacol.* 4, 139–147. doi: 10.2174/157015906776359577

Nimmrich, V., and Eckert, A. (2013). Calcium channel blockers and dementia. *Br. J. Pharmacol.* 169, 1203–1210. doi: 10.1111/bph.12240

Nishida, K., Yasuda, E., Nagasawa, K., and Fujimoto, S. (2008). Altered levels of oxidation and phospholipase C isozyme expression in the brains of theanine-administered rats. *Biol. Pharm. Bull.* 31, 857–860. doi: 10.1248/bpb.31.857

Nishiyama, N., Chu, P. J., and Saito, H. (1995). Beneficial effects of Biota, a traditional Chinese herbal medicine on learning impairment induced by basal forebrain-lesion in mice. *Biol. Pharm. Bull.* 28, 1513–1517.

Olin, J., and Schneider, L. (2002). Galantamine for Alzheimer's disease. *Cochrane database Syst. Rev.* 3:CD001747. doi: 10.1002/14651858.CD001747

Ortiz de Montellano, B. R. (1990). *Aztec Medicine, Health and Nutrition*. New Brunswick: Rutgers University Press.

Owen, G. N., Parnell, H., De Bruin, E. A., and Rycroft, J. A. (2008). The combined effects of L-theanine and caffeine on cognitive performance and mood. *Nutr. Neurosci.* 11, 193–198. doi: 10.1179/147683008X301513

Paganelli, R. A., Benetoli, A., and Milani, H. (2006). Sustained neuroprotection and facilitation of behavioral recovery by the *Ginkgo biloba* extract, EGb 761, after transient forebrain ischemia in rats. *Behav. Brain Res.* 174, 70–77. doi: 10.1016/j.bbr.2006.07.005

Parle, M., Dhingra, D., and Kulkarni, S. K. (2004). Memory-strengthening activity of Glycyrrhiza glabra in exteroceptive and interoceptive behavioral models. *J. Med. Food* 7, 462–466. doi: 10.1089/jmf.2004.7.462

Pasqualetti, G., Brooks, D. J., and Edison, P. (2015). The role of neuroinflammation in dementias. *Curr. Neurol. Neurosci. Rep.* 15:17. doi: 10.1007/s11910-015-0531-7

Pastor, P., Roe, C. M., Villegas, A., Bedoya, G., Chakraverty, S., Garcia, G., et al. (2003). Apolipoprotein Eepsilon4 modifies Alzheimer's disease onset in an E280A PS1 kindred. *Ann. Neurol.* 54, 163–169. doi: 10.1002/ana.10636

Pathak, L., Agrawal, Y., and Dhir, A. (2013). Natural polyphenols in the management of major depression. *Expert Opin. Investig. Drugs* 22, 863–880. doi: 10.1517/13543784.2013.794783

Perry, E., and Howes, M. R. (2011). Medicinal plants and dementia therapy: herbal hopes for brain aging? *CNS Neurosci. Ther.* 17, 683–698. doi: 10.1111/j.1755-5949.2010.00202.x

Perry, E. K., Pickering, A. T., Wang, W. W., Houghton, P., and Perry, N. S. L. (1998). Medicinal plants and Alzheimer's disease: integrating ethnobotanical and contemporary scientific evidence. *J. Altern. Complement. Med.* 4, 419–428.

Pohl, S., Zobel, J., and Moffat, A. (2010). "Extended boolean retrieval for systematic biomedical reviews," in *Proceedings of the Thirty-Third Australasian Conferenc on Computer Science - Volume 102* ACSC'10. (Darlinghurst, NSW: Australian Computer Society, Inc.), 117–126. Available online at: http://dl.acm.org/citation.cfm?id=1862199.1862212

Popovich, D. G., and Kitts, D. D. (2004). Generation of ginsenosides Rg3 and Rh2 from North American ginseng. *Phytochemistry* 65, 337–344. doi: 10.1016/j.phytochem.2003.11.020

Power, M. C., Adar, S. D., Yanosky, J. D., and Weuve, J. (2016). Exposure to air pollution as a potential contributor to cognitive function, cognitive decline, brain imaging, and dementia: a systematic review of epidemiologic research. *Neurotoxicology* 56, 235–253. doi: 10.1016/j.neuro.2016.06.004

Price, S., and Price, L. (1995). *Aromatherapy for Health Professionals*. Edinburgh: Churchill Livingston.

Prince, M., Comas-Herrera, A., Knapp, M., Guerchet, M., and Karagiannidou, M. (2016). *World Alzheimer Report 2016: Improving Healthcare for People Living with Dementia: Coverage, Quality and Costs Now and in the Future*. London: Personal Social Services Research Unit; London School of Economics and Political Science.

Qiao, X., Ji, S., Yu, S.-W., Lin, X.-H., Jin, H.-W., Duan, Y.-K., et al. (2014). Identification of key licorice constituents which interact with cytochrome P450: evaluation by LC/MS/MS cocktail assay and metabolic profiling. *AAPS J.* 16, 101–113. doi: 10.1208/s12248-013-9544-9

Qiu, C., Kivipelto, M., and von Strauss, E. (2009). Epidemiology of Alzheimer's disease: occurrence, determinants, and strategies toward intervention. *Dialogues Clin. Neurosci.* 11, 111–128.

Quaglio, G., Brand, H., and Dario, C. (2016). Fighting dementia in Europe: the time to act is now. *Lancet Neurol.* 15, 452–454. doi: 10.1016/S1474-4422(16)00079-X

Rabinovici, G. D., and Miller, B. L. (2010). Frontotemporal lobar degeneration: epidemiology, pathophysiology, diagnosis and management. *CNS Drugs* 24, 375–398. doi: 10.2165/11533100-000000000-00000

Raina, A. K., Zhu, X., Rottkamp, C. A., Monteiro, M., Takeda, A., and Smith, M. A. (2000). Cyclin' toward dementia: cell cycle abnormalities and abortive oncogenesis in Alzheimer disease. *J. Neurosci. Res.* 61, 128–133. doi: 10.1002/1097-4547(20000715)61:2<128::AID-JNR2>3.0.CO;2-H

Ramkumar, M., Rajasankar, S., Gobi, V. V., Dhanalakshmi, C., Manivasagam, T., Justin Thenmozhi, A., et al. (2017). Neuroprotective effect of Demethoxycurcumin, a natural derivative of Curcumin on rotenone induced neurotoxicity in SH-SY 5Y Neuroblastoma cells. *BMC Complement. Altern. Med.* 17, 217. doi: 10.1186/s12906-017-1720-5

Rastogi, M., Ojha, R. P., Sagar, C., Agrawal, A., and Dubey, G. P. (2014). Protective effect of curcuminoids on age-related mitochondrial impairment in female Wistar rat brain. *Biogerontology* 15, 21–31. doi: 10.1007/s10522-013-9466-z

Reddy, A. P., and Reddy, P. H. (2017). mitochondria-targeted molecules as potential drugs to treat patients with Alzheimer's disease. *Prog. Mol. Biol. Transl. Sci.* 146, 173–201. doi: 10.1016/bs.pmbts.2016.12.010

Rezai-Zadeh, K., Arendash, G. W., Hou, H., Fernandez, F., Jensen, M., Runfeldt, M., et al. (2008). Green tea epigallocatechin-3-gallate (EGCG) reduces beta-amyloid mediated cognitive impairment and modulates tau pathology in Alzheimer transgenic mice. *Brain Res.* 1214, 177–187. doi: 10.1016/j.brainres.2008.02.107

Rhein, V., Giese, M., Baysang, G., Meier, F., Rao, S., Schulz, K. L., et al. (2010). *Ginkgo biloba* extract ameliorates oxidative phosphorylation performance and rescues abeta-induced failure. *PLoS ONE* 5:e12359. doi: 10.1371/journal.pone.0012359

Ribeiro, M. L., Moreira, L. M., Arcari, D. P., Dos Santos, L. F., Marques, A. C., Pedrazzoli, J. J., et al. (2016). Protective effects of chronic treatment with a standardized extract of *Ginkgo biloba* L. in the prefrontal cortex and dorsal hippocampus of middle-aged rats. *Behav. Brain Res.* 313, 144–150. doi: 10.1016/j.bbr.2016.06.029

Ridley, N. J., Draper, B., and Withall, A. (2013). Alcohol-related dementia: an update of the evidence. *Alzheimers. Res. Ther.* 5, 3. doi: 10.1186/alzrt157

Rivas-Arancibia, S., Hernández-Zimbrón, L. F., Rodríguez-Martínez, E., Borgonio-Pérez, G., Velumani, V., and Durán-Bedolla, J. (2013). Chronic exposure to low doses of ozone produces a state of oxidative stress and blood-brain barrier damage in the hippocampus of rat. *Adv. Biosci. Biotechnol.* 4:24. doi: 10.4236/abb.2013.411A2004

Roeder, B.A. (1988). *Chicano Folk Medicine from Los Angeles*. Berkeley; Los Angeles: CA: University of California Press.

Romero, A., Egea, J., Garcia, A. G., and Lopez, M. G. (2010). Synergistic neuroprotective effect of combined low concentrations of galantamine and melatonin against oxidative stress in SH-SY5Y neuroblastoma cells. *J. Pineal Res.* 49, 141–148. doi: 10.1111/j.1600-079X.2010.00778.x

Ross, I. A. (2001). *Medicinal Plants of the World: Chemical Constituents, Traditional and Modern Medicinal Uses*. New York, NY: Humana Press.

Ruttkay-Nedecky, B., Nejdl, L., Gumulec, J., Zitka, O., Masarik, M., Eckschlager, T., et al. (2013). The role of metallothionein in oxidative stress. *Int. J. Mol. Sci.* 14, 6044–6066. doi: 10.3390/ijms14036044

Saharan, S., and Mandal, P. K. (2014). The emerging role of glutathione in Alzheimer's disease. *J. Alzheimers. Dis.* 40, 519–529. doi: 10.3233/JAD-132483

Sahne, F., Mohammadi, M., Najafpour, G. D., and Moghadamnia, A. A. (2017). Enzyme-assisted ionic liquid extraction of bioactive compound from turmeric (*Curcuma longa* L.): isolation, purification and analysis of curcumin. *Ind. Crops Prod.* 95, 686–694. doi: 10.1016/j.indcrop.2016.11.037

Sama, D. M., and Norris, C. M. (2013). Calcium dysregulation and neuroinflammation: discrete and integrated mechanisms for age-related synaptic dysfunction. *Ageing Res. Rev.* 12, 982–995. doi: 10.1016/j.arr.2013.05.008

Savelev, S. U., Okello, E. J., and Perry, E. K. (2004). Butyryl-and acetyl-cholinesterase inhibitory activities in essential oils of Salvia species and their constituents. *Phyther. Res.* 18, 315–324. doi: 10.1002/ptr.1451

Schultes, R. E. (1993). Plants in treating senile dementia in the Northwest Amazon. *J. Ethnopharmacol.* 38, 121–128. doi: 10.1016/0378-8741(93)90007-R

Schultes, R. E. (1994). *Amazonian Ethnobotany and the Search for New Drugs BT - Ciba Foundation Symposium 185*. Chichester: Wiley.

Schulz, R., McGinnis, K. A., Zhang, S., Martire, L. M., Hebert, R. S., Beach, S. R., et al. (2008). Dementia patient suffering and caregiver depression. *Alzheimer Dis. Assoc. Disord.* 22, 170–176. doi: 10.1097/WAD.0b013e31816653cc

Schwarzkopf, T. M., Koch, K. A., and Klein, J. (2013). Neurodegeneration after transient brain ischemia in aged mice: beneficial effects of bilobalide. *Brain Res.* 1529, 178–187. doi: 10.1016/j.brainres.2013.07.003

Schweitzer de Palacios, D. (1994). *Cambiashun. Las prácticas médicas tradicionales y sus expertos en San Miguel del Común, una comuna indígena en los alrededores de Quito*. Berlin: Holos-Verlag; Free University of Berlin.

Sfikas, G. (1980). *Heilpflanzen Griechenlands. P. Efstathiadis & Söhne AG*. Athen.

Shankar, G. M., and Walsh, D. M. (2009). Alzheimer's disease: synaptic dysfunction and Aβ. *Mol. Neurodegener.* 4:48. doi: 10.1186/1750-1326-4-48

Sirirugsa, P., Larsen, K., and Maknoi, C. (2007). The genus *Curcuma* L.(zingiberaceae): distribution and classification with reference to species diversity in Thailand. *Gard. Bull. Singapore* 59, 203–320.

Solfrizzi, V., and Panza, F. (2015). Plant-based nutraceutical interventions against cognitive impairment and dementia: meta-analytic evidence of efficacy of a standardized Gingko biloba extract. *J. Alzheimers. Dis.* 43, 605–611. doi: 10.3233/JAD-141887

Song, L., Xu, M.-B., Zhou, X.-L., Zhang, D.-P., Zhang, S.-L., and Zheng, G.-Q. (2017). A Preclinical systematic review of ginsenoside-Rg1 in experimental Parkinson's disease. *Oxid. Med. Cell. Longev.* 2017:2163053. doi: 10.1155/2017/2163053

Spano, M., Signorelli, M., Vitaliani, R., Aguglia, E., and Giometto, B. (2015). The possible involvement of mitochondrial dysfunctions in

Lewy body dementia: a systematic review. *Funct. Neurol.* 30, 151–158. doi: 10.11138/FNeur/2015.30.3.151

Stackman, R. W., Eckenstein, F., Frei, B., Kulhanek, D., Nowlin, J., and Quinn, J. F. (2003). Prevention of age-related spatial memory deficits in a transgenic mouse model of Alzheimer's disease by chronic *Ginkgo biloba* treatment. *Exp. Neurol.* 184, 510–520. doi: 10.1016/S0014-4886(03)00399-6

Stafford, G. I., Pedersen, M. E., van Staden, J., and Jäger, A. K. (2008). Review on plants with CNS-effects used in traditional South African medicine against mental diseases. *J. Ethnopharmacol.* 119, 513–537. doi: 10.1016/j.jep.2008.08.010

Sun, M., Ye, Y., Xiao, L., Duan, X., Zhang, Y., and Zhang, H. (2017). Anticancer effects of ginsenoside Rg3 (Review). *Int. J. Mol. Med.* 39, 507–518. doi: 10.3892/ijmm.2017.2857

Sun, S., Wang, C.-Z., Tong, R., Li, X.-L., Fishbein, A., Wang, Q., et al. (2010). Effects of steaming the root of Panax notoginseng on chemical composition and anticancer activities. *Food Chem.* 118, 307–314. doi: 10.1016/j.foodchem.2009.04.122

Sun, Z.-K., Yang, H.-Q., and Chen, S.-D. (2013). Traditional Chinese medicine: a promising candidate for the treatment of Alzheimer's disease. *Transl. Neurodegener.* 2:6. doi: 10.1186/2047-9158-2-6

Swerdlow, R. H., Burns, J. M., and Khan, S. M. (2010). The Alzheimer's disease mitochondrial cascade hypothesis. *J. Alzheimers. Dis.* 20(Suppl. 2), S265–S279. doi: 10.3233/JAD-2010-100339

Swerdlow, R. H., Koppel, S., Weidling, I., Hayley, C., Ji, Y., and Wilkins, H. M. (2017). mitochondria, cybrids, aging, and Alzheimer's disease. *Prog. Mol. Biol. Transl. Sci.* 146, 259–302. doi: 10.1016/bs.pmbts.2016.12.017

Tabernaemontanus, D. I. T. (1987). *Kräuterbuch, Johann Ludwig König/Johann Brandmüller.* Basel.

Takuma, K., Hoshina, Y., Arai, S., Himeno, Y., Matsuo, A., Funatsu, Y., et al. (2007). *Ginkgo biloba* extract EGb 761 attenuates hippocampal neuronal loss and cognitive dysfunction resulting from chronic restraint stress in ovariectomized rats. *Neuroscience* 149, 256–262. doi: 10.1016/j.neuroscience.2007.07.042

Tanaka, A., Arai, Y., Kim, S.-N., Ham, J., and Usuki, T. (2011). Synthesis and biological evaluation of bilobol and adipostatin A. *J. Asian Nat. Prod. Res.* 13, 290–296. doi: 10.1080/10286020.2011.554828

Taylor, L. (1998). *Herbal Secrets of the Rainforest: The Healing Power of over 50 Medicinal Plants You Should Know About.* Rocklin, CA: Prima Publishing.

Tayyem, R. F., Heath, D. D., Al-Delaimy, W. K., and Rock, C. L. (2006). Curcumin content of turmeric and curry powders. *Nutr. Cancer* 55, 126–131. doi: 10.1207/s15327914nc5502_2

Tewari, D., Mocan, A., Parvanov, E. D., Sah, A. N., Nabavi, S. M., Huminiecki, L., et al. (2017). Ethnopharmacological approaches for therapy of jaundice: Part II. Highly used plant species from Acanthaceae, Euphorbiaceae, Asteraceae, Combretaceae, and Fabaceae families. *Front. Pharmacol.* 8:519. doi: 10.3389/fphar.2017.00518

Tian, J., Zhang, S., Li, G., Liu, Z., and Xu, B. (2009). 20(S)-ginsenoside Rg3, a neuroprotective agent, inhibits mitochondrial permeability transition pores in rat brain. *Phytother. Res.* 23, 486–491. doi: 10.1002/ptr.2653

Tripathi, M., and Vibha, D. (2009). Reversible dementias. *Indian J. Psychiatry* 51, S52.

Tsvetkova, D., Obreshkova, D., Zheleva-Dimitrova, D., and Saso, L. (2013). Antioxidant activity of galantamine and some of its derivatives. *Curr. Med. Chem.* 20, 4595–4608. doi: 10.2174/09298673113209990148

Tzvetkov, N. T., and Antonov, L. (2017). Subnanomolar indazole-5-carboxamide inhibitors of monoamine oxidase B (MAO-B) continued: indications of iron binding, experimental evidence for optimised solubility and brain penetration. *J. Enzyme Inhib. Med. Chem.* 32, 960–967. doi: 10.1080/14756366.2017.1344980

van Horssen, J., van Schaik, P., and Witte, M. (2017). Inflammation and mitochondrial dysfunction: a vicious circle in neurodegenerative disorders? *Neurosci. Lett.* doi: 10.1016/j.neulet.2017.06.050. [Epub ahead of print].

Waldemar, G., Dubois, B., Emre, M., Georges, J., McKeith, I. G., Rossor, M., et al. (2007). Recommendations for the diagnosis and management of Alzheimer's disease and other disorders associated with dementia: EFNS guideline. *Eur. J. Neurol.* 14, e1–e26. doi: 10.1111/j.1468-1331.2006.01605.x

Walsh, C., Barrow, S., Voronina, S., Chvanov, M., Petersen, O. H., and Tepikin, A. (2009). Modulation of calcium signalling by mitochondria. *Biochim. Biophys. Acta* 1787, 1374–1382. doi: 10.1016/j.bbabio.2009.01.007

Waltenberger, B., Mocan, A., Smejkal, K., Heiss, E. H., and Atanasov, A. G. (2016). Natural Products to counteract the epidemic of cardiovascular and metabolic disorders. *Molecules* 21, 1–33. doi: 10.3390/molecules21060807

Wan, W., Cao, L., Liu, L., Kalionis, B., Chen, C., Tai, X., et al. (2014). EGb761 provides a protective effect against Aβ(1-42) oligomer-induced cell damage and blood-brain barrier disruption in an *in vitro* bEnd.3 endothelial model. *PLoS ONE* 9:e113126. doi: 10.1371/journal.pone.0113126

Wang, C., and Wang, B. (2016). *Ginkgo biloba* extract attenuates oxidative stress and apoptosis in mouse cochlear neural stem cells. *Phytother. Res.* 30, 774–780. doi: 10.1002/ptr.5572

Wang, C., and Youle, R. J. (2009). The Role of Mitochondria in Apoptosis. *Annu. Rev. Genet.* 43, 95–118. doi: 10.1146/annurev-genet-102108-134850

Wang, D.-S., Dickson, D. W., and Malter, J. S. (2006). beta-Amyloid degradation and Alzheimer's disease. *J. Biomed. Biotechnol.* 2006:58406. doi: 10.1155/JBB/2006/58406

Wang, P., Su, C., Li, R., Wang, H., Ren, Y., Sun, H., et al. (2014). Mechanisms and effects of curcumin on spatial learning and memory improvement in APPswe/PS1dE9 mice. *J. Neurosci. Res.* 92, 218–231. doi: 10.1002/jnr.23322

Wang, Y.-H., and Du, G.-H. (2009). Ginsenoside Rg1 inhibits beta-secretase activity *in vitro* and protects against Abeta-induced cytotoxicity in PC12 cells. *J. Asian Nat. Prod. Res.* 11, 604–612. doi: 10.1080/10286020902843152

Wang, Y., Huang, L., Tang, X., and Zhang, H. (2010). Retrospect and prospect of active principles from Chinese herbs in the treatment of dementia. *Acta Pharmacol. Sin.* 31, 649–664. doi: 10.1038/aps.2010.46

Wang, Y., Yang, G., Gong, J., Lu, F., Diao, Q., Sun, J., et al. (2016). Ginseng for Alzheimer's disease: a systematic review and meta-analysis of randomized controlled trials. *Curr. Top. Med. Chem.* 16, 529–536. doi: 10.2174/1568026615666150813143753

Weksler, M. E., Szabo, P., Relkin, N. R., Reidenberg, M. M., Weksler, B. B., and Coppus, A. M. W. (2013). Alzheimer's disease and Down's syndrome: treating two paths to dementia. *Autoimmun. Rev.* 12, 670–673. doi: 10.1016/j.autrev.2012.10.013

Winblad, B., Amouyel, P., Andrieu, S., Ballard, C., Brayne, C., Brodaty, H., et al. (2016). Defeating Alzheimer's disease and other dementias: a priority for European science and society. *Lancet Neurol.* 15, 455. doi: 10.1016/S1474-4422(16)00062-4

Wolters, B. (1994). *Drogen, Pfeilgift und Indianermedizin: Arzneipflanzen aus Südamerika.* Greifenberg: Urs Freud Verlag GmbH.

Xiong, Z., Hongmei, Z., Lu, S., and Yu, L. (2011). Curcumin mediates presenilin-1 activity to reduce beta-amyloid production in a model of Alzheimer's Disease. *Pharmacol. Rep.* 63, 1101–1108. doi: 10.1016/S1734-1140(11)70629-6

Yamada, T., Terashima, T., Honma, H., Nagata, S., Okubo, T., Juneja, L. R., et al. (2008). Effects of theanine, a unique amino acid in tea leaves, on memory in a rat behavioral test. *Biosci. Biotechnol. Biochem.* 72, 1356–1359. doi: 10.1271/bbb.70669

Yan, D., Zhang, Y., Liu, L., and Yan, H. (2016). Pesticide exposure and risk of Alzheimer's disease: a systematic review and meta-analysis. *Sci. Rep.* 6:32222. doi: 10.1038/srep32222

Yan, F.-L., Zheng, Y., and Zhao, F.-D. (2008). Effects of *Ginkgo biloba* extract EGb761 on expression of RAGE and LRP-1 in cerebral microvascular endothelial cells under chronic hypoxia and hypoglycemia. *Acta Neuropathol.* 116, 529–535. doi: 10.1007/s00401-008-0435-6

Yan, J., Hu, J., Liu, A., He, L., Li, X., and Wei, H. (2017). Design, synthesis, and evaluation of multitarget-directed ligands against Alzheimer's disease based on the fusion of donepezil and curcumin. *Bioorg. Med. Chem.* 25, 2946–2955. doi: 10.1016/j.bmc.2017.02.048

Yanagisawa, D., Taguchi, H., Yamamoto, A., Shirai, N., Hirao, K., and Tooyama, I. (2011). Curcuminoid binds to amyloid-beta1-42 oligomer and fibril. *J. Alzheimers. Dis.* 24(Suppl. 2), 33–42. doi: 10.3233/JAD-2011-102100

Yang, E.-J., Min, J. S., Ku, H.-Y., Choi, H.-S., Park, M., Kim, M. K., et al. (2012). Isoliquiritigenin isolated from Glycyrrhiza uralensis protects neuronal cells against glutamate-induced mitochondrial dysfunction. *Biochem. Biophys. Res. Commun.* 421, 658–664. doi: 10.1016/j.bbrc.2012.04.053

Yang, L., Hao, J., Zhang, J., Xia, W., Dong, X., Hu, X., et al. (2009). Ginsenoside Rg3 promotes beta-amyloid peptide degradation by enhancing gene expression of neprilysin. *J. Pharm. Pharmacol.* 61, 375–380. doi: 10.1211/jpp.61.03.0013

Ye, J., and Zhang, Y. (2012). Curcumin protects against intracellular amyloid toxicity in rat primary neurons. *Int. J. Clin. Exp. Med.* 5, 44–49.

Ye, R., Zhang, X., Kong, X., Han, J., Yang, Q., Zhang, Y., et al. (2011). Ginsenoside Rd attenuates mitochondrial dysfunction and sequential apoptosis after transient focal ischemia. *Neuroscience* 178, 169–180. doi: 10.1016/j.neuroscience.2011.01.007

Yim, S. B., Park, S. E., and Lee, C. S. (2007). Protective effect of glycyrrhizin on 1-methyl-4-phenylpyridinium-induced mitochondrial damage and cell death in differentiated PC12 cells. *J. Pharmacol. Exp. Ther.* 321, 816–822. doi: 10.1124/jpet.107.119602

Yin, S. Y., Kim, H. J., and Kim, H.-J. (2013). A comparative study of the effects of whole red ginseng extract and polysaccharide and saponin fractions on influenza A (H1N1) virus infection. *Biol. Pharm. Bull.* 36, 1002–1007. doi: 10.1248/bpb.b13-00123

Yokota, T., Nishio, H., Kubota, Y., and Mizoguchi, M. (1998). The inhibitory effect of glabridin from licorice extracts on melanogenesis and inflammation. *Pigment cell Res.* 11, 355–361. doi: 10.1111/j.1600-0749.1998.tb00494.x

Yun, T. K. (2001). Brief introduction of Panax ginseng C.A. Meyer. *J. Korean Med. Sci.* 16(Suppl.) S3–S5. doi: 10.3346/jkms.2001.16.S.S3

Zhang, L., Fang, Y., Xu, Y., Lian, Y., Xie, N., Wu, T., et al. (2015). Curcumin improves amyloid beta-peptide (1-42) induced spatial memory deficits through BDNF-ERK signaling pathway. *PLoS ONE* 10:e0131525. doi: 10.1371/journal.pone.0131525

Zhang, L., Fiala, M., Cashman, J., Sayre, J., Espinosa, A., Mahanian, M., et al. (2006). Curcuminoids enhance amyloid-beta uptake by macrophages of Alzheimer's disease patients. *J. Alzheimers. Dis.* 10, 1–7. doi: 10.3233/JAD-2006-10101

Zhou, J.-S., Wang, J.-F., He, B.-R., Cui, Y.-S., Fang, X.-Y., Ni, J.-L., et al. (2014). Ginsenoside Rd attenuates mitochondrial permeability transition and cytochrome c release in isolated spinal cord mitochondria: involvement of kinase-mediated pathways. *Int. J. Mol. Sci.* 15, 9859–9877. doi: 10.3390/ijms15069859

Zhou, S., Lim, L. Y., and Chowbay, B. (2004). Herbal modulation of P-glycoprotein. *Drug Metab. Rev.* 36, 57–104. doi: 10.1081/DMR-120028427

Zhou, X., Cui, G., Tseng, H. H. L., Lee, S. M.-Y., Leung, G. P. H., Chan, S. W., et al. (2016a). Vascular contributions to cognitive impairment and treatments with traditional chinese medicine. *Evid. Based. Complement. Alternat. Med.* 2016, 9627258. doi: 10.1155/2016/9627258

Zhou, X., Seto, S. W., Chang, D., Kiat, H., Razmovski-Naumovski, V., Chan, K., et al. (2016b). Synergistic effects of chinese herbal medicine: a comprehensive review of methodology and current research. *Front. Pharmacol.* 7:201. doi: 10.3389/fphar.2016.00201

Zhou, X., Wang, H.-Y., Wu, B., Cheng, C.-Y., Xiao, W., Wang, Z.-Z., et al. (2017). Ginkgolide K attenuates neuronal injury after ischemic stroke by inhibiting mitochondrial fission and GSK-3beta-dependent increases in mitochondrial membrane permeability. *Oncotarget* 8, 44682–44693. doi: 10.18632/oncotarget.17967

Zhu, X., Chen, C., Ye, D., Guan, D., Ye, L., Jin, J., et al. (2012). Diammonium glycyrrhizinate upregulates PGC-1α and protects against Aβ 1–42-induced neurotoxicity. *PLoS ONE* 7:e35823. doi: 10.1371/journal.pone.0035823

Zhu, X., Perry, G., Smith, M. A., and Wang, X. (2013). Abnormal mitochondrial dynamics in the pathogenesis of Alzheimer's disease. *J. Alzheimers. Dis.* 33(Suppl. 1), S253–S262. doi: 10.3233/JAD-2012-129005

Zlokovic, B., V (2011). Neurovascular pathways to neurodegeneration in Alzheimer's disease and other disorders. *Nat. Rev. Neurosci.* 12, 723–738. doi: 10.1038/nrn3114

Zupancic, M., Mahajan, A., and Handa, K. (2011). Dementia with lewy bodies: diagnosis and management for primary care providers. *Prim. Care Companion CNS Disord.* 13:PCC.11r01190.

11

Application of Ferulic Acid for Alzheimer's Disease: Combination of Text Mining and Experimental Validation

Guilin Meng [1,2†], Xiulin Meng [3†], Xiaoye Ma [1], Gengping Zhang [4], Xiaolin Hu [5], Aiping Jin [1], Yanxin Zhao [1] and Xueyuan Liu [1*]*

[1]Shanghai Tenth People's Hospital, Tongji University School of Medicine, Shanghai, China, [2]School of Computer Science and Informatics, Indiana University, Bloomington, IN, United States, [3]Houma People's Hospital, Linfen, China, [4]Library of Tongji University, Shanghai, China, [5]School of Life Sciences, Tsinghua University, Beijing, China

***Correspondence:**
Yanxin Zhao
287594350@qq.com
Xueyuan Liu
1510922@tongji.edu.cn

†Co-first authors.

Alzheimer's disease (AD) is an increasing concern in human health. Despite significant research, highly effective drugs to treat AD are lacking. The present study describes the text mining process to identify drug candidates from a traditional Chinese medicine (TCM) database, along with associated protein target mechanisms. We carried out text mining to identify literatures that referenced both AD and TCM and focused on identifying compounds and protein targets of interest. After targeting one potential TCM candidate, corresponding protein-protein interaction (PPI) networks were assembled in STRING to decipher the most possible mechanism of action. This was followed by validation using Western blot and co-immunoprecipitation in an AD cell model. The text mining strategy using a vast amount of AD-related literature and the TCM database identified curcumin, whose major component was ferulic acid (FA). This was used as a key candidate compound for further study. Using the top calculated interaction score in STRING, BACE1 and MMP2 were implicated in the activity of FA in AD. Exposure of SHSY5Y-APP cells to FA resulted in the decrease in expression levels of BACE-1 and APP, while the expression of MMP-2 and MMP-9 increased in a dose-dependent manner. This suggests that FA induced BACE1 and MMP2 pathways maybe novel potential mechanisms involved in AD. The text mining of literature and TCM database related to AD suggested FA as a promising TCM ingredient for the treatment of AD. Potential mechanisms interconnected and integrated with Aβ aggregation inhibition and extracellular matrix remodeling underlying the activity of FA were identified using *in vitro* studies.

Keywords: Alzheimer disease, BACE1, curcumin, ferulic acid, MMP2, STRING, text mining

INTRODUCTION

Alzheimer's disease (AD) is a chronic neurodegenerative disease that usually progresses from short memory loss to dementia, and accounts for 50%–70% of dementia cases (Burns and Iliffe, 2009). According to the World Alzheimer Report (Prince, 2015), 46.8 million people worldwide are living with dementia, and this number is estimated to reach 131.5 million by 2050, which will result in an increasing burden on society and families. In addition, the cost of long-term care, home services, and non-professional caregivers is greater than the cost of direct medical care (Bullock, 2004; Winblad et al., 2016; Yokoyama et al., 2016).

Despite enormous financial and research investments, appropriate interventions to prevent the progress of AD are lacking (Iqbal and Grundke-Iqbal, 2011; Selkoe, 2013). Based on the failure of a number of novel AD drugs, investigators are increasingly convinced that AD is not a single but rather a multifactorial disease (Iqbal et al., 2013), and hence, drugs that target one node on the classical pathway have little effect on the AD disease network. Since AD is a multifactorial disease, drugs that modulate systemic or multiple targets are of interest.

Traditional Chinese medicine (TCM) compositions usually exert systemic impact and can be a source of drug repositioning efforts (Wang et al., 2011). TCM treatments are natural herbs discovered by the ancient Chinese and evolved through at least 3000 years of clinical practice. TCM is gaining increasing attention with the emergence of integrative and personalized medicine, characterized by pattern differentiation on individual variance and treatments based on natural herbal synergism (Wang and Wei, 2009). With the growing popularity and promising approach of TCM applicability, the ever-increasing demand for understanding the pharmacological mechanisms and potential drug efficacy are the major issues that need to be addressed.

In this study, we sought to shed light on TCM for AD. What typical TCM treatments could be effective for AD, and what are the underlying target-based mechanisms? How can we integrate systemic and target-based understandings of the disease and treatments (Cho et al., 2006)? With the overwhelming amount of biomedical knowledge recorded in texts, text mining is essential for identifying, extracting, managing, integrating and exploiting this information to discover new, hidden, or unsuspected information. Text mining is a computer-based discovery of new, previously unknown information, which automatically extracts information from different written resources (Ding et al., 2013), drawing on information retrieval, statistics, and computational linguistics. It has considerable potential for drug target discovery and re-labeling of existing drugs. Some typical proven drug repositioning cases are available for text mining, such as the beneficial effect of estrogen on human memory discovered by Smalheiser and Swanson (1996), thalidomide for treating acute pancreatitis extracted by Weeber et al. (2003), and the association of migraine with AMPA receptors identified using Litlinker (Yetisgen-Yildiz and Pratt, 2006).

Herein, we report an approach for finding an appropriate TCM for AD through the utilization of text-mining from literature database, exploring the underlying therapeutic mechanisms followed by searching for protein-protein interactions (PPI) using the STRING platform, and finally using the SHSY5Y-APP AD cell line model for validation.

MATERIALS AND METHODS

Our first aim was to select a TCM candidate from the extensive literature collection. The study workflow is shown in **Figure 1**.

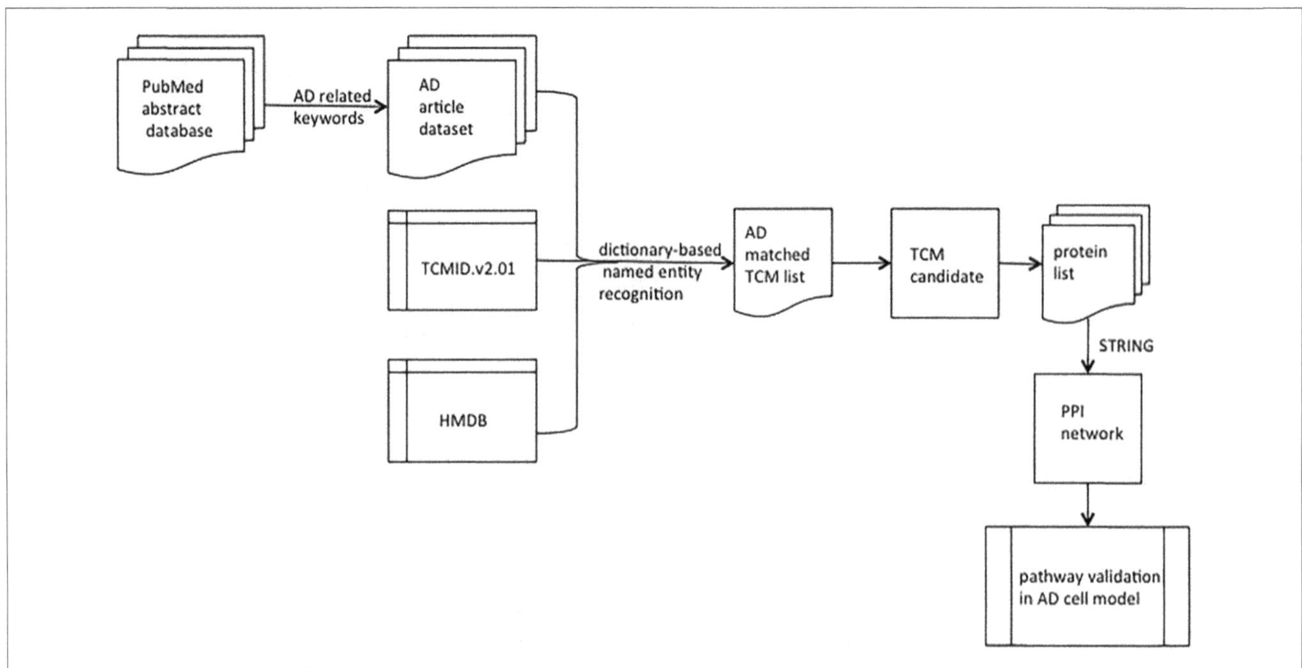

FIGURE 1 | Flowchart for selecting TCM candidates for validation. AD, Alzheimer's disease; TCM, traditional Chinese medicine; TCMID.v2.01, a TCM database; HMDB, human metabolomics database; STRING, a platform of protein-protein interaction (PPI).

Data Collection and Extraction to Find a TCM Candidate for AD

First, we assembled an AD literature dataset by retrieving articles from PubMed using AD-related keywords: "Alzheimer or Mild cognitive impairment or Dementia or Significant memory concern or Subjective memory complaint," a resource for extracting and defining TCM candidates. The TCM database, TCMID.v2.01 (Chen et al., 2006), was then utilized, which included names, stitch_id, PubChem_id, synonyms, formula, SMILES strings, and the source of the involved chemicals. The TCM terminologies, mentioned in the abstracts of the retrieved articles were then extracted using dictionary-based named entity recognition (i.e., simple word matching) provided by LingPipe[1]. Using this method, the selection of the TCM for AD was retrieved in a relatively short duration.

Furthermore, we matched the PubChem ID of TCM and the origin ontology in the human metabolome database (HMDB; Southan et al., 2013) to determine the optimal TCM candidates. After focusing on a possible lead TCM candidate, we retrieved articles in the AD dataset, and extracted protein names that co-occurred with the candidate TCM using the dictionary-based entity recognition from NCBI protein list[2]. This gave us with a list of possible proteins affected by the TCM candidate.

Inferring Possible PPI (Li et al., 2017) Networks of the TCM Candidate Using STRING

STRING presents a specific and productive functional relationship between two proteins into a combined interaction confidence score, which is derived from the co-expression score, experimentally determined interaction score, and the automated text mining score. In this system, the automated text mining score is higher than or approximately equal to the experimentally determined interaction score since it is integrated from these scores. However, if the text mining score was lower than the experimentally determined interaction, there were two possibilities: (1) the experimentally determined interaction score was a false positive; (2) only a few studies are available related to these two proteins; however, experimental validation could be conducted.

We deposited the protein list mentioned above in the multiple protein column in the search webpage of STRING[3] and acquired the PPI network after deleting results with co-expression scores >0 (already validated PPI), or experimentally determined interaction score × automated text mining score = 0 (little relevance). In the next step, we rearranged the PPI network according to text mining scores and obtained the top proteins in the network, which were most likely related to candidate mechanisms in AD.

[1] http://alias-i.com/lingpipe/index.html
[2] https://www.ncbi.nlm.nih.gov/protein/
[3] https://string-db.org/

Validation of Protein Expression and PPI in an AD Cell Line Model

In order to generate strong evidence not only in the data level, we validated the possible mechanisms mined from STRING using AD cell lines.

Cell Culture and Treatment With TCM Candidate for AD

SHSY5Y-APP cells, a classic cell line for AD research, were a kind gift from Shanghai Jiao Tong University. The cells were cultured in MEM supplemented with 10% heat-inactivated fetal bovine serum (FBS), 100 units/mL penicillin, and 100 μg/mL streptomycin (Invitrogen, Carlsbad, CA, USA) at 95% humidity, 37°C, and 5% CO_2 in an incubator. The cells were passaged by trypsinization every 2–3 days. The SHSY5Y-APP cells were treated with different doses of the TCM candidate for 24 h. In the existing researches, the effective ferulic acid (FA) concentrations vary from 10 nM to 1 mM without toxic reactions in a variety of cell lines, in accordance with the point that FA is highly safe for daily and long-term consumption (Thakkar et al., 2015; Sompong et al., 2017; Zhang et al., 2017). In line with a previous study using the same cell line (Cui et al., 2013), micromolar (μM) was chosen as the unit for FA concentration and upgraded in steps of 0 μM, 15 μM, 30 μM and 60 μM.

Co-immunoprecipitation Assays (co-IP)

Cell lysates were centrifuged (10,000× *g*) at 4°C for 15 min. Proteins were then immunoprecipitated with the relevant antibodies to determine interactions. The precleared Protein A/G Plus-Agarose beads (Merck KGaA, Darmstadt, Germany) were incubated with the immunocomplexes for 2 h and washed four times with phosphate-buffered saline. The immunoprecipitates were subjected to sodium dodecyl sulfate-polyacrylamide gel electrophoresis (SDS-PAGE; Merck KGaA, Darmstadt, Germany), followed by transfer to polyvinylidene difluoride (PVDF) membrane (Amresco, OH, USA). The antibody-antigen complexes were visualized using the UPV software according to the manufacturer's instructions. The immunoreactive bands were quantified to confirm the appropriate levels of proteins.

Western Blot

Preparation of Protein Samples

After TCM candidate exposure for 24 h, SHSY5Y-APP cells were washed with pre-cooled 4°C PBS, and then the wash solution was discarded. The above procedure was repeated twice. PMSF was added to lyse the cells on ice with frequent shaking for 30 min. After lysis, the cells were scraped with a clean scraper, and then the cell debris and lysate were transferred and centrifuged at 12,000 rpm for 5 min at 4°C. The supernatant after centrifugation was stored at −20°C.

Determination of Protein Concentration

The standard BCA assay procedure was done as previously described (Huang et al., 2010). After blocking, the membranes were probed with the following primary antibodies (Cell

Signaling, Beverly, MA, USA) using different dilutions: rabbit anti-MMP2 (92 kDa, Abcam ab92539, 1:2000), rabbit anti-MMP9 (92 kDa, Abcam ab38898, 1:2000), rabbit anti-BACE1 (68 kDa, Abcam ab183612, 1:1000), rabbit anti-APP (87 kDa, Abcam ab15272, 1:600), and mouse anti-beta-actin (42 kDa, Boster, BM0627, 1:200). All experiments were performed at least three times.

Electrophoresis

We prepared the 12% separation gel, 10% separation gel and 5% concentration gel. The prepared protein sample and the maker were added to 40 μg. After the sample was added, constant 80 V electrophoresis was performed until the bromophenol blue indicator was linear at the junction of the concentrated gel and the separation gel, and the pressure was changed to constant 120 V. This process took about 1.5 h. Next, we removed the gel and the target band according to the Marker. The PVDF membrane was soaked in methanol for several seconds and soaked in the electroporation buffer together with the filter paper. The transfer membrane conditions were as below: β-actin 200 mA 90 min, BACE1 200 mA 120 min, APP, MMP2 and MMP9 250 mA 120 min.

Immunoblotting and Analysis

The PVDF membrane was soaked in TBST containing 5% skimmed milk powder and shaken at room temperature for 2 h. We mixed the ECL reagent with the stable peroxidase solution in a ratio of 1:1, added the solution onto the PVDF membrane. X-ray film was placed in the solution, flushed, dried, scanned, and finally analyzed grayscale value with BandScan 5.0 software (NIH, USA). Statistical analysis was performed using SPSS 20.0 software (SPSS, Chicago, IL, USA). Quantitative data are presented as mean ± standard deviation (SD) of triplicates in an independent experiment that was repeated three times. Data were compared using Student's unpaired t-test for direct comparison between two-groups and the Tukey-Kramer test after a significant one-way analysis of variance (ANOVA), and F-test for multiple-group comparisons. $P < 0.05$ was considered as statistically significant.

RESULTS

Text Mining Using AD Literature and the TCM Database

We retrieved 195,882 articles from PubMed using AD-related keywords and assembled an AD article dataset.

After matching TCMID.v2.01 ingredients to the AD article database, we extracted a list of AD-related TCM ingredients with PubChem IDs, which was checked for origin ontology in HMDB.

We ranked the TCM ingredients by the number of mentions and focused on the top 20 frequent terms after deleting common words, such as "protein," "glucose," "amino acid," and others (**Table 1**).

Next, we checked the origin ontology of all the 20 components. In **Table 1**, a total of 12 endogenous ingredients, including Tau, Acetylcholine, Dopamine, Melatonin, Glutathione, Aspartate, Serotonin, Tyrosine, Serine, Levodopa, Estradiol and Creatine were selected. These endogenous ingredients could not only be absorbed from the environment but also produced and synthesized within the organism or system. Cholinesterase does not have an origin result in HMDB, and hence, our list was narrowed down to Glutamate, Choline, Nicotine, Scopolamine, Curcumin, Methionine and Physostigmine, of which Glutamate, Choline, Methionine and Physostigmine could be extracted from a broad list of drug and food options, in which includes Nicotine, Scopolamine and Curcumin. Literature suggested that Scopolamine induced retrograde amnesia, or an inability to recall events prior to its administration (Colettis et al., 2014), and hence, it was

TABLE 1 | TCM ingredients' AD-matched list in PubMed.

No.	Frequency	TCM ingredients	PubChem ID	Origin ontology in HMDB
1	41288	Tau	156615	Endogenous
2	5431	Glutamate	5128032	Bacteria and beans
3	3609	Cholinesterase	4460501	Not available
4	3557	Acetylcholine	5315629	Endogenous
5	3453	Dopamine	681	Endogenous
6	2824	Choline	305	Many plants and animal organs
7	1999	Nicotine	89594	Tobacco
8	1973	Melatonin	896	Endogenous
9	1898	Glutathione	124886	Drug metabolite and Endogenous
10	1722	Aspartate	5460541	Endogenous
11	1718	Serotonin	5202	Endogenous
12	1593	Tyrosine	6057	Endogenous
13	1534	Scopolamine	5184	Solanaceae
14	1432	Serine	5951	Endogenous
15	1372	*Curcumin*	969516	*Curcuma longa*
16	1089	Levodopa	6047	Endogenous
17	939	Estradiol	5757	Drug, Endogenous, Food
18	931	Methionine	6137	Drug metabolite and Food
19	788	Creatine	586	Endogenous
20	785	Physostigmine	5983	Drug

TCM, traditional Chinese medicine; HMDB, human metabolome database.

deleted from our list. Compared to the double-edged function of Nicotine, Curcumin has not been shown to cause any toxicity despite its daily consumption for centuries in Asian countries (Maheshwari et al., 2006). Thus, we first focused on Curcumin in the candidate list, an obvious TCM component that is extracted from Curcuma longa, a common plant in China.

In order to confirm its effect, we extracted all the sentences that contained "curcumin" from the AD article database. From the 107 retrieved sentences, one sentence inferred that Curcumin was suitable for treating AD; whereas, FA appeared in the same sentence with Curcumin at a high frequency. Three representative sentences are shown in **Table 2.**

Curcumin and FA share some similarities, and as a major metabolite of curcumin, FA has better bioavailability and metabolic stability than curcumin, thus rendering it as a better candidate (Badavath et al., 2016). Thus, we re-assigned our TCM target from curcumin to FA. FA also denoted as 3-(4-hydroxy-3-methoxyphenyl)-2-propenoic acid, has the following chemical structure:

O
MeO
OH
HO

After selecting FA as our TCM target, the next step was to understand the possible mechanism of FA in AD. Given the apparent complexity of the FA mechanism network, understanding its involvement in the underlying AD pathological pathways was a challenge.

We retrieved 178,725 articles using FA-related keywords "Curcumin, or FA, or Sodium Ferulate" in PubMed. From these articles, we extracted a list of proteins that was co-mentioned with FA, using the dictionary-based entity recognition. This resulted in 178 proteins that were ranked by the number of times mentioned with links to sentence sources in PubMed. After deleting a large number of false positives using the auto stop list (Fenner, 2008) of drug abbreviations, experimental test abbreviations, cell lines, synonyms of other genes, and common serum proteins, we reduced the list of proteins to 20, which are listed below:

APOB, BACE1, BCL2, CCNB1, CCND1, ERBB2, GAPDH, GSR, HMOX1, MMP2, MYB, NOS1, PCNA, PEA15, PIK3CA, PPARA, PTGS2, RAF1, TXN and VEGFA.

Potential PPI Network in STRING

Next, we entered these proteins into STRING in order to obtain direct as well as indirect protein associations (**Figure 2**).

The PPI scores were also exported into **Table 3**. The BACE1 and MMP2 combined score ranked on top among the interactions, however it had a lower automated text mining score than in the experimentally determined interaction score. We selected BACE1-MMP2 interaction as the target PPI. The edges connecting BACE1 and MMP2 (**Figure 1**) are and , which indicates that BACE1 and MMP2 may interact with each other. However, when we searched for *in-silico* evidence, the two words occurred in the full-text of some experimental articles, albeit without any direct correlation, such that the experimentally determined interaction was a false positive with a high validation possibility.

Novel Hypothesis for the FA Related Mechanism in AD

Based on the above results, we hypothesized that BACE1 and MMP2 were closely linked to the mechanism of FA. The two possibilities are as follows: these two proteins interacted directly, which could be validated by co-IP; in addition to proteolytic cleaving of the amyloid precursor protein (APP), the extracellular matrix proteins may also have a role in the AD pathological pathways, and these two pathways were always concurrent in AD.

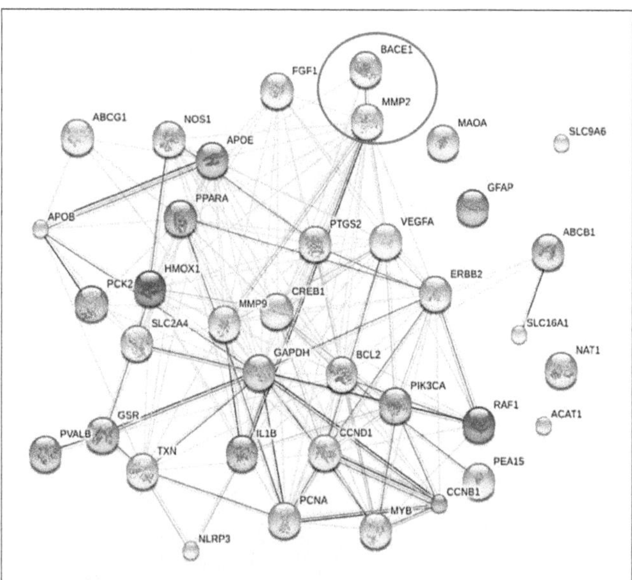

FIGURE 2 | PP1 map generated by STRING showing the interactions of the selected 20 proteins Edges represent protein-protein associations, interactions from experimentally determined, text mining, known interactions from curated databases, gene fusions, gene co-occurrence, co-expression and protein homology.

TABLE 2 | Sentences retrieved from the literature based on the entities' biomedical researches.

PMID	Sentences retrieved from literature
16387689	Because it can modulate the expression of these targets, curcumin is now being used to treat cancer, arthritis, diabetes, Crohn's disease, cardiovascular diseases, osteoporosis, Alzheimer's disease, psoriasis and other pathologies.
17127365	Food supplementation with curcumin and ferulic acid is considered a nutritional approach to reduce oxidative damage and amyloid pathology in Alzheimer's disease.
26592858	Ferulic acid has structural similarity with curcumin, which is known for its monoamine oxidase (MAO) inhibitory activity.

TABLE 3 | Ranking scores of protein interactions in STRING.

Node 1	Node 2	Co-expression	Experimentally determined interaction	Automated text mining	Combined score
BACE1	MMP2	0	0.534	0.149	0.586
PPARA	APOB	0.053	0	0.578	0.583
CCND1	MMP2	0	0	0.575	0.575
NOS1	BCL2	0.048	0	0.566	0.569
APOB	GAPDH	0	0.179	0.491	0.564
BCL2	PPARA	0	0.377	0.304	0.548
MYB	GAPDH	0.061	0	0.517	0.527
RAF1	GAPDH	0.059	0	0.503	0.512
TXN	BCL2	0	0	0.507	0.507
PCNA	PTGS2	0	0	0.507	0.507
PCNA	TXN	0.2	0.102	0.367	0.506
PCNA	MMP2	0	0	0.506	0.506
PPARA	GAPDH	0	0.042	0.501	0.501
NOS1	GAPDH	0.084	0	0.476	0.5
ERBB2	RAF1	0	0.292	0.76	0.487
BACE1	GAPDH	0.053	0	0.465	0.472
ERBB2	CCNB1	0	0	0.454	0.454
BCL2	GSR	0.048	0	0.446	0.45
NOS1	MMP2	0.055	0	0.442	0.45
TXN	VEGFA	0	0	0.442	0.442
PCNA	MYB	0.058	0	0.426	0.436
VEGFA	CCNB1	0	0	0.432	0.432
TXN	APOB	0	0	0.417	0.416
MYB	PIK3CA	0.055	0.104	0.349	0.401

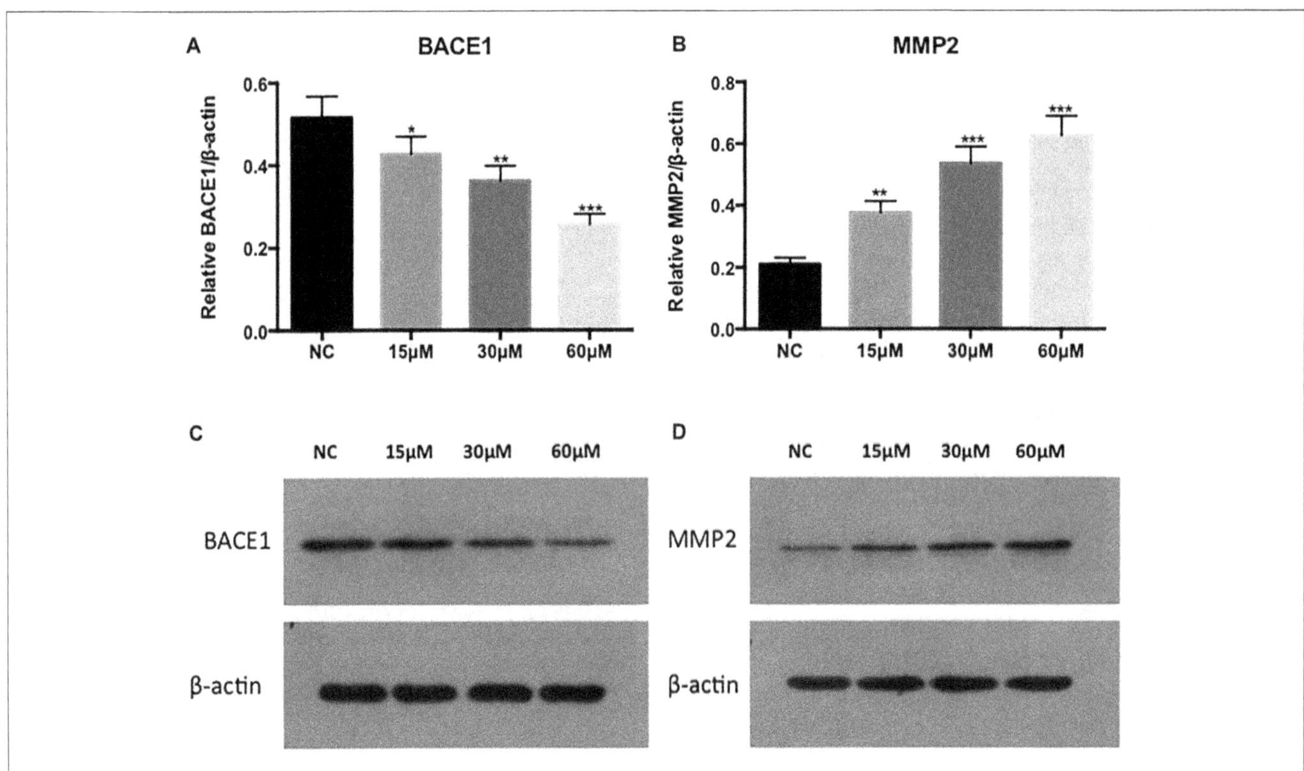

FIGURE 3 | Protein expression of BACE-1 and MMP-2 after exposure to 0, 15, 30 and 60 μM ferulic acid (FA). **(A,B)** are the expression analysis results of **(C,D)**. Statistical significance is denoted by $^{*}p < 0.05$, $^{**}p < 0.01$, $^{***}p < 0.001$ (one-way ANOVA; N = NC).

The SHSY5Y-APP cell lines were passaged every 2–3 days by trypsinization, and treated with 0, 15, 30 and 60 μM FA (Yuanmu Tech, China) for 24 h. After FA exposure for 24 h, the BACE-1 expression decreased and MMP-2 expression increased in a dose-dependent manner (**Figure 3**).

We next tested the expression of APP, another dominant protein in the Aβ aggregation pathway, which is positively correlated with BACE1. After exposure to FA, the proteolytic cleavage of APP and APP enzymolysis is decreased, thereby improving the AD process. In addition, we tested MMP9, another protein in the extracellular matrix pathway. We observed that extracellular matrix protein expression was increased after FA exposure and contributes to the pathological process of AD (**Figure 4**).

DISCUSSION

TCM Candidate Selection for AD Using Data Mining

In this study, we used text mining to select a TCM candidate for subsequent validation. FA was selected and *in vitro* validation was performed to understand the potential mechanisms involved in AD. Furthermore, the current study used the information-medicine integrated system to map TCM for AD research. In addition, text mining was coupled to the experimental validation to assess the drug selection outcomes. This offset the information gap and maximized the utilization of existing knowledge to select the optimal TCM candidate to study.

Drug discovery for AD is no longer a game of chance or just limited to the availability of new technology. Societal expectations about drug efficacy are rising; thus, early-stage drug discovery necessitates accessible, standardized data sets to generate a complete scenario of the physiological function and disease relevance. Some pioneering studies have focused on drug repurposing, such as systematic "omics" data mining of genome-wide association studies (GWAS), HMDB, epigenomics and proteomics data (Zhang et al., 2016; Pimplikar, 2017). These studies suggested drugs that were applicable for other diseases having novel anti-AD indications. These attempts were very logical however these studies did not consider TCM as a source of information for AD research. TCM is a good source for drug discovery. The uniqueness of the TCM system is based on the philosophical logic underlying daily practices (Ho et al., 2011), which was accumulated over thousands of years of empirical studies and provides a unique view of the relationships between the human body and the universe (Gu and Chen, 2014). Therefore, a better understanding of TCM and key learning from the past with appropriate strategies for the future is essential to make a significant difference. These theories render the proposed approach useful in identifying novel relationships between diseases and drugs that have a high probability of being physiologically effective. On the other hand, existing TCM drug mining primarily focuses on the assessment of ancient classic literature, with less analysis of herbal components (May et al., 2014; Pae et al., 2016), and thus may affect knowledge dissemination. Our study is the first to combine well-known TCM database with text mining approaches. This led us to select FA as a lead candidate for experimental validation for AD.

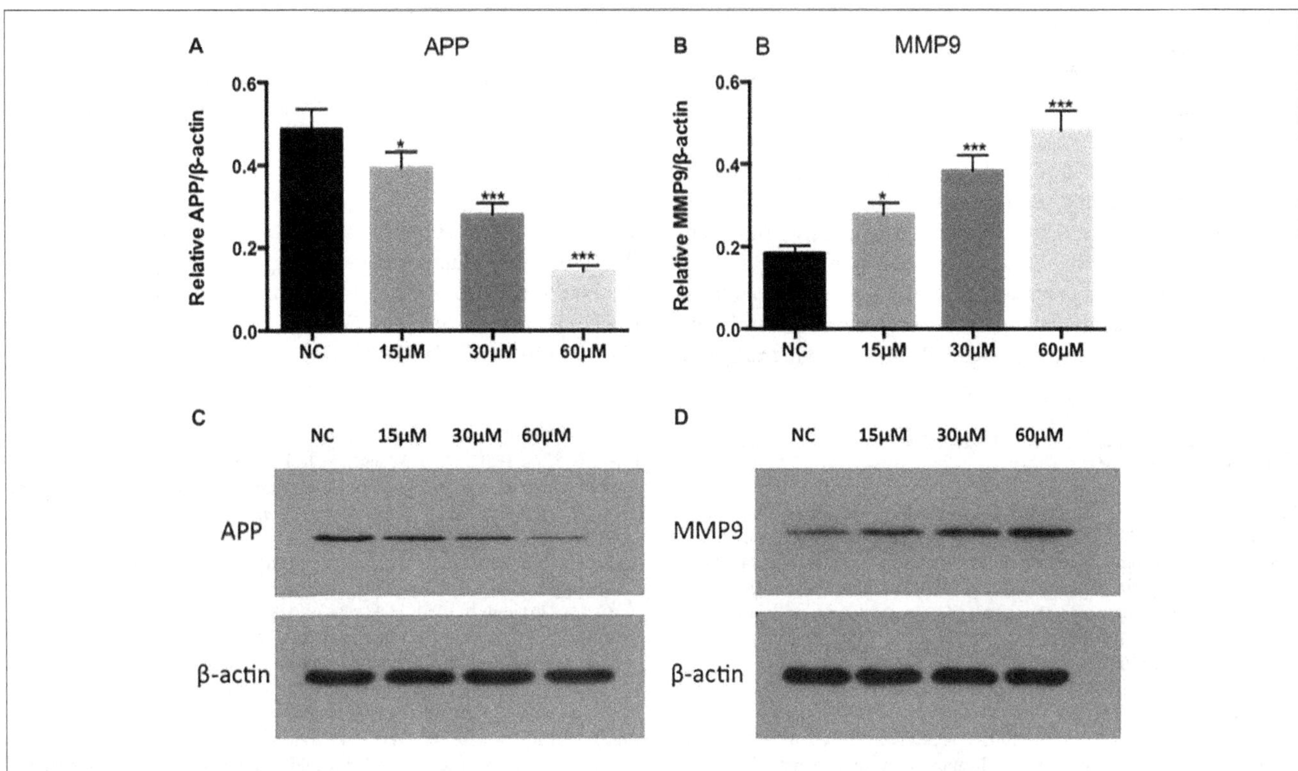

FIGURE 4 | Protein expression of APP and MMP9 after exposure to 0, 15, 30 and 60 μM FA. **(A,B)** are the expression analysis results of **(C,D)**. Statistical significance is denoted by $^*p < 0.05$, $^{***}p < 0.001$ (one-way ANOVA; N = NC).

MMP2-BACE1 Mechanisms of FA in AD

Our findings suggested that FA might be a promising multi-targeted TCM with a therapeutic potential for AD (Jung et al., 2016). We evaluated the APP and BACE1 inhibitory activities, which inhibit Ab aggregation; in addition, the matrix clearance properties of MMP-2 and MMP-9 implicated FA was actively involved in the alteration of matrix proteins and that it played a major role in *in vitro* extracellular matrix remodeling. As shown in a previous *in situ* proximity ligation assay (*in situ* PLA), which is a new technique to monitor PPI with high specificity and sensitivity, it was found that APP, MMP2 and MMP9 all interacted with TGFB1, and the interaction of MMP2 and BACE1 was also positive (Chen et al., 2014). Furthermore, from the Human Protein Reference Database (HPRD) in the STRING platform (Higashi and Miyazaki, 2003), the COOH-terminal parts of APP were found to interact with the extracellular matrix and highly selectively inhibit MMP2, in which the decapeptide region of APP was likely an active site-directed inhibitor toward MMP2.

The pathways of PPI at the molecular level include cellular transduction and biological function. Hence, the two pathways of Aβ aggregation inhibition and extracellular matrix remodeling were interconnected and integrated to the biological function-signaling map for AD. The results of these analyses might have potential application in exploring FA mechanism because they can be used as rational targets to inhibit the function of pathways essential to AD. In the multi-targeted AD model, APP cleavage, inhibition of Aβ deposition, and extracellular matrix remodeling are co-operative interactions involved in AD pathology, which could be attractive therapeutics with respect to pharmacokinetics and pharmacodynamics when compared to a specific highly specific single target molecule. These results highlight the prospective beneficial effects of FA as a therapeutic agent against AD pathology.

One limitation of this study was that no animal model was validated, and the experimental validation in the AD cell model was not sufficient to make a conclusive statement regarding the potential efficacy and benefit of FA. However, we found evidence in previous study of FA's protective effects on different animal models of intra-cerebroventricular (i.c.v.) injection of Aß1–42 in mice and APP/PS1 mutant transgenic mice (Jung et al., 2016), which shows potent anti-oxidant and anti-inflammatory activities. Future studies should discuss the in-depth mechanisms of FA together with the physiological data to evaluate FA efficacy and involvement in an AD animal model. These include: What are the safety implications of the different doses of FA for AD? What biomarkers exist for FA metabolites? In addition, understanding the role of FA within the system, the pathways and networks of the different protein interactions are invaluable.

CONCLUSION

In summary, we demonstrate that the combination of text mining and professional medical knowledge is an effective approach for finding new mechanisms underlying the clinical therapeutics for AD. Equipped with this data, the clinical scientist can obtain information in a short period of time without searching large volumes of articles. Moreover, using *in vitro* studies for validation, the data-driven results were based on not only a hypothesis but also true novel findings of potential mechanisms interconnected and integrated by Aβ aggregation inhibition and extracellular matrix remodeling underlying the activity of FA. The present study strongly supported text mining of the ever-increasing volume of literature and TCM database as a drug repositioning approach for elucidating FA as a promising TCM ingredient for treating AD.

AUTHOR CONTRIBUTIONS

GM, YZ and XMeng designed the study. XMa and AJ performed experiments and prepared figures. XMa, GZ and XH analyzed the data. GM and XMeng wrote and discussed all sections of the manuscript. All authors reviewed and approved the manuscript.

FUNDING

This study was supported by the International Exchange Program for Graduate Students, Tongji University (2016020033), the National Natural Science Foundation of China (81571033, 81771131) and the Shanghai Science and Technology Committee (17411950100, 17411950101).

REFERENCES

Badavath, V. N., Baysal, I., Uçar, G., Mondal, S. K., Sinha, B. N., and Jayaprakash, V. (2016). Monoamine oxidase inhibitory activity of ferulic acid amides: curcumin-based design and synthesis. *Arch. Pharm.* 349, 9–19. doi: 10.1002/ardp.201500317

Bullock, R. (2004). The needs of the caregiver in the long-term treatment of Alzheimer disease. *Alzheimer Dis. Assoc. Disord.* 18, S17–S23. doi: 10.1097/01.wad.0000127493.65032.9a

Burns, A., and Iliffe, S. (2009). Alzheimer's disease. *BMJ* 338:b158. doi: 10.1136/bmj.b158

Chen, T. C., Lin, K. T., Chen, C. H., Lee, S. A., Lee, P. Y., Liu, Y. W., et al. (2014). Using an in situ proximity ligation assay to systematically profile endogenous protein-protein interactions in a pathway network. *J. Proteome Res.* 13, 5339–5346. doi: 10.1021/pr5002737

Chen, X., Zhou, H., Liu, Y. B., Wang, J. F., Li, H., Ung, C. Y., et al. (2006). Database of traditional Chinese medicine and its application to studies of mechanism and to prescription validation. *Br. J. Pharmacol.* 149, 1092–1103. doi: 10.1038/sj.bjp.0706945

Cho, C. R., Labow, M., Reinhardt, M., van Oostrum, J., and Peitsch, M. C. (2006). The application of systems biology to drug discovery. *Curr. Opin. Chem. Biol.* 10, 294–302. doi: 10.1016/j.cbpa.2006.06.025

Colettis, N. C., Snitcofsky, M., Kornisiuk, E. E., Gonzalez, E. N., Quillfeldt, J. A., and Jerusalinsky, D. A. (2014). Amnesia of inhibitory avoidance by scopolamine is overcome by previous open-field exposure. *Learn. Mem.* 21, 634–645. doi: 10.1101/lm.036210.114

Cui, L., Zhang, Y., Cao, H., Wang, Y., Teng, T., Ma, G., et al. (2013). Ferulic acid inhibits the transition of amyloid-β42 monomers to oligomers but accelerates the transition from oligomers to fibrils. *J. Alzheimers Dis.* 37, 19–28. doi: 10.3233/JAD-130164

Ding, Y., Song, M., Han, J., Yu, Q., Yan, E., Lin, L., et al. (2013). Entitymetrics: measuring the impact of entities. *PLoS One* 8:e71416. doi: 10.1371/journal.pone.0071416

Fenner, M. (2008). Duplication: stop favouring applicant with longest list. *Nature* 452:29. doi: 10.1038/452029a

Gu, P., and Chen, H. (2014). Modern bioinformatics meets traditional Chinese medicine. *Brief. Bioinform.* 15, 984–1003. doi: 10.1093/bib/bbt063

Higashi, S., and Miyazaki, K. (2003). Identification of a region of β-amyloid precursor protein essential for its gelatinase A inhibitory activity. *J. Biol. Chem.* 278, 14020–14028. doi: 10.1074/jbc.M212264200

Ho, Y. S., So, K. F., and Chang, R. C. (2011). Drug discovery from Chinese medicine against neurodegeneration in Alzheimer's and vascular dementia. *Chin. Med.* 6:15. doi: 10.1186/1749-8546-6-15

Huang, T., Long, M., and Huo, B. (2010). Competitive binding to cuprous ions of protein and BCA in the bicinchoninic acid protein assay. *Open Biomed. Eng. J.* 4, 271–278. doi: 10.2174/1874120701004010271

Iqbal, K., Flory, M., and Soininen, H. (2013). Clinical symptoms and symptom signatures of Alzheimer's disease subgroups. *J. Alzheimers Dis.* 37, 475–481. doi: 10.3233/JAD-130899

Iqbal, K., and Grundke-Iqbal, I. (2011). Opportunities and challenges in developing Alzheimer disease therapeutics. *Acta Neuropathol.* 122, 543–549. doi: 10.1007/s00401-011-0878-z

Jung, J. S., Yan, J. J., Li, H. M., Sultan, M. T., Yu, J., Lee, H. S., et al. (2016). Protective effects of a dimeric derivative of ferulic acid in animal models of Alzheimer's disease. *Eur. J. Pharmacol.* 782, 30–34. doi: 10.1016/j.ejphar.2016.04.047

Li, T., Wernersson, R., Hansen, R. B., Horn, H., Mercer, J., Slodkowicz, G., et al. (2017). A scored human protein-protein interaction network to catalyze genomic interpretation. *Nat. Methods* 14, 61–64. doi: 10.1038/nmeth.4083

Maheshwari, R. K., Singh, A. K., Gaddipati, J., and Srimal, R. C. (2006). Multiple biological activities of curcumin: a short review. *Life Sci.* 78, 2081–2087. doi: 10.1016/j.lfs.2005.12.007

May, B. H., Zhang, A., Lu, Y., Lu, C., and Xue, C. C. (2014). The systematic assessment of traditional evidence from the premodern Chinese medical literature: a text-mining approach. *J. Altern. Complement. Med.* 20, 937–942. doi: 10.1089/acm.2013.0372

Pae, S. B., Yun, B. C., Han, Y. K., Choi, B. T., Shin, H. K., and Baek, J. U. (2016). Cognitive-enhancing herbal formulae in korean medicine: identification of candidates by text mining and literature review. *J. Altern. Complement. Med.* 22, 413–418. doi: 10.1089/acm.2015.0257

Pimplikar, S. W. (2017). Multi-omics and Alzheimer's disease: a slower but surer path to an efficacious therapy? *Am. J. Physiol. Cell Physiol.* 313, C1–C2. doi: 10.1152/ajpcell.00109.2017

Prince, M. J. (2015). World Alzheimer Report 2015: the global impact of dementia: an analysis of prevalence, incidence, cost and trends. Available online at: http://www.alz.co.uk/research/world-report-2015

Selkoe, D. J. (2013). The therapeutics of Alzheimer's disease: where we stand where we are heading. *Ann. Neurol.* 74, 328–336. doi: 10.1002/ana.24001

Smalheiser, N. R., and Swanson, D. R. (1996). Linking estrogen to Alzheimer's disease: an informatics approach. *Neurology* 47, 809–810. doi: 10.1212/WNL.47.3.809

Sompong, W., Cheng, H., and Adisakwattana, S. (2017). Ferulic acid prevents methylglyoxal-induced protein glycation, DNA damage, and apoptosis in pancreatic β-cells. *J. Physiol. Biochem.* 73, 121–131. doi: 10.1007/s13105-016-0531-3

Southan, C., Sitzmann, M., and Muresan, S. (2013). Comparing the chemical structure and protein content of ChEMBL, DrugBank, human metabolome database and the therapeutic target database. *Mol. Inform.* 32, 881–897. doi: 10.1002/minf.201300103

Thakkar, A., Chenreddy, S., Wang, J., and Prabhu, S. (2015). Ferulic acid combined with aspirin demonstrates chemopreventive potential towards pancreatic cancer when delivered using chitosan-coated solid-lipid nanoparticles. *Cell Biosci.* 5:46. doi: 10.1186/s13578-015-0041-y

Wang, H., Ding, Y., Tang, J., Dong, X., He, B., Qiu, J., et al. (2011). Finding complex biological relationships in recent PubMed articles using Bio-LDA. *PLoS One* 6:e17243. doi: 10.1371/journal.pone.0017243

Wang, J. F., and Wei, D. Q. (2009). Role of structural bioinformatics and traditional Chinese medicine databases in pharmacogenomics. *Pharmacogenomics* 10, 1213–1215. doi: 10.2217/pgs.09.81

Weeber, M., Vos, R., Klein, H., De Jong-Van Den Berg, L. T., Aronson, A. R., and Molema, G. (2003). Generating hypotheses by discovering implicit associations in the literature: a case report of a search for new potential therapeutic uses for thalidomide. *J. Am. Med. Inform. Assoc.* 10, 252–259. doi: 10.1197/jamia.m1158

Winblad, B., Amouyel, P., Andrieu, S., Ballard, C., Brayne, C., Brodaty, H., et al. (2016). Defeating Alzheimer's disease and other dementias: a priority for European science and society. *Lancet Neurol.* 15, 455–532. doi: 10.1016/S1474-4422(16)00062-4

Yetisgen-Yildiz, M., and Pratt, W. (2006). Using statistical and knowledge-based approaches for literature-based discovery. *J. Biomed. Inform.* 39, 600–611. doi: 10.1016/j.jbi.2005.11.010

Yokoyama, J. S., Wang, Y., Schork, A. J., Thompson, W. K., Karch, C. M., Cruchaga, C., et al. (2016). Association between genetic traits for immune-mediated diseases and Alzheimer disease. *JAMA Neurol* 73, 691–697. doi: 10.1001/jamaneurol.2016.0150

Zhang, M., Schmitt-Ulms, G., Sato, C., Xi, Z., Zhang, Y., Zhou, Y., et al. (2016). Drug repositioning for Alzheimer's disease based on systematic 'omics' data mining. *PLoS One* 11:e0168812. doi: 10.1371/journal.pone.0168812

Zhang, X. D., Wu, Q., and Yang, S. H. (2017). Ferulic acid promoting apoptosis in human osteosarcoma cell lines. *Pak. J. Med. Sci.* 33, 127–131. doi: 10.12669/pjms.331.12066

12

Repetitive Transcranial Magnetic Stimulation (rTMS) Modulates Lipid Metabolism in Aging Adults

Weicong Ren [1,2,3†], *Jiang Ma* [4†], *Juan Li* [3], *Zhijie Zhang* [1,2*] *and Mingwei Wang* [2,5*]

[1] Department of Psychology, Hebei Normal University, Shijiazhuang, China, [2] Key Laboratory of Brain Aging and Cognitive Neuroscience of Hebei Province, Hebei Medical University, Shijiazhuang, China, [3] Center on Aging Psychology, Key Laboratory of Mental Health, Institute of Psychology, Chinese Academy of Sciences, Beijing, China, [4] Department of Rehabilitation, First Hospital of Shijiazhuang, Shijiazhuang, China, [5] Department of Neurology, First Hospital of Hebei Medical University, Shijiazhuang, China

***Correspondence:**
Zhijie Zhang
zhangzhj2002@sina.com
Mingwei Wang
mwei99@yahoo.com

† These authors have contributed equally to this work.

Hyperlipidemia, one of the cardiovascular (CV) risk factors, is associated with an increase in the risk for dementia. Repetitive transcranial magnetic stimulation (rTMS) was applied over the right dorsolateral prefrontal cortex (DLPFC) to modulate serum lipid levels in older adults. Participants received 10 sessions of rTMS or sham stimulation intervention within 2 weeks. The serum lipid and thyroid hormone-related endocrine levels were assessed before and after the treatment. We found that rTMS significantly decreased serum lipid levels, including the total cholesterol (CHO) and triglyceride (TG); meanwhile, it also increased the thyroid-stimulating hormone (TSH) as well as thyroxine (T4) levels. This suggests that rTMS modulated the serum lipid metabolism by altering activity in the hypothalamo-pituitary-thyroid (HPT) axis. The trial was registered on the website of Chinese Clinical Trial Registry (http://www.chictr.org.cn).

Keywords: rTMS, older adults, cardiovascular disease, lipid metabolism, HPT axis

INTRODUCTION

Cardiovascular (CV) risk factors, such as hyperlipidemia, diabetes and hypertension, are associated with increased risk of dementia in older adults (Chuang et al., 2014). Longitudinal population-based studies have been used to assess the incidence of dementia in relation to CV diseases (CVD). Kloppenborg et al. (2008) reviewed the evidence for the association of CVD risk factors, including dyslipidemia, obesity, diabetes and hypertension with dementia. They found that these risk factors were indeed associated with an increased risk of dementia. Notably, for older adults, dyslipidemia appears to convey high risk of dementia.

Previous studies showed that cholesterol plays an important role in Alzheimer's disease (AD) as it forms the core of neuritic plaques that characterize AD (Puglielli et al., 2003). Moreover, it has been suggested that blood lipids are promising AD biomarkers. For example, epidemiological studies proposed that high total serum cholesterol in midlife is linked to sporadic AD in old age (Notkola et al., 1998). Lipid measures, such as high-density lipoproteins (HDL) and total cholesterol (Kivipelto et al., 2006; Reitz et al., 2010), are currently used as assessment tools to evaluate the risk of AD and dementia (Wang H. L. et al., 2016). This suggests that vascular risk factors, especially blood lipids, should be regarded as a major target for preventive measures later in life.

It has been suggested that non-invasive brain stimulation (NIBS) is a promising therapeutic tool for CVD (Cogiamanian et al., 2010; Makovac et al., 2017). In a series of meta-analyses, it was demonstrated that NIBS, especially repetitive transcranial magnetic stimulation (rTMS), was effective in reducing the heart rate (HR) and enhancing the HR variability (HRV; Makovac et al., 2017), which are the risk factors for CVD.

George et al. (1996) applied rTMS over the prefrontal cortex (PFC) and found that stimulation of PFC was associated with increases in serum thyroid-stimulating hormone (TSH). Furthermore, in a case study, Trojak et al. (2011) applied rTMS to a patient with depression and demonstrated that serum TSH remained increased during the whole rTMS period. This suggests that rTMS may influence the hypothalamo-pituitary-thyroid (HPT) axis. In cross-sectional studies, serum TSH levels in the upper part of the reference range have been associated with low levels of HDL cholesterol (Boekholdt et al., 2010; Ittermann et al., 2012, 2013). In an 11-year prospective population-based study, it was demonstrated that high TSH levels within the reference range might be associated with decreased serum lipids (Åsvold et al., 2013). In animal studies, it was found that rTMS applied to aged mice could reverse the metabolic abnormalities of cholesterol levels (Wang et al., 2013). It can be speculated, from the above studies, that rTMS might alter the serum lipid level by modulating the HPT axis.

In the present study, we aimed to directly examine the aforementioned hypothesis. Specifically, we investigated the effect of rTMS on the serum lipid level, with rTMS applied over the right PFC. The total cholesterol (CHO), triglyceride (TG), high density lipoprotein cholesterol (HDL-C) and low density lipoprotein cholesterol (LDL-C) were measured as indexes of lipid level. Additionally, TSH, as well as thyroxine (T4), and triiodothyronine (T3), were assessed before and after the treatment. It is expected that lipid levels would be decreased after the session of rTMS treatment, along with alterations of thyroid-related hormones.

MATERIALS AND METHODS

Participants

The participants met the following inclusion criteria: (1) age ≥60 years; (2) education ≥8 years; (3) a score of ≥21 on the Beijing Version of the Montreal cognitive assessment (MoCA; Yu et al., 2012); (4) right-handed; (5) a score of ≥2 on the Chinese memory symptoms scale (CMSS; Lam et al., 2005); (6) eligible for TMS procedures (Rossi et al., 2009). The exclusion criteria were: (1) history of neurological or psychiatric diseases; (2) history of brain damage; (3) history of thyroid disease; (4) dropout from the experiment because of bodily discomfort. All 30 elderly subjects, who were recruited and screened were randomly assigned into the rTMS group (n = 14) or the control (sham) group (n = 16) according to the random number table method.

This research is registered in the Chinese Clinical Trial Registry (ChiCTR-IOR-15006731). This study was carried out in accordance with the recommendations of the institutional review board of the Institute of Psychology, Chinese Academy of Sciences with written informed consent from all subjects. All subjects gave written informed consent in accordance with the Declaration of Helsinki. The protocol was approved by the review board of the First Hospital of Hebei Medical University, as well as the institutional review board of the Institute of Psychology, Chinese Academy of Sciences.

Procedure

Participants were randomly assigned into the rTMS or control group. Both groups participated in rTMS or sham stimulation protocol for 2 weeks, including five sessions every week. The baseline assessment occurred the day before the first stimulation session. The post-intervention assessment occurred 1 day after the final stimulation session. All participants had blood drawn at 8:00 am. Blood samples were collected to detect blood lipids and thyroid hormones. Participants were kept blind to the study hypothesis.

rTMS Protocol

The rTMS was applied with the MagPro X100 stimulator (MagVenture) and figure-of-eight coil (MFC-B65). The right dorsolateral PFC (DLPFC) was the target site, which was defined as the F4 region of the international 10-20 system for electroencephalography. The motor threshold was determined before the stimulation. It was defined as the minimum stimulator output value required to generate contraction of the abductor pollicis brevis for at least 5 of 10 consecutive pulses, and was measured via EMG by means of the Biopac MP100, using a contraction threshold of 50 mV (Moscatelli et al., 2016a,b,c). In each session, 10 Hz of rTMS was applied at 90% motor threshold to the stimulation location. In each stimulation block, rTMS pulses were present for 2 s and absent for 28 s; there were 40 blocks in total. Subjects in the sham stimulation group received the same stimulation protocol applied in the same manner, except that the coil was held at an angle of 90° (Kim et al., 2012).

Output Measures

Hematological Examination

All subjects fasted prior to having blood drawn at 8:00 am before receiving rTMS intervention and the day after the intervention. Blood was drawn using right elbow flexion, routine disinfection and at about 10 ml for each patient. The venous blood was extracted into the coagulation vacuum tube and left at about 25°C for 1 h. The serum was separated with 3000 rotations/min centrifugal force (LODZ-1.2, Beijing centrifuge factory) for 10 min and was kept in a −70°C refrigerator. Before the experiment, serum samples were removed from the refrigerator and were re-dissolved in a water-bath at 37°C water. After the second centrifugation, supernatant was used to measure the indexes. Throughout the whole process, the instrument maintained a good working state, and the quality was controlled in strict accordance with the reagent manual for testing.

Blood Lipids

CHO, TG, HDL-C and LDL-C were measured using the enzyme method. The reagents were sealed away from light, stored at 2–8°C, and could not be inverted.

Thyroid-Related Hormones

T3, T4 and TSH were measured using the electrochemical luminescence method (Roche company cobas e601 automatic immunoassay). The reagents we used were: roche reagents T3 detection kit, Roche reagent T4 detection kit, and Roche reagent thyrotropin detection kit. Reagents were stored at 2–8°C away from light and not inverted.

T3 measurement steps (competition law principle)

1. Take 30 μl of the specimen; mix it with anti-T3 antibody (ruthenium mark) and 8-Anilino-1-naphthalenesulfonic acid (ANS) following the instructions; the ANS release combined T3.
2. Add streptavidin-coated microparticles and biotinylated T3. Biotinylated T3 occupies the relevant binding site on the labeled antibody (still in a free state).
3. Add the mixture to the measurement cell (immune complex), and adsorb the particles to the electrode through the magnet. Form the electrochemical luminescence by adding voltage to the electrode. Use the photomultiplier to detect T3 content.

T4 measurement steps (competition law principle)

1. Take 15 μl of the specimen; mix it with anti-T4 antibody (ruthenium) and ANS following the instructions; the ANS release combined T4.
2. Add streptavidin-coated microparticles and biotinylated T4. Biotinylated T4 occupies the relevant binding site on the labeled antibody (still in a free state).
3. Add the mixture to the measurement cell (immune complex), and adsorb the particles to the electrode through the magnet. Form the electrochemical luminescence by adding voltage to the electrode. Use the photomultiplier to detect T4 content.

TSH assay procedure (double antibody sandwich principle)

1. Take 50 μl of the sample; mix the anti-TSH monoclonal antibody (biotinylated antibody) and anti-TSH monoclonal antibody (ruthenium).
2. Add streptavidin-coated particles to the microparticles, and combine the mixture in step 1 with the microparticles. This combination uses the reaction between biotin and streptavidin.
3. Add the mixture to the measurement cell (immune complex), and adsorb the particles to the electrode through the magnet. Form the electrochemical luminescence by adding voltage to the electrode. Use the photomultiplier to detect TSH content.

Data Analysis

The two-sample two-tailed Student's *t*-test was used to assess the baseline characteristics (age, years of education, scores of CMSS and MoCA) of participants in both groups, and the Chi-squared test was used to assess the gender difference between group. Paired sample *t*-test was used to examine the effect of rTMS/sham stimulation on the serum lipid metabolism activity, as well as on the endocrine activity related to the thyroid. All statistical analyses were conducted using SPSS 19.0 (IBM Corporation, Somers, NY, USA). The absolute effect size, Cohen's d (Cohen, 1988), were calculated to assess the effect of the rTMS intervention.

RESULTS

Demographic Characteristics

No significant differences at baseline were found between the two groups in age, gender, education, memory complaint and MoCA ($p > 0.05$), as shown in **Table 1**.

Effect of rTMS on Lipid Levels

The blood lipid levels between the two groups had no statistical difference at baseline ($p > 0.05$). As shown in **Table 2**, the CHO and TG levels were significantly lower after rTMS intervention ($p < 0.05$). Cohen's d for CHO was 0.54, and that for TG was 0.31. While in the sham group, no significant differences were found between baseline and post-treatment assessments ($p > 0.05$).

Effect of rTMS on Endocrine Activity Related to the Thyroid Gland

Serum thyroid hormone levels between the two groups had no statistical differences at baseline assessment ($p > 0.05$). As shown in **Table 3**, after rTMS intervention, the TSH and T4 levels were found to be significantly higher than those at baseline ($p < 0.05$). Cohen's d for T4 was 0.40, and that for TSH was 0.27. In the sham group, no significant differences were found between pre- and post-assessments ($p > 0.05$).

DISCUSSION

In this study, 10 Hz of rTMS was applied to healthy older adults with normal baseline lipid levels. After 10 sessions of stimulation, CHO and TG levels were significantly decreased, accompanied by increased TSH and T4, compared with the baseline condition, while no significant differences were found in the control group.

TABLE 1 | Characteristics of repetitive transcranial magnetic stimulation (rTMS) and sham groups.

Group	Age (years)	Gender		Education (years)	CMSS	MoCA
		M	F			
rTMS group (n = 14)	65.71 ± 5.08	3	11	12.21 ± 2.75	3.79 ± 1.81	28.07 ± 1.49
Sham group (n = 16)	66.62 ± 5.19	5	11	11.94 ± 3.04	4.25 ± 1.61	28 ± 2.07
p	>0.05[a]	>0.05[b]		>0.05[a]	>0.05[a]	>0.05[a]

Note: CMSS, the Chinese Memory Symptoms Scale; MoCA, the Beijing Version of the Montreal cognitive assessment. [a]The p value was obtained using a two-sample two-tailed t test. [b]The p value was obtained using a two-tailed Pearson chi-square test. Data are shown as mean ± SD.

TABLE 2 | Comparison of lipid levels (mmol/L) between rTMS and sham groups.

Group	Test	CHO	TG	HDL-C	LDL-C
rTMS (n = 14)	Pre	6.23 ± 1.82	1.94 ± 1.49	1.43 ± 0.80	3.68 ± 0.79
	Post	5.37 ± 1.33	1.54 ± 1.10	1.19 ± 0.40	3.15 ± 1.28
	t	2.682*	2.513*	1.552	1.636
Sham (n = 16)	Pre	5.26 ± 1.25	1.45 ± 1.06	1.17 ± 0.33	3.25 ± 0.89
	Post	5.76 ± 1.70	1.68 ± 1.03	1.3 ± 0.52	3.48 ± 0.97
	t	−1.704	−1.706	−1.273	−1.519

*Note: CHO, the total cholesterol; TG, triglyceride; HDL-C, high density lipoprotein cholesterol; LDL-C, low density lipoprotein cholesterol. *$p < 0.05$, two-tailed. Data are shown as mean ± SD.*

TABLE 3 | Comparison of thyroid hormone levels (nmol/L) between rTMS and sham groups.

Test	rTMS (n = 14)			Sham (n = 16)		
	T3	T4	TSH	T3	T4	TSH
Pre	1.65 ± 0.19	93.63 ± 14.24	3.45 ± 2.76	1.79 ± 0.25	102.53 ± 12.23	3.45 ± 2.35
Post	1.70 ± 0.25	99.14 ± 13.18	4.31 ± 3.56	1.75 ± 0.26	102.05 ± 10.55	3.32 ± 2.24
t	1.744	3.248**	2.379*	−0.428	−0.099	−0.181

*Note: T3, triiodothyronine; T4, thyroxine; TSH, the thyroid-stimulating hormone. *$p < 0.05$, **$p < 0.01$, two-tailed. Data are shown as mean ± SD.*

Our results indicate that rTMS may be effective for CVD risk factors. Previous studies confirmed the effect of rTMS on CV systems indexed by HR and HRV. In this study, we investigated the effect of rTMS on endocrine activity related to CVD risk factors and found that decreased serum lipid levels resulted from rTMS, suggesting rTMS influence on endocrine activity. In an animal study, Wang et al. (2013) explored the metabolic mechanism underlying the effects of rTMS. They observed that in mature mice, rTMS could reverse the metabolic abnormalities of cholesterol levels, to a degree similar to the young mice, showing that the rTMS could improve the metabolic profiles in PFC. Combining the present study with previous studies shows that rTMS could modulate the lipid metabolic activity associated with CVD.

The effect of rTMS on the serum lipid metabolic activity might result from its influence on the HPT axis. George et al. (1996) found that rTMS, applied over regions within the PFC, was associated with increases in serum TSH. Furthermore, Trojak et al. (2011) reported a significant increase in plasma TSH, above normal range, during low frequency rTMS (1 Hz) treatment. In addition, Osuch et al. (2009) demonstrated an increase in plasma T4 during treatment of anxiety disorders using low frequency rTMS. Thus, it can be inferred that rTMS may have significant effects on the pituitary-thyroid axis, which may potentially induce hyperthyroidism. Similar to previous studies, our study found significantly elevated TSH after rTMS, along with increased T4. Furthermore, in this study, we directly observed the alteration of serum lipid levels, suggesting that rTMS may influence the HPT axis and then affect the serum lipid levels.

Based on animal studies, we had confirmed that both normal aging (Wang et al., 2014) and pathological aging (Han et al., 2016; Wang J. et al., 2016; Shen et al., 2017) lead to metabolic abnormalities and that rTMS treatment could ameliorate metabolic abnormalities (Wang H. L. et al., 2016). For example, rTMS normalized prefrontal dysfunctions and cognitive-related metabolic profiling in aged mice (Wang H. L. et al., 2016). Besides, Lee et al. (2012) found that the effects of rTMS are related to changes in the brain lipids. In human studies, it also has been found that rTMS affects cortical metabolism (Bohning et al., 1999; Kimbrell et al., 2002). In the present study, we found that rTMS applied over the right DLPFC could alter the endocrine activity in normal aging adults. Combined evidence suggested that there is a pathway between the PFC and the hypothalamus, through which the PFC could modulate the endocrine activity.

As a non-invasive tool for the electrical stimulation of neural tissue (Barker et al., 1985), rTMS has the potential to modify excitability of the cerebral cortex at the stimulated site and at remote areas along functional anatomical connections (for a review, see Rossini et al., 2010). The PFC is linked to the thalamus (Alexander et al., 1986; Jones, 2007; Bolkan et al., 2017), and as a result, rTMS applied to the DLPFC might modulate the neural activity in the thalamus, which would then have an effect on the activity of the hypothalamus. The hypothalamus links the nervous system to the endocrine system, via the pituitary gland, in order to modulate the serum metabolic activity. It can be speculated that the PFC-thalamus pathway might play an important role in the present study to influence the HPT axis, and finally to modulate the serum metabolic activity of lipid levels.

Previous studies showed that CVD risk factors could be reduced with aerobic exercises. In a meta-analysis, Kodama et al. (2007) demonstrated that regular aerobic exercise could increase HDL-C level, which is associated with decreased risk of CVD (Maron, 2000). Alternative to physical exercise, in this study, the non-invasive rTMS is demonstrated as another promising tool for modulating CVD risk factors, specifically lipid levels, suggesting that rTMS is effective in minimizing CVD prevalence. Aerobic exercise may influence CV fitness, which results in changes to endocrine activity. While the effect of rTMS on endocrine activity might result from the altered excitability of the neuron, which may influence the signaling pathway of the HPT axis. This suggests that there is a pathway that underlies the transmission between electric signal and chemical signal. Future research on this issue is of great importance.

CONCLUSION

rTMS of the PFC is associated with increases in the TSH and T4 levels and decreases in the serum CHO and TG levels. rTMS might alter the serum lipid levels by modulating the activity of the HPT axis. It is a promising tool for the modulation of lipid metabolism in older adults, and it reduces the risk for AD. In future studies, more indexes related to lipid metabolism and the activity of the HPT axis need to be assessed to clarify the effect of rTMS on the risk for CVD and to examine the direct relationship between lipid metabolism and the activity of the HPT axis following rTMS.

AUTHOR CONTRIBUTIONS

WR designed the work and drafted the manuscript. JM collected and analyzed the data. JL guided the research project. ZZ and MW revised the work and agreed to be accountable for all aspects of the work.

REFERENCES

Alexander, G. E., DeLong, M. R., and Strick, P. L. (1986). Parallel organization of functionally segregated circuits linking basal ganglia and cortex. *Annu. Rev. Neurosci.* 9, 357–381. doi: 10.1146/annurev.neuro.9.1.357

Åsvold, B. O., Bjøro, T., and Vatten, L. J. (2013). Associations of TSH levels within the reference range with future blood pressure and lipid concentrations: 11-year follow-up of the HUNT study. *Eur. J. Endocrinol.* 169, 73–82. doi: 10.1530/EJE-13-0087

Barker, A. T., Jalinous, R., and Freeston, I. L. (1985). Non-invasive magnetic stimulation of human motor cortex. *Lancet* 325, 1106–1107. doi: 10.1016/s0140-6736(85)92413-4

Boekholdt, S. M., Titan, S. M., Wiersinga, W. M., Chatterjee, K., Basart, D. C., Luben, R., et al. (2010). Initial thyroid status and cardiovascular risk factors: the EPIC-Norfolk prospective population study. *Clin. Endocrinol.* 72, 404–410. doi: 10.1111/j.1365-2265.2009.03640.x

Bohning, D., Shastri, A., McConnell, K., Nahas, Z., Lorberbaum, J., Roberts, D., et al. (1999). A combined TMS/fMRI study of intensity-dependent TMS over motor cortex. *Biol. Psychiatry* 45, 385–394. doi: 10.1016/s0006-3223(98)00368-0

Bolkan, S. S., Stujenske, J. M., Parnaudeau, S., Spellman, T. J., Rauffenbart, C., Abbas, A. I., et al. (2017). Thalamic projections sustain prefrontal activity during working memory maintenance. *Nat. Neurosci.* 20, 987–996. doi: 10.1038/nn.4568

Chuang, Y. F., Eldreth, D., Erickson, K. I., Varma, V., Harris, G., Fried, L. P., et al. (2014). Cardiovascular risks and brain function: a functional magnetic resonance imaging study of executive function in older adults. *Neurobiol. Aging* 35, 1396–1403. doi: 10.1016/j.neurobiolaging.2013.12.008

Cogiamanian, F., Brunoni, A. R., Boggio, P. S., Fregni, F., Ciocca, M., and Priori, A. (2010). Non-invasive brain stimulation for the management of arterial hypertension. *Med. Hypotheses* 74, 332–336. doi: 10.1016/j.mehy.2009.08.037

Cohen, J. (1988). *Statistical Power Analysis for the Behavioral Sciences.* 2nd Edn. Hillsdale, NJ: Lawrence Earlbam Associates.

George, M. S., Wassermann, E. M., Williams, W. A., Steppel, J., Pascual-Leone, A., Basser, P., et al. (1996). Changes in mood and hormone levels after rapid-rate transcranial magnetic stimulation (rTMS) of the prefrontal cortex. *J. Neuropsychiatry Clin. Neurosci.* 8, 172–180. doi: 10.1176/jnp.8.2.172

Han, B., Yu, L., Geng, Y., Shen, L., Wang, H., Wang, Y., et al. (2016). Chronic stress aggravates cognitive impairment and suppresses insulin associated signaling pathway in APP/PS1 mice. *J. Alzheimers Dis.* 53, 1539–1552. doi: 10.3233/JAD-160189

Ittermann, T., Thamm, M., Wallaschofski, H., Rettig, R., and Völzke, H. (2012). Serum thyroid-stimulating hormone levels are associated with blood pressure in children and adolescents. *J. Clin. Endocrinol. Metab.* 97, 828–834. doi: 10.1210/jc.2011-2768

Ittermann, T., Tiller, D., Meisinger, C., Agger, C., Nauck, M., Rettig, R., et al. (2013). High serum thyrotropin levels are associated with current but not with incident hypertension. *Thyroid* 23, 955–963. doi: 10.1089/thy.2012.0626

Jones, E. G. (2007). *The Thalamus.* 2nd Edn. Cambridge, MA: Cambridge University Press.

Kim, S. H., Han, H. J., Ahn, H. M., Kim, S. A., and Kim, S. E. (2012). Effects of five daily high-frequency rTMS on Stroop task performance in aging individuals. *Neurosci. Res.* 74, 256–260. doi: 10.1016/j.neures.2012.08.008

Kimbrell, T. A., Dunn, R. T., George, M. S., Danielson, A. L., Willis, M. W., Repella, J. D., et al. (2002). Left prefrontal-repetitive transcranial magnetic stimulation (rTMS) and regional cerebral glucose metabolism in normal volunteers. *Psychiatry Res.* 115, 101–113. doi: 10.1016/s0925-4927(02)00041-0

Kivipelto, M., Ngandu, T., Laatikainen, T., Winblad, B., Soininen, H., and Tuomilehto, J. (2006). Risk score for the prediction of dementia risk in 20 years among middle aged people: a longitudinal, population-based study. *Lancet Neurol.* 5, 735–741. doi: 10.1016/s1474-4422(06)70537-3

Kloppenborg, R. P., van den Berg, E., Kappelle, L. J., and Biessels, G. J. (2008). Diabetes and other vascular risk factors for dementia: which factor matters most? A systematic review. *Eur. J. Pharmacol.* 585, 97–108. doi: 10.1016/j.ejphar.2008.02.049

Kodama, S., Tanaka, S., Saito, K., Shu, M., Sone, Y., Onitake, F., et al. (2007). Effect of aerobic exercise training on serum levels of high-density lipoprotein cholesterol: a meta-analysis. *Arch. Int. Med.* 167, 999–1008. doi: 10.1001/archinte.167.10.999

Lam, L. C. W., Lui, V. W. C., Tam, C. W. C., and Chiu, H. F. K. (2005). Subjective memory complaints in Chinese subjects with mild cognitive impairment and early Alzheimer's disease. *Int. J. Geriatr. Psychiatry* 20, 876–882. doi: 10.1002/gps.1370

Lee, L. H. W., Tan, C. H., Lo, Y. L., Farooqui, A. A., Shui, G., Wenk, M. R., et al. (2012). Brain lipid changes after repetitive transcranial magnetic stimulation: potential links to therapeutic effects? *Metabolomics* 8, 19–33. doi: 10.1007/s11306-011-0285-4

Makovac, E., Thayer, J. F., and Ottaviani, C. (2017). A meta-analysis of non-invasive brain stimulation and autonomic functioning: implications for brain-heart pathways to cardiovascular disease. *Neurosci. Biobehav. Rev.* 74, 330–341. doi: 10.1016/j.neubiorev.2016.05.001

Maron, D. J. (2000). The epidemiology of low levels of high-density lipoprotein cholesterol in patients with and without coronary artery disease. *Am. J. Cardiol.* 86, 11L–14L. doi: 10.1016/s0002-9149(00)01462-4

Moscatelli, F., Messina, G., Valenzano, A., Monda, V., Viggiano, A., Messina, A., et al. (2016a). Functional assessment of corticospinal system excitability in karate athletes. *PLoS One* 11:e0155998. doi: 10.1371/journal.pone.0155998

Moscatelli, F., Messina, G., Valenzano, A., Petito, A., Triggiani, A. I., Messina, A., et al. (2016b). Differences in corticospinal system activity and reaction response between karate athletes and non-athletes. *Neurol. Sci.* 37, 1947–1953. doi: 10.1007/s10072-016-2693-8

Moscatelli, F., Valenzano, A., Petito, A., Triggiani, A. I., Ciliberti, M. A. P., Luongo, L., et al. (2016c). Relationship between blood lactate and cortical excitability between taekwondo athletes and non-athletes after hand-grip exercise. *Somatosensory Mot. Res.* 33, 137–144. doi: 10.1080/08990220.2016.1203305

Notkola, I. L., Sulkava, R., Pekkanen, J., Erkinjuntti, T., Ehnholm, C., Kivinen, P., et al. (1998). Serum total cholesterol, apolipoprotein E {FC12}e4 allele, and Alzheimer's disease. *Neuroepidemiology* 17, 14–20. doi: 10.1159/000026149

Osuch, E. A., Benson, B. E., Luckenbaugh, D. A., Geraci, M., Post, R. M., and McCann, U. (2009). Repetitive TMS combined with exposure therapy for

PTSD: a preliminary study. *J. Anxiety Disord.* 23, 54–59. doi: 10.1016/j.janxdis.2008.03.015

Puglielli, L., Tanzi, R. E., and Kovacs, D. M. (2003). Alzheimer's disease: the cholesterol connection. *Nat. Neurosci.* 6, 345–351. doi: 10.1038/nn0403-345

Reitz, C., Tang, M., Schupf, N., Manly, J. J., Mayeux, R., and Luchsinger, J. A. (2010). A summary risk score for the prediction of alzheimer disease in elderly persons. *Arch. Neurol.* 67, 835–841. doi: 10.1001/archneurol.2010.136

Rossi, S., Hallett, M., Rossini, P. M., and Pascual-Leone, A. (2009). Safety, ethical considerations, and application guidelines for the use of transcranial magnetic stimulation in clinical practice and research. *Clin. Neurophysiol.* 120, 2008–2039. doi: 10.1016/j.clinph.2009.08.016

Rossini, P. M., Rossini, L., and Ferreri, F. (2010). Brain-behavior relations: transcranial magnetic stimulation: a review. *IEEE Eng. Med. Biol. Mag.* 29, 84–96. doi: 10.1109/MEMB.2009.935474

Shen, L., Han, B., Geng, Y., Wang, J., Wang, Z., and Wang, M. (2017). Amelioration of cognitive impairments in APPswe/PS1dE9 mice is associated with metabolites alteration induced by total salvianolic acid. *PLoS One* 12:e0174763. doi: 10.1371/journal.pone.0174763

Trojak, B., Chauvet-Gelinier, J.-C., Vergès, B., and Bonin, B. (2011). Significant increase in plasma thyroid-stimulating hormone during low-frequency repetitive transcranial magnetic stimulation. *J. Neuropsychiatry Clin. Neurosci.* 23:E12. doi: 10.1176/appi.neuropsych.23.1.e12

Wang, H., Geng, Y., Han, B., Qiang, J., Li, X., Sun, M., et al. (2013). Repetitive transcranial magnetic stimulation applications normalized prefrontal dysfunctions and cognitive-related metabolic profiling in aged mice. *PLoS One* 8:e81482. doi: 10.1371/journal.pone.0081482

Wang, H., Lian, K., Han, B., Wang, Y., Kuo, S. H., Geng, Y., et al. (2014). Age-related alterations in the metabolic profile in the hippocampus of the senescence-accelerated mouse prone 8: a spontaneous Alzheimer's disease mouse model. *J. Alzheimers Dis.* 39, 841–848. doi: 10.3233/JAD-131463

Wang, H. L., Wang, Y. Y., Liu, X. G., Kuo, S. H., Liu, N., Song, Q. Y., et al. (2016). Cholesterol, 24-hydroxycholesterol, and 27-hydroxycholesterol as surrogate biomarkers in cerebrospinal fluid in mild cognitive impairment and Alzheimer's disease: a meta-analysis. *J. Alzheimers Dis.* 51, 45–55. doi: 10.3233/JAD-150734

Wang, J., Yuan, J., Pang, J., Ma, J., Han, B., Geng, Y., et al. (2016). Effects of chronic stress on cognition in male SAMP8 mice. *Cell. Physiol. Biochem.* 39, 1078–1086. doi: 10.1159/000447816

Yu, J., Li, J., and Huang, X. (2012). The Beijing version of the montreal cognitive assessment as a brief screening tool for mild cognitive impairment: a community-based study. *BMC Psychiatry* 12:156. doi: 10.1186/1471-244X-12-156

13

Dissecting Endoplasmic Reticulum Unfolded Protein Response (UPR^{ER}) in Managing Clandestine Modus Operandi of Alzheimer's Disease

*Safikur Rahman[1], Ayyagari Archana[2], Arif Tasleem Jan[3] and Rinki Minakshi[4]**

[1]*Department of Medical Biotechnology, Yeungnam University, Gyeongsan, South Korea,* [2]*Department of Microbiology, Swami Shraddhanand College, University of Delhi, New Delhi, India,* [3]*School of Biosciences and Biotechnology, Baba Ghulam Shah Badshah University, Rajouri, India,* [4]*Institute of Home Economics, University of Delhi, New Delhi, India*

***Correspondence:**
Rinki Minakshi
rinki.minakshi@hotmail.com;
minakshi4050@gmail.com

Alzheimer's disease (AD), a neurodegenerative disorder, is most common cause of dementia witnessed among aged people. The pathophysiology of AD develops as a consequence of neurofibrillary tangle formation which consists of hyperphosphorylated microtubule associated tau protein and senile plaques of amyloid-β (Aβ) peptide in specific brain regions that result in synaptic loss and neuronal death. The feeble buffering capacity of endoplasmic reticulum (ER) proteostasis in AD is evident through alteration in unfolded protein response (UPR), where UPR markers express invariably in AD patient's brain samples. Aging weakens UPR^{ER} causing neuropathology and memory loss in AD. This review highlights molecular signatures of UPR^{ER} and its key molecular alliance that are affected in aging leading to the development of intriguing neuropathologies in AD. We present a summary of recent studies reporting usage of small molecules as inhibitors or activators of UPR^{ER} sensors/effectors in AD that showcase avenues for therapeutic interventions.

Keywords: Alzheimer disease, neurodegenerative diseases, endoplasmic reticulum stress (ER), aging, UPR (unfolded protein response)

INTRODUCTION

Alzheimer's disease (AD), the most common form of dementia faced by more than 40 million people worldwide, significantly affect morbidity and mortality in aged people (Alzheimer's Association, 2016; Fiest et al., 2016; Scheltens et al., 2016; Cass, 2017). The most vulnerable group falling as target is above 65 years, which puts aging as the crucial risk factor associated with development of the disease (Alzheimer's Association, 2016; Fiest et al., 2016; Scheltens et al., 2016; Cass, 2017). AD is a progressively neurodegenerative disorder, characterized by cognitive alterations and behavioral changes that owe to synaptic impairment and loss of neurons (Alzheimer's Association, 2016; Scheltens et al., 2016). Mutations in genes encoding APP (amyloid precursor protein), presenilin 1 and 2 (PS1 and PS2 respectively), as well as ε4 allele of Apolipoprotein E are reported to be linked to rare familial and early development of AD (Selkoe, 2001a,b; Scheltens et al., 2016). AD leads to the formation of neurofibrillary tangles having hyperphosphorylated microtubule associated tau protein and senile plaques of amyloid-β (Aβ) peptide in specific brain regions, result in brain inflammation, astrogliosis and microglial proliferation (Citron, 2002; Selkoe, 2004a,b; Cleary et al., 2005; Haass and Selkoe, 2007; Atwood and Bowen, 2015; Minter et al., 2016; Sami et al., 2017). Gradual accumulation of Aβ peptide attributed to β- and γ-secretases action on the APP, results in synaptic loss and neuronal death (Chyung et al., 2005; Tatarnikova et al., 2015).

The expression pattern of neurodegenerative pathologies shows distinct molecular signatures, such as misfolded Aβ aggregation and tau protein hyperphosphorylation in the brain (Jiang et al., 2010; Atwood and Bowen, 2015; Sami et al., 2017). How this load of protein aggregates disrupt the neuronal function is still a mystery to medical science? In this review, we have tried to focus on the role of ER stress and the ensuing unfolded protein response (UPR^{ER}) imposed on the neuronal cell due to misfolded protein aggregates. Also, we have discussed various therapeutic interventions targeting the molecules involved in UPR pathways aiming at averting the neuropathologies of AD.

ER STRESS AND UPR^{ER}

Adversities in the endoplasmic reticulum (ER) microenvironment like nutrient deprivation, changes in redox potential, calcium homeostasis, hypoxia and accumulation of unfolded/misfolded protein triggers the UPR^{ER} (Schroder and Kaufman, 2005; Moneim, 2015). UPR^{ER} is a highly conserved signaling cascade in all eukaryotes involved in the cellular homeostasis (Ellgaard and Helenius, 2003; Mori, 2009; Walter and Ron, 2011) through transcriptional remodeling of ER proteostasis pathways (Lee et al., 2003; Yamamoto et al., 2007; Shoulders et al., 2013; Genereux et al., 2015). The ER lumen harbors various molecular chaperones like the Glucose Regulated Protein 78 kDa (GRP78) that are recruited to misfolded nascent peptides for aiding in their proper folding (Bertolotti et al., 2000; Shen et al., 2002). A plethora of studies have reported UPR^{ER} upregulation in the brain samples of Alzheimer's patients (Hamos et al., 1991; Hoozemans et al., 2005, 2009).

The UPR^{ER} embodies a complex network comprised of three stress-responsive transmembrane proteins, Protein Kinase RNA like ER kinase (PERK), Inositol Requiring Element 1 (IRE1) and Activating Transcription Factor 6 (ATF6; **Figure 1**; Schroder and Kaufman, 2005; Walter and Ron, 2011; Minakshi et al., 2017; Rahman et al., 2017). PERK, a type 1 transmembrane kinase protein, gets trans-autophosphorylated and homodimerized after activation, thereby promoting phosphorylation of serine residues on cytoplasmic eIF2α (eukaryotic initiation factor 2 alpha; Harding et al., 1999; Bertolotti et al., 2000; Ma et al., 2002; Marciniak et al., 2006). Despite the general translational halt induced by the phosphorylated eIF2α (eIF2α-P), certain specific mRNAs bearing internal ribosome entry site (IRES), like the Activating Transcription Factor 4 (ATF4) mRNAs continues to be translated (Harding et al., 2000a; Baumeister et al., 2005). ATF4 regulates genes for various foldases, chaperones, regulatory proteins of the redox and autophagy, cholesterol metabolism etc. (Harding et al., 2003; Fusakio et al., 2016). CCAAT enhancer-binding (C/EBP) protein homologous protein (CHOP) is also a direct target of ATF4 and represents the pro-apoptotic component of the UPR^{ER} (Han et al., 2013). In a study, wild type mice subjected to tunicamycin injection showed higher degrees of apoptosis in their renal epithelium as compared to CHOP knockout mice (Marciniak et al., 2004; Onuki et al., 2004). PERK also induces the activation of another transcription factor nuclear factor (erythroid derived 2)-like 2 (Nrf2) independent of eIF2α, which regulates the antioxidant response (Cullinan et al., 2003; Cullinan and Diehl, 2004).

IRE1 is the most evolutionarily conserved ER stress transducer (Tirasophon et al., 1998), which upon activation, undergoes dimerization and trans-autophosphorylation, leading to the activation of its cytosolic endoribonuclease activity that splices a 26-nucleotide intron from the mRNA encoding transcription factor X box binding protein 1 (XBP1) forming XBP1(S) (Yoshida et al., 2001, 2003). The XBP1(S) upregulates genes involved in ER protein maturation and ER-associated degradation (ERAD; Lee et al., 2003; Acosta-Alvear et al., 2007). Cells lacking XBP1 are more sensitive to hypoxia-induced apoptosis (Romero-Ramirez et al., 2004). Upon activation, IRE1 also activates c-Jun N-terminal kinase (JNK) through tumor necrosis factor receptor-associated factor 2 (TRAF2); Zeng et al., 2015). IRE1-mediated JNK activation has been demonstrated to trigger autophagy under ER-stress (Urano et al., 2000).

ATF6 is a type II transmembrane protein, with a basic leucine zipper (bZIP) domain (Yoshida et al., 1998). During the imposed stress, luminal domain of ATF6 loses its association with GRP78, triggering the translocation of ATF6 into the Golgi apparatus where two intramembrane Golgi specific proteases, site 1 protease (S1P) and site 2 protease (S2P), process it. The N-terminal cleaved product p50ATF6 of full length ATF6 (p90ATF), then acts as a transcription factor, which upregulates several genes, including GRP78, Protein Disulfide Isomerase (PDI), XBP1 and CHOP (Haze et al., 1999; Walter and Ron, 2011).

UPR^{ER} IN ALZHEIMER'S DISEASE

In neuronal pathophysiology, the activation of UPR^{ER} can have paradoxical affects. During stress condition, activation of UPR^{ER} could reactivate proteostasis; thereby rescuing the neurons by escalating the rate of protein folding through molecular chaperones, or may trigger neurodegeneration and neuronal collapse through the expression of apoptotic markers.

Evidences support the presence of abundant hyperphosphorylated tau protein and ER stress markers in the neurons of the cortex in postmortem brain samples of AD patients (Scheper and Hoozemans, 2015). It is presumed that ER stress is a cell death mechanism triggered by Aβ, and is linked to changes in ER calcium homeostasis (Cornejo and Hetz, 2013). Under the influence of Aβ imposed ER stress, Ca^{2+} leaching from ER is taken up by mitochondria leading to activation of apoptotic death of neurons (Fonseca et al., 2013). The presenilins are responsible for passive ER Ca^{2+} outflow. Documents support that aging neurons fail to maintain tight Ca^{2+} homeostasis across plasma membrane and ER

(Supnet and Bezprozvanny, 2010). Such effects paved the way for "calcium hypothesis of brain aging and AD" (Khachaturian, 1989). Rise in prolonged imbalanced Ca^{2+} invites ROS accumulation and mitochondrial dysfunction resulting in neuronal death (Supnet and Bezprozvanny, 2010). ER stress may display binary role in AD, firstly modulating the production kinetics of amyloid plaques and secondly altering the cognitive functions in a distinct way (Halliday and Mallucci, 2015). Neurons of AD patients were also characterized by GRP78 induction in temporal cortex and hippocampus and phosphorylation of PERK (p-PERK; Hoozemans et al., 2005).

Active protein synthesis is a hallmark feature of synaptic plasticity and consolidation of memory (Costa-Mattioli et al., 2009). PERK signaling and protein translation control was linked to the cognitive impairment observed in AD models (Devi and Ohno, 2013, 2014). Impairment of cognitive functions due to the reduction in synaptic protein synthesis is displayed during increased phosphorylation of eIF2α (Costa-Mattioli et al., 2005, 2009; Jiang et al., 2010). Mitigating the expression of PERK improves cognitive function and synaptic plasticity in an AD model (Devi and Ohno, 2014). Moreover, targeting other eIF2α kinases like General Control Nonderepressible-2 (GCN2) and dsRNA-dependent protein kinase R (PKR) was also witnessed not only to improve learning and memory processes (Devi and Ohno, 2013), but also reduced inflammation (Lourenco et al., 2013). These results significantly indicate that genetic manipulation of PERK improved cognitive ability of cells to survive under stress conditions induced by Aβ deposition.

The activation of UPR^{ER} in early stages of AD could be protective through activation of autophagy. However, sustained UPR^{ER} activation may be detrimental to the neurons (Hoozemans et al., 2005; Nijholt et al., 2011). The expression of XBP1 in *Drosophila* where the AD-associated Aβ peptide was expressed in neurons, led to reduced neurotoxicity, supporting the cytoprotective role of XBP1 (Casas-Tinto et al., 2011). In *Caenorhabditis elegans* (*C. elegans*) models expressing aggregation-prone mutant tau variants, XBP-1 was identified to be playing a similar protective role (Kraemer et al., 2006; Loewen and Feany, 2010). However, reports also suggest that IRE1 interacts with PS1 leading to activation of proapoptotic signaling by JNK (Shoji et al., 2000). The JNK3 (member of JNK family) localized in brain, is highly expressed in brain tissue and cerebrospinal fluid sample from AD patients (Gourmaud et al., 2015) and the activation of JNK3 exacerbates stress perpetuating AD pathology (Yoon and Jo, 2012).

AGING, UPR^{ER} AND ALZHEIMER'S DISEASE

Aging is the single most important risk factor for AD. Decline in the UPR^{ER} with advancing age marked by the oxidative damage of ER chaperones, leads to disempowering of protein folding capacity (Rabek et al., 2003; Nuss et al., 2008). Studies report that the levels of GRP78 were low in murine cortex, in rat hippocampus, cortex, cerebellum, as well as in a multitude of organs (Paz Gavilán et al., 2006; Hussain and Ramaiah, 2007; Naidoo et al., 2008). Transcription of PERK mRNA were lowered in the aging rat hippocampus, while an increment was reported in the expression of growth arrest and DNA damage protein 34 (GADD34), because it escapes the effect of eIF2α-P translational inhibition (Paz Gavilán et al., 2006). Studies on *C. elegans* revealed that the activation of IRE1 branch of the UPR^{ER} diminishes during the fertile period of adulthood, manifesting in lowered immunity against ER stress (Taylor and Dillin, 2013). The implication of IRE1/XBP1 tier in aging was proven in *C. elegans* where IRE1 defect reduced life span (Chen et al., 2009).

MITOCHONDRIA, OXIDATIVE STRESS AND ALZHEIMER'S DISEASE

Under the imposed stress, apart from UPR^{ER} coming to the rescue, the herald of mitochondrial UPR (UPR^{mt}) ensuing after accumulation of unfolded peptide load is well documented. The pathway focuses on invigorating folding and degradation of misfolded peptides in mitochondrial matrix through the execution of retrograde transcriptional activation (Arnould et al., 2015). AD being a multifactorial malady, the accumulation of Aβ not only affects ER but also mitochondria. There are accumulating evidences, which support deposition of Aβ in mitochondrial matrix disrupting signaling of the organelle thereby leading to neurodegeneration (Kawamata and Manfredi, 2017). Impairment in the production and functionalities of metabolic enzymes preferentially of TCA cycle disturbs energy metabolism of the brain. Mitochondrial dysfunction causes depletion of cellular ATP pool and enhanced ROS production, which is well implicated in the pathogenesis of AD (Swerdlow et al., 2014; Hoekstra et al., 2016). Besides, impairment of mitochondrial turnover and function in brain, aging potentiates oxidative stress, leading to significant decrease in the cytochrome C oxidase activity that is associated with rise in oxygen radicals in different regions of postmortem AD brain (**Figure 2**; Hirai et al., 2001; Mosconi et al., 2007; Krishnan et al., 2012). A strong correlation of the cognitive decline with increase in oxidative stress is observed in AD patients (Revel et al., 2015). Incidence of aberrant Aβ processing ensues after the oxidation of mitochondrial DNA (mtDNA) under stressful circumstances (Volgyi et al., 2015).

Aberrations in mtDNA have been well studied in AD. In an elegant study by Aliev et al. (2013) mtDNA-proliferation and deletion has been reported in AD tissues. Furthermore, the report also illustrates abnormal mitochondrial function in damaged hippocampal neurons in human AD as well as transgenic AD models. In another study using *in situ* hybridization, Aliev et al. (2008) detected a 5 kB deletion in mtDNA under oxidative stress in abnormal neurons. Such mitochondrial anomalies were also reported to help in AD pathogenesis in Aβ transgenic mice (Aliev et al., 2008).

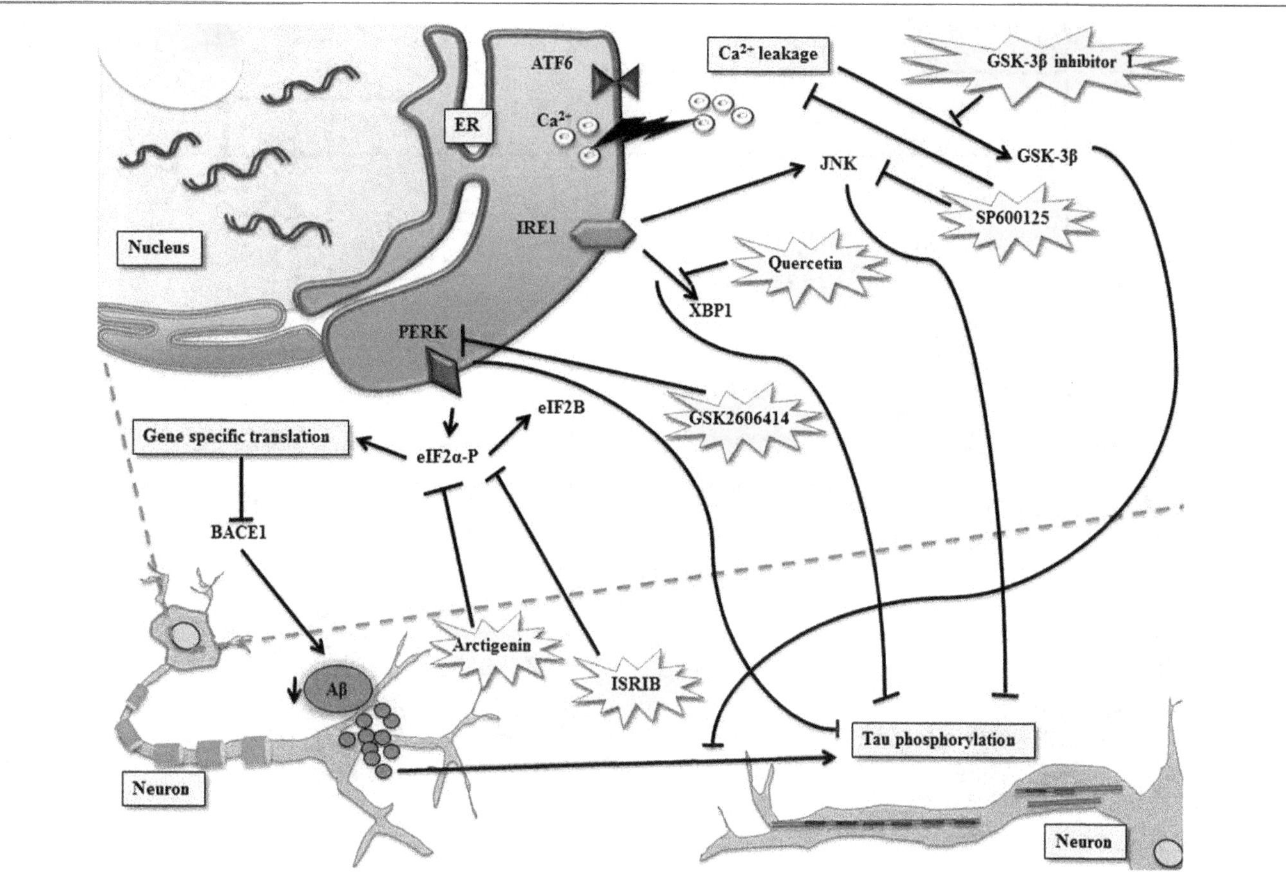

FIGURE 1 | Targeting unfolded protein response (UPR) to manage Alzheimer's disease (AD) with specific molecules. *PERK/eIF2α*: the phosphorylation of eIF2α shuts down global translation in the cell but for gene-specific translation upregulation of mRNA with internal ribosome entry site (IRES), for example β-site APP cleaving enzyme-1 (BACE1), the β-secretase enzyme (Ohno, 2014). Arctigenin, targets eIF2α-P thereby downregulating BACE1, consequently protects neurons from amyloid-β (Aβ) toxicity. ISRIB, affects eIF2B leading to inhibition of eIF2α-P, which comprehensively restores protein translation and hence enhances long term memory. PERK can be directly inhibited by GSK2606414, leading to halt in tau phosphorylation. Ca^{2+} leakage induced activation of glycogen synthase kinase-3β (GSK-3β) can be checked by GSK-3β inhibitor I, which prevents Aβ induced phosphorylation of tau. *IRE1/XBP1*: Quercetin, activates endoribonuclease activity of IRE1 inhibiting tau hyperphosphorylation. The c-Jun N-terminal kinase (JNK) inhibitor, SP600125, inhibits Ca^{2+} leakage and inhibits Aβ-induced c-Jun phosphorylation.

In a study proving the existence of interlink between mitochondrial dysfunction and AD, the pharmacological/genetic targeting of mitochondrial translation process not only increased life span of GMC101 (model of Aβ proteotoxicity), but also showed reduction in beta-amyloid aggregation in worms and transgenic mouse models of AD (Sorrentino et al., 2017). Treatment of the mitochondrial division inhibitor-1 (mdiv-1) that inhibits mitochondrial fragmentation, thereby rescuing mitochondrial distribution, improves mitochondrial function in CRND8 (AD mouse model) neurons (Reddy et al., 2017; Wang et al., 2017). Treatment with mdivi-1 also causes a decrease in extracellular amyloid deposition and Aβ1–42/Aβ1–40 ratio (Wang et al., 2017). Additionally, SIRT-3, a sirtuin localized to inner mitochondrial membrane, has been found associated with enhancement in the levels of glutathione (Onyango et al., 2002; Someya et al., 2010). As downregulation of SIRT-3 was found to be having a retrograde effect on p53 mediated mitochondrial and neuronal damage in AD, its modulation by therapeutics was found to ameliorate mitochondrial pathology and neurodegeneration in AD (Lee et al., 2018).

DERANGEMENT OF GLUCOSE METABOLISM IN ALZHEIMER'S DISEASE: THE FALLIBLE UPR^{ER}

Among the many observed hallmarks of AD, positron emission tomography (PET) revealed a deranged glucose metabolism in brain regions. Aging registers diminished brain glucose utilization that surges in AD (Ivançević et al., 2000). Various reports suggest that UPR^{ER} is linked to abnormal glucose metabolism and insulin resistance (Hetz et al., 2015). Type 2 diabetes mellitus (T2DM) has been mechanistically linked to AD pathogenesis, where higher insulin resistance poses a greater risk of AD with reduced glucose uptake in the brain

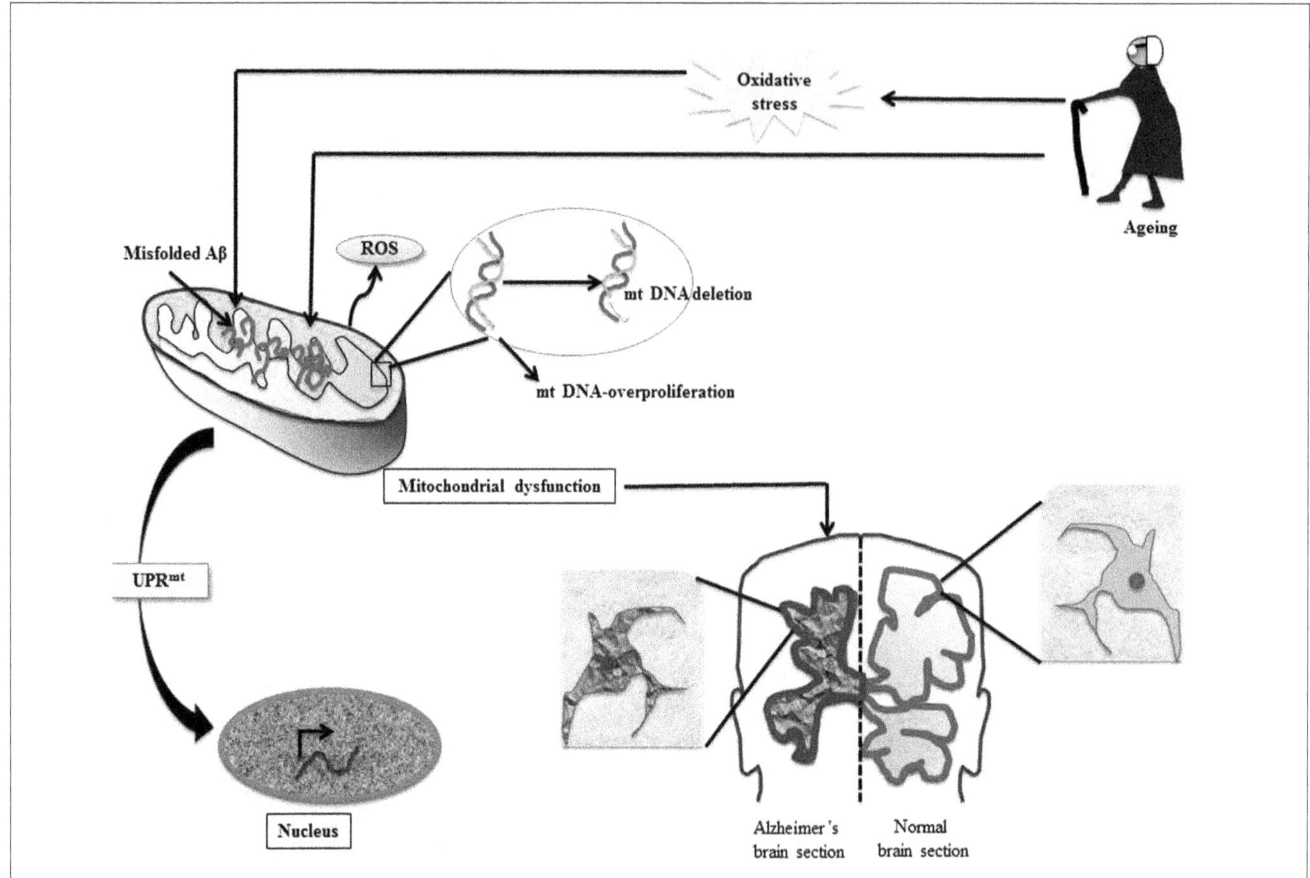

FIGURE 2 | Mitochondrial dysfunction in AD: various stress insults like aging and oxidative stress disrupt client protein folding in mitochondria thereby invoking mitochondrial UPR (UPR^{mt}). Numerous events line up; there is mitochondrial DNA (mtDNA) proliferation and deletion, misfolded Aβ overload and ROS generation. This leads to the condition of mitochondrial dysfunction and to rescue the ailing cell UPR^{mt} is stimulated. The effect of mitochondrial dysfunction leads to development of neuropathologies associated with AD (Aliev et al., 2008, 2013; Onyango et al., 2016).

as well as memory loss (Willette et al., 2015; Wijesekara et al., 2017). In addition, there is decline in key neuronal glucose transporters, GLUT1 and GLUT3, as shown in AD mouse models (Ding et al., 2013). The exact molecular mechanism underlying the effect of glucose uptake in AD model is not completely understood, but evidences suggest a close link between AD and insulin signaling. Apart from controlling glucose metabolism, insulin also regulates neural development with respect to learning and memory (Ying et al., 2017).

The lowering in glucose concentration due to lack of active transporters (GLUT1 and GLUT3) instates mitigating effect on hexosamine pathway (HBP), due to which O-GlcNAcylation is compromised with hyperphosphorylation on tau protein (Liu et al., 2009). XBP1(S) is shown to directly target the rate limiting enzyme of HBP, glutamine fructose-6-phosphate aminotransferase (GFAT1; Wang et al., 2014), as XBP1(S) transgenics showed rise in O-GlcNAcylation (Wang et al., 2014). The situation of insulin resistance established in aging has also been shown to increase HBP flux (Einstein et al., 2008). A gain-of-function mutation in GFAT1 of *C. elegans* showed significant induction of ERAD and autophagy favoring longevity (Denzel et al., 2014).

Protein aggregation is a consequence of AD which is a result of abnormal proteostasis in the cell (Kaushik and Cuervo, 2015). An increase in the UPR^{ER} driven protein homeostasis was observed with the overexpression of GLUT1 as this promoted downregulation of expression of GRP78. GRP78, being the negative regulator of the UPR^{ER}, binds ATF6 and IRE1 thereby continuing them in an inactive state. One interesting study showed that flies (with increased glucose transport) when fed with the drug metformin showed mitigated levels of GRP78 with ensuing gain in lifespan, additionally the expression of GLUT1 and its association with the beginning of UPR^{ER} exerted neuroprotective effect (Niccoli et al., 2016).

TARGETING UPR^{ER} TO MANAGE AD

The involvement of ER stress and hence the UPR^{ER} in neuropathologies exposes the molecules of the pathway as attractive targets for therapeutic interventions. Here, we have compiled reports from studies that have targeted molecules of UPR^{ER} for managing the deterioration caused by AD (**Figure 1**).

eIF2α and PERK in AD

There are accumulating evidences that support increased phosphorylation of PERK and eIF2α in AD (Chang et al., 2002; Page et al., 2006; Kim et al., 2007). The processing of highly expressed single-pass transmembrane protein in brain, the amyloid precursor protein, leads to the generation of neurotoxic Aβ during neuropathogenesis. Reports suggest that the secretase β-site APP cleaving enzyme-1 (BACE1), increases APP cleavage as a result of eIF2α phosphorylation leading to the production of Aβ in neurons (O'Connor et al., 2008). The PERK tier of UPR when suppressed leads to the alleviation of synaptic plasticity and memory loss in AD (Ma et al., 2013). The administration of arctigenin, a bioactive product from *Arctium lappa* (L.), has been known to inhibit BACE1 translation through dephosphorylation of eIF2α-P (Zhu et al., 2013). The phosphorylation of eIF2α is central to integrated stress response (ISR) that modulates UPR (Harding et al., 2000b) and formation of memory proteins (Costa-Mattioli et al., 2005). ISR inhibitor (ISRIB) interferes with ISR by affecting eIF2B activity whose competitive inhibitor is eIF2α-P (Krishnamoorthy et al., 2001; Sekine et al., 2015; Bogorad et al., 2017). This comprehensively reverses the effect of eIF2α-P, which resulted in the restoration of translation and hence long term memory enhancement in rodents (Sidrauski et al., 2013, 2015). The genetic deletion of eIF2 kinases, PERK, GCN2 and dsRNA-dependent protein kinase (PKR) ameliorate synaptic plasticity and memory in AD models (Ma et al., 2013). The transient translational halt induced by PERK-P/eIF2α-P was challenged by GSK2606414, a PERK inhibitor, because of which tau phosphorylation could be checked, resulting in the amelioration of neurodegeneration (Axten et al., 2012; Radford et al., 2015). The development of AD manifested by Aβ accumulation forces tau hyper phosphorylation in sync with increased activity of glycogen synthase kinase-3β (GSK-3β) in the cortical neurons (Takashima et al., 1993, 1996; Tomidokoro et al., 2001; De Felice et al., 2008; Resende et al., 2008). Resende et al. (2008) showed that Aβ oligomers cause ER stress linked calcium leakage which in turn leads to GSK-3β activation, the later when inhibited by GSK-3β inhibitor I, led to the prevention of Aβ induced phosphorylation of tau.

IRE1/XBP1 in AD

The advantageous effects of XBP1 on memory was proven in neural-specific XBP1 knockout mice featuring impaired learning and synaptic plasticity deficit, where injections of adeno-associated viruses delivered XBP1(S) resulted in establishing long-term hippocampus memory (Martínez et al., 2016). In accordance with this finding, another study reinforced the neuro-protective role of XBP1 in AD mice (Casas-Tinto et al., 2011; Cisse et al., 2017). Nonetheless, a flavonol, called quercetin, activated endoribonuclease activity of IRE1 and inhibited tau hyperphosphorylation (de Boer et al., 2006; Suganthy et al., 2016). In cases of familial AD, deletions or mutations in presenilin genes accentuate ER Ca^{2+} leakage. The JNK inhibitor, SP600125, when challenged in PS1/PS2 double knockout mouse embryonic fibroblast, caused inhibition of Ca^{2+} leakage (Das et al., 2012). The neuroinflammation exhibited in AD through tau phosphorylation mediated by the kinase activity of JNK was inhibited by SP600125, consequently inhibiting Aβ-induced c-Jun phosphorylation (Vukic et al., 2009; Zhou et al., 2015).

FUTURE DIRECTIONS AND CONCLUDING REMARKS

ER, being a central organelle in nerve cells, coordinates with the cellular homeostasis by managing translation/modification of proteins and Ca^{2+} equilibrium, thereby maintains the proper signaling in brain. The disruption in neuronal physiology is quite evident in age-related AD where ER dysfunctions are prominently expressed in the form of imbalance in proteostasis. Advancements in studies based on AD models have clearly shown how we can intervene the molecular pillars of UPR^{ER} and its associated signaling cascades to manage neurodegeneration in age-related AD. The present review is an attempt to revise functional relevance of the studies conducted in the field of management of age-related AD through therapeutic interventions on the UPR^{ER} pathway and its associate's molecules. Studies reinforce that the strategies where intervening the molecules, which are involved in transposing effects of aging on neurodegeneration, will cause reduction in probability of AD pathology. The manifestation of ER proteostasis is a direct indication of healthy nervous system. Progression in AD witnesses glucose hypo-metabolism in brain, reduction in glucose transporters in neurons and endothelial cells of blood brain barrier in direct proportion with the amount of neurofibrillary tangles. Type 2 diabetics with higher insulin resistance are at a greater risk of AD. Recent reports elucidate that managing UPR^{ER} can exert neuroprotective effect in AD (Smith and Mallucci, 2016). Additionally, as evidenced in the study by Sorrentino et al. (2017), the recapitulation of mitochondrial function through activation of UPR^{mt} can impede plaque formation. Aliev et al., also demonstrated link between cancer and AD where mtDNA over-proliferation and deletion induces cell cycle dysregulation prompting oncogenic pathway (Aliev et al., 2013). We have supporting literature that underpins the reversal of AD pathology by anticancer drugs (Cramer et al., 2012). Aiming at therapeutic intervention, the ailing mitochondria can be challenged with specific antioxidants like MitoQ, acetyl-L-carnitine and R-alpha lipoic acid to alleviate AD (Aliev et al., 2011; Volgyi et al., 2015). One remarkable study on astrocytes underpins the protective role of conditioned medium of human mesenchymal stem cells (CM-hMSCA) sourced from adipose tissue against neuropathologies (Baez-Jurado et al., 2017). The state of astrocyte mitochondrial dysfunction has been proven to be a start point for neuronal death (Baez et al., 2016). Pharmacological targeting of astrocytes has been proposed to be a potential way in therapeutics of AD (Baez et al.,

2016). A transcriptomic analysis in astrocytes has put forward a conglomeration of various algorithms for strategic approaches in therapeutics of neuropathologies (Barreto et al., 2017).

We still need extensive and efficient model systems where the molecular intricacies of weakened UPR^{ER} in aging-induced neuropathology in AD can be ventured upon, so that pharmacological as well as genetic tools could underscore the significance of UPR^{ER} as well as UPR^{mt} in aged brain.

AUTHOR CONTRIBUTIONS

SR and RM conceived the idea. SR, ATJ, AA and RM contributed to writing of the manuscript.

ACKNOWLEDGMENTS

Authors extend their thanks to colleagues for their criticism that helped to improve the quality of contents in the perspective of broader audience. No funding was availed to carry out the study.

REFERENCES

Acosta-Alvear, D., Zhou, Y., Blais, A., Tsikitis, M., Lents, N. H., Arias, C., et al. (2007). XBP1 controls diverse cell type- and condition-specific transcriptional regulatory networks. *Mol. Cell* 27, 53–66. doi: 10.1016/j.molcel.2007.06.011

Aliev, G., Gasimov, E., Obrenovich, M. E., Fischbach, K., Shenk, J. C., Smith, M. A., et al. (2008). Atherosclerotic lesions and mitochondria DNA deletions in brain microvessels: implication in the pathogenesis of Alzheimer's disease. *Vasc. Health Risk Manag.* 4, 721–730. doi: 10.2147/vhrm.s2608

Aliev, G., Li, Y., Palacios, H. H., and Obrenovich, M. E. (2011). Oxidative stress induced mitochondrial DNA deletion as a hallmark for the drug development in the context of the cerebrovascular diseases. *Recent Pat. Cardiovasc. Drug Discov.* 6, 222–241. doi: 10.2174/157489011797376942

Aliev, G., Obrenovich, M. E., Tabrez, S., Jabir, N. R., Reddy, V. P., Li, Y., et al. (2013). Link between cancer and Alzheimer disease via oxidative stress induced by nitric oxide-dependent mitochondrial DNA overproliferation and deletion. *Oxid. Med. Cell. Longev.* 2013:962984. doi: 10.1155/2013/962984

Alzheimer's Association. (2016). 2016 Alzheimer's disease facts and figures. *Alzheimers Dement.* 12, 459–509. doi: 10.1016/j.jalz.2016.03.001

Arnould, T., Michel, S., and Renard, P. (2015). Mitochondria retrograde signaling and the UPR mt: where are we in mammals? *Int. J. Mol. Sci.* 16, 18224–18251. doi: 10.3390/ijms160818224

Atwood, C. S., and Bowen, R. L. (2015). A unified hypothesis of early- and late-onset Alzheimer's disease pathogenesis. *J. Alzheimers Dis.* 47, 33–47. doi: 10.3233/JAD-143210

Axten, J. M., Medina, J. R., Feng, Y., Shu, A., Romeril, S. P., Grant, S. W., et al. (2012). Discovery of 7-methyl-5-(1-[3-(trifluoromethyl)phenyl]acetyl-2,3-dihydro- 1*H*-indol-5-yl)-7H-p yrrolo[2,3-*d*]pyrimidin-4-amine (GSK2606414), a potent and selective first-in-class inhibitor of protein kinase R (PKR)-like endoplasmic reticulum kinase (PERK). *J. Med. Chem.* 55, 7193–7207. doi: 10.1021/jm300713s

Baez, E., Echeverria, V., Cabezas, R., Ávila-Rodriguez, M., Garcia-Segura, L. M., and Barreto, G. E. (2016). Protection by neuroglobin expression in brain pathologies. *Front. Neurol.* 7:146. doi: 10.3389/fneur.2016.00146

Baez-Jurado, E., Hidalgo-Lanussa, O., Guio-Vega, G., Ashraf, G. M., Echeverria, V., Aliev, G., et al. (2017). Conditioned medium of human adipose mesenchymal stem cells increases wound closure and protects human astrocytes following scratch assay *in vitro*. *Mol. Neurobiol.* doi: 10.1007/s12035-017-0771-4 [Epub ahead of print].

Barreto, G. E., Gomez, R. M., Bustos, R. H., Forero, D. A., Aliev, G., Tarasov, V. V., et al. (2017). Approaches of the transcriptomic analysis in astrocytes: potential pharmacological targets. *Curr. Pharm. Des.* 23, 4189–4197. doi: 10.2174/1381612823666170406113501

Baumeister, P., Luo, S., Skarnes, W. C., Sui, G., Seto, E., Shi, Y., et al. (2005). Endoplasmic reticulum stress induction of the Grp78/BiP promoter: activating mechanisms mediated by YY1 and its interactive chromatin modifiers. *Mol. Cell. Biol.* 25, 4529–4540. doi: 10.1128/mcb.25.11.4529-4540.2005

Bertolotti, A., Zhang, Y., Hendershot, L. M., Harding, H. P., and Ron, D. (2000). Dynamic interaction of BiP and ER stress transducers in the unfolded-protein response. *Nat. Cell Biol.* 2, 326–332. doi: 10.1038/35014014

Bogorad, A. M., Lin, K. Y., and Marintchev, A. (2017). Novel mechanisms of eIF2B action and regulation by eIF2α phosphorylation. *Nucleic Acids Res.* 45, 11962–11979. doi: 10.1093/nar/gkx845

Casas-Tinto, S., Zhang, Y., Sanchez-Garcia, J., Gomez-Velazquez, M., Rincon-Limas, D. E., and Fernandez-Funez, P. (2011). The ER stress factor XBP1s prevents amyloid-β neurotoxicity. *Hum. Mol. Genet.* 20, 2144–2160. doi: 10.1093/hmg/ddr100

Cass, S. P. (2017). Alzheimer's disease and exercise: a literature review. *Curr. Sports Med. Rep.* 16, 19–22. doi: 10.1249/JSR.0000000000000332

Chang, R. C., Wong, A. K., Ng, H. K., and Hugon, J. (2002). Phosphorylation of eukaryotic initiation factor-2α (eIF2α) is associated with neuronal degeneration in Alzheimer's disease. *Neuroreport* 13, 2429–2432. doi: 10.1097/00001756-200212200-00011

Chen, D., Thomas, E. L., and Kapahi, P. (2009). HIF-1 modulates dietary restriction-mediated lifespan extension via IRE-1 in Caenorhabditis elegans. *PLoS Genet.* 5:e1000486. doi: 10.1371/journal.pgen.1000486

Chyung, J. H., Raper, D. M., and Selkoe, D. J. (2005). γ-secretase exists on the plasma membrane as an intact complex that accepts substrates and effects intramembrane cleavage. *J. Biol. Chem.* 280, 4383–4392. doi: 10.1074/jbc.M409272200

Cisse, M., Duplan, E., Lorivel, T., Dunys, J., Bauer, C., Meckler, X., et al. (2017). The transcription factor XBP1s restores hippocampal synaptic plasticity and memory by control of the Kalirin-7 pathway in Alzheimer model. *Mol. Psychiatry* 22, 1562–1575. doi: 10.1038/mp.2016.152

Citron, M. (2002). Alzheimer's disease: treatments in discovery and development. *Nat. Neurosci.* 5, 1055–1057. doi: 10.1038/nn940

Cleary, J. P., Walsh, D. M., Hofmeister, J. J., Shankar, G. M., Kuskowski, M. A., Selkoe, D. J., et al. (2005). Natural oligomers of the amyloid-β protein specifically disrupt cognitive function. *Nat. Neurosci.* 8, 79–84. doi: 10.1038/nn1372

Cornejo, V. H., and Hetz, C. (2013). The unfolded protein response in Alzheimer's disease. *Semin. Immunopathol.* 35, 277–292. doi: 10.1007/s00281-013-0373-9

Costa-Mattioli, M., Gobert, D., Harding, H., Herdy, B., Azzi, M., Bruno, M., et al. (2005). Translational control of hippocampal synaptic plasticity and memory by the eIF2α kinase GCN2. *Nature* 436, 1166–1173. doi: 10.1038/nature03897

Costa-Mattioli, M., Sossin, W. S., Klann, E., and Sonenberg, N. (2009). Translational control of long-lasting synaptic plasticity and memory. *Neuron* 61, 10–26. doi: 10.1016/j.neuron.2008.10.055

Cramer, P. E., Cirrito, J. R., Wesson, D. W., Lee, C. Y., Karlo, J. C., Zinn, A. E., et al. (2012). ApoE-directed therapeutics rapidly clear β-amyloid and reverse deficits in AD mouse models. *Science* 335, 1503–1506. doi: 10.1126/science.1217697

Cullinan, S. B., and Diehl, J. A. (2004). PERK-dependent activation of Nrf2 contributes to redox homeostasis and cell survival following endoplasmic reticulum stress. *J. Biol. Chem.* 279, 20108–20117. doi: 10.1074/jbc.M314219200

Cullinan, S. B., Zhang, D., Hannink, M., Arvisais, E., Kaufman, R. J., and Diehl, J. A. (2003). Nrf2 is a direct PERK substrate and effector of PERK-dependent cell survival. *Mol. Cell. Biol.* 23, 7198–7209. doi: 10.1128/mcb.23.20.7198-7209.2003

Das, H. K., Tchedre, K., and Mueller, B. (2012). Repression of transcription of presenilin-1 inhibits γ-secretase independent ER Ca^{2+} leak that is impaired by FAD mutations. *J. Neurochem.* 122, 487–500. doi: 10.1111/j.1471-4159.2012.07794.x

de Boer, V. C., de Goffau, M. C., Arts, I. C., Hollman, P. C., and Keijer, J. (2006). SIRT1 stimulation by polyphenols is affected by their stability and metabolism. *Mech. Aging Dev.* 127, 618–627. doi: 10.1016/j.mad.2006.02.007

De Felice, F. G., Wu, D., Lambert, M. P., Fernandez, S. J., Velasco, P. T., Lacor, P. N., et al. (2008). Alzheimer's disease-type neuronal tau hyperphosphorylation induced by Aβ oligomers. *Neurobiol. Aging* 29, 1334–1347. doi: 10.1016/j.neurobiolaging.2007.02.029

Denzel, M. S., Storm, N. J., Gutschmidt, A., Baddi, R., Hinze, Y., Jarosch, E., et al. (2014). Hexosamine pathway metabolites enhance protein quality control and prolong life. *Cell* 156, 1167–1178. doi: 10.1016/j.cell.2014.01.061

Devi, L., and Ohno, M. (2013). Deletion of the eIF2α Kinase GCN2 fails to rescue the memory decline associated with Alzheimer's disease. *PLoS One* 8:e77335. doi: 10.1371/journal.pone.0077335

Devi, L., and Ohno, M. (2014). PERK mediates eIF2α phosphorylation responsible for BACE1 elevation, CREB dysfunction and neurodegeneration in a mouse model of Alzheimer's disease. *Neurobiol. Aging* 35, 2272–2281. doi: 10.1016/j.neurobiolaging.2014.04.031

Ding, F., Yao, J., Rettberg, J. R., Chen, S., and Brinton, R. D. (2013). Early decline in glucose transport and metabolism precedes shift to ketogenic system in female aging and Alzheimer's mouse brain: implication for bioenergetic intervention. *PLoS One* 8:e79977. doi: 10.1371/journal.pone.0079977

Einstein, F. H., Fishman, S., Bauman, J., Thompson, R. F., Huffman, D. M., Atzmon, G., et al. (2008). Enhanced activation of a "nutrient-sensing" pathway with age contributes to insulin resistance. *FASEB J.* 22, 3450–3457. doi: 10.1096/fj.08-109041

Ellgaard, L., and Helenius, A. (2003). Quality control in the endoplasmic reticulum. *Nat. Rev. Mol. Cell Biol.* 4, 181–191. doi: 10.1038/nrm1052

Fiest, K. M., Roberts, J. I., Maxwell, C. J., Hogan, D. B., Smith, E. E., Frolkis, A., et al. (2016). The prevalence and incidence of dementia due to Alzheimer's disease: a systematic review and meta-analysis. *Can. J. Neurol. Sci.* 43, S51–S82. doi: 10.1017/cjn.2016.36

Fonseca, A. C., Ferreiro, E., Oliveira, C. R., Cardoso, S. M., and Pereira, C. F. (2013). Activation of the endoplasmic reticulum stress response by the amyloid-β 1–40 peptide in brain endothelial cells. *Biochim. Biophys. Acta* 1832, 2191–2203. doi: 10.1016/j.bbadis.2013.08.007

Fusakio, M. E., Willy, J. A., Wang, Y., Mirek, E. T., Al Baghdadi, R. J., Adams, C. M., et al. (2016). Transcription factor ATF4 directs basal and stress-induced gene expression in the unfolded protein response and cholesterol metabolism in the liver. *Mol. Biol. Cell* 27, 1536–1551. doi: 10.1091/mbc.E16-01-0039

Genereux, J. C., Qu, S., Zhou, M., Ryno, L. M., Wang, S., Shoulders, M. D., et al. (2015). Unfolded protein response-induced ERdj3 secretion links ER stress to extracellular proteostasis. *EMBO J.* 34, 4–19. doi: 10.15252/embj.201488896

Gourmaud, S., Paquet, C., Dumurgier, J., Pace, C., Bouras, C., Gray, F., et al. (2015). Increased levels of cerebrospinal fluid JNK3 associated with amyloid pathology: links to cognitive decline. *J. Psychiatry Neurosci.* 40, 151–161. doi: 10.1503/jpn.140062

Haass, C., and Selkoe, D. J. (2007). Soluble protein oligomers in neurodegeneration: lessons from the Alzheimer's amyloid β-peptide. *Nat. Rev. Mol. Cell Biol.* 8, 101–112. doi: 10.1038/nrm2101

Halliday, M., and Mallucci, G. R. (2015). Modulating the unfolded protein response to prevent neurodegeneration and enhance memory. *Neuropathol. Appl. Neurobiol.* 41, 414–427. doi: 10.1111/nan.12211

Hamos, J. E., Oblas, B., Pulaski-Salo, D., Welch, W. J., Bole, D. G., and Drachman, D. A. (1991). Expression of heat shock proteins in Alzheimer's disease. *Neurology* 41, 345–350. doi: 10.1212/WNL.41.3.345

Han, J., Back, S. H., Hur, J., Lin, Y.-H., Gildersleeve, R., Shan, J., et al. (2013). ER-stress-induced transcriptional regulation increases protein synthesis leading to cell death. *Nat. Cell Biol.* 15, 481–490. doi: 10.1038/ncb2738

Harding, H. P., Novoa, I., Zhang, Y., Zeng, H., Wek, R., Schapira, M., et al. (2000a). Regulated translation initiation controls stress-induced gene expression in mammalian cells. *Mol. Cell* 6, 1099–1108. doi: 10.1016/s1097-2765(00)00108-8

Harding, H. P., Zhang, Y., Bertolotti, A., Zeng, H., and Ron, D. (2000b). Perk is essential for translational regulation and cell survival during the unfolded protein response. *Mol. Cell* 5, 897–904. doi: 10.1016/s1097-2765(00)80330-5

Harding, H. P., Zhang, Y., and Ron, D. (1999). Protein translation and folding are coupled by an endoplasmic-reticulum-resident kinase. *Nature* 397, 271–274. doi: 10.1038/16729

Harding, H. P., Zhang, Y., Zeng, H., Novoa, I., Lu, P. D., Calfon, M., et al. (2003). An integrated stress response regulates amino acid metabolism and resistance to oxidative stress. *Mol. Cell* 11, 619–633. doi: 10.1016/s1097-2765(03)00105-9

Haze, K., Yoshida, H., Yanagi, H., Yura, T., and Mori, K. (1999). Mammalian transcription factor ATF6 is synthesized as a transmembrane protein and activated by proteolysis in response to endoplasmic reticulum stress. *Mol. Biol. Cell* 10, 3787–3799. doi: 10.1091/mbc.10.11.3787

Hetz, C., Chevet, E., and Oakes, S. A. (2015). Proteostasis control by the unfolded protein response. *Nat. Cell Biol.* 17, 829–838. doi: 10.1038/ncb3184

Hirai, K., Aliev, G., Nunomura, A., Fujioka, H., Russell, R. L., Atwood, C. S., et al. (2001). Mitochondrial abnormalities in Alzheimer's disease. *J. Neurosci.* 21, 3017–3023.

Hoekstra, J. G., Hipp, M. J., Montine, T. J., and Kennedy, S. R. (2016). Mitochondrial DNA mutations increase in early stage Alzheimer disease and are inconsistent with oxidative damage. *Ann. Neurol.* 80, 301–306. doi: 10.1002/ana.24709

Hoozemans, J. J., van Haastert, E. S., Nijholt, D. A., Rozemuller, A. J., Eikelenboom, P., and Scheper, W. (2009). The unfolded protein response is activated in pretangle neurons in Alzheimer's disease hippocampus. *Am. J. Pathol.* 174, 1241–1251. doi: 10.2353/ajpath.2009.080814

Hoozemans, J. J., Veerhuis, R., Van Haastert, E. S., Rozemuller, J. M., Baas, F., Eikelenboom, P., et al. (2005). The unfolded protein response is activated in Alzheimer's disease. *Acta Neuropathol.* 110, 165–172. doi: 10.1007/s00401-005-1038-0

Hussain, S. G., and Ramaiah, K. V. (2007). Reduced eIF2α phosphorylation and increased proapoptotic proteins in aging. *Biochem. Biophys. Res. Commun.* 355, 365–370. doi: 10.1016/j.bbrc.2007.01.156

Ivançević, V., Alavi, A., Souder, E., Mozley, P. D., Gur, R. E., Bénard, F., et al. (2000). Regional cerebral glucose metabolism in healthy volunteers determined by fluordeoxyglucose positron emission tomography: appearance and variance in the transaxial, coronal, and sagittal planes. *Clin. Nucl. Med.* 25, 596–602. doi: 10.1097/00003072-200008000-00005

Jiang, X. Y., Litkowski, P. E., Taylor, A. A., Lin, Y., Snider, B. J., and Moulder, K. L. (2010). A role for the ubiquitin-proteasome system in activity-dependent presynaptic silencing. *J. Neurosci.* 30, 1798–1809. doi: 10.1523/JNEUROSCI.4965-09.2010

Kaushik, S., and Cuervo, A. M. (2015). Proteostasis and aging. *Nat. Med.* 21, 1406–1415. doi: 10.1038/nm.4001

Kawamata, H., and Manfredi, G. (2017). Proteinopathies and OXPHOS dysfunction in neurodegenerative diseases. *J. Cell Biol.* 216, 3917–3929. doi: 10.1083/jcb.201709172

Khachaturian, Z. S. (1989). Calcium, membranes, aging, and Alzheimer's disease. Introduction and overview. *Ann. N Y Acad. Sci.* 568, 1–4. doi: 10.1111/j.1749-6632.1989.tb12485.x

Kim, H. S., Choi, Y., Shin, K. Y., Joo, Y., Lee, Y. K., Jung, S. Y., et al. (2007). Swedish amyloid precursor protein mutation increases phosphorylation of eIF2α *in vitro* and *in vivo*. *J. Neurosci. Res.* 85, 1528–1537. doi: 10.1002/jnr.21267

Kraemer, B. C., Burgess, J. K., Chen, J. H., Thomas, J. H., and Schellenberg, G. D. (2006). Molecular pathways that influence human tau-induced pathology in Caenorhabditis elegans. *Hum. Mol. Genet.* 15, 1483–1496. doi: 10.1093/hmg/ddl067

Krishnamoorthy, T., Pavitt, G. D., Zhang, F., Dever, T. E., and Hinnebusch, A. G. (2001). Tight binding of the phosphorylated α subunit of initiation factor 2 (eIF2α) to the regulatory subunits of guanine nucleotide exchange factor eIF2B is required for inhibition of translation initiation. *Mol. Cell. Biol.* 21, 5018–5030. doi: 10.1128/mcb.21.15.5018-5030.2001

Krishnan, K. J., Ratnaike, T. E., De Gruyter, H. L., Jaros, E., and Turnbull, D. M. (2012). Mitochondrial DNA deletions cause the biochemical defect observed in Alzheimer's disease. *Neurobiol. Aging* 33, 2210–2214. doi: 10.1016/j.neurobiolaging.2011.08.009

Lee, A. H., Iwakoshi, N. N., and Glimcher, L. H. (2003). XBP-1 regulates a subset of endoplasmic reticulum resident chaperone genes in the unfolded protein response. *Mol. Cell. Biol.* 23, 7448–7459. doi: 10.1128/mcb.23.21.7448-7459.2003

Lee, J., Kim, Y., Liu, T., Hwang, Y. J., Hyeon, S. J., Im, H., et al. (2018). SIRT3 deregulation is linked to mitochondrial dysfunction in Alzheimer's disease. *Aging Cell* 17:e12679. doi: 10.1111/acel.12679

Liu, F., Shi, J., Tanimukai, H., Gu, J., Grundke-Iqbal, I., Iqbal, K., et al. (2009). Reduced O-GlcNAcylation links lower brain glucose metabolism and tau pathology in Alzheimer's disease. *Brain* 132, 1820–1832. doi: 10.1093/brain/awp099

Loewen, C. A., and Feany, M. B. (2010). The unfolded protein response protects from tau neurotoxicity *in vivo*. *PLoS One* 5:e13084. doi: 10.1371/journal.pone.0013084

Lourenco, M. V., Clarke, J. R., Frozza, R. L., Bomfim, T. R., Forny-Germano, L., Batista, A. F., et al. (2013). TNF-α mediates PKR-dependent memory impairment and brain IRS-1 inhibition induced by Alzheimer's β-amyloid oligomers in mice and monkeys. *Cell Metab.* 18, 831–843. doi: 10.1016/j.cmet.2013.11.002

Ma, T., Trinh, M. A., Wexler, A. J., Bourbon, C., Gatti, E., Pierre, P., et al. (2013). Suppression of eIF2α kinases alleviates Alzheimer's disease-related plasticity and memory deficits. *Nat. Neurosci.* 16, 1299–1305. doi: 10.1038/nn.3486

Ma, K., Vattem, K. M., and Wek, R. C. (2002). Dimerization and release of molecular chaperone inhibition facilitate activation of eukaryotic initiation factor-2 kinase in response to endoplasmic reticulum stress. *J. Biol. Chem.* 277, 18728–18735. doi: 10.1074/jbc.M200903200

Marciniak, S. J., Garcia-Bonilla, L., Hu, J., Harding, H. P., and Ron, D. (2006). Activation-dependent substrate recruitment by the eukaryotic translation initiation factor 2 kinase PERK. *J. Cell Biol.* 172, 201–209. doi: 10.1083/jcb.200508099

Marciniak, S. J., Yun, C. Y., Oyadomari, S., Novoa, I., Zhang, Y., Jungreis, R., et al. (2004). CHOP induces death by promoting protein synthesis and oxidation in the stressed endoplasmic reticulum. *Genes Dev.* 18, 3066–3077. doi: 10.1101/gad.1250704

Martínez, G., Vidal, R. L., Mardones, P., Serrano, F. G., Ardiles, A. O., Wirth, C., et al. (2016). Regulation of memory formation by the transcription factor XBP1. *Cell Rep.* 14, 1382–1394. doi: 10.1016/j.celrep.2016.01.028

Minakshi, R., Rahman, S., Jan, A. T., Archana, A., and Kim, J. (2017). Implications of aging and the endoplasmic reticulum unfolded protein response on the molecular modality of breast cancer. *Exp. Mol. Med.* 49:e389. doi: 10.1038/emm.2017.215

Minter, M. R., Taylor, J. M., and Crack, P. J. (2016). The contribution of neuroinflammation to amyloid toxicity in Alzheimer's disease. *J. Neurochem.* 136, 457–474. doi: 10.1111/jnc.13411

Moneim, A. E. (2015). Oxidant/Antioxidant imbalance and the risk of Alzheimer's disease. *Curr. Alzheimer Res.* 12, 335–349. doi: 10.2174/1567205012666150325182702

Mori, K. (2009). Signalling pathways in the unfolded protein response: development from yeast to mammals. *J. Biochem.* 146, 743–750. doi: 10.1093/jb/mvp166

Mosconi, L., Brys, M., Switalski, R., Mistur, R., Glodzik, L., Pirraglia, E., et al. (2007). Maternal family history of Alzheimer's disease predisposes to reduced brain glucose metabolism. *Proc. Natl. Acad. Sci. U S A* 104, 19067–19072. doi: 10.1073/pnas.0705036104

Naidoo, N., Ferber, M., Master, M., Zhu, Y., and Pack, A. I. (2008). Aging impairs the unfolded protein response to sleep deprivation and leads to proapoptotic signaling. *J. Neurosci.* 28, 6539–6548. doi: 10.1523/JNEUROSCI.5685-07.2008

Niccoli, T., Cabecinha, M., Tillmann, A., Kerr, F., Wong, C. T., Cardenes, D., et al. (2016). Increased glucose transport into neurons rescues Aβ toxicity in Drosophila. *Curr. Biol.* 26, 2291–2300. doi: 10.1016/j.cub.2016.07.017

Nijholt, D. A., de Graaf, T. R., van Haastert, E. S., Oliveira, A. O., Berkers, C. R., Zwart, R., et al. (2011). Endoplasmic reticulum stress activates autophagy but not the proteasome in neuronal cells: implications for Alzheimer's disease. *Cell Death Differ.* 18, 1071–1081. doi: 10.1038/cdd.2010.176

Nuss, J. E., Choksi, K. B., Deford, J. H., and Papaconstantinou, J. (2008). Decreased enzyme activities of chaperones PDI and BiP in aged mouse livers. *Biochem. Biophys. Res. Commun.* 365, 355–361. doi: 10.1016/j.bbrc.2007.10.194

O'Connor, T., Sadleir, K. R., Maus, E., Velliquette, R. A., Zhao, J., Cole, S. L., et al. (2008). Phosphorylation of the translation initiation factor eIF2α increases BACE1 levels and promotes amyloidogenesis. *Neuron* 60, 988–1009. doi: 10.1016/j.neuron.2008.10.047

Ohno, M. (2014). Roles of eIF2α kinases in the pathogenesis of Alzheimer's disease. *Front. Mol. Neurosci.* 7:22. doi: 10.3389/fnmol.2014.00022

Onuki, R., Bando, Y., Suyama, E., Katayama, T., Kawasaki, H., Baba, T., et al. (2004). An RNA-dependent protein kinase is involved in tunicamycin-induced apoptosis and Alzheimer's disease. *EMBO J.* 23, 959–968. doi: 10.1038/sj.emboj.7600049

Onyango, P., Celic, I., McCaffery, J. M., Boeke, J. D., and Feinberg, A. P. (2002). SIRT3, a human SIR2 homologue, is an NAD-dependent deacetylase localized to mitochondria. *Proc. Natl. Acad. Sci. U S A* 99, 13653–13658. doi: 10.1073/pnas.222538099

Onyango, I. G., Dennis, J., and Khan, S. M. (2016). Mitochondrial dysfunction in Alzheimer's disease and the rationale for bioenergetics based therapies. *Aging Dis.* 7, 201–214. doi: 10.14336/AD.2015.1007

Page, G., Rioux Bilan, A., Ingrand, S., Lafay-Chebassier, C., Pain, S., Perault Pochat, M. C., et al. (2006). Activated double-stranded RNA-dependent protein kinase and neuronal death in models of Alzheimer's disease. *Neuroscience* 139, 1343–1354. doi: 10.1016/j.neuroscience.2006.01.047

Paz Gavilán, M., Vela, J., Castaño, A., Ramos, B., del Río, J. C., Vitorica, J., et al. (2006). Cellular environment facilitates protein accumulation in aged rat hippocampus. *Neurobiol. Aging* 27, 973–982. doi: 10.1016/j.neurobiolaging.2005.05.010

Rabek, J. P., Boylston, W. H. III., and Papaconstantinou, J. (2003). Carbonylation of ER chaperone proteins in aged mouse liver. *Biochem. Biophys. Res. Commun.* 305, 566–572. doi: 10.1016/s0006-291x(03)00826-x

Radford, H., Moreno, J. A., Verity, N., Halliday, M., and Mallucci, G. R. (2015). PERK inhibition prevents tau-mediated neurodegeneration in a mouse model of frontotemporal dementia. *Acta Neuropathol.* 130, 633–642. doi: 10.1007/s00401-015-1487-z

Rahman, S., Jan, A. T., Ayyagari, A., Kim, J., Kim, J., and Minakshi, R. (2017). Entanglement of UPRER in aging driven neurodegenerative diseases. *Front. Aging Neurosci.* 9:341. doi: 10.3389/fnagi.2017.00341

Reddy, P. H., Manczak, M., and Yin, X. (2017). Mitochondria-division inhibitor 1 protects against amyloid-β induced mitochondrial fragmentation and synaptic damage in Alzheimer's disease. *J. Alzheimers Dis.* 58, 147–162. doi: 10.3233/JAD-170051

Resende, R., Ferreiro, E., Pereira, C., and Oliveira, C. R. (2008). ER stress is involved in Aβ-induced GSK-3β activation and tau phosphorylation. *J. Neurosci. Res.* 86, 2091–2099. doi: 10.1002/jnr.21648

Revel, F., Gilbert, T., Roche, S., Drai, J., Blond, E., Ecochard, R., et al. (2015). Influence of oxidative stress biomarkers on cognitive decline. *J. Alzheimers Dis.* 45, 553–560. doi: 10.3233/JAD-141797

Romero-Ramirez, L., Cao, H., Nelson, D., Hammond, E., Lee, A. H., Yoshida, H., et al. (2004). XBP1 is essential for survival under hypoxic conditions and is required for tumor growth. *Cancer Res.* 64, 5943–5947. doi: 10.1158/0008-5472.can-04-1606

Sami, N., Rahman, S., Kumar, V., Zaidi, S., Islam, A., Ali, S., et al. (2017). Protein aggregation, misfolding and consequential human neurodegenerative diseases. *Int. J. Neurosci.* 127, 1047–1057. doi: 10.1080/00207454.2017.1286339

Scheltens, P., Blennow, K., Breteler, M. M., de Strooper, B., Frisoni, G. B., Salloway, S., et al. (2016). Alzheimer's disease. *Lancet* 388, 505–517. doi: 10.1016/S0140-6736(15)01124-1

Scheper, W., and Hoozemans, J. J. (2015). The unfolded protein response in neurodegenerative diseases: a neuropathological perspective. *Acta Neuropathol.* 130, 315–331. doi: 10.1007/s00401-015-1462-8

Schroder, M., and Kaufman, R. J. (2005). The mammalian unfolded protein response. *Annu. Rev. Biochem.* 74, 739–789. doi: 10.1146/annurev.biochem.73.011303.074134

Sekine, Y., Zyryanova, A., Crespillo-Casado, A., Fischer, P. M., Harding, H. P., and Ron, D. (2015). Stress responses. Mutations in a translation initiation factor identify the target of a memory-enhancing compound. *Science* 348, 1027–1030. doi: 10.1126/science.aaa6986

Selkoe, D. J. (2001a). Alzheimer's disease results from the cerebral accumulation and cytotoxicity of amyloid β-protein. *J. Alzheimers Dis.* 3, 75–80. doi: 10.3233/jad-2001-3111

Selkoe, D. J. (2001b). Alzheimer's disease: genes, proteins, and therapy. *Physiol. Rev.* 81, 741–766. doi: 10.1152/physrev.2001.81.2.741

Selkoe, D. J. (2004a). Alzheimer disease: mechanistic understanding predicts novel therapies. *Ann. Intern. Med.* 140, 627–638. doi: 10.7326/0003-4819-140-8-200404200-00047

Selkoe, D. J. (2004b). Cell biology of protein misfolding: the examples of Alzheimer's and Parkinson's diseases. *Nat. Cell Biol.* 6, 1054–1061. doi: 10.1038/ncb1104-1054

Shen, J., Chen, X., Hendershot, L., and Prywes, R. (2002). ER stress regulation of ATF6 localization by dissociation of BiP/GRP78 binding and unmasking of Golgi localization signals. *Dev. Cell* 3, 99–111. doi: 10.1016/s1534-5807(02)00203-4

Shoji, M., Iwakami, N., Takeuchi, S., Waragai, M., Suzuki, M., Kanazawa, I., et al. (2000). JNK activation is associated with intracellular β-amyloid accumulation. *Brain Res. Mol. Brain Res.* 85, 221–233. doi: 10.1016/s0169-328x(00)00245-x

Shoulders, M. D., Ryno, L. M., Genereux, J. C., Moresco, J. J., Tu, P. G., Wu, C., et al. (2013). Stress-independent activation of XBP1s and/or ATF6 reveals three functionally diverse ER proteostasis environments. *Cell Rep.* 3, 1279–1292. doi: 10.1016/j.celrep.2013.03.024

Sidrauski, C., Acosta-Alvear, D., Khoutorsky, A., Vedantham, P., Hearn, B. R., Li, H., et al. (2013). Pharmacological brake-release of mRNA translation enhances cognitive memory. *Elife* 2:e00498. doi: 10.7554/eLife.00498

Sidrauski, C., McGeachy, A. M., Ingolia, N. T., and Walter, P. (2015). The small molecule ISRIB reverses the effects of eIF2α phosphorylation on translation and stress granule assembly. *Elife* 4:e05033. doi: 10.7554/eLife.05033

Smith, H. L., and Mallucci, G. R. (2016). The unfolded protein response: mechanisms and therapy of neurodegeneration. *Brain* 139, 2113–2121. doi: 10.1093/brain/aww101

Someya, S., Yu, W., Hallows, W. C., Xu, J., Vann, J. M., Leeuwenburgh, C., et al. (2010). Sirt3 mediates reduction of oxidative damage and prevention of age-related hearing loss under caloric restriction. *Cell* 143, 802–812. doi: 10.1016/j.cell.2010.10.002

Sorrentino, V., Romani, M., Mouchiroud, L., Beck, J. S., Zhang, H., D'Amico, D., et al. (2017). Enhancing mitochondrial proteostasis reduces amyloid-β proteotoxicity. *Nature* 552, 187–193. doi: 10.1038/nature25143

Suganthy, N., Devi, K. P., Nabavi, S. F., Braidy, N., and Nabavi, S. M. (2016). Bioactive effects of quercetin in the central nervous system: focusing on the mechanisms of actions. *Biomed. Pharmacother.* 84, 892–908. doi: 10.1016/j.biopha.2016.10.011

Supnet, C., and Bezprozvanny, I. (2010). The dysregulation of intracellular calcium in Alzheimer disease. *Cell Calcium* 47, 183–189. doi: 10.1016/j.ceca.2009.12.014

Swerdlow, R. H., Burns, J. M., and Khan, S. M. (2014). The Alzheimer's disease mitochondrial cascade hypothesis: progress and perspectives. *Biochim. Biophys. Acta* 1842, 1219–1231. doi: 10.1016/j.bbadis.2013.09.010

Takashima, A., Noguchi, K., Michel, G., Mercken, M., Hoshi, M., Ishiguro, K., et al. (1996). Exposure of rat hippocampal neurons to amyloid β peptide (25–35) induces the inactivation of phosphatidyl inositol-3 kinase and the activation of tau protein kinase I/glycogen synthase kinase-3 β. *Neurosci. Lett.* 203, 33–36. doi: 10.1016/s0006-3495(96)79570-x

Takashima, A., Noguchi, K., Sato, K., Hoshino, T., and Imahori, K. (1993). Tau protein kinase I is essential for amyloid β-protein-induced neurotoxicity. *Proc. Natl. Acad. Sci. U S A* 90, 7789–7793. doi: 10.1073/pnas.90.16.7789

Tatarnikova, O. G., Orlov, M. A., and Bobkova, N. V. (2015). β-amyloid and tau-protein: structure, interaction, and prion-like properties. *Biochemistry (Mosc)* 80, 1800–1819. doi: 10.1134/S000629791513012X

Taylor, R. C., and Dillin, A. (2013). XBP-1 is a cell-nonautonomous regulator of stress resistance and longevity. *Cell* 153, 1435–1447. doi: 10.1016/j.cell.2013.05.042

Tirasophon, W., Welihinda, A. A., and Kaufman, R. J. (1998). A stress response pathway from the endoplasmic reticulum to the nucleus requires a novel bifunctional protein kinase/endoribonuclease (Ire1p) in mammalian cells. *Genes Dev.* 12, 1812–1824. doi: 10.1101/gad.12.12.1812

Tomidokoro, Y., Ishiguro, K., Harigaya, Y., Matsubara, E., Ikeda, M., Park, J. M., et al. (2001). Aβ amyloidosis induces the initial stage of tau accumulation in APP(Sw) mice. *Neurosci. Lett.* 299, 169–172. doi: 10.1016/s0304-3940(00)01767-5

Urano, F., Wang, X., Bertolotti, A., Zhang, Y., Chung, P., Harding, H. P., et al. (2000). Coupling of stress in the ER to activation of JNK protein kinases by transmembrane protein kinase IRE1. *Science* 287, 664–666. doi: 10.1126/science.287.5453.664

Volgyi, K., Juhász, G., Kovacs, Z., and Penke, B. (2015). Dysfunction of endoplasmic reticulum (ER) and mitochondria (MT) in Alzheimer's disease: the role of the ER-MT cross-talk. *Curr. Alzheimer Res.* 12, 655–672. doi: 10.2174/1567205012666150710095035

Vukic, V., Callaghan, D., Walker, D., Lue, L. F., Liu, Q. Y., Couraud, P. O., et al. (2009). Expression of inflammatory genes induced by β-amyloid peptides in human brain endothelial cells and in Alzheimer's brain is mediated by the JNK-AP1 signaling pathway. *Neurobiol. Dis.* 34, 95–106. doi: 10.1016/j.nbd.2008.12.007

Walter, P., and Ron, D. (2011). The unfolded protein response: from stress pathway to homeostatic regulation. *Science* 334, 1081–1086. doi: 10.1126/science.1209038

Wang, Z. V., Deng, Y., Gao, N., Pedrozo, Z., Li, D. L., Morales, C. R., et al. (2014). Spliced X-box binding protein 1 couples the unfolded protein response to hexosamine biosynthetic pathway. *Cell* 156, 1179–1192. doi: 10.1016/j.cell.2014.01.014

Wang, W., Yin, J., Ma, X., Zhao, F., Siedlak, S. L., Wang, Z., et al. (2017). Inhibition of mitochondrial fragmentation protects against Alzheimer's disease in rodent model. *Hum. Mol. Genet.* 26, 4118–4131. doi: 10.1093/hmg/ddx299

Wijesekara, N., Ahrens, R., Sabale, M., Wu, L., Ha, K., Verdile, G., et al. (2017). Amyloid-β and islet amyloid pathologies link Alzheimer disease and type 2 diabetes in a transgenic model. *FASEB J.* 31, 5409–5418. doi: 10.1096/fj.201700431R

Willette, A. A., Bendlin, B. B., Starks, E. J., Birdsill, A. C., Johnson, S. C., Christian, B. T., et al. (2015). Association of insulin resistance with cerebral glucose uptake in late middle-aged adults at risk for Alzheimer disease. *JAMA Neurol.* 72, 1013–1020. doi: 10.1001/jamaneurol.2015.0613

Yamamoto, K., Sato, T., Matsui, T., Sato, M., Okada, T., Yoshida, H., et al. (2007). Transcriptional induction of mammalian ER quality control proteins is mediated by single or combined action of ATF6α and XBP1. *Dev. Cell* 13, 365–376. doi: 10.1016/j.devcel.2007.07.018

Ying, M., Sui, X., Zhang, Y., Sun, Q., Qu, Z., Luo, X., et al. (2017). Identification of novel key molecules involved in spatial memory impairment in triple transgenic mice of Alzheimer's disease. *Mol. Neurobiol.* 54, 3843–3858. doi: 10.1007/s12035-016-9959-2

Yoon, S. S., and Jo, S. A. (2012). Mechanisms of amyloid-β peptide clearance: potential therapeutic targets for Alzheimer's disease. *Biomol. Ther. (Seoul)* 20, 245–255. doi: 10.4062/biomolther.2012.20.3.245

Yoshida, H., Haze, K., Yanagi, H., Yura, T., and Mori, K. (1998). Identification of the cis-acting endoplasmic reticulum stress response element responsible for transcriptional induction of mammalian glucose-regulated proteins. Involvement of basic leucine zipper transcription factors. *J. Biol. Chem.* 273, 33741–33749. doi: 10.1074/jbc.273.50.33741

Yoshida, H., Matsui, T., Hosokawa, N., Kaufman, R. J., Nagata, K., and Mori, K. (2003). A time-dependent phase shift in the mammalian unfolded protein response. *Dev. Cell* 4, 265–271. doi: 10.1016/s1534-5807(03)00022-4

Yoshida, H., Matsui, T., Yamamoto, A., Okada, T., and Mori, K. (2001). XBP1 mRNA is induced by ATF6 and spliced by IRE1 in response to ER stress to produce a highly active transcription factor. *Cell* 107, 881–891. doi: 10.1016/s0092-8674(01)00611-0

Zeng, T., Peng, L., Chao, H., Xi, H., Fu, B., Wang, Y., et al. (2015). IRE1α-TRAF2-ASK1 complex-mediated endoplasmic reticulum stress and mitochondrial dysfunction contribute to CXC195-induced apoptosis in human bladder carcinoma T24 cells. *Biochem. Biophys. Res. Commun.* 460, 530–536. doi: 10.1016/j.bbrc.2015.03.064

Zhou, Q., Wang, M., Du, Y., Zhang, W., Bai, M., Zhang, Z., et al. (2015). Inhibition of c-Jun N-terminal kinase activation reverses Alzheimer disease phenotypes in APPswe/PS1dE9 mice. *Ann. Neurol.* 77, 637–654. doi: 10.1002/ana.24361

Zhu, Z., Yan, J., Jiang, W., Yao, X. G., Chen, J., Chen, L., et al. (2013). Arctigenin effectively ameliorates memory impairment in Alzheimer's disease model mice targeting both β-amyloid production and clearance. *J. Neurosci.* 33, 13138–13149. doi: 10.1523/JNEUROSCI.4790-12.2013

14

Tai Chi Chuan and Baduanjin Mind-Body Training Changes Resting-State Low-Frequency Fluctuations in the Frontal Lobe of Older Adults: A Resting-State fMRI Study

Jing Tao [1,2,3], Xiangli Chen [4], Jiao Liu [1], Natalia Egorova [3], Xiehua Xue [5], Weilin Liu [1,2], Guohua Zheng [1], Ming Li [5], Jinsong Wu [1], Kun Hu [1], Zengjian Wang [3,6], Lidian Chen [1,2] and Jian Kong [3]**

[1]College of Rehabilitation Medicine, Fujian University of Traditional Chinese Medicine, Fuzhou, China, [2]Fujian Key Laboratory of Rehabilitation Technology, Fujian University of Traditional Chinese Medicine, Fuzhou, China, [3]Department of Psychiatry, Massachusetts General Hospital and Harvard Medical School, Charlestown, MA, United States, [4]Department of Rehabilitation Psychology and Special Education, University of Wisconsin-Madison, Madison, WI, United States, [5]Affiliated Rehabilitation Hospital, Fujian University of Traditional Chinese Medicine, Fuzhou, China, [6]Developmental and Educational Psychology, South China Normal University, Guangzhou, China

***Correspondence:**
Lidian Chen
cld@fjtcm.edu.cn
Jian Kong
kongj@nmr.mgh.harvard.edu*

Age-related cognitive decline is a significant public health concern. Recently, non-pharmacological methods, such as physical activity and mental training practices, have emerged as promising low-cost methods to slow the progression of age-related memory decline. In this study, we investigated if Tai Chi Chuan (TCC) and Baduanjin modulated the fractional amplitude of low-frequency fluctuations (fALFF) in different frequency bands (low-frequency: 0.01–0.08 Hz; slow-5: 0.01–0.027 Hz; slow-4: 0.027–0.073 Hz) and improved memory function. Older adults were recruited for the randomized study. Participants in the TCC and Baduanjin groups received 12 weeks of training (1 h/day for 5 days/week). Participants in the control group received basic health education. Each subject participated in memory tests and fMRI scans at the beginning and end of the experiment. We found that compared to the control group: (1) TCC and Baduanjin groups demonstrated significant improvements in memory function; (2) TCC increased fALFF in the dorsolateral prefrontal cortex (DLPFC) in the slow-5 and low-frequency bands; and (3) Baduanjin increased fALFF in the medial PFC in the slow-5 and low-frequency bands. This increase was positively associated with memory function improvement in the slow-5 and low-frequency bands across the TCC and Baduanjin groups.

Abbreviations: AD, Alzheimer's disease; ALFF, amplitude of low frequency fluctuations; aMCI, amnestic mild cognitive impairment; BDI, Beck depression inventory; CCN, cognitive control network; CSF, cerebrospinal fluid; DLPFC, dorsolateral prefrontal cortex; DPARSF, Data Processing Assistant for Resting-State fMRI; fALFF, fractional amplitude of low-frequency fluctuations; FWHM, full-width at half maximum; LFF, low frequency fluctuations; MCI, mild cognitive impairment; MDD, major depressive disorder; MMSE, Mini-Mental State Exam; mPFC, medial prefrontal cortex; MPRAGE, magnetization-prepared rapid gradient echo; PD, Parkinson's Disease; SAD, social anxiety disorder; TCC, Tai Chi Chuan; WMS-CR, Wechsler Memory Scale–Chinese Revision.

Our results suggest that TCC and Baduanjin may work through different brain mechanisms to prevent memory decline due to aging.

Keywords: mind-body exercise, memory, aging, fractional amplitude of low-frequency fluctuations (fALFF), resting-state functional magnetic resonance imaging (fMRI), frequency bands

INTRODUCTION

Age is the main risk factor for most common neurodegenerative diseases, such as mild cognitive impairment (MCI) and Alzheimer's disease (AD). Memory dysfunction is the primary cognitive symptom in MCI and AD and has a profound impact on those whom it affects (McKhann et al., 2011). Nevertheless, pharmaceutical treatments for age-related memory decline remain unsatisfactory.

Recently, non-pharmacological methods, such as physical activity and mental training practices, have emerged as promising low-cost methods to slow the progression of age-related memory decline (Hillman et al., 2008; Erickson et al., 2011, 2014; Killgore et al., 2013; Makizako et al., 2013; Voss et al., 2013; Kelly et al., 2014; Tang and Posner, 2014; Tamura et al., 2015). For instance, Ruscheweyh et al. (2011) found that a 6 months intervention of low-intensity physical activity can improve episodic memory performance in healthy elderly individuals, and this improvement is associated with increases in local gray matter volume in the prefrontal and cingulate cortex, and Brain-derived neurotrophic factor (BDNF) levels. Innes et al. (2017) also reported that 12 min/day for 3 months of Kirtan Kriya meditation training can significantly improve memory and cognitive performance. Unlike pharmaceutical treatments, these methods usually lack serious side effects.

Tai Chi Chuan (TCC) and Baduanjin are popular mind-body practices (Wang et al., 2010; Zheng et al., 2014; Tao et al., 2015). Both of these practices combine meditation with slow movements, deep breathing, and relaxation to smooth vital energy (or qi) flow in the body (Wang et al., 2010). However, these practices are also different from each other; TCC involves more complicated body movements and requires moving one's trunk and all four limbs (Wei et al., 2013), whereas the movement involved in Baduanjin is much simpler and is characterized by eight fixed movements (Xiong et al., 2015). Accumulating evidence has shown that TCC and Baduanjin practice improves cognitive performance and memory function (Wang, 2007; Chang et al., 2010; Lam et al., 2011; Tsai et al., 2013; Fong et al., 2014; Li F. et al., 2014; Wayne et al., 2014; Yin et al., 2014; Zheng et al., 2015). Nevertheless, the mechanisms underlying TCC and Baduanjin are still poorly understood.

In recent years, spontaneous fluctuations in brain activity during rest have drawn the attention of neuroimaging researchers. Investigators believe that these slow-frequency fluctuations may provide information about the intrinsic functional organization of the brain (Fox and Raichle, 2007). Furthermore, studies suggest that the human brain is a complex system that can generate a multitude of oscillatory waves, with different oscillatory classes carrying different dimensions of brain integration. The coupling of different bands of oscillators can provide enhanced combinatorial opportunities for storing complex temporal patterns to accomplish specific functions (Knyazev, 2007).

The low frequency fluctuations (LFF) between 0.01 Hz and 0.08 Hz are of particular relevance to resting state fMRI (rs-fMRI; Biswal et al., 1995). This low frequency range has been further divided into several distinct bands (Buzsáki and Draguhn, 2004), such as slow-4 (0.027–0.073 Hz) and slow-5 (0.01–0.027 Hz), which may indicate the modulation of cortical excitability and neuronal synchronization (Hoptman et al., 2010; Zuo et al., 2010). Recently, investigators have analyzed resting-state fMRI data filtered at the slow-4 and slow-5 bands separately to investigate AD (Liu et al., 2014), MCI (Han et al., 2012; Zhao et al., 2015), social anxiety disorder (SAD; Zhang et al., 2015), Parkinson's Disease (PD; Esposito et al., 2013), and schizophrenia (Hoptman et al., 2010). Studies have found characteristic differences between these specific bands, further endorsing the value of distinguishing the slow-4 and slow-5 bands.

There are many methods that can be used to investigate the brain's resting state spontaneous fluctuations. One such method is to characterize the regional spontaneous neuronal activity using the fractional amplitude of low frequency fluctuations (fALFF; Zang et al., 2007; Zou et al., 2008). As a normalized index of amplitude of low frequency fluctuations (ALFF), fALFF is defined as the total power within the low-frequency range divided by the total power in the entire detectable frequency range (Zuo et al., 2010). This method significantly suppresses non-specific signal components in resting state MRI and increases sensitivity to regional spontaneous brain activity (Zuo et al., 2010).

Alterations in fALFF have been found in several diseases. For instance, Sui et al. (2015) reported that in schizophrenic patients, increased cognitive performance was associated with higher fALFF in the striatum and decreased cognitive performance was associated with higher fALFF in the dorsolateral prefrontal cortex (DLPFC). McGill et al. (2014) reported decreased fALFF in the (PFC) and thalamus in patients with idiopathic generalized epilepsy. Additionally, Han et al. (2011) found that MCI is associated with decreased ALFF/fALFF values in the PCC/PCu, mPFC, hippocampus/PHG and prefrontal regions and increased ALFF/fALFF values in the occipital and temporal regions.

In this study, we investigated changes in spontaneous brain activity using fALFF in older adults following 3-months of TCC or Baduanjin practice. We hypothesized that 3-months of TCC and Baduanjin practice would improve memory function and modulate spontaneous brain activity in the brain regions associated with memory. In addition, we hypothesized that the modulatory effects of TCC and Baduanjin might vary in different low frequency bands.

MATERIALS AND METHODS

In this study, we applied a data driven method to investigate fALFF changes before and after TCC and Baduanjin as compared to a control group. Although, the data has been used previously to investigate the resting state functional connectivity changes of the hippocampus (Tao et al., 2016) and DLPFC (Tao et al., 2017a) and brain structure changes (Tao et al., 2017b) following TCC and Baduanjin practice, we have never reported the results published in this manuscript. Please also see these published studies for more details on the experimental procedure.

Participants

The study was approved by the Medical Ethics Committee of Affiliated Rehabilitation Hospital, Fujian University of Traditional Chinese Medicine and registered in the Chinese Clinical Trial Registry (ChiCTR[1], ChiCTR-IPR-15006131). All participants were informed and signed a written consent.

Two cohorts of older adults from one community were recruited independently and randomized into a TCC or control group in one cohort and a Baduanjin or control group in the other cohort. We recruited the two cohorts separately to avoid potential cross practicing between TCC and Baduanjin. The randomized treatment assignments were sealed in opaque envelopes and opened each time when new participants were included. Outcome raters were blind to the group allocation.

Inclusion criteria were: (1) 50–70 years old; (2) right-handed; and (3) no regular physical exercise for at least 1 year (the minimal standard for regular physical exercise was defined as 30 min 3–4 times per week for the past 3 months). Exclusion criteria were: (1) history of stroke; (2) suffered from severe cerebrovascular disease, musculoskeletal system disease, or other contraindications caused by sports injury; (3) a score of Beck depression inventory (BDI-II) $\geq$ 14 (Beck et al., 1996); and (4) a score on the Mini-Mental State Exam (MMSE) $<$ 24 (Zhang et al., 1990).

Intervention

Two professional instructors with more than 5 years of training experience from Fujian University of Traditional Chinese Medicine were responsible for TCC and Baduanjin exercise training. To guarantee research quality, two staff members monitored the whole training procedure.

Tai Chi Chuan Exercise Group

TCC exercise, which was based on Yang-style 24-form (China National Sports Commission, 1983), was conducted for 60 min per session, 5 days per week for 12 weeks. Each session consisted of a warm-up and review of Tai Chi principles, TCC exercises, breathing technique training, and relaxation.

[1]http://www.chictr.org.cn/index.aspx

Baduanjin Exercise Group

The Baduanjin training regimen was in accordance with "Health Qigong—Baduanjin", published by the General Administration of Sport of China. Each Baduanjin session consisted of a warm-up, eight fixed movements, and ending posture. The frequency of the Baduanjin exercise was the same as the TCC group, i.e. 60 min per session, one session per day, 5 days per week for 12 weeks.

Control Group

Participants in the control group received basic health education at the beginning of the experiment (Hughes et al., 2014). For the next 12 weeks, they were instructed to keep their original physical activity habits. At the end of the experiment (after the second MRI scan), free TCC or Baduanjin training was offered.

Behavioral Measurement

The Wechsler Memory Scale–Chinese Revision (WMS-CR) was used to assess the memory function of each participant. The WMS-CR is designed to assess memory function (Gong and Wang, 1989; Woodard and Axelrod, 1995) and is one of the most frequently used clinical assessments. It consists of ten subtests: information, orientation, mental control, picture, recognition, visual reproduction, associative learning, touch, comprehension memory, and digit span. It also provides an overall memory quotient (MQ). Two licensed WMS-CR raters who were blinded to the randomization distribution administered the WMS-CR.

MRI Acquisition

All MRI scans were acquired on a 3.0T magnetic resonance scanner (General Electric SignaHDxt, Milwaukee, WI, USA) with an 8-channel phased-array head coil. For the rs-fMRI, the scans were acquired with TR = 2100 ms, TE = 30 ms, flip angle = 90°, slice thickness = 3 mm, gap = 0.6 mm, acquisition matrix = 64 $\times$ 64, voxel size = 3.125 $\times$ 3.125 $\times$ 3.6 mm^3, 42 axial slices, FOV = 200 $\times$ 200 mm, phases per location = 160. The scan lasted for 5 min and 36 s, and participants were required to stay awake with their eyes closed and ears plugged during the rs-fMRI scanning. In addition, magnetization-prepared rapid gradient echo (MPRAGE) T1-weighted images were collected.

Statistical Analysis

Behavioral Analysis

Baseline characteristics were compared by one-way analysis of variance (ANOVA) and Chi square tests using SPSS 18.0 Software (SPSS Inc., Chicago, IL, USA). During the analysis, all control participants from the two cohorts were combined into one group to increase the power. In order to estimate the effects of TCC and Baduanjin, ANCOVA analysis was applied to compare the change of MQ and the subtests across the three groups with age (years), with gender and education (years) included as covariates in the model. *Post hoc* analysis (Sidak corrected) was applied to explore the between-group differences.

Resting State Data Analysis

The fMRI data preprocessing was performed using Data Processing Assistant for Resting-State fMRI (DPARSF) Software (available at: http://rfmri.org/DPARSF; Chao-Gan and Yu-Feng, 2010) in MATLAB (Mathworks Inc., Natick, MA, USA). The software is based on Statistical Parametric Mapping (SPM8)[2] and the Resting-State fMRI Data Analysis Toolkit[3] (Song et al., 2011).

The first 10 volumes of functional data for each subject were discarded for signal equilibrium and participants' adaptation to the imaging noise. The remaining volumes were slice timing corrected, within-subject spatially realigned, co-registered to the respective structural images for each subject, and then segmented. Subjects were excluded if head movement exceeded 3 mm on any axis or if head rotation was greater than 3°. To perform subject-level correction of head motion, the Friston 24-parameter model (6 head motion parameters, 6 head motion parameters one time point before, and the 12 corresponding squared items; Friston et al., 1996; Yan et al., 2013) was used. Images were normalized using structural image unified segmentation and then re-sampled to 3-mm cubic voxels. After smoothing with a 6 mm full-width at half maximum (FWHM) Gaussian kernel, the linear and quadric trends of the time courses were removed. Similar to previous studies (Han et al., 2011), no temporal filtering was implemented during preprocessing so that the entire frequency band could be calculated. In this study, we applied three frequency bands: slow-5 (0.01–0.027 Hz), slow-4 (0.027–0.073 Hz), and the traditionally used low-frequency (0.01–0.08 Hz) bands.

Group analysis was performed with a random effects model using SPM8. To explore the difference between TCC and Baduanjin after longitudinal treatment, we used a full factorial module in SPM8 with two factors for group analysis. The first factor had three levels (TCC, Baduanjin, control group) and the second factor had two levels (pre- and post-treatment). Age, gender and years of education were also included in the analysis as covariates of non-interest. A threshold of a voxel-wise $p < 0.001$ uncorrected and cluster-level $p < 0.05$ family-wise error corrected based on the random Gaussian field theory base (Lindquist et al., 2009) was applied.

[2]http://www.fil.ion.ucl.ac.uk/spm
[3]http://www.restfmri.net

RESULTS

102 older adults between 50–70 years old were screened for this study. Of the 90 participants who were qualified for the study and finished baseline scans, 62 participants completed all study procedures (21 in the TCC group, 16 in the Baduanjin group, and 25 in the control group). Four participants in the TCC group dropped out (1 due to relocation, 1 due to unwillingness to get the second MRI scan, and 2 due to scheduling conflicts). Nine participants in the Baduanjin group dropped out (8 due to scheduling conflicts and 1 due to unwillingness to participate in the MRI scan). Fifteen participants in the control group dropped out (11 due to scheduling conflicts and 4 due to inability to participate in post-treatment MRI scans). One subject in the Baduanjin group was excluded from fALFF analysis due to excessive head movement (exceeded 3.0 mm).

Behavioral Results

Group characteristics are shown in **Table 1**. Age, gender, handedness, average years of education, MMSE score, and BDI score did not significantly differ among the three groups ($P > 0.05$). Average attendance rates were 95% in the TCC group (ranging from 88% to 100%) and 97% in the Baduanjin group (ranging from 92% to 100%).

MQ scores before and after exercise are presented in **Table 1**. No significant differences were found among the three groups at baseline. ANCOVA analysis of change between the baseline and post-treatment MQ scores showed a significant difference among the three groups ($F = 25.45$, $p < 0.001$). *Post hoc* Sidak correction analysis showed that compared with the control group, MQ scores significantly increased in the TCC and Baduanjin groups (Baduanjin: $p < 0.001$, TCC: $p < 0.001$). There were no significant differences between the TCC and Baduanjin groups ($p = 0.233$). The comparisons of the subscores of WMS-CR showed TCC significantly increased visual reproduction subscores compared to controls. Baduanjin produced greater improvement in mental control, recognition, visual reproduction, touch and comprehension memory subscores compared to controls after bonferroni correction ($p < 0.0063$). Baduanjin also produced greater improvements in touch subscores compared to TCC after bonferroni correction ($p < 0.0063$). Please also see our previous

TABLE 1 | Demographics of study participants and clinical outcome measurements.

Characteristics	Control (n = 25) Mean (SD)	Tai Chi Chuan (n = 21) Mean (SD)	Baduanjin (n = 15) Mean (SD)	Between-group difference: Tai Chi Chuan vs. Control P value	Baduanjin vs. Control p value	Tai Chi Chuan vs. Baduanjin p value
Age†	59.76 (4.83)	62.38 (4.55)	62.33 (3.88)	0.055	0.087	0.975
Gender (female/male)‡	19/6	13/8	9/6		0.473	
Handedness (right/left)	25/0	21/0	15/0	-	-	-
Average years of education†	8.52 (3.65)	9.61 (3.02)	9.13 (2.69)	0.255	0.563	0.658
MQ_Pre treatment†	99.08 (14.59)	105.81 (10.24)	99.20 (9.30)	0.065	0.976	0.112
MQ_Post treatment†††	97.76 (13.92)	123.57 (11.42)	124.86 (11.21)	<0.001	<0.001	0.907

†p values were calculated with one-way analysis of variance, ‡p values were calculated with the chi-square test, †††p values were calculated with mixed-model regression.

publications on subscore changes across different treatment (Tao et al., 2017b).

Resting-State fMRI Data Analysis Results

fALFF in Low-Frequency Band (0.01–0.08 Hz)

Pre- and post-treatment comparison of fALFF in the low-frequency band (0.01–0.08 Hz) among the three groups showed that after 12 weeks, fALFF was significantly increased in the right DLPFC in the TCC group compared to the control group (**Table 2**, **Figure 1A**). In the Baduanjin group, there was a significant increase in fALFF in the bilateral medial prefrontal cortex (mPFC) compared to the control group (**Table 2**, **Figure 1B**). No significant difference was observed between the TCC and Baduanjin groups at the threshold we set.

To explore the difference between Tai Chi vs. Baduanjin intervention, we also applied a relatively less conservative threshold of voxel-wise $p < 0.005$ uncorrected with 10 continuous voxels. We found that compared to the Baduanjin group, there was a significant increase in fALFF in the periaqueductal gray, bilateral DLPFC, and temporoparietal junction in the TCC group. Compared with the TCC group, the Baduanjin group was associated with a significant fALFF increase in the left mPFC and left precuneus.

To explore the association between the fALFF changes observed above and behavioral outcomes, we also extracted the average fALFF values of the significant clusters (DLPFC and mPFC) and performed a multiple regression analysis including age, gender, and education as covariates. Results showed a significant association between the fALFF changes at mPFC and corresponding MQ ($r = 0.48$, $p = 0.005$ significant after Bonferroni correction (0.025 (0.05/2); **Figure 1C**), as well as a marginal association between the fALFF changes at DLPFC and corresponding MQ changes ($p = 0.048$, not significant after Bonferroni correction across the TCC and Baduanjin groups).

fALFF in Slow-5 Band

Pre- and post-treatment comparison of fALFF in the slow-5 band among the three groups is shown in **Table 2** and **Figure 1**. After 12 weeks, participants in the TCC group showed significant increases in the right DLPFC compared with participants in the control group (**Figure 1D**). Participants in the Baduanjin group showed significant increases in the bilateral mPFC compared with participants in the control group (**Figure 1E**). No significant difference was found between the TCC and Baduanjin groups at the threshold we set.

To further explore the difference between Tai Chi vs. Baduanjin comparisons, we applied a relatively less conservative threshold of voxel-wise $p < 0.005$ uncorrected with 10 continuous voxels. We found that compared to the Baduanjin group, there was a significant fALFF increase in the right lateral prefrontal cortex and periaqueductal gray/pon, and a significant fALFF decrease in the left DLPFC in the TCC group.

To explore the association between the fALFF changes observed above and behavioral outcomes, we also extracted the average fALFF values of the significant clusters and performed multiple regression analysis respectively including age, gender and education as covariates across the participants in TCC and Baduanjin group. Results showed a significant association between the mPFC fALFF changes and corresponding MQ changes ($r = 0.40$, $p = 0.02$, significant after after Bonferroni correction (0.025 (0.05/2; **Figure 1F**). There was no significant association between DLPFC fALFF changes and corresponding MQ changes ($p = 0.078$).

fALFF in Slow-4 Band

No significant differences among the three groups (two exercise groups and one control group) were observed. When we applied a relatively less conservative threshold of voxel-wise $p < 0.001$ uncorrected with 10 continuous voxels, we

TABLE 2 | Comparisons of fractional amplitude of low-frequency fluctuations (fALFF) at different bands between groups.

Contrast	Brain regions	Cluster size	Peak *z*-value	Cluster effect size	MNI coordinates *X*	*Y*	*Z*
Low-frequency band							
TaiChiChuan > control	R DLPFC	60	5.45	3.02	51	18	39
Baduanjin > control	L mPFC	33	4.64	1.68	−12	12	66
	R mPFC	34	4.23	1.59	12	54	36
Control > Tai Chi Chuan			No brain region above the threshold				
Control > Baduanjin			No brain region above the threshold				
Tai Chi Chuan > Baduanjin			No brain region above the threshold				
Baduanjin > Tai Chi Chuan			No brain region above the threshold				
Slow-5 band							
Tai Chi Chuan > control	R DLPFC	65	5.1	2.17	48	15	42
Baduanjin > control	R mPFC	167	4.51	1.67	9	57	36
	L mPFC		4.41		−6	60	39
Control > Tai Chi Chuan			No brain region above the threshold				
Control > Baduanjin			No brain region above the threshold				
Tai Chi Chuan > Baduanjin			No brain region above the threshold				
Baduanjin > Tai Chi Chuan			No brain region above the threshold				

L, left; R, right; DLPFC, dorsolateral prefrontal cortex; mPFC, medial prefrontal cortex.

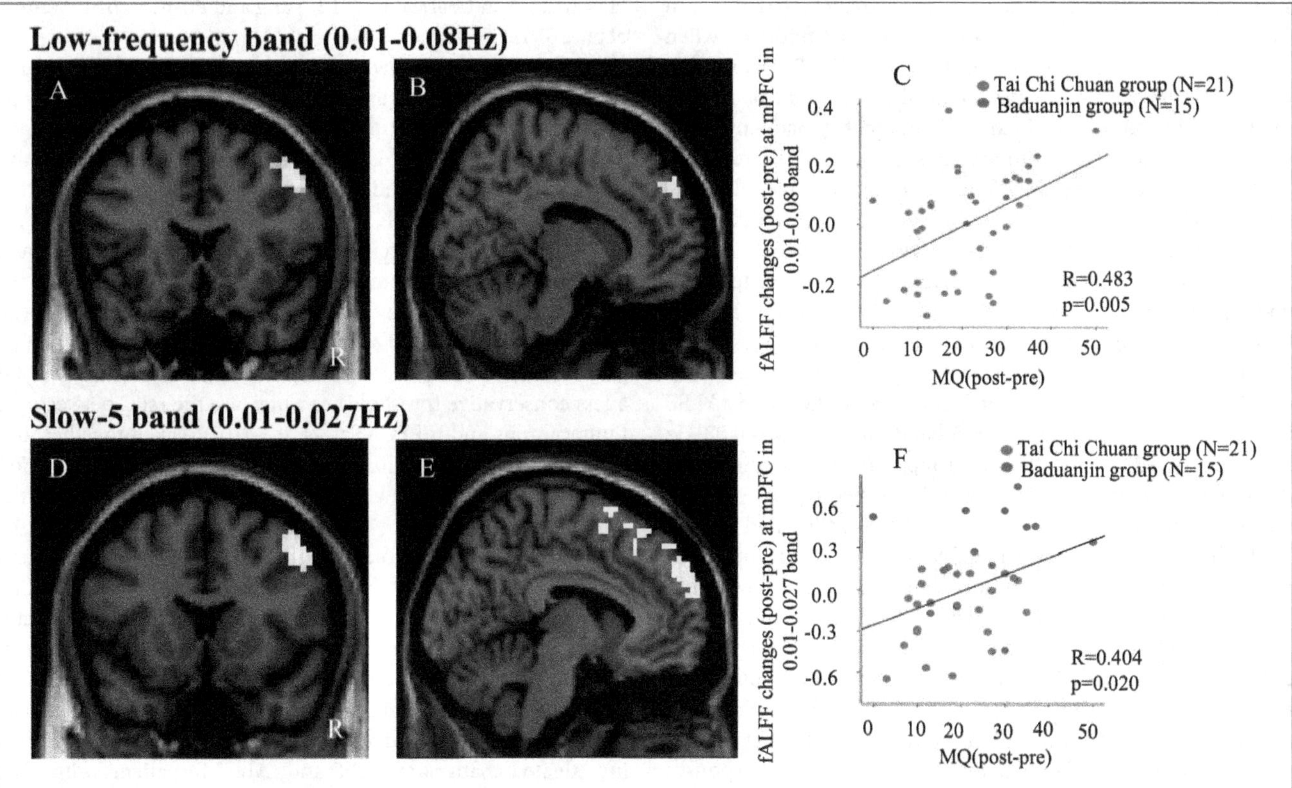

FIGURE 1 | (A) Increased fractional amplitude of low-frequency fluctuations (fALFF) in the 0.01–0.08 Hz band in the Tai Chi Chuan (TCC) group compared with the control group. **(B)** Increased fALFF in the 0.01–0.08 Hz band in the Baduanjin group compared with the control group. **(D)** Increased fALFF in the 0.01–0.027 Hz band in the TCC group compared with the control group. **(E)** Increased fALFF in the 0.01–0.027 Hz band in the Baduanjin group compared with the control group. **(C,F)** Scatter plots showing the association between the prefrontal cortex fALFF value of the significant cluster and improvements in memory across the TCC and Baduanjin groups, corrected for age, gender, years of education (**C**: $r = 0.483$, $p = 0.005$; **F**: $r = 0.404$, $p = 0.02$). R: right.

also did not find any significant results between the three groups.

DISCUSSION

In this study, we investigated the effects of 12 weeks of TCC and Baduanjin exercise on fALFF changes and clinical outcome measures in older adults. We found that: (1) MQ significantly increased in both TCC and Baduanjin groups compared with the control group; (2) TCC increased fALFF in the right DLPFC in the slow-5 band and the 0.01–0.08 Hz band; and (3) Baduanjin increased fALFF in the bilateral mPFC in the slow-5 band and the 0.01–0.08 Hz band following exercise. fALFF changes at the mPFC in the slow-5 and 0.01–0.08 Hz bands showed a significant positive association with corresponding MQ changes.

Both TCC and Baduanjin are mind-body exercises consisting of meditation, breathing, and gentle movements. From the viewpoint of physical exercise, both TCC and Baduanjin are safe aerobic activities (Li R. et al., 2014; Wayne et al., 2014). Aerobic exercise has been shown to improve memory function (Flöel et al., 2010; Erickson et al., 2011; Li L. et al., 2014; Seo et al., 2014). In addition to the physical component, TCC and Baduanjin also include sustained attention, focus, and multi-tasking. Thus, the mind-body exercise component may also have positive effects on cognitive function. Our finding of a significant improvement in general memory function after 3 months of TCC and Baduanjin practice is consistent with previous studies (Chang et al., 2010; Miller and Taylor-Piliae, 2014; Zheng et al., 2015) showing positive cognitive benefits of TCC in older adults. Our study demonstrates the power of TCC and Baduanjin practice in helping older adults improve memory.

We found that compared to controls, participants in the TCC group had increased fALFF in the right DLPFC, while the participants in the Baduanjin group had increased fALFF in the bilateral mPFC in the slow-5 band and the 0.01–0.08 Hz band. Although TCC and Baduanjin are associated with different patterns compared to controls, we did not find significant differences between the TCC and Baduanjin groups at this threshold we set. However, at a less conservative threshold of voxel-wise $p < 0.005$ uncorrected with 10 continuous voxels, there was a significant fALFF increase in the bilateral DLPFC, and decrease in the left mPFC and left precuneus in the TCC group compared to Baduanjin group in the 0.01–0.08 band. We also found that compared to the Baduanjin group, there was a significant fALFF increase in right lateral prefrontal cortex compared to the Baduanjin group in the slow-5 band. These significant difference activity pattern between TCC and Baduanjin is consistent with the findings when comparing: (1) Tai Chi vs. Control; and (2) Baduanjin vs. Control. Furthermore, we also found that TCC and Baduanjin modulate the subtests of WMS-CR differently, Baduanjin can significantly increase the touch subscore compared to TCC, which further suggests that different mechanism may underlying Tai Chi Quan and Baduanjin. We speculate this difference may due to different exercise characteristics associated with the two mind-body interactions. TCC involves more complicated body movements and requires moving the trunk and all four limbs, whereas the movement involved in Baduanjin is much simpler.

In this study, we found that TCC exercise increased fALFF in the right DLPFC in the slow-5 band and the 0.01–0.08 Hz band compared to the control group. Previous studies have demonstrated that the DLPFC, a task positive region, is a key area in the cognitive control network (CCN; Miller and Cohen, 2001; Cieslik et al., 2013). The CCN is important in top-down modulation of attention–memory interactions (Corbetta and Shulman, 2002; Cole and Schneider, 2007; Chiu and Yantis, 2009; Spreng et al., 2010; Kong et al., 2013; Hwang et al., 2015; Rosen et al., 2016). Recent studies have shown that non-invasive brain stimulation techniques such as repetitive transcranial magnetic stimulation and transcranial direct current stimulation of the DLPFC enhanced memory-guided responses in a visuospatial working memory task (Balconi and Ferrari, 2012; Brunoni and Vanderhasselt, 2014; Giglia et al., 2014). These findings further confirm the DLPFC's role in memory function.

Previous studies (Baron Short et al., 2010) found significantly increased DLPFC activation during meditation in comparison to a control task. In a recent study, investigators found that compared with control participants, TCC experts show greater functional homogeneity in the right post-central gyrus and lower functional homogeneity in the right DLPFC and the left anterior cingulate cortex. The gain in functional integration was significantly correlated with cognitive performance in TCC experts (Wei et al., 2014). In another study, investigators found that multimodal intervention including TCC exercise enhanced the ALFF in the right middle frontal gyrus/DLPFC in older adults (Yin et al., 2014). In a more recent study, we found that TCC practice significantly modulates the rsFC between the CCN and the superior frontal gyrus and ACC, and that Baduanjin modulates the rsFC between the CCN and the putamen and insula (Tao et al., 2017a). Our results are partially consistent with these findings.

We also found fALFF increases in the slow-5 band and the 0.01–0.08 Hz band in the Baduanjin group at the mPFC. This change was significantly associated with memory function changes. The mPFC is associated with the highest baseline metabolic activity at rest (Gusnard et al., 2001) and is a key region in the default mode network (DMN; Li L. et al., 2014). The mPFC identified in the present study overlaps with the findings observed in previous studies on the impact of physical activity and meditation on cognitive functions (Flöel et al., 2010; Hasenkamp and Barsalou, 2012; Tang and Posner, 2014; Tamura et al., 2015).

The mPFC is known to undergo both structural and functional changes with aging (Gutchess et al., 2007; Hurtz et al., 2014; van de Vijver et al., 2014). Research suggests that the mPFC's function is related to different aspects of social cognitive processing (Amodio and Frith, 2006), which involves action monitoring (Barch et al., 2001), self-knowledge (Macrae et al., 2004), person perception, mentalization (Grèzes et al., 2004), and outcome monitoring (Camille et al., 2004). Studies also found the mPFC is involved in the encoding and retrieval of memory (van Kesteren et al., 2010, 2012; Brod et al., 2013). In a previous study based on the same data, we found that TCC and Baduanjin (at a less conservative threshold) can increase the rsFC between the hippocampus and mPFC (Tao et al., 2016). Taken together, our result suggests that Baduanjin may improve memory function through the mPFC and associated brain networks, such as the hippocampus.

In this study, we found that the slow-5 frequency band and the low-frequency band (0.01–0.08 Hz) showed fALFF changes after TCC and Baiduanjin practice, while no significant differences were observed in the slow-4 band. This suggests that the memory-relevant changes induced by 3 months of TCC and Baduanjin practice are specifically reflected difference low-frequency band. In a previous study, Han et al. (2011) investigated changes of ALFF and fALFF in patients with MCI between the slow-4 and slow-5 bands. They found significant differences in fALFF between MCI patients and controls only in the slow-5 band. The pattern of intrinsic functional connectivity is sensitive to specific frequency bands. Chao-Gan and Yu-Feng (2010) found that the low-frequency range (0.01–0.08 Hz) may better reveal the DMN. Zuo et al. (2010) also shown that Slow-5 (0.01–0.027 Hz) amplitudes at low frequency were more dominant within ventromedial prefrontal cortices. Consistent with these results, our findings also predominantly locate at the frontal area in Slow-5 band and low-frequency range. Further studies are needed to confirm and expand our findings.

The current study has several limitations. First, the sample size is relatively small. Second, both TCC and Baduanjin are considered mind-body exercises. Therefore, our design could not disentangle the effect of physical activity vs. mental exercise, and was unable to identify the crucial components of the exercise affecting memory improvement and brain functional fluctuation changes. Further research is needed to compare the effects of exercise, meditation, TCC and Baduanjin directly. Third, we did not record the participants' original physical activity habits, and only gave them an introduction to keep their original physical activity habits throughout the duration of the experiment. Further study should record the participants original physical activity habits for more accurate documentation of their activity intensity.

CONCLUSION

In this study, we found that 12 weeks of intensive group TCC/Baduanjin practice can significantly modulate fALFF in different frequency bands and improve memory function. TCC increased fALFF in the slow-5 band and the 0.01–0.08 Hz band in the DLPFC, and Baduanjin increased fALFF in the slow-5 band and the 0.01–0.08 Hz band in the mPFC. fALFF changes in the mPFC in the slow-5 band and 0.01–0.08 Hz band were also correlated with general memory improvement. Our results imply that TCC and Baduanjin may work through different brain mechanisms due to differences in the characteristics and complexity of their respective regimens, but both exercises may hold the potential to prevent age-related memory decline.

ETHICS STATEMENT

The Medical Ethics Committee in the Affiliated Rehabilitation Hospital of Fujian University of Traditional Chinese Medicine approved all study procedures. The experiment was performed in accordance with approved guidelines. All participants signed a written consent. This study was registered on the Chinese Clinical Trial Registry (ChiCTR-IPR-15006131).

AUTHOR CONTRIBUTIONS

LC: experimental design; JK: analysis and manuscript preparation; JT: experimental design, data analysis and manuscript preparation; GZ: data analysis; JL and XX: data collection and data analysis; WL, JW, ML, ZW and KH: data collection; XC and NE: manuscript preparation. All authors contributed to manuscript draft and have read and approved the final manuscript.

FUNDING

This study is supported by the Special Scientific Research Fund of Public Welfare Profession of China (Grant No. 201307004), Ministry of Science and Technology and Ministry of Finance of the People's Republic of China. It is also supported by the National Rehabilitation Research Center of Traditional Chinese Medicine, Fujian rehabilitation industrial institution and Fujian Rehabilitation Tech Co-innovation Center (Grant No. X2012007-Collaboration). JK is supported by R01AT006364, R01AT008563, R61AT009310, R21AT008707 and P01 AT006663 from NIH/NCCIH.

ACKNOWLEDGMENTS

We thank two professional instructors from the Fujian University of Traditional Chinese Medicine Hongmei Yi and Tingjin Duan, for their training in Tai Chi Chuan and Baduanjin exercise. We thank Sharon Sun, Courtney Lang and Joel Park for editing the English.

REFERENCES

Amodio, D. M., and Frith, C. D. (2006). Meeting of minds: the medial frontal cortex and social cognition. *Nat. Rev. Neurosci.* 7, 268–277. doi: 10.1038/nrn1884

Balconi, M., and Ferrari, C. (2012). rTMS stimulation on left DLPFC increases the correct recognition of memories for emotional target and distractor words. *Cogn. Affect. Behav. Neurosci.* 12, 589–598. doi: 10.3758/s13415-012-0090-1

Barch, D. M., Braver, T. S., Akbudak, E., Conturo, T., Ollinger, J., and Snyder, A. (2001). Anterior cingulate cortex and response conflict: effects of response modality and processing domain. *Cereb. Cortex* 11, 837–848. doi: 10.1093/cercor/11.9.837

Baron Short, E., Kose, S., Mu, Q., Borckardt, J., Newberg, A., George, M. S., et al. (2010). Regional brain activation during meditation shows time and practice effects: an exploratory FMRI study. *Evid. Based Complement. Alternat. Med.* 7, 121–127. doi: 10.1093/ecam/nem163

Beck, A. T., Steer, R. A., and Brown, G. K. (1996). *Manual for the Beck Depression Inventory-II.* San Antonio, TX: Psychological Corporation.

Biswal, B., Yetkin, F. Z., Haughton, V. M., and Hyde, J. S. (1995). Functional connectivity in the motor cortex of resting human brain using echo-planar MRI. *Magn. Reson. Med.* 34, 537–541. doi: 10.1002/mrm.1910340409

Brod, G., Werkle-Bergner, M., and Shing, Y. L. (2013). The influence of prior knowledge on memory: a developmental cognitive neuroscience perspective. *Front. Behav. Neurosci.* 7:139. doi: 10.3389/fnbeh.2013.00139

Brunoni, A. R., and Vanderhasselt, M. A. (2014). Working memory improvement with non-invasive brain stimulation of the dorsolateral prefrontal cortex: a systematic review and meta-analysis. *Brain Cogn.* 86, 1–9. doi: 10.1016/j.bandc.2014.01.008

Buzsáki, G., and Draguhn, A. (2004). Neuronal oscillations in cortical networks. *Science* 304, 1926–1929. doi: 10.1126/science.1099745

Camille, N., Coricelli, G., Sallet, J., Pradat-Diehl, P., Duhamel, J. R., and Sirigu, A. (2004). The involvement of the orbitofrontal cortex in the experience of regret. *Science* 304, 1167–1170. doi: 10.1126/science.1094550

Chang, Y.-K., Nien, Y.-H., Tsai, C.-L., and Etnier, J. L. (2010). Physical activity and cognition in older adults: the potential of Tai Chi Chuan. *J. Aging Phys. Act.* 18, 451–472. doi: 10.1123/japa.18.4.451

Chao-Gan, Y., and Yu-Feng, Z. (2010). DPARSF: a MATLAB toolbox for 'Pipeline' data analysis of resting-state fMRI. *Front. Syst. Neurosci.* 4:13. doi: 10.3389/fnsys.2010.00013

China National Sports Commission. (1983). *Simplified Taijiquan.* Beijing: People's Sports Press.

Chiu, Y. C., and Yantis, S. (2009). A domain-independent source of cognitive control for task sets: shifting spatial attention and switching categorization rules. *J. Neurosci.* 29, 3930–3938. doi: 10.1523/jneurosci.5737-08.2009

Cieslik, E. C., Zilles, K., Caspers, S., Roski, C., Kellermann, T. S., Jakobs, O., et al. (2013). Is there "One" DLPFC in cognitive action control? Evidence for heterogeneity from co-activation-based parcellation. *Cereb. Cortex* 23, 2677–2689. doi: 10.1093/cercor/bhs256

Cole, M. W., and Schneider, W. (2007). The cognitive control network: integrated cortical regions with dissociable functions. *Neuroimage* 37, 343–360. doi: 10.1016/j.neuroimage.2007.03.071

Corbetta, M., and Shulman, G. L. (2002). Control of goal-directed and stimulus-driven attention in the brain. *Nat. Rev. Neurosci.* 3, 201–215. doi: 10.1038/nrn755

Erickson, K. I., Leckie, R. L., and Weinstein, A. M. (2014). Physical activity, fitness, and gray matter volume. *Neurobiol. Aging* 35, S20–S28. doi: 10.1016/j.neurobiolaging.2014.03.034

Erickson, K. I., Voss, M. W., Prakash, R. S., Basak, C., Szabo, A., Chaddock, L., et al. (2011). Exercise training increases size of hippocampus and improves memory. *Proc. Natl. Acad. Sci. U S A* 108, 3017–3022. doi: 10.1073/pnas.1015950108

Esposito, F., Tessitore, A., Giordano, A., De Micco, R., Paccone, A., Conforti, R., et al. (2013). Rhythm-specific modulation of the sensorimotor network in drug-naive patients with Parkinson's disease by levodopa. *Brain* 136, 710–725. doi: 10.1093/brain/awt007

Flöel, A., Ruscheweyh, R., Krüger, K., Willemer, C., Winter, B., Völker, K., et al. (2010). Physical activity and memory functions: are neurotrophins and cerebral gray matter volume the missing link? *Neuroimage* 49, 2756–2763. doi: 10.1016/j.neuroimage.2009.10.043

Fong, D.-Y., Chi, L.-K., Li, F., and Chang, Y.-K. (2014). The benefits of endurance exercise and Tai Chi Chuan for the task-switching aspect of executive function in older adults: an ERP study. *Front. Aging Neurosci.* 6:295. doi: 10.3389/fnagi.2014.00295

Fox, M. D., and Raichle, M. E. (2007). Spontaneous fluctuations in brain activity observed with functional magnetic resonance imaging. *Nat. Rev. Neurosci.* 8, 700–711. doi: 10.1038/nrn2201

Friston, K. J., Williams, S., Howard, R., Frackowiak, R. S., and Turner, R. (1996). Movement-related effects in fMRI time-series. *Magn. Reson. Med.* 35, 346–355. doi: 10.1002/mrm.1910350312

Giglia, G., Brighina, F., Rizzo, S., Puma, A., Indovino, S., Maccora, S., et al. (2014). Anodal transcranial direct current stimulation of the right dorsolateral prefrontal cortex enhances memory-guided responses in a visuospatial working memory task. *Funct. Neurol.* 29, 189–193. doi: 10.11138/FNeur/2014.29.3.189

Gong, Y., and Wang, D. J. (1989). *Handbook of Wechsler Memory Scale-Revised (WMS-RC), Chinese Version.* Changsha: Bulletin of Hunan Medical College.

Grèzes, J., Frith, C., and Passingham, R. E. (2004). Brain mechanisms for inferring deceit in the actions of others. *J. Neurosci.* 24, 5500–5505. doi: 10.1523/jneurosci.0219-04.2004

Gusnard, D. A., Akbudak, E., Shulman, G. L., and Raichle, M. E. (2001). Medial prefrontal cortex and self-referential mental activity: relation to a default mode of brain function. *Proc. Natl. Acad. Sci. U S A* 98, 4259–4264. doi: 10.1073/pnas.071043098

Gutchess, A. H., Kensinger, E. A., and Schacter, D. L. (2007). Aging, self-referencing, and medial prefrontal cortex. *Soc. Neurosci.* 2, 117–133. doi: 10.1080/17470910701399029

Han, Y., Lui, S., Kuang, W., Lang, Q., Zou, L., and Jia, J. (2012). Anatomical and functional deficits in patients with amnestic mild cognitive impairment. *PLoS One* 7:e28664. doi: 10.1371/journal.pone.0028664

Han, Y., Wang, J., Zhao, Z., Min, B., Lu, J., Li, K., et al. (2011). Frequency-dependent changes in the amplitude of low-frequency fluctuations in amnestic mild cognitive impairment: a resting-state fMRI study. *Neuroimage* 55, 287–295. doi: 10.1016/j.neuroimage.2010.11.059

Hasenkamp, W., and Barsalou, L. W. (2012). Effects of meditation experience on functional connectivity of distributed brain networks. *Front. Hum. Neurosci.* 6:38. doi: 10.3389/fnhum.2012.00038

Hillman, C. H., Erickson, K. I., and Kramer, A. F. (2008). Be smart, exercise your heart: exercise effects on brain and cognition. *Nat. Rev. Neurosci.* 9, 58–65. doi: 10.1038/nrn2298

Hoptman, M. J., Zuo, X. N., Butler, P. D., Javitt, D. C., D'Angelo, D., Mauro, C. J., et al. (2010). Amplitude of low-frequency oscillations in schizophrenia: a resting state fMRI study. *Schizophr. Res.* 117, 13–20. doi: 10.1016/j.schres.2009.09.030

Hughes, T. F., Flatt, J. D., Fu, B., Butters, M. A., Chang, C. C., and Ganguli, M. (2014). Interactive video gaming compared with health education in older adults with mild cognitive impairment: a feasibility study. *Int. J. Geriatr. Psychiatry* 29, 890–898. doi: 10.1002/gps.4075

Hurtz, S., Woo, E., Kebets, V., Green, A. E., Zoumalan, C., Wang, B., et al. (2014). Age effects on cortical thickness in cognitively normal elderly individuals. *Dement. Geriatr. Cogn. Dis. Extra* 4, 221–227. doi: 10.1159/000362872

Hwang, J. W., Egorova, N., Yang, X. Q., Zhang, W. Y., Chen, J., Yang, X. Y., et al. (2015). Subthreshold depression is associated with impaired resting-state functional connectivity of the cognitive control network. *Transl. Psychiatry* 5:e683. doi: 10.1038/tp.2015.174

Innes, K. E., Selfe, T. K., Khalsa, D. S., and Kandati, S. (2017). Meditation and music improve memory and cognitive function in adults with subjective cognitive decline: a pilot randomized controlled trial. *J. Alzheimers Dis.* 56, 899–916. doi: 10.3233/JAD-160867

Kelly, M. E., Loughrey, D., Lawlor, B. A., Robertson, I. H., Walsh, C., and Brennan, S. (2014). The impact of exercise on the cognitive functioning of healthy older adults: a systematic review and meta-analysis. *Ageing Res. Rev.* 16, 12–31. doi: 10.1016/j.arr.2014.05.002

Killgore, W. D., Olson, E. A., and Weber, M. (2013). Physical exercise habits correlate with gray matter volume of the hippocampus in healthy adult humans. *Sci. Rep.* 3:3457. doi: 10.1038/srep03457

Knyazev, G. G. (2007). Motivation, emotion, and their inhibitory control mirrored in brain oscillations. *Neurosci. Biobehav. Rev.* 31, 377–395. doi: 10.1016/j.neubiorev.2006.10.004

Kong, J., Jensen, K., Loiotile, R., Cheetham, A., Wey, H. Y., Tan, Y., et al. (2013). Functional connectivity of the frontoparietal network predicts cognitive modulation of pain. *Pain* 154, 459–467. doi: 10.1016/j.pain.2012.12.004

Lam, L. C., Chau, R. C., Wong, B. M., Fung, A. W., Lui, V. W., Tam, C. C., et al. (2011). Interim follow-up of a randomized controlled trial comparing chinese style mind body (Tai Chi) and stretching exercises on cognitive function in subjects at risk of progressive cognitive decline. *Int. J. Geriatr. Psychiatry* 26, 733–740. doi: 10.1002/gps.2602

Li, F., Harmer, P., Liu, Y., and Chou, L. S. (2014). Tai Ji Quan and global cognitive function in older adults with cognitive impairment: a pilot study. *Arch. Gerontol. Geriatr.* 58, 434–439. doi: 10.1016/j.archger.2013.12.003

Li, R., Jin, L., Hong, P., He, Z.-H., Huang, C.-Y., Zhao, J.-X., et al. (2014). The effect of baduanjin on promoting the physical fitness and health of adults. *Evid. Based Complement. Alternat. Med.* 2014:784059. doi: 10.1155/2014/784059

Li, L., Men, W. W., Chang, Y. K., Fan, M. X., Ji, L., and Wei, G. X. (2014). Acute aerobic exercise increases cortical activity during working memory: a functional MRI study in female college students. *PLoS One* 9:e99222. doi: 10.1371/journal.pone.0099222

Lindquist, M. A., Meng Loh, J., Atlas, L. Y., and Wager, T. D. (2009). Modeling the hemodynamic response function in fMRI: efficiency, bias and mis-modeling. *Neuroimage* 45, S187–S198. doi: 10.1016/j.neuroimage.2008.10.065

Liu, X., Wang, S., Zhang, X., Wang, Z., Tian, X., and He, Y. (2014). Abnormal amplitude of low-frequency fluctuations of intrinsic brain activity in Alzheimer's disease. *J. Alzheimers Dis.* 40, 387–397. doi: 10.3233/JAD-131322

Macrae, C. N., Moran, J. M., Heatherton, T. F., Banfield, J. F., and Kelley, W. M. (2004). Medial prefrontal activity predicts memory for self. *Cereb. Cortex* 14, 647–654. doi: 10.1093/cercor/bhh025

Makizako, H., Shimada, H., Doi, T., Park, H., Yoshida, D., and Suzuki, T. (2013). Six-minute walking distance correlated with memory and brain volume in older adults with mild cognitive impairment: a voxel-based morphometry study. *Dement. Geriatr. Cogn. Dis. Extra* 3, 223–232. doi: 10.1159/000354189

McGill, M. L., Devinsky, O., Wang, X., Quinn, B. T., Pardoe, H., Carlson, C., et al. (2014). Functional neuroimaging abnormalities in idiopathic generalized epilepsy. *Neuroimage Clin.* 6, 455–462. doi: 10.1016/j.nicl.2014.10.008

McKhann, G. M., Knopman, D. S., Chertkow, H., Hyman, B. T., Jack, C. R. Jr., Kawas, C. H., et al. (2011). The diagnosis of dementia due to Alzheimer's disease: recommendations from the national institute on aging- Alzheimer's association workgroups on diagnostic guidelines for Alzheimer's disease. *Alzheimers Dement.* 7, 263–269. doi: 10.1016/j.jalz.2011.03.005

Miller, E. K., and Cohen, J. D. (2001). An integrative theory of prefrontal cortex function. *Annu. Rev. Neurosci.* 24, 167–202. doi: 10.1146/annurev.neuro.24.1.167

Miller, S. M., and Taylor-Piliae, R. E. (2014). Effects of Tai Chi on cognitive function in community-dwelling older adults: a review. *Geriatr. Nurs.* 35, 9–19. doi: 10.1016/j.gerinurse.2013.10.013

Rosen, M. L., Stern, C. E., Michalka, S. W., Devaney, K. J., and Somers, D. C. (2016). Cognitive control network contributions to memory-guided visual attention. *Cereb. Cortex* 26, 2059–2073. doi: 10.1093/cercor/bhv028

Ruscheweyh, R., Willemer, C., Krüger, K., Duning, T., Warnecke, T., Sommer, J., et al. (2011). Physical activity and memory functions: an interventional study. *Neurobiol. Aging* 32, 1304–1319. doi: 10.1016/j.neurobiolaging.2009.08.001

Seo, T. B., Kim, T. W., Shin, M. S., Ji, E. S., Cho, H. S., Lee, J. M., et al. (2014). Aerobic exercise alleviates ischemia-induced memory impairment by enhancing cell proliferation and suppressing neuronal apoptosis in hippocampus. *Int. Neurourol. J.* 18, 187–197. doi: 10.5213/inj.2014.18.4.187

Song, X. W., Dong, Z. Y., Long, X. Y., Li, S. F., Zuo, X. N., Zhu, C. Z., et al. (2011). REST: a toolkit for resting-state functional magnetic resonance imaging data processing. *PLoS One* 6:e25031. doi: 10.1371/journal.pone.0025031

Spreng, R. N., Stevens, W. D., Chamberlain, J. P., Gilmore, A. W., and Schacter, D. L. (2010). Default network activity, coupled with the frontoparietal control network, supports goal-directed cognition. *Neuroimage* 53, 303–317. doi: 10.1016/j.neuroimage.2010.06.016

Sui, J., Pearlson, G. D., Du, Y., Yu, Q., Jones, T. R., Chen, J., et al. (2015). In search of multimodal neuroimaging biomarkers of cognitive deficits in schizophrenia. *Biol. Psychiatry* 78, 794–804. doi: 10.1016/j.biopsych.2015.02.017

Tamura, M., Nemoto, K., Kawaguchi, A., Kato, M., Arai, T., Kakuma, T., et al. (2015). Long-term mild-intensity exercise regimen preserves prefrontal cortical volume against aging. *Int. J. Geriatr. Psychiatry* 30, 686–694. doi: 10.1002/gps.4205

Tang, Y.-Y., and Posner, M. I. (2014). Training brain networks and states. *Trends. Cogn. Sci.* 18, 345–350. doi: 10.1016/j.tics.2014.04.002

Tao, J., Chen, X., Egorova, N., Liu, J., Xue, X., Wang, Q., et al. (2017a). Tai Chi Chuan and baduanjin practice modulates functional connectivity of the cognitive control network in older adults. *Sci. Rep.* 7:41581. doi: 10.1038/srep41581

Tao, J., Liu, J., Liu, W., Huang, J., Xue, X., Chen, X., et al. (2017b). Tai Chi Chuan and baduanjin increase grey matter volume in older adults: a brain imaging study. *J. Alzheimers Dis.* 60, 389–400. doi: 10.3233/JAD-170477

Tao, J., Liu, J., Egorova, N., Chen, X., Sun, S., Xue, X., et al. (2016). Increased hippocampus-medial prefrontal cortex resting state functional connectivity and memory function after Tai Chi Chuan practice in elder adults. *Front. Aging Neurosci.* 8:25. doi: 10.3389/fnagi.2016.00025

Tao, J., Rao, T., Lin, L., Liu, W., Wu, Z., Zheng, G., et al. (2015). Evaluation of Tai Chi yunshou exercises on community-based stroke patients with balance dysfunction: a study protocol of a cluster randomized controlled trial. *BMC Complement. Altern. Med.* 15:31. doi: 10.1186/s12906-015-0555-1

Tsai, P. F., Chang, J. Y., Beck, C., Kuo, Y. F., and Keefe, F. J. (2013). A pilot cluster-randomized trial of a 20-week Tai Chi program in elders with cognitive impairment and osteoarthritic knee: effects on pain and other health outcomes. *J. Pain Symptom Manage.* 45, 660–669. doi: 10.1016/j.jpainsymman.2012.04.009

van de Vijver, I., Cohen, M. X., and Ridderinkhof, K. R. (2014). Aging affects medial but not anterior frontal learning-related theta oscillations. *Neurobiol. Aging* 35, 692–704. doi: 10.1016/j.neurobiolaging.2013.09.006

van Kesteren, M. T., Rijpkema, M., Ruiter, D. J., and Fernández, G. (2010). Retrieval of associative information congruent with prior knowledge is related to increased medial prefrontal activity and connectivity. *J. Neurosci.* 30, 15888–15894. doi: 10.1523/JNEUROSCI.2674-10.2010

van Kesteren, M. T., Ruiter, D. J., Fernández, G., and Henson, R. N. (2012). How schema and novelty augment memory formation. *Trends Neurosci.* 35, 211–219. doi: 10.1016/j.tins.2012.02.001

Voss, M. W., Heo, S., Prakash, R. S., Erickson, K. I., Alves, H., Chaddock, L., et al. (2013). The influence of aerobic fitness on cerebral white matter integrity and cognitive function in older adults: results of a one- year exercise intervention. *Hum. Brain Mapp.* 34, 2972–2985. doi: 10.1002/hbm.22119

Wang, S. T. (2007). Effect of baduanjin on physiological age of intelligence for old people. *J. Clin. Rehabil. Tissue Eng. Res.* 11, 7910–7913.

Wang, C., Schmid, C. H., Rones, R., Kalish, R., Yinh, J., Goldenberg, D. L., et al. (2010). A randomized trial of Tai Chi for fibromyalgia. *N. Engl. J. Med.* 363, 743–754. doi: 10.1056/NEJMoa0912611

Wayne, P. M., Walsh, J. N., Taylor-Piliae, R. E., Wells, R. E., Papp, K. V., Donovan, N. J., et al. (2014). Effect of Tai Chi on cognitive performance in older adults: systematic review and meta-analysis. *J. Am. Geriatr. Soc.* 62, 25–39. doi: 10.1111/jgs.12611

Wei, G. X., Dong, H. M., Yang, Z., Luo, J., and Zuo, X. N. (2014). Tai Chi Chuan optimizes the functional organization of the intrinsic human brain architecture in older adults. *Front. Aging Neurosci.* 6:74. doi: 10.3389/fnagi.2014.00074

Wei, G.-X., Xu, T., Fan, F.-M., Dong, H.-M., Jiang, L.-L., Li, H.-J., et al. (2013). Can taichi reshape the brain? a brain morphometry study. *PLoS One* 8:e61038. doi: 10.1371/journal.pone.0061038

Woodard, J. L., and Axelrod, B. N. (1995). Parsimonious prediction of wechsler memory scale—revised memory indices. *Psychol. Assess.* 7, 445–449. doi: 10.1037//1040-3590.7.4.445

Xiong, X., Wang, P., Li, S., Zhang, Y., and Li, X. (2015). Effect of baduanjin exercise for hypertension: a systematic review and meta-analysis of randomized controlled trials. *Maturitas* 80, 370–378. doi: 10.1016/j.maturitas.2015.01.002

Yan, C. G., Cheung, B., Kelly, C., Colcombe, S., Craddock, R. C., Di Martino, A., et al. (2013). A comprehensive assessment of regional variation in the impact of head micromovements on functional connectomics. *Neuroimage* 76, 183–201. doi: 10.1016/j.neuroimage.2013.03.004

Yin, S., Zhu, X., Li, R., Niu, Y., Wang, B., Zheng, Z., et al. (2014). Intervention-induced enhancement in intrinsic brain activity in healthy older adults. *Sci. Rep.* 4:7309. doi: 10.1038/srep07309

Zang, Y. F., He, Y., Zhu, C. Z., Cao, Q. J., Sui, M. Q., Liang, M., et al. (2007). Altered baseline brain activity in children with ADHD revealed by resting-state functional MRI. *Brain Dev.* 29, 83–91. doi: 10.1016/j.braindev.2006.07.002

Zhang, M. Y., Katzman, R., Salmon, D., Jin, H., Cai, G. J., Wang, Z. Y., et al. (1990). The prevalence of dementia and Alzheimer's disease in shanghai, china: impact of age, gender, and education. *Ann. Neurol.* 27, 428–437. doi: 10.1002/ana.410270412

Zhang, Y., Zhu, C., Chen, H., Duan, X., Lu, F., Li, M., et al. (2015). Frequency-dependent alterations in the amplitude of low-frequency fluctuations in social anxiety disorder. *J. Affect. Disord.* 174, 329–335. doi: 10.1016/j.jad.2014.12.001

Zhao, Z.-L., Fan, F.-M., Lu, J., Li, H.-J., Jia, L.-F., Han, Y., et al. (2015). Changes of gray matter volume and amplitude of low-frequency oscillations in amnestic MCI: an integrative multi-modal MRI study. *Acta Radiol.* 56, 614–621. doi: 10.1177/0284185114533329

Zheng, G., Chen, B., Fang, Q., Yi, H., Lin, Q., Chen, L., et al. (2014). Primary prevention for risk factors of ischemic stroke with baduanjin exercise intervention in the community elder population: study protocol for a randomized controlled trial. *Trials* 15:113. doi: 10.1186/1745-6215-15-113

Zheng, G., Liu, F., Li, S., Huang, M., Tao, J., and Chen, L. (2015). Tai Chi and the protection of cognitive ability. *Am. J. Prev. Med.* 49, 89–97. doi: 10.1016/j.amepre.2015.01.002

Zou, Q. H., Zhu, C. Z., Yang, Y., Zuo, X. N., Long, X. Y., Cao, Q. J., et al. (2008). An improved approach to detection of amplitude of low-frequency fluctuation (ALFF) for resting-state fMRI: fractional ALFF. *J. Neurosci. Methods* 172, 137–141. doi: 10.1016/j.jneumeth.2008.04.012

Zuo, X. N., Di Martino, A., Kelly, C., Shehzad, Z. E., Gee, D. G., Klein, D. F., et al. (2010). The oscillating brain: complex and reliable. *Neuroimage* 49, 1432–1445. doi: 10.1016/j.neuroimage.2009.09.037

15

Subregional Structural Alterations in Hippocampus and Nucleus Accumbens Correlate with the Clinical Impairment in Patients with Alzheimer's Disease Clinical Spectrum: Parallel Combining Volume and Vertex-Based Approach

Xiuling Nie[1†], Yu Sun[1,2†], Suiren Wan[1†], Hui Zhao[3], Renyuan Liu[4], Xueping Li[4], Sichu Wu[4], Zuzana Nedelska[5,6], Jakub Hort[5,6], Zhao Qing[4], Yun Xu[3] and Bing Zhang[4]*

[1]State Key laboratory of Bioelectronics, School of Biological Sciences and Medical Engineering, Southeast University, Nanjing, China, [2]Institute of Cancer and Genetic Science, University of Birmingham, Birmingham, United Kingdom, [3]Department of Neurology, Affiliated Drum Tower Hospital of Nanjing University Medical School, Nanjing, China, [4]Department of Radiology, Affiliated Drum Tower Hospital of Nanjing University Medical School, Nanjing, China, [5]Department of Neurology, Memory Clinic, 2nd Faculty of Medicine, Charles University in Prague, Motol University Hospital, Prague, Czechia, [6]International Clinical Research Center, St. Anne's University Hospital Brno, Brno, Czech Republic

Correspondence:
Bing Zhang
zhangbing_nanjing@vip.163.com

[†]Cofirst author: these authors have contributed equally to this work.

Deep gray matter structures are associated with memory and other important functions that are impaired in Alzheimer's disease (AD) and mild cognitive impairment (MCI). However, systematic characterization of the subregional atrophy and deformations in these structures in AD and MCI still need more investigations. In this article, we combined complex volumetry- and vertex-based analysis to investigate the pattern of subregional structural alterations in deep gray matter structures and its association with global clinical scores in AD (n = 30) and MCI patients (n = 30), compared to normal controls (NCs, n = 30). Among all seven pairs of structures, the bilateral hippocampi and nucleus accumbens showed significant atrophy in AD compared with NCs ($p < 0.05$). But only the subregional atrophy in the dorsal–medial part of the left hippocampus, the ventral part of right hippocampus, and the left nucleus accumbens, the posterior part of the right nucleus accumbens correlated with the worse clinical scores of MMSE and MOCA ($p < 0.05$). Furthermore, the medial–ventral part of right thalamus significantly shrank and correlated with clinical scores without decreasing in its whole volume ($p > 0.05$). In conclusion, the atrophy of these four subregions in bilateral hippocampi and nucleus accumbens was associated with cognitive impairment of patients, which might be potential target regions of treatment in AD. The surface analysis could provide additional information to volume comparison in finding the early pathological progress in deep gray matter structures.

Keywords: Alzheimer's disease, mild cognitive impairment, deep gray matter structures, surface alteration, vertex analysis

INTRODUCTION

Alzheimer's disease (AD) is the most prevalent form of age-related dementia (1, 2) and is usually preceded by a stage of cognitive decline. This clinical state of cognitive decline is conceptualized as mild cognitive impairment (MCI) (3, 4). Previous studies showed that MRI-based assessments of brain volume, such as hippocampal atrophy, can provided additional information for diagnosis of AD (5). Specifically deep gray matter structures, including bilateral nucleus accumbens (NAc), amygdala, caudate nucleus, hippocampus, pallidum, putamen, and thalamus, are associated with memory, emotional learning, shifting attention, and spatial working memory (6, 7), which were typically impaired in AD stage. Previous studies have focused on these regions and reported that there was atrophy on hippocampus and entorhinal cortex (8–12). Besides, it also suggested that other deep gray matter structures, like amygdala, putamen, and thalamus also showed significantly reduced volume, even in MCI (10, 13–15).

However, the subregions of deep gray matter structures may have different function and their impairment in AD may also have subregional specificity (9, 15–17). Therefore, it is very informative to explore the changes of deep gray matter structures on the subregional level in the AD and MCI. Previous studies have reported shape abnormalities in multiple deep gray matter structures, such as the dorsal–medial part of thalamus (15), the anterior hippocampus (9, 17), and the basolateral complex of amygdala (16, 17) in AD patients compared to controls. However, there is still lack of a systematic investigation of all deep gray matter structures.

In the current study, we unitized the automated software package, FMRIB's Integrated Registration and Segmentation Tool (FIRST) (16, 18, 19), which provided a powerful tool to analyze subregional atrophy and shape alterations within seven pairs of deep gray matter structures. The volumes of each deep gray matter structure and the vertex-wised distortion were compared among clinically normal controls (NCs) as well as MCI and AD patients. We hypothesized that the pattern of atrophy on subregional level would differ among the three mentioned groups, and the specific pattern of more profound atrophy or shape alterations would correlate with poorer scores of global clinical scores.

MATERIALS AND METHODS

Subjects

Ninety consecutive subjects were recruited from the memory clinic of Affiliated Drum Tower Hospital of Nanjing University Medical School. All subjects underwent a clinical evaluation using Mini-Mental State Examination (MMSE) (20) and Montreal Cognitive Assessment (MOCA) (21). Written consent was obtained from all subjects or their proxies after a detailed explanation of the study procedures, which was approved by the local Ethics Committee.

The MCI patients (n = 30) were diagnosed based on the following criteria (22): (a) memory complaint, preferably confirmed by an informant; (b) objective memory impairment, adjusted for age, and education; (c) normal or near-normal performance on general cognitive functioning and no or minimum impairment of daily life activities; and (d) not meeting the criteria for dementia. AD patients (n = 30) met NINCDS-ADRDA criteria (23). For comparison, we included NC (n = 30) who (a) had no cognitive complaints, (b) scored normally on global cognitive scales such as MMSE and MOCA, and (c) had no evidence of any structural abnormality on a conventional MRI scan.

Exclusion criteria were history of any significant medical, psychiatric, or neurological illness other than MCI or AD; history of brain injury; alcohol or drug abuse of alcohol; and missing clinical assessments.

MRI Acquisition

Images were acquired on a 3.0-T MR scanner (Achieva 3.0T TX dual Medical Systems; Philips Medical Systems, Eindhoven, Netherlands) using a three-dimensional turbo fast echo (3D-TFE) T_1-weighted pulse sequence with TR = 9.7 ms, TE = 4.6 ms, flip angle = 8°, slice thickness = 1 mm, slice gap = 1 mm, FOV = 256 mm × 256 mm, and matrix = 192.

Image Processing

The flowchart of image processing is shown in **Figure 1**. MRI volume were processed using FMRIB Software Library (FSL, Version 5.0, http://www.fmrib.ox.ac.uk/fsl) (18, 24). Briefly, brain extraction was performed on 3D T1-weighted MR images using Brain Extraction Tool (25), which uses a deformable model that evolves to fit the brain's surface by the application of a set of locally adaptive model forces (25).

FMRIB's Integrated Registration and Segmentation Tool (16) was applied to perform the segmentation and to measure volumes and vertexes in seven deep gray matter structures bilaterally, including NAc, amygdala, caudate nucleus, hippocampus, pallidum, putamen, and thalamus. FIRST initially performed a two-stage linear registration using 12 degrees of freedom, and the registration was performed by FLIRT (26). In the first stage, an affine registration of the whole-head to a standard space template (MNI template), with 1 mm × 1 mm × 1 mm resolution, was implemented. In the second stage, a subcortical mask was used to exclude regions outside the deep gray matter structures. Finally, a boundary correction was used to determine whether boundary voxels belong to this structure or not.

Based on this deep gray matter segmentation, the volume of each region was first extracted. The boundary of each region was reconstructed into a vertex-based surface, and the vertex locations from each subject (at a corresponding anatomical point) were projected onto the surface normal of the average shape of all

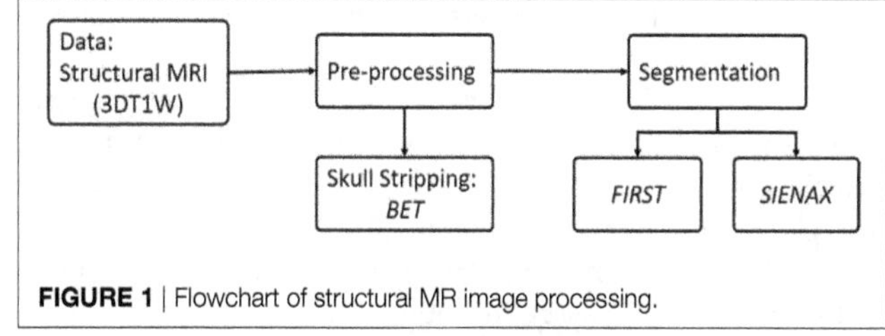

FIGURE 1 | Flowchart of structural MR image processing.

the subjects. The projections were scalar values representing the signed, perpendicular distance from the average surface, where a positive value was outside the surface and a negative value was inside. Therefore, these scalar values of the vertex-based projection represented the shape information of each subjects and were used in the analysis of vertex-level group difference and to evaluate the shape deformation.

To reduce the influence of variation in head size, all volumes were scaled by normalized brain volume (NBV) estimated using SIENAX-FSL tool (24, 27). The segmentation result of each subject was visually checked and no error was observed. In the following statistical analysis, the volumes of each structure for each individual subject were corrected for NBV.

Statistical Analysis

Volume-Based Analysis

After calculating the volumes, we used SPSS v 21.0 to analyze the data, including two statistical methods: analysis of covariance (ANCOVA) and linear regression. To correct the differences in head size among individual participants, volumes of each structure were scaled by NBV using the following equation:

$$V_{\text{standard}} = \left(V_{\text{roi}} / V_{\text{NBV}}\right) \times 10^6$$

where V_{standard} means the standardized volume corrected with NBV, V_{roi} means the absolute volume of each segmented structure, and V_{NBV} means NBV.

Analysis of covariance model was used to evaluate group-wise differences in volume measures between AD, MCI and NC, with controlling for age and gender. In this model, volumes of deep gray matter structures were included as dependent factors and diagnosis as independent factors. A correction for multiple comparisons was carried out using the false discovery rate (FDR) correction at $p < 0.05$. Subsequently, *post hoc* pair-wise comparisons were applied to identify between-group differences with p-value ≤ 0.05, which is considered as significant. Second, a linear regression model was applied to measure the associations between global clinical scores (MMSE and MOCA score) and volumes of each structure among all of the subjects. In the linear regression model, global clinical scores were included as the dependent variables and the volumes of deep gray matter structure were included as independent variables. Age, gender and NBV were included as covariates. A collinearity test was also performed to rule out multicollinearity between age and the volumes of deep gray matter structure.

Vertex-Based Analysis

To carry out the vertex analysis, we used FSL dedicated tools, generalized linear model (18) to design the statistical matrix and Randomize (28) to perform permutation inference. Two statistical models were also designed in the vertex analysis.

First, ANCOVA was applied to determine the subregional changes within the deep gray matter structures across AD, MCI, and NC groups. Second, we correlated local subregional changes with global clinical scores at p-value ≤ 0.05 across all subjects. Age and gender were taken into as covariates in both of the ANCOVA and correlational analyses. We applied the FDR ($q = 0.05$) to correct for the multiple comparisons. The MNI coordinates of the center of gravity (COG) (18) at subregional alterations were also calculated for a better awareness of the locations where subregional changes occurred.

RESULTS

Group Characteristics

Demographic and clinical characteristics of three groups are listed in **Table 1**. The AD, MCI, and NC groups did not differ in NBV ($p = 0.052$) and gender ($p = 0.194$), but differ in age ($p = 0.028$). As expected, the pathological alteration among groups led to the significant difference in the scores of MMSE and MOCA among patients with AD, MCI, and NC ($p < 0.001$).

Deep Gray Matter Structures Volumes in AD and MCI Groups

Group-wise differences in volumes of the deep gray matter structure are displayed in **Table 2**. Volumes of bilateral NAc and bilateral hippocampi (Hipp) were smaller in AD, compared to NC group (L_Hipp: $p = 0.001$, R_Hipp: $p = 0.001$, L_NAc: $p = 0.003$, R_NAc: $p = 0.003$). MCI had smaller left hippocampus ($p = 0.020$), right NAc ($p = 0.010$), and left putamen ($p = 0.038$) volumes, compared to the NC group. Only right hippocampus showed a smaller volume in AD, compared to MCI group ($p = 0.012$).

Associations between Volumes and Clinical Rating Scales

We did not find a multicollinearity among the selected variables: age and volumes of deep gray matter structures. After controlling age, gender, and NBV, the p-values and β-regression coefficient of the correlations between volumes of deep gray matter structures and the global clinical scores across all subjects are displayed in **Table 3**. The volumes of bilateral NAc, bilateral hippocampi, which also showed significant atrophy in AD, compared to NC, were significantly correlated with MMSE and MOCA scores ($p \leq 0.05$). The volumes of other deep gray matter structures did not show significant correlations with clinical scores ($p > 0.05$).

TABLE 1 | Study sample characteristics.

Group	AD (n = 30)	MCI (n = 30)	NC (n = 30)	p-Value
Age (years; SD)	74.1 ± 10.5	74.6 ± 9.6	68.0 ± 11.0	0.028*
Gender (M/F)	13:17	17:13	20:10	0.194
NBV (cm³; SD)	1,154.6 ± 114.9	1,225.6 ± 116.6	1,183.5 ± 102.9	0.052
MMSE (SD)	16.5 ± 5.5	25.4 ± 2.1	29.0 ± 1.2	<0.001**
MOCA (SD)	11.9 ± 4.7	21.9 ± 2.1	26.9 ± 2.1	<0.001**

*$p \leq 0.05$.
**$p \leq 0.01$.
Demographic data are presented as means ± SDs for continuous and proportions for categorical variables.
AD, Alzheimer's disease; MCI, mild cognitive impairment; NC, normal controls; NBV, normalized brain volume; MMSE, Mini-Mental State Examination; MOCA, Montreal Cognitive Assessment; M, male; F, female.

TABLE 2 | Group-wise differences in the deep gray matter structures.

Structure	AD, mean ± SD	MCI, mean ± SD	NC, mean ± SD	*t*-Test (*p*-value)		
				AD-MCI	AD-NC	MCI-NC
L_NAc	316.5 ± 135.0	355.9 ± 126.2	443.3 ± 89.2	0.171	**0.003****	0.078
R_ NAc	215.7 ± 104.5	228.1 ± 105.0	322.6 ± 83.2	0.585	**0.003****	**0.010****
L_Hipp	2,583.5 ± 591.0	2,724.7 ± 544.9	3,166.8 ± 374.9	0.283	**0.001****	**0.020***
R_Hipp	2,652.4 ± 625.7	2,988.9 ± 493.7	3,283.6 ± 386.3	**0.012***	**0.001****	0.240
L_Put	3,395.1 ± 804.1	3,409.9 ± 466.9	3,923.5 ± 618.7	0.853	0.062	**0.038***
R_Put	3,415.8 ± 770.5	3,461.3 ± 591.0	3,847.9 ± 604.6	0.981	0.276	0.277
L_Thal	5,100.6 ± 650.5	5,033.1 ± 773.1	5,466.3 ± 534.6	0.592	0.352	0.145
R_Thal	4,833.0 ± 570.8	4,754.2 ± 687.0	5,152.1 ± 516.8	0.515	0.367	0.125

$*p \leq 0.05$; $**p \leq 0.01$ using ANCOVA; FDR corrected for t-test and adjusted for normalized brain volume, age, and gender.
Significant across and between-group differences are in bold.
L, left; R, right; NAc, nucleus accumbens; Hipp, hippocampus; Put, putamen; Thal, thalamus.

TABLE 3 | Association between volumes in deep gray matter structures and global clinical scores.

Structure	MMSE	MOCA
L_NAc	0.359 (0.002**)	0.382 (0.001**)
R_NAc	0.277 (0.024*)	0.324 (0.007**)
L_Hipp	0.389 (0.001**)	0.359 (0.001**)
R_Hipp	0.383 (0.001**)	0.369 (0.001**)
L_Put	0.103 (0.377)	0.078 (0.493)
R_Put	0.174 (0.139)	0.139 (0.232)
L_Thal	0.074 (0.522)	0.008 (0.945)
R_Thal	0.016 (0.888)	0.000 (0.998)

Results are presented as β-coefficient (p-values) based on linear regression model.
$*p \leq 0.05$.
$**p \leq 0.01$.

Vertex Analysis of Deep Gray Matter Structures

The results from vertex analysis are illustrated as probabilistic images that show the significant shape abnormalities within deep gray matter structures with $1 - p \geq 0.95$ ($p \leq 0.05$) in **Figure 2**. After controlling for age and gender, the surface abnormalities were located within bilateral hippocampi and NAc in AD, compared to NC group, and only shape alterations in the right hippocampus were found in AD, compared to MCI group. Specifically, significant shape differences were detected in the ventral part of left NAc (left ventral NAc) and right hippocampus (right ventral hippocampus), posterior part of right NAc (right posterior NAc), the dorsal–medial part of left hippocampus (left dorsal–medial hippocampus), and medial–ventral part of right thalamus (right medial–ventral thalamus) in AD when compared to NC. Less surface alterations were found in left hippocampus, right NAc, and left putamen in MCI, compared to NC without correction for the multiple comparisons, while these alterations did not survive under FDR correction. **Figure 3** shows the location of shape abnormalities using MNI coordinates of COG (colored in yellow).

Relationship between Regional Shape Alterations and Clinical Measures

Figure 4 shows correlations between shape alterations of deep gray matter structures and clinical measures of MMSE and MOCA within the whole sample. MMSE scores were associated with shape abnormalities in bilateral hippocampi, left NAc, and right thalamus, whereas MOCA scores were associated with shape abnormalities in bilateral hippocampi, NAc, and thalami. The localization of subregional alterations and their correlation with MMSE and MOCA scores is shown in **Table 4**. It can be observed that the left dorsal–medial hippocampus, the right ventral hippocampus, the left ventral NAc, and the right medial–ventral thalamus significantly correlated with MMSE and MOCA, while the right posterior NAc and the medial–ventral part of the left thalamus only correlated with MOCA. Notably, compared with NC, these results are quite consistent with the atrophy regions found in AD groups, which are shown in **Figures 2** and **3**.

DISCUSSION

In this study, we assessed the pattern of subregional structural alterations in deep gray matter structures in AD and MCI patients. Compared with NC, we found that among all seven pairs of structures, the bilateral hippocampi and NAc showed significant atrophy in AD. But only the atrophy in the left dorsal-medial hippocampus, the right ventral hippocampus, the left ventral NAc and the right posterior NAc correlated with the worse global clinical scores. These results suggested that the atrophy of these four subregions in bilateral hippocampi and NAc was associated with clinical impairment in MCI and AD patients, which might be useful in diagnosis, evaluation and management of AD. Furthermore, compared with NC, the volume of bilateral thalami did not significantly decrease in AD patients, but the significant atrophy was observed in the right medial-ventral thalamus and correlated with global clinical scores by using surface analysis. These results implied that the surface analysis could provide additional information for volume comparison in finding the early pathological progress.

It is well known that hippocampus plays an important role in spatial, semantic, and episodic memory, which are generally impaired in AD and MCI patients (29–32). Numerous studies indicated that hippocampal atrophy contributes to memory impairment in patients with AD (33–38). Recent studies in AD found that obvious atrophy in hippocampal CA1, especially in MCI patients who converted to AD over time (37, 38). In the current study, we found that hippocampal atrophy and its

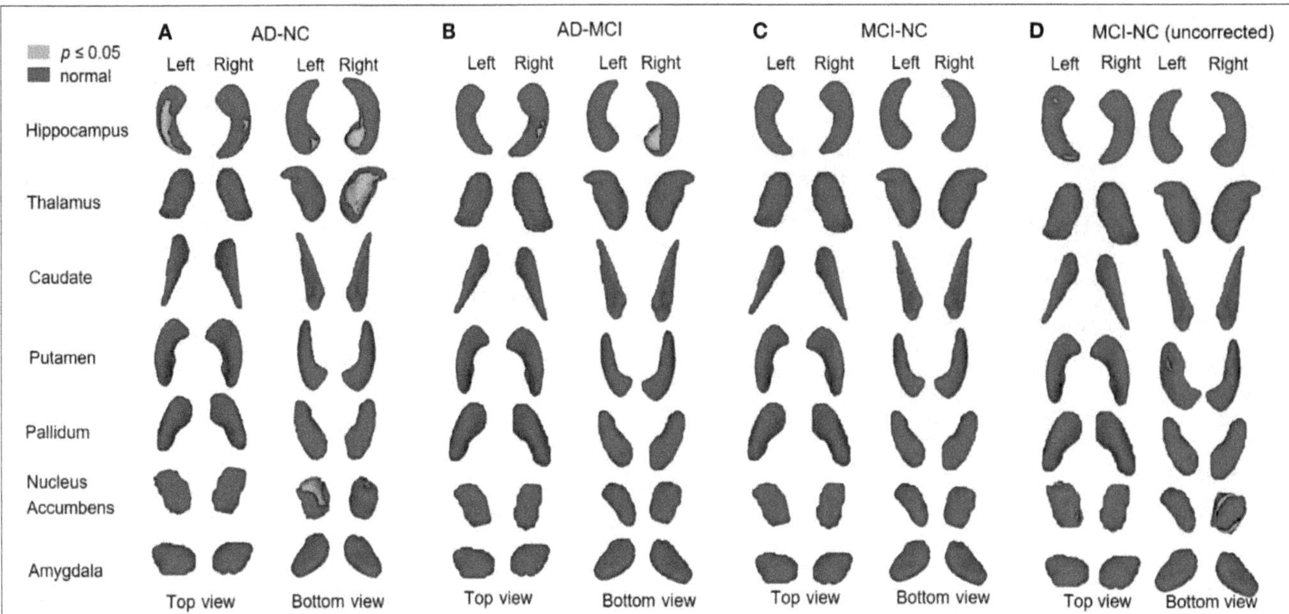

FIGURE 2 | Analysis of covariance (ANCOVA) of between-group shape differences. 3D rendering of 1 – *p* value images with vertex analysis between-group comparisons showing the subregional changes (yellow color coded) of deep gray matter structures [adjusted for age and gender; *p*-value corrected for multiple comparisons using false discovery rate (FDR)]. Shape alterations are seen in Alzheimer's disease (AD) compared to normal control (NC) **(A)** in bilateral hippocampi, bilateral nucleus accumbens (NAc), right thalamus; AD compared to mild cognitive impairment (MCI) **(B)** in right hippocampus; MCI showed no significant alteration compared to NC after FDR corrected **(C)**, while there are alterations found in left hippocampus, right NAc, and left putamen before FDR corrected **(D)**.

correlation with global clinical scores. Moreover, vertex analysis showed a alteration in the right ventral hippocampus and the left dorsal-medial hippocampus. This result is in line with a previous report that hippocampal atrophy is not homogeneous across the various hippocampal subregions during the progression of AD (5, 39). The dorsal hippocampus has been studied extensively for its significant role in spatial working memory, especially when processing the short-term spatial memory (40). Fanselow and Dong reported that the dorsal hippocampus performs primarily cognitive functions, while the ventral hippocampus relates to stress, emotion, and affect (41). Other studies also indicated that loss of neurogenesis in the dorsal and ventral hippocampus was associated with the impaired cognitive function (42), and the ventral hippocampus supported working memory for odor information (43). Experiments in rats showed that dorsal-medial hippocampus plays a role in flexible, adaptive behavior, and cognitive processing, and rats with dorsal-medial hippocampus lesions suffered significant working memory deficits (44). In line with the previous studies, the significant correlation between the dorsal/ventral hippocampal shape distortion and the global clinical scores in our study also emphasized the critical role of these two hippocampal subregions in cognitive impairment in AD process. Besides, the subregional level atrophy in hippocampi, which is slightly in MCI patients, but dramatically deteriorated in AD, further supporting the concept that AD is generally converted from MCI. Therefore, treatment on dorsal/ventral hippocampus may be effective to prevent the progression of AD. Drug treatment upon reduction of memory consolidation in rats with impaired dorsal hippocampus indicated that morphine may prevent impairment of memory consolidation (45). Yiu et al. also reported that targeting CREB in the CA1 region of dorsal hippocampus may be a useful therapeutic strategy in treating humans with AD (46). The role of the ventral hippocampus in AD is still not clear. Since the stress management related to the ventral hippocampus is suggested as a useful intervention in early AD and MCI (47), the treatment on ventral hippocampus for AD still need to be explored. The measurement in hippocampal subregion might be useful in monitoring the effect of treatment or intervention on subregional level.

In addition to hippocampus, NAc participates in integrating the information involved in learning and executive function and is also related to the cognitive processing of aversion, motivation, pleasure, reward, and reinforcement learning (48, 49). NAc is part of the striatum and has close connections with both limbic structures of the hippocampus, the amygdala, and the prefrontal cortex. One previous research about late-onset Alzheimer's disease patients showed the significant reductions in NAc volumes (50). Some previous studies have shown that atrophy of NAc occurred in patients with AD (51, 52), while they failed to reveal its function in cognitive decline. In our study, our results were on par with these previous studies that the bilateral NAc were more atrophied in AD and MCI patients compared to NCs. Furthermore, we found the atrophy in NAc was correlated with MMSE and MOCA scores. These results suggested that in addition to hippocampus, the atrophy in bilateral NAc may also play an important role in clinical impairment in AD and MCI. The localized atrophy in NAc has been confirmed to be associated with apathy in Parkinson's disease, and the severity of apathy was correlated with morphological changes in this region (53). Comparably, the vertex analyses in our study found

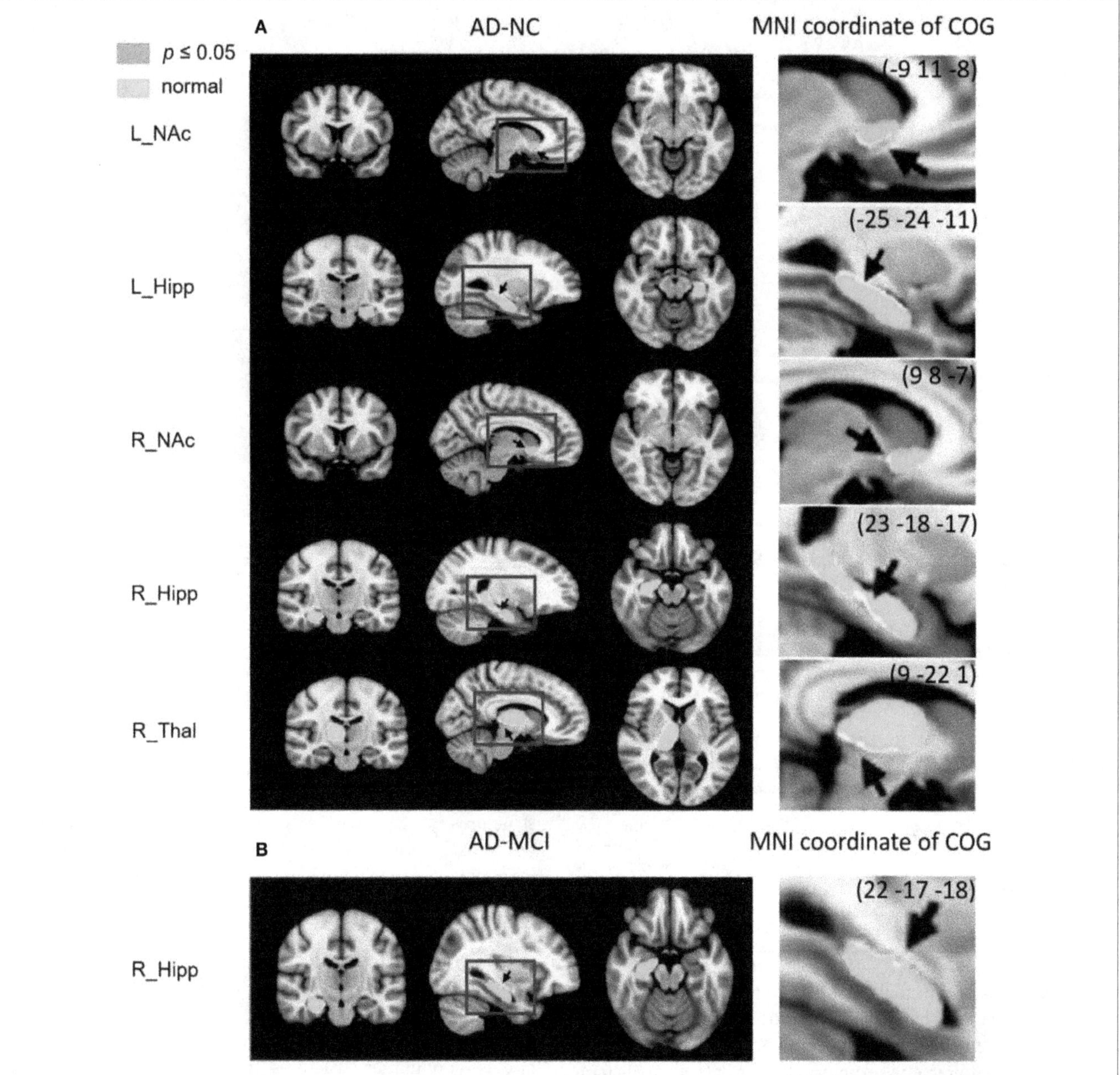

FIGURE 3 | Subregional surface alterations in hippocampus, nucleus accumbens (NAc), and thalamus, indicating the MNI coordinates of subregions where shape changes occurred (marked with an arrow). COG, center of gravity. **(A)** AD-NC and **(B)** AD-MCI.

that the atrophy of NAc and its association with clinical scores were both constrained within the ventral and posterior aspects in AD. Our results suggested that the ventral/posterior parts of NAc may involve in AD progression. However, few studies have explored the function of NAc in subregional level, especially its functions in AD or MCI, which need to be investigated in the future. A previous study reported that the deep brain stimulation of NAc could be a new treatment strategies to addiction (54). In the future, treatment like deep brain stimulation on subregional level of NAc may be considered for intervention in AD patients.

Some studies have revealed that other deep gray matter structures, such as amygdala, basal nuclei, and thalamus, also suffer atrophy in AD patients (55). Shape changes of ventricle system were reported in ventricular regions adjacent to amygdala, caudate nucleus, and thalamus in AD patients (56). MRI study showed strongly reduced volumes of putamen and thalamus in AD patients and this atrophy may contribute to cognitive impairment (10). Volumes of caudate and thalamus in familial AD reduced at a presymptomatic stage (57). It is well recognized that thalamus is essential for generating attention (58) and is involved as a subcortical hub in many different neuronal pathways related to emotional, motivational and cognitive abilities that are impaired in AD (6). To our knowledge, few studies have investigated the subregional atrophy and its relationship with

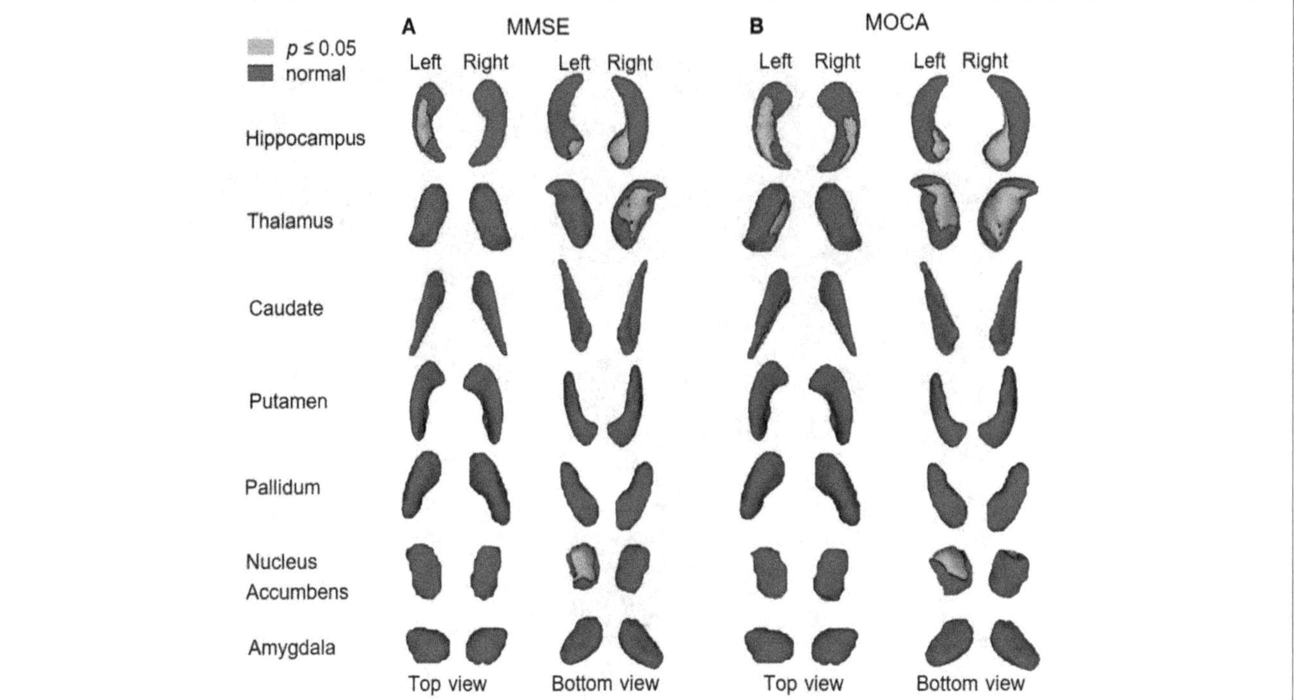

FIGURE 4 | Correlations between subregional shape alterations and global clinical scores. This 3D rendering of $1 - p$ value images shows the correlations (yellow color coded) between subregional atrophy and clinical scores (adjusted for age and gender; FDR corrected). Across the whole data cohort, correlations were observed **(A)** in hippocampi, left NAc, and right thalamus and MMSE scores; **(B)** in hippocampi, NAc, and thalami and MOCA scores.

TABLE 4 | Associations between subregional shape alterations and clinical measures (corresponding to the yellow areas in **Figure 4**).

Structure	L_NAc	R_NAc	L_Hipp	R_Hipp	L_Thal	R_Thal
MMSE	Ventral	–	Dorsal–medial	Ventral	–	Medial–ventral
MOCA	Ventral	Posterior	Dorsal–medial	Ventral	Medial–ventral	Medial–ventral

global clinical scores in thalami. Significant bilateral volumetric and subregional atrophy in the dorsal-medial part of the thalamus in AD patients has already been reported (10, 15). Another study found the subregional atrophy in the medial part of bilateral thalami (59), but not explored the relationship with clinical scores. Our study revealed significant shape abnormalities in the right medial-ventral thalamus in AD patients, but not found smaller volumes in bilateral thalami. Furthermore, the atrophy in right medial-ventral thalamus significantly correlated with MMSE and MOCA, suggesting that some parts of thalamus may be more vulnerable in AD and MCI. Our results suggest a specific atrophy pattern of the thalamus in AD and MCI, and also indicated that vertex-based (shape) analysis may provide additional and valuable information to popular volumetric analysis.

The main limitation of our study is that, although we adjusted our analysis for age, gender, and NBV, relatively small group samples may have reduced the statistical power. Therefore, some counterintuitive results were also need to be further validated in the future. For example, the putamen volume was significantly different between MCI and NC, but not between AD and NC. Furthermore, this was a cross-sectional study, and so it was difficult to judge whether atrophy of specific deep gray matter structures was a primary or secondary phenomenon to the hippocampal or entorhinal cortex. Therefore, further and preferable longitudinal investigations are needed to confirm the relationship between clinical and cognitive decline and the subregional atrophy patterns.

CONCLUSION

Based both on volumetric and vertex-based (shape) analysis of deep gray matter structures, this study showed that atrophy of deep gray matter structures in AD and MCI patients occurs at subregional level even when the volume of the whole given structure is not reduced. And this subregional atrophy within hippocampi and NAc correlates with worse global clinical scores. Atrophy measurement on subregional level may be useful in early diagnosis and management of AD patients or in evaluation of the treatment strategies.

AUTHOR CONTRIBUTIONS

XLN, YS, and SRW contributed to this article equally, being responsible for the image procession, data analysis, and writing the article. HZ, RYL, XPL, and SCW are responsible for the MRI acquisition and data collection; ZN, JH, ZQ, and YX give advice on how to do the data analysis and modify the article. BZ put forward the research ideas and guide the whole study.

ACKNOWLEDGMENTS

This work was supported by the National Natural Science Foundation of China (91649116, 81571040, and 81471643), Jiangsu province key medical talents, "13th Five-Year" health promotion project of Jiangsu province (BZ.2016-2020), Social development project of science and technology project in Jiangsu Province (BE2016605), the National and Provincial postdoctoral project (BE179 and 1501076A, BZ), the key project of Nanjing Health Bureau (ZKX14027, BZ), Nanjing science and technology development program (NE179, BZ), Jiangsu Provincial Key Medical Discipline (Laboratory) (ZDXKA2016020, XY), and Jiangsu Provincial KeyMedical Discipline (Laboratory) (ZDXKA2016020). ZN and JH are supported by the project no. LQ1605 from the National Program of Sustainability II (MEYS CR) and ZN is supported by "Nadani" Foundation and Czech Alzheimer Foundation. The funders had no role in study design, data collection and analysis, decision to publish, or preparation of the manuscript.

REFERENCES

Schott J, Kennedy J, Fox N. New developments in mild cognitive impairment and Alzheimer's disease. *Curr Opin Neurol* (2006) 19:552–8. doi:10.1097/01.wco.0000247611.44106.76

Yaari R, Corey-Bloom J. Alzheimer's disease. *Semin Neurol* (2007) 27:32–41. doi:10.1055/s-2006-956753

Petersen RC, Doody R, Kurz A, Mohs R, Morris J, Rabins P, et al. Current concepts in mild cognitive impairment. *Arch Neurol* (2001) 58:1985–92. doi:10.1001/archneur.58.12.1985

Peterson RC. Mild cognitive impairment: current research and clinical implications. *Semin Neurol* (2007) 27:22–31. doi:10.1055/s-2006-956752

Carlesimo GA, Piras F, Orfei MD, Iorio M, Caltagirone C, Spalletta G. Atrophy of presubiculum and subiculum is the earliest hippocampal anatomical marker of Alzheimer's disease. *Alzheimers Dement* (2015) 1:24–32. doi:10.1016/j.dadm.2014.12.001

Herrero MT, Barcia C, Navarro JM. Functional anatomy of thalamus and basal ganglia. *Childs Nerv Syst* (2002) 18:386–404. doi:10.1007/s00381-002-0604-1

Rugg MD, Yonelinas AP. Human recognition memory: a cognitive neuroscience perspective. *Trends Cogn Sci* (2003) 7:313–9. doi:10.1016/S1364-6613(03)00131-1

Fox NC, Freeboroug PA. Brain atrophy progression measured from registered serial MRI: validation and application to Alzheimer's disease. *J Magn Reson Imaging* (1997) 7:1069–75. doi:10.1002/jmri.1880070620

Gerardin E, Chételat G, Chupin M, Cuingnet R, Desgranges B, Kim H, et al. Multidimensional classification of hippocampal shape features discriminates Alzheimer's disease and mild cognitive impairment from normal aging. *Neuroimage* (2009) 47:1476–86. doi:10.1016/j.neuroimage.2009.05.036

de Jong LW, van der Hiele K, Veer IM, Houwing JJ, Westendorp RG, Bollen EL, et al. Strongly reduced volumes of putamen and thalamus in Alzheimer's disease: an MRI study. *Brain* (2008) 131:3277–85. doi:10.1093/brain/awn278

Scheltens P, Leys D, Barkhof F, Huglo D, Weinstein H, Vermersch P, et al. Atrophy of medial temporal lobes on MRI in "probable" Alzheimer's disease and normal ageing: diagnostic value and neuropsychological correlates. *J Neurol Neurosurg Psychiatry* (1992) 55:967–72. doi:10.1136/jnnp.55.10.967

Stoub TR, Bulgakova M, Leurqans S, Bennett DA, Fleischman D, Turner DA, et al. MRI predictors of risk of incident Alzheimer disease: a longitudinal study. *Neurology* (2005) 64:1520–4. doi:10.1212/01.WNL.0000160089.43264.1A

Alves GS, O'Dwyer L, Jurcoane A, Oertel-Knöchel V, Knöchel C, Prvulovic D, et al. Different patterns of white matter degeneration using multiple diffusion indices and volumetric data in mild cognitive impairment and Alzheimer patients. *PLoS One* (2012) 7:e52859. doi:10.1371/journal.pone.0052859

Cheng WC, Cheng PE, Liou M. Group factor analysis for Alzheimer's disease. *Comput Math Methods Med* (2013) 2013:1–8. doi:10.1155/2013/830237

Zarei M, Patenaude B, Damoiseaux J, Morgese C, Smith S, Matthews PM, et al. Combining shape and connectivity analysis: an MRI study of thalamic degeneration in Alzheimer's disease. *Neuroimage* (2010) 49:1–8. doi:10.1016/j.neuroimage.2009.09.001

Patenaude B, Smith SM, Kennedy DN, Jenkinson M. A Bayesian model of shape and appearance for subcortical brain segmentation. *Neuroimage* (2011) 56:907–22. doi:10.1016/j.neuroimage.2011.02.046

Qiu A, Fennema-Notestine C, Dale AM, Miller MI. Regional shape abnor- malities in mild cognitive impairment and Alzheimer's disease. *Neuroimage* (2009) 45:656–61. doi:10.1016/j.neuroimage.2009.01.013

Jenkinson M, Beckmann CF, Behrens TEJ, Woolrich MW, Smith SM. FSL. *Neuroimage* (2012) 62:782–90. doi:10.1016/j.neuroimage.2011.09.015

Nugent AC, Luckenbaugh DA, Wood SE, Bogers W, Zarate CA, Drevets WC. Automated subcortical segmentation using FIRST: test-retest reliability, interscanner reliability, and comparison to manual segmentation. *Hum Brain Mapp* (2013) 34:2313–29. doi:10.1002/hbm.22068

Folstein MF, Folstein SE, McHugh PR. Mini-mental state: a practical method for grading the cognitive state of patients for the clinician. *J Psychiatr Res* (1975) 12:189–98. doi:10.1016/0022-3956(75)90026-6

Smith T, Gildeh N, Holmes C. The Montreal Cognitive Assessment: validity and utility in a memory clinic setting. *Can J Psychiatry* (2007) 52:329–32. doi:10.1177/070674370705200508

Winblad B, Palmer K, Kivipelto M, Jelic V, Fratiglioni L, Wahlund LO, et al. Mild cognitive impairment-beyond controversies, towards a consensus: report of the International Working Group on mild cognitive impairment. *J Intern Med* (2004) 256:240–6. doi:10.1111/j.1365-2796.2004.01380.x

McKhann G, Drachman D, Folstein M, Katzman R, Price D, Stadlan EM. Clinical diagnosis of Alzheimer's disease: report of the NINCDS–ADRDA work group under the auspices of department of health and human services task force on Alzheimer's disease. *Neurology* (1984) 34:939–44. doi:10.1212/WNL.34.7.939

Smith SM, Jenkinson M, Woolrich MW, Beckmann CF, Behrens TEJ, Johansen-Berg H, et al. Advances in functional and structural MR image analysis and implementation as FSL. *Neuroimage* (2004) 23:S208–19. doi:10.1016/j.neuroimage.2004.07.051

Smith SM. Fast robust automated brain extraction. *Hum Brain Mapp* (2002) 17:143–55. doi:10.1002/hbm.10062

Jenkinson MBP, Brady M, Smith S. Improved optimization for the robust and accurate linear registration and motion correction of brain images. *Neuroimage* (2002) 17:825–41. doi:10.1006/nimg.2002.1132

Smith SM, Zhang Y, Jenkinson M, Chen J. Accurate, robust and automated longitudinal and cross-sectional brain change analysis. *Neuroimage* (2002) 17:479–89. doi:10.1006/nimg.2002.1040

Winkler AM, Ridgway GR, Webster MA, Smith SM, Nichols TE. Permutation inference for the general linear model. *Neuroimage* (2014) 92:381–97. doi:10.1016/j.neuroimage.2014.01.060

Cohen NJ, Eichenbaum H. *Memory, Amnesia, and the Hippocampal System*. Massachusetts: MIT Press (1993).

Squire LR, Schacter DL. *The Neuropsychology of Memory*. New York: Guilford Press (2002).

Mavrogiorgou P, Gertz HJ, Ferszt R, Wolf R, Bär KJ, Juckel G. Are routine methods good enough to stain senile plaques and neurofibrillary tangles in different brain regions of demented patients. *Psychiatr Danub* (2011) 23:334–9.

Wood R, Chan D. The hippocampus, spatial memory and Alzheimer's disease. *ACNR* (2015) 15:5–7.

Dubois B, Feldman HH, Jacova C, Dekosky ST, Barberger-Gateau P, Cummings J, et al. Research criteria for the diagnosis of Alzheimer's disease: revising the NINCDS-ADRDA criteria. *Lancet Neurol* (2007) 6:734–46. doi:10.1016/S1474-4422(07)70178-3

Chetelat G, Baron JC. Early diagnosis of Alzheimer's disease: contribution of structural neuroimaging. *Neuroimage* (2003) 18:525–41. doi:10.1016/S1053-8119(02)00026-5

de Leon MJ, Convit A, DeSanti S, Golomb J, Tarshish C, Rusinek H, et al. The hippocampus in aging and Alzheimer's disease. *Neuroimag Clin N Am* (1995) 5:1–17.

Laakso MP, Soininen H, Partanen K, Helkala EL, Hartikainen P, Vainio P, et al. Volumes of hippocampus, amygdala and frontal lobes in the MRI-based diagnosis of early Alzheimer's disease: correlation with memory functions. *J Neural Transm Park Dis Dement Sect* (1995) 9:73–86. doi:10.1007/BF02252964

Tang X, Holland D, Dale AM, Younes L, MI M. The diffeomorphometry of regional shape change rates and its relevance to cognitive deterioration in mild cognitive impairment and Alzheimer's disease. *Hum Brain Mapp* (2015) 36:2093–117. doi:10.1002/hbm.22758

Tang X, Holland D, Dale AM, Younes L, Miller M. Shape abnormalities of subcortical and ventricular structures in mild cognitive impairment and Alzheimer's disease: detecting, quantifying, and predicting. *Hum Brain Mapp* (2014) 35:3701–25. doi:10.1002/hbm.22431

Wachinger C, Salat DH, Weiner M, Reuter M. Whole-brain analysis reveals increased neuroanatomical asymmetries in dementia for hippocampus and amygdala. *Brain* (2016) 139:3253–66. doi:10.1093/brain/aww243

Lee I, Kesner RP. Time-dependent relationship between the dorsal hippocampus and the prefrontal cortex in spatial memory. *J Neurosci* (2003) 23:1517–23.

Fanselow MS, Dong HW. Are the dorsal and ventral hippocampus functionally distinct structures. *Neuron* (2010) 65:7–19. doi:10.1016/j.neuron.2009.11.031

Vetreno RP, Crews FT. Binge ethanol exposure during adolescence leads to a persistent loss of neurogenesis in the dorsal and ventral hippocampus that is associated with impaired adult cognitive functioning. *Front Neurosci* (2015) 9:35. doi:10.3389/fnins.2015.00035

Kesner R, Hunsaker M, Ziegler W. The role of the dorsal and ventral hippocampus in olfactory working memory. *Neurobiol Learn Mem* (2011) 96:361–6. doi:10.1016/j.nlm.2011.06.011

Sahina H. *Lesions of the Dorsal Medial Hippocampus Induce Different Forms of Repetitive Behaviour in the Rat.* New Zealand: University of Canterbury (2015).

Zarrindast MR, Navaeian M, Nasehi M. Influence of three-day morphine- treatment upon impairment of memory consolidation induced by cannabi- noid infused into the dorsal hippocampus in rats. *Neurosci Res* (2011) 69:51–9. doi:10.1016/j.neures.2010.09.007

Yiu AP, Rashid AJ, Josselyn SA. Increasing CREB function in the CA1 region of dorsal hippocampus rescues the spatial memory deficits in a mouse model of Alzheimer's disease. *Neuropsychopharmacology* (2011) 36:2169–86. doi:10.1038/npp.2011.107

Lombardo NBE, Wu B, Volicer L, Martin A, Serper LL, Zhang XW. Evidence based nutrition, exercise, cognitive rehabilitation & stress management inter- ventions for Alzheimer's disease: treatment or prevention? *Neurobiol Aging* (2004) 25:S206–7. doi:10.1016/S0197-4580(04)80692-4

Nestler E, Hyman S, Malenka R. *Molecular Neuropharmacology: A Foundation for Clinical Neuroscience.* 2nd ed. New York, NY: McGraw-Hill Professional (2015).

Wenzel JM, Rauscher NA, Cheer JF, Oleson EB. A role for phasic dopamine release within the nucleus accumbens in encoding aversion: a review of the neurochemical literature. *ACS Chem Neurosci* (2015) 6:16–26. doi:10.1021/cn500255p

Pievani M, Bocchetta M, Boccardi M, Cavedo E, Bonetti M, Thompson PM, et al. Striatal morphology in early-onset and late-onset Alzheimer's disease: a preliminary study. *Neurobiol Aging* (2013) 34:1728–39. doi:10.1016/j.neurobiolaging.2013.01.016

Hilal S, Amin SM, Venketasubramanian N, Niessen WJ, Vrooman H, Wong TY, et al. Subcortical atrophy in cognitive impairment and dementia. *J Alzheimer Dis* (2015) 48:813–23. doi:10.3233/JAD-150473

Möller C, Dieleman N, van der Flier WM, Versteeg A, Pijnenburg Y, Scheltens P, et al. More atrophy of deep gray matter structures in frontotemporal dementia compared to Alzheimer's disease. *J Alzheimers Dis* (2015) 44(2):635–47. doi:10.3233/JAD-141230

Carriere N, Besson P, Dujardin K, Duhamel A, Defebvre L, Delmaire C, et al. Apathy in Parkinson's disease is associated with nucleus accumbens atrophy: a magnetic resonance imaging shape analysis. *Mov Disord* (2014) 29:897–903. doi:10.1002/mds.25904

de Leon MJ, George AE, Stylopoulos LA, Smith G, Miller DC. Early marker for Alzheimer's disease: the atrophic hippocampus. *Lancet* (1989) 2:672–3. doi:10.1016/S0140-6736(89)90911-2

Cherubini A, Péran P, Spoletini I, Di Paola M, Di Iulio F, Hagberg GE, et al. Combined volumetry and DTI in subcortical structures of mild cog- nitive impairment and Alzheimer's disease patients. *J Alzheimers Dis* (2010) 19:1273–82. doi:10.3233/JAD-2010-091186

Ferrarini L, Palm WM, Olofsen H, van Buchem MA, Reiber JH, Admiraal- Behloul F. Shape differences of the brain ventricles in Alzheimer's disease. *Neuroimage* (2006) 32:1060–9. doi:10.1016/j.neuroimage.2006.05.048

Ryan NS, Keihaninejad S, Shakespeare TJ, Lehmann M, Crutch SJ, Malone IB, et al. Magnetic resonance imaging evidence for presymptomatic change in thalamus and caudate in familial Alzheimer's disease. *Brain* (2013) 136: 1399–414. doi:10.1093/brain/awt065

Newman J. Thalamic contributions to attention and consciousness. *Conscious Cogn* (1995) 4:172–93. doi:10.1006/ccog.1995.1024

Cho H, Kim J, Kim C, Ye B, Kim H, Yoon C, et al. Shape changes of the basal ganglia and thalamus in Alzheimer's disease: a three-year longitudinal study. *J Alzheimers Dis* (2014) 40:285–95. doi:10.3233/JAD-132072

16

Metabolic Abnormalities of Erythrocytes as a Risk Factor for Alzheimer's Disease

Elena A. Kosenko[1], Lyudmila A. Tikhonova[1], Carmina Montoliu[2], George E. Barreto[3,4], Gjumrakch Aliev[5]* and Yury G. Kaminsky[1]*

[1] Institute of Theoretical and Experimental Biophysics, Russian Academy of Sciences, Pushchino, Russia, [2] Fundación Investigación Hospital Clínico, INCLIVA Instituto Investigación Sanitaria, Valencia, Spain, [3] Departamento de Nutrición y Bioquímica, Facultad de Ciencias, Pontificia Universidad Javeriana, Bogotá, Colombia, [4] Instituto de Ciencias Biomédicas, Universidad Autónoma de Chile, Santiago, Chile, [5] GALLY International Biomedical Research Institute Inc., San Antonio, TX, United States

***Correspondence:**
Elena A. Kosenko
eakos@rambler.ru
Gjumrakch Aliev
aliev03@gmail.com

Alzheimer's disease (AD) is a slowly progressive, neurodegenerative disorder of uncertain etiology. According to the amyloid cascade hypothesis, accumulation of non-soluble amyloid β peptides (Aβ) in the Central Nervous System (CNS) is the primary cause initiating a pathogenic cascade leading to the complex multilayered pathology and clinical manifestation of the disease. It is, therefore, not surprising that the search for mechanisms underlying cognitive changes observed in AD has focused exclusively on the brain and Aβ-inducing synaptic and dendritic loss, oxidative stress, and neuronal death. However, since Aβ depositions were found in normal non-demented elderly people and in many other pathological conditions, the amyloid cascade hypothesis was modified to claim that intraneuronal accumulation of soluble Aβ oligomers, rather than monomer or insoluble amyloid fibrils, is the first step of a fatal cascade in AD. Since a characteristic reduction of cerebral perfusion and energy metabolism occurs in patients with AD it is suggested that capillary distortions commonly found in AD brain elicit hemodynamic changes that alter the delivery and transport of essential nutrients, particularly glucose and oxygen to neuronal and glial cells. Another important factor in tissue oxygenation is the ability of erythrocytes (red blood cells, RBC) to transport and deliver oxygen to tissues, which are first of all dependent on the RBC antioxidant and energy metabolism, which finally regulates the oxygen affinity of hemoglobin. In the present review, we consider the possibility that metabolic and antioxidant defense alterations in the circulating erythrocyte population can influence oxygen delivery to the brain, and that these changes might be a primary mechanism triggering the glucose metabolism disturbance resulting in neurobiological changes observed in the AD brain, possibly related to impaired cognitive function. We also discuss the possibility of using erythrocyte biochemical aberrations as potential tools that will help identify a risk factor for AD.

Keywords: Alzheimer's disease, amyloid β, erythrocytes, metabolic dysfunction, multilayered pathology, clinical manifestation

INTRODUCTION

Alzheimer's disease (AD) is a slowly progressing, systemic neurodegenerative disorder of uncertain etiology. Clinical manifestation of this disorder usually consists of cognitive deficits in memory in the elderly. Some estimates suggest that 50% of the population over the age of 80 years suffers from this type of dementia. With increases in life expectancy of our population, AD is already approaching epidemic proportions with no cure or preventative therapy yet available. Now, AD affects ~24 million people worldwide with 4.6 million new cases of dementia every year (one new case every 7 s), and if existing trends continue, 115 million individuals worldwide will have Alzheimer's disease (AD) by 2050 (Wimo and Prince, 2010; Fita et al., 2011).

AD develops sporadically in 95–98% of the AD population (Bird, 2005; Reddy, 2006; Kaminsky et al., 2010). However, the genetic-linked cases have provided a great deal of biochemical insights in the disease process. The research field has been focused on the role of Aβ in the brain stemming from the fact that accumulation of these peptides results in aggregation and formation of insoluble plaques, which trigger a cascade of deleterious changes, leading to neuronal death and thus causing AD. This train of events has been called the amyloid-cascade hypothesis of AD (Hardy and Higgins, 1992). It is significant that accumulation of aggregated Aβ is the primary abnormality in AD and that its deposition is required for postmortem diagnosis. Now, however, a large body of evidence exists, and new data continues to accumulate indicating that the number of Aβ deposits in the brain does not correlate well with the degree of cognitive impairment (Braak and Braak, 1991; Terry et al., 1991; Giannakopoulos et al., 2003; Guillozet et al., 2003). Indeed, Aβ deposition may occur in normal non-demented elderly people (Joachim et al., 1989; Mann et al., 1992; Lue et al., 1999; Schmitt et al., 2000; Pike et al., 2007), that is in agree with the fact that virtually all humans start to accumulate Aβ in the brain upon aging (Funato et al., 1998; Wang et al., 1999; Morishima-Kawashima et al., 2000). Besides, amyloid plaques are not specific for Alzheimer's disease and have been found in many other pathological conditions, including transmissible spongiform encephalopathies (Liberski, 2004), Down's syndrome (Glenner and Wong, 1984), Lewy body in Parkinson's disease (Arai et al., 1992), acute traumatic brain injury with diffuse axonal damage (Smith et al., 2003) and chronic traumatic brain injury associated with boxing (Roberts et al., 1990; Jordan, 2000) and football (Omalu et al., 2005). What is clear from these studies is that the presence of brain plaques alone is insufficient to produce cognitive decline in AD (Jack et al., 2009) and that such studies support the basis for the formation of a new hypothesis.

Recently, a modified Aβ-cascade hypothesis has been formulated that predicts intraneuronal accumulation of soluble Aβ oligomers, but not monomer or insoluble amyloid fibrils, as the first step of a fatal cascade in AD (McLean et al., 1999; Wirths et al., 2004; Selkoe, 2007). The amyloid oligomerization is observed to occur intracellularly (Connolly and Volpe, 1990) and $A\beta_{1-42}$ oligomers turn out to be potent neurotoxins in animal brain and neuronal cultures where they are able to disrupt glutamatergic synaptic function (Lambert et al., 1998; Hsia et al., 1999; Klein et al., 2001; Hardy and Selkoe, 2002; Kamenetz et al., 2003; Walsh and Selkoe, 2004; Roselli et al., 2005) and neuronal calcium homeostasis (Bapat et al., 1983; Mattson et al., 1992; Demuro et al., 2005), promote abnormal release of glutamate in hippocampal neurons (Brito-Moreira et al., 2011), induce oxidative stress (De Felice et al., 2007), incite tau hyperphosphorylation (De Felice et al., 2008), and synapse loss (Lue et al., 1999; Selkoe, 2008), inhibit long-term potentiation in the hippocampus (Walsh et al., 2002), which is required for memory formation, and in turn leads to the cognitive deficits in the animal. Using oligomer-sensitive immunoassay, the soluble Aβ oligomers have been found in brains of AD patients (Kuo et al., 1996; Lue et al., 1999; Gong et al., 2003). This confirms the prediction that soluble oligomeric Aβ-forms are characteristic of AD pathology. However, the soluble Aβ burden displayed considerable individual variation in the brain of AD patients. Thus, the mean level of soluble Aβ can increase 3-fold (McLean et al., 1999), 6-fold, 12-fold (Kuo et al., 1996), and 70-fold (Gong et al., 2003) in brain of AD patients compared to age-matched control, at that, the majority of soluble peptides was $A\beta_{1-42}$ (Kuo et al., 1996). On the other hand, it was found that the levels of soluble $A\beta_{1-42}$ were smallest in the AD brain (0.7%) and that the soluble pools of $A\beta_{1-40}$ and $A\beta_{1-42}$ were the largest fractions of total Aβ in the normal brain (50 and 23% respectively, Wang et al., 1999). Other authors also showed that the $A\beta_{1-42}$ levels were found in the brains of normal elderly subjects (Tabaton and Piccini, 2005) and that in subjects with AD these concentrations increased slightly compared with the age-matched control (Lue et al., 1999). These studies suggest that within individual AD subjects, the areas with greater numbers of soluble Aβ oligomers did not, as a rule, and whether the levels of these "concentration-jumping" oligomers correlate with the memory decline in AD remains to be determined. Indeed, previous studies have shown that these Aβ forms were observed in the brains of patients with Down's syndrome (DS) (Teller et al., 1996; Gyure et al., 2001; Tabaton and Gambetti, 2006) indicating that the accumulation of soluble oligomers are not specific for AD. Moreover, in brains of patients with DS, increased levels of oxidative damage occur prior to the onset of Aβ deposition (Nunomura et al., 2000). Hence, the formation of diffuse amyloid plaques may be considered as the message talking about the disruption of brain homeostasis or as a compensatory response to remove reactive oxygen species (Atwood et al., 2003). Thus, these facts provide the opportunity to investigate the pathological conditions that precede the formation of the Aβ deposits in the human brain.

It is well known that a characteristic reduction of cerebral perfusion and metabolism occurs in patients with AD (de la Torre, 2000b; Aliev et al., 2003a). It was suggested that capillary distortions commonly found in the AD brain elicit hemorheological changes that altered the delivery and transport of essential nutrients, particularly glucose, and oxygen required for its aerobic oxidation in brain cells (de la Torre and Mussivand, 1993; de la Torre, 2002a; Chang et al., 2007; Aliev, 2011) resulting in an energy metabolic breakdown of the biosynthetic and synaptic pathways, subsequently leading to the death of neurons as a consequence of cognitive deterioration. In fact, it was proposed that AD may originate as a vascular disorder with the resultant impairment of oxygen delivery to the brain with the plaques and tangles found in the brain secondary to the effects of the vascular pathology (de la Torre, 2002a). Another important factor in tissue oxygenation is the ability of red blood cells (RBC) to the binding, transport and delivery of oxygen to tissues that depends, first of all, on RBC energy metabolism and antioxidant status (Brewer et al., 1974) that is extremely important for the functioning and regulation of oxygen affinity to hemoglobin (van Wijk and van Solinge, 2005).

Surprisingly, despite the main role of RBC metabolism in the delivery of oxygen to the tissues, no systematic programs of research have examined the relationship between the breach of the energy metabolism of these cells in destabilization of glucose metabolism in the brain pathology and this relationship is still not sufficiently discussed in the literature. Therefore, our current hypothesis is that RBC metabolism plays a key role in AD brain disorders. We propose that the long-term lack of sufficient energy, disturbance of glycolytic, antioxidant RBSs pathways, and sodium potassium pump in oldest subjects [caused by different reasons and also in contact with Aβ, which is located on the luminal surfaces of cerebral microvessels (Grammas et al., 2002; Michaud et al., 2013)] can cause a decrease in the ability of RBC to transfer oxygen to tissue, leading to inadequate oxygenation and can result in abnormal glucose/energy metabolism, oxidative stress and, thereby, increase the susceptibility of neurons to damage, and reduce mental capacity as a consequence thereof. We have called this chain of events as *"the erythrocytic hypothesis of Alzheimer disease"* (Kosenko et al., 2016). In support of this hypothesis we also believe that erythrocyte biochemical aberrations might be used as potential tools in the early detection of the brain pathology development. This hypothesis provides ideas for the development of innovative personalized medical technologies allowing recovering the energy metabolism and the system of antioxidant defense in erythrocytes.

BRAIN GLUCOSE METABOLISM, GLUTAMATE TOXICITY, AND Aβ ACCUMULATION: CAUSE OR EFFECT?

The brain is normally dependent on glucose for oxidative metabolism and function, therefore it is extremely sensitive to fluctuation in the blood glucose concentration, and since no satisfactory brain endogenous substitute exists. In spite of the fact that under certain conditions such as starvation or diabetes the ketone bodies can supply up to 50% of the brain's energy needs, the rest of the energy anyway must come from glucose. Therefore, within even just a few minutes glucose and oxygen deprivation induces significant dysfunction, and a longer time period can ultimately result in cell death (Blass, 2002). In addition to ATP production, the oxidation of glucose can produce other important intermediate such as lactate, which does not enter necessarily in the tricarboxylic acid cycle, but rather can be released and transported by the circulation into the liver for glucose synthesis de novo. Glucose also can be incorporated into lipids, proteins, and glycogen, and it is also the precursor of certain neurotransmitters such as γ-aminobutyric acid (GABA) (Plum and Posner, 1972), glutamate (Hamberger et al., 1979), and acetylcholine (Gibson et al., 1975). Thus, circulating glucose regulates many brain functions, including brain vitality, activity, learning, and memory (Korol and Gold, 1998).

Whereas the cerebral energy status is only slightly decreased during the normal aging process, glucose metabolism, and cellular ATP production are severely reduced in sporadic AD (Kyles et al., 1993; Hoyer, 1996). Certain neuronal populations are especially vulnerable to cut glucose oxidation, specifically neurons in the CA1, subiculum, and dentate gyrus of the hippocampus, and neurons in the outer layers of the cortex (Auer and Siesjö, 1993). A substantial proportion of neurons in these regions is glutamatergic and evidence suggests that hypoglycemic injury in these neurons is initiated almost entirely by hyperactivation of glutamate receptor (Auer et al., 1985), followed by the glutamate cascade and oxidative stress. The numerous studies have provided conclusive proof that glutamate becomes neurotoxic via the NMDA receptor when intracellular energy levels are reduced (Novelli et al., 1988; Beal et al., 1991; Albin and Greenamyre, 1992; Beal, 1992; Storey et al., 1992; Kosenko et al., 1994; Gonzalez et al., 2015). On the other hand, there is a direct relationship between disturbances in energy metabolism and mental disorder. For example, in 1932 Quastel J. first put forward a general suggestion that disturbances in energy metabolism would impair the neurological function, including particularly cognition (Quastel, 1932). During the past decades, a lot of work has proved Quastel's theory to be prescient and showed that the cause-effect relation is nonspecific as impairing cerebral energy metabolism can induce mental disorders to varying degrees (confusion, mental fatigue, agnosia, or dementia) in different pathological situations. Thus, impaired mental function has been reported in association with hypoglycemia (Bruce et al., 2009), inadequate transportation of glucose across the blood-brain barrier (Klepper and Voit, 2002; Pascual et al., 2004), defective astroglial glutamate transportation (Rönnbäck and Hansson, 2004), hypoxia (Gibson et al., 1981), diabetes (Richardson, 1990), heart failure (Riegel et al., 2002), reduced glucose tolerance (Vanhanen et al., 1997), bradycardia, hypotension (Ackerman, 1974), high intracranial pressure (Yoshida et al., 1996), stroke (van der Zwaluw et al., 2011), hypothermia, alcohol intoxication, thiamine and vitamin C deficiency, sedative-hypnotic drugs, opioids consumption (Martindale et al., 2010), general anesthesia (Parikh and Chung, 1995; Xie et al., 2006b), hypocapnia (Dodds and Allison, 1998), chronic stress (Conrad et al., 1996; Conrad, 2006), chronic noise stress (Arnsten and Goldman-Rakic, 1998; Manikandan et al., 2006), mixed brain pathologies (Schneider et al., 2007), hepatic encephalopathy (Butterworth, 2003), hyperammonemia (Llansola et al., 2007), trauma (Brooks et al., 2000), and so forth. Interestingly, after trauma, a large number of Aβ positive neurons appeared in human (Chen et al., 2004; Uryu et al., 2007) and animal brain (Kamal et al., 2001; Kasa et al., 2001; Papp et al., 2002; Hamberger et al., 2003). APP (amyloid precursor protein) accumulation is also observed following rat (Li et al., 1995) and human spinal cord injury (Ahlgren et al., 1996; Cornish et al.,

2000). Long-term presence of APP and accumulation of Aβ in the rat thalamus were observed after middle cerebral artery occlusion (van Groen et al., 2005) and in cultured cells that had been treated with spirochetes or bacterial lipopolysaccharide (LPS) (Miklossy et al., 2006) and other infectious agents (Balin and Appelt, 2001).

A number of studies have also demonstrated that abnormal activation of β-adrenergic receptors (β-ARs), which mediate the effect of stress, might contribute to Aβ peptides production resulting in accelerating amyloid plaque formation *in vitro* and *in vivo* by enhancing γ-secretase activity (Ni et al., 2006) and that blocking β-ARs attenuates acute stress-induced Aβ peptide production (Yu et al., 2010). Indeed, the common inhalation anesthetic isoflurane has been reported to increase brain Aβ protein levels *in vitro* (Xie et al., 2006a) and *in vivo* (Xie et al., 2008; Zhang et al., 2008; Dong et al., 2009). Hypocapnia can also increase Aβ production in H4 human neuroglioma cells (Xie et al., 2004). Nanoscale particulates, a major component airborne pollution, inducing the blood-brain barrier disruption and neuroinflammation (Murr et al., 2006), result in AD-associated $A\beta_{1-42}$, accumulation in the brains of children living in the high-pollution area (Calderón-Garcidueñas et al., 2008a,b). Upon careful analysis of these pathologies, one can see that there is a steady disruption of brain aerobic metabolism and the subsequent increase in APP processing and the formation of amyloids (Gabuzda et al., 1994; Webster et al., 1998; Velliquette et al., 2005). Thus, according to positron emission tomography (PET), isoflurane anesthesia can cause a 50% decrease in the rate of glucose uptake by the brain (Alkire et al., 1995, 1997), which leads to a sharp inhibition of aerobic oxidation in the cells and development of severe hypoxia, decreased neuronal activity (Hodes et al., 1985), and the appearance of amyloid in the brain 6-24 h after application of the anesthetic (Xie et al., 2006a, 2008). In ischemia-reperfusion, in addition to increasing oxidative stress, there is a decrease in the rate of blood flow, since migration of neutrophils to the site damaged by hypoxia can cause blockage of capillaries (Simpson et al., 1988), which impairs the entry of glucose and oxygen into the brain and promotes the formation of amyloids in damaged brain structures (van Groen et al., 2005; Tesco et al., 2007). In hypoglycemia, the limited supply of glucose from the blood to the brain also contributes to the accumulation of amyloids in the brain (Shi et al., 1997).

Altogether, these findings suggest that a transient insult, e.g., trauma, ischemia, neuroinflammation, anesthesia, or infectious agents could lead to secondary and persistent brain injuries and that the initial production of Aβ and its precursor, perhaps, are associated with physiological compensatory mechanisms for repair or protection of neurons exposed to significant disturbances in homeostasis (Smith et al., 2000; Lee et al., 2004). These facts are consistent with the numerous data showing that amyloid exhibits trophic and neuroprotective (Whitson et al., 1989; Koo et al., 1993; Singh et al., 1994; Luo et al., 1996), antioxidant (Smith et al., 1998, 2002a; Kontush et al., 2001; Atwood et al., 2002) properties and accumulates in the tissue after impairment of the energy metabolism with non-specific stimulus (Gabuzda et al., 1994; Webster et al., 1998; Velliquette et al., 2005), while under physiological conditions the diurnal fluctuation of brain Aβ levels is strictly regulated (Kang et al., 2009). Additionally, scores obtained on mini-mental state examination in AD subjects correlate highly with reductions of glucose metabolism (Blass, 2003), suggesting that the metabolic lesion precedes the development of neuropsychological abnormalities (Gibson and Huang, 2002) and support the conclusion that sporadic AD is a hypometabolic disorder which is provoked by a dysfunctional cerebral energy metabolism (Hoyer et al., 1988; Blass and Gibson, 1991; Meier-Ruge and Bertoni-Freddari, 1996; Perry et al., 1998; Smith et al., 2002b; Aliev et al., 2003b, 2004; Zhu et al., 2007). Obviously, the detection of mechanisms of disturbance of aerobic glucose metabolism in the brain is one of the most pressing tasks which will facilitate further progress on to determine not only to the midlife AD risk factor, but also on the lifespan of the older persons. Therefore, any pharmacological intervention, directed at correcting the chronic hypoperfusion state would possibly change the natural course of development of dementing neurodegeneration (Aliev et al., 2003a).

THE POSSIBLE ROLE OF RBC IN PATHOGENESIS OF AD

The pathologic causes of brain glucose metabolism disorders in AD may vary in signs and symptoms, which are as follows: desensitization of the neuronal insulin receptor (Hoyer, 2000), a decrease in the enzymes of the tricarbonic acid cycle activities (Meier-Ruge et al., 1984; Marcus et al., 1989; Marcus and Freedman, 1997; Bubber et al., 2005), impaired glucose transporter at the blood-brain barrier (Kalaria and Harik, 1989), depressed glucose transport into neurons (Simpson and Davies, 1994; Simpson et al., 1994), hippocampal region atrophy (Jobst et al., 1992; Villain et al., 2008) neuronal loss in the affected areas (McGeer et al., 1990), NO-dependent endothelial dysfunction and degeneration (De Jong et al., 1999; de la Torre, 2000a, 2002b) in brain capillaries that affect the capillary blood flow and optimal delivery of glucose and oxygen to neuronal cells (de la Torre, 2000b; Aliev et al., 2003a).

Another important factor in tissue oxygenation is the ability of RBC to bind, transport and release oxygen to tissues. For this, the RBC requires several essential metabolic pathways such as (i) anaerobic glycolysis, which is the only source of energy (ATP production) for sustaining cell structure and function; (ii) maintenance of the electrolyte gradient between plasma and red cell cytoplasm through the activity of adenosine triphosphate (ATP)-driven membrane pumps; (iii) pentose phosphate shunt (PPS) that controls the anti-oxidant pathways by produced NADPH, which plays an important role in maintaining glutathione in the reduced state; (iv) antioxidant pathways necessary for the protection of RBC proteins and hemoglobin against oxidation; and (v) nucleotide metabolism for the maintenance of the purine and pyrimidine homeostasis. Moreover, erythrocytes possess a unique glycolytic bypass, Rapoport-Luebering shunt to produce 2,3-diphosphoglycerate (2,3-DPG), a crucial metabolite in the regulation of hemoglobin affinity for oxygen (Cho et al., 2008). Thus, the mature erythrocyte retains a strictly regulated system of soluble enzymes, structural proteins, carbohydrates, lipids, anions, cations, cofactors, metabolites, antioxidants all of which are required in balance for effective metabolism and functioning of the cell. A change of at least one component of this system will lead to an imbalance and loss of RBC functional capacity. Indeed, a significant loss in ATP (Rabini et al., 1997), Mg^{2+}, Na^{+}, and ATP-ase activity (Ajmani and Rifkind, 1998) all of which may decrease erythrocyte deformability (Sakuta, 1981; Kucukatay et al., 2009), changes morphology (Gov and Safran, 2005) and increases RBC volume (Kowluru et al., 1989; Kucukatay et al., 2009). Extensive diminution of intracellular antioxidant GSH promotes oxidative damage of protein and lipids and compromises structural integrity of the RBC (Morris et al., 2008). Decreased 2,3-DPG, operating as a regulator of the oxygen affinity of RBC (Duhm, 1971) reduces the ability of RBC to release oxygen, resulting in tissue hypoxia (MacDonald, 1977; Nakamura et al., 1995; **Figure 1**). Considering the cause-effect relationship between various intracellular metabolic pathways and RBC function, it may be inferred that intact biochemical intracellular pathways are a major factor controlling the paramount RBC function associated with the ability to bind, transport, and release oxygen to tissues.

Recently, we measured some parameters of adenine nucleotide metabolism, glycolysis, pentose phosphate pathway, 2,3-DPG shunt (Kaminsky et al., 2013), oxidant and antioxidant enzymes and metabolites (Kosenko et al., 2012) in RBCs samples from Alzheimer's subjects (AD) and non-Alzheimer's dementia (NA) patients. We found that activities of all glycolytic, pentose phosphate pathway and 2,3-DPG shunt enzymes, Na^{+}, K^{+}-ATPase, as well as NAD/NADH ratio, pyruvate and lactate levels evidently decreased in aging and increased equally in AD and NA to levels or above levels of the YC (young controls) group indicating an increase in RBC glycolysis and ion fluxes. Elevated Na^{+}, K^{+}-ATPase activity and decreased ATP levels imply that ATP loss was mostly based on energy-expending redistribution of Na^{+} and K^{+} across the plasma membrane in erythrocytes from AD patients. These results confirm the fact that in AD, as in certain other diseases the balance between ATP formation and ion pumping may be disordered resulting in a decrease in intercellular energy charge, and an increase in lactate formation and catabolism of adenylates (Ronquist and Waldenström, 2003). These defects were accompanied by a significant decrease [relatively to both age-matched controls (AMC) and young adult controls (YC)] in the 2,3-DPG concentration that was accompanied by increases in the activity of diphosphoglycerate phosphatase (DPGP-ase), an enzyme that converts 2,3-DPG to 3PG (Kosenko et al., 2016). Of course, other factors besides of 2,3-DPG may affect the affinity of oxygen to hemoglobin (Samaja et al., 2003), but the relationship between the 2,3-DPG concentration in RBC as a biological indicator of tissue hypoxia in diabetic neuropathy (Nakamura et al., 1995), as well as in preterm infants with perinatal problems (Tsirka et al., 1990; Cholevas et al., 2008), in patients with the nondeletion genotype of hemoglobinopathy (Papassotiriou et al., 1998), with hypertension (Resnick et al., 1994), in experimental endotoxin shock (Matsumoto, 1995), severe hypophosphatemia (Larsen et al., 1996), and some types of glycolytic enzymes disturbances (McCully et al., 1999) was well established. Thus, the results generated the hypothesis that chronic enhancement in the rate of active transport in AD (Ronquist and Waldenström, 2003) leading to the increase in ATP and 2,3-DPG hydrolysis and can increase in Hb affinity to oxygen, loss of adequate oxygen delivery to tissues that may be one of the factors contributing to brain hypoxia (Aliev et al., 2004), glucose hypometabolism, and memory dysfunction in AD. It should be noted, however, that RBC of even cognitively stable aging persons (AMC) was characterized by a slight but significant decrease in 2,3-DPG when compared with the young adult control group. The tendency for the ATP production, adenylate energy charge, adenine nucleotide pool size, and ATP/ADP ratio (Kosenko et al., 2016) was a decrease in aging with no notable changes in dementia. There were no differences between AMC, AD, and NA groups in GSH levels, as well as in GSSG levels and the GSH/GSSG ratio in RBCs (Kosenko et al., 2012). Activities of calpain and caspase-3 in RBCs from aged subjects, on the contrary, were three times higher than those in young controls and were equally high in both dementia types (Kaminsky et al., 2012). The trend for the hydroperoxide generation was an increase in aging with no dramatic changes in dementia. There were no significant differences between AC, AD, and NA subjects in H_2O_2, organic hydroperoxide and the sum of H_2O_2 plus organic hydroperoxides content of RBC (Kaminsky et al., 2013). The results suggest that oxidative stress to some extent is already present in the RBC of the AMC subjects (Kosenko et al., 2012) and that together with the disturbances of glycolytic and transport processes and proteolysis increasing are a general feature of aging and not a feature of dementia. This view is supported by data comparing AD with normal aging, where was documented the same profile of damage (Smith et al., 1991; Moreira et al., 2006) suggesting that RBC oxidative damage is no longer an end stage but rather a signal of underlying changes of state (Moreira et al., 2006).

Although endogenous oxidative stress may damage the RBC itself the mass effect of large quantities of free radicals leaving the red cell has a prodigious potential to damage other components of the circulation (Johnson et al., 2005) including endothelial cells resulting in the microvascular pathology (Kiefmann et al., 2008). The combined effects of these damages most likely contribute to the morphological changes in oldster subjects (Richards et al., 2007), which may result in decreased erythrocyte deformability (Kuypers et al., 1990) and alter rheology and reduce the threshold for the development of neuropathology (Ajmani et al., 2003). We propose that the long-term lack of sufficient energy, disturbances of glycolytic pathway and sodium/potassium pump in aged subjects can decrease the ability of RBC to transfer oxygen, leading to inadequate tissue oxygenation and abnormal glucose metabolism in the brain and thereby reducing mental capacity and cognition. Thus, the reduced mental capacity may be, to a large extent, due to the imbalance in the metabolic processes in RBC. Obviously, other factors may be operative, but the role of RBC biochemical alterations as possible preclinical indicator of mental disorders must be critically examined. During the last 10 years, numerous biochemical abnormalities in RBC of subjects suffering from various mental disturbances have been detected

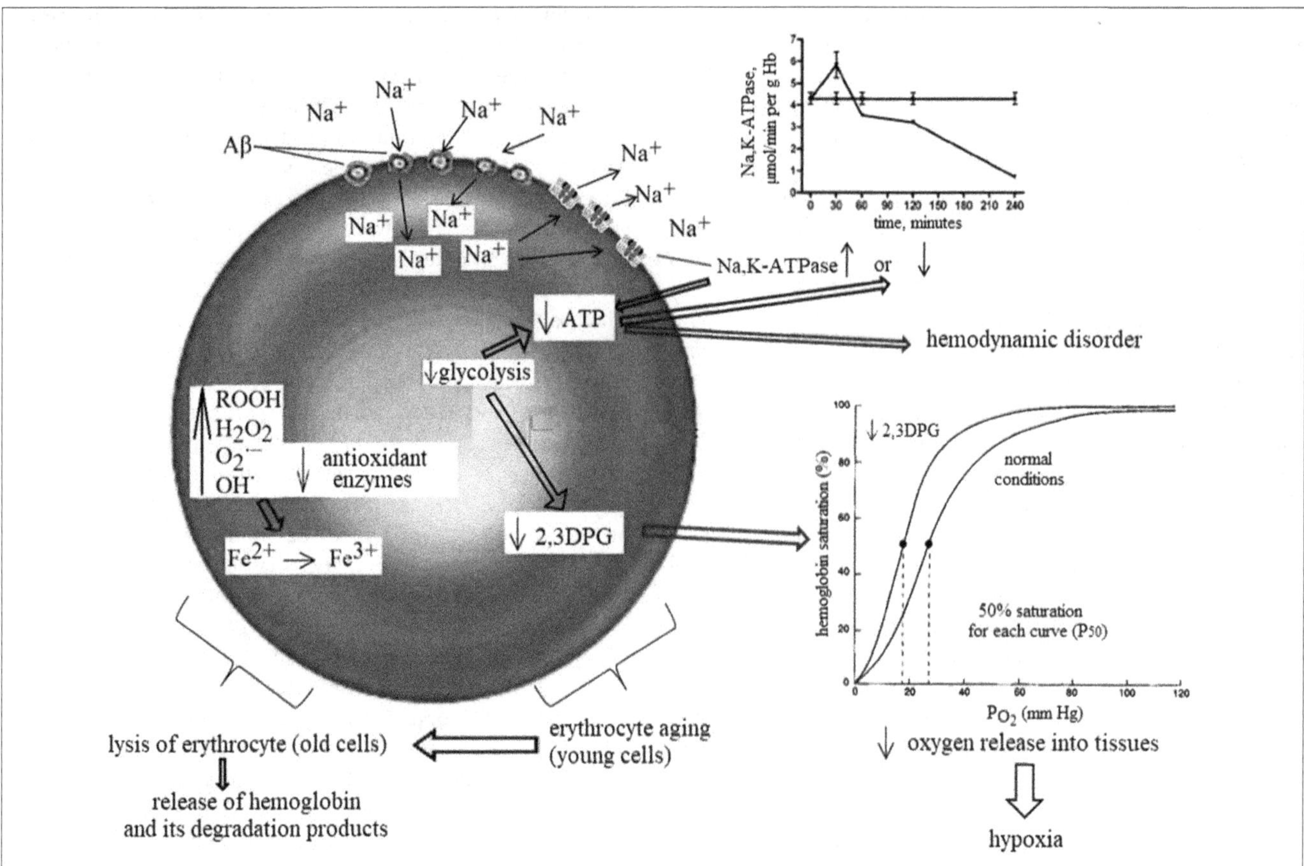

FIGURE 1 | Normal aging diminishes RBC functions, including a detectable decrease in the activity of glycolytic and antioxidant enzymes. The combined effects of these damage together with a slight but significant decrease in 2,3-DPG are most likely contributor to the morphological changes in oldster subject which may result in decreased erythrocyte deformability, alter rheology, loss of adequate oxygen delivery and reduce the threshold for the development of neuropathology. The left part of the scheme: Amyloids possess gramicidin D-like action and upon contact with erythrocytes rapidly increase the concentration of sodium in the cells causing rapid activation of the Na^+, K^+-ATPase leading to the increase in ATP and 2,3DPG hydrolysis and can increase in Hb affinity to oxygen, that may be one of the factors contributing to brain hypoxia which lead to glucose hypometabolism and memory dysfunction in AD. The right part of the scheme: Prolonged contact with erythrocytes depletes ATP stores, causing Na^+, K^+-ATPase pumps and Na^+- dependent ion channels to stop working and, consequently, the erythrocytes to swell and lyse. RBCs release hemoglobin, which is a source of iron. In turn, this metal catalyses the formation of toxic reactive oxygen species that mediate neuronal injury.

(Danon et al., 1992; Rifkind et al., 1999; Ponizovsky et al., 2003; Pankowska et al., 2005; Lang et al., 2015; Pretorius et al., 2016). We believe that obligatory measurement of RBC biochemical parameters in peoples older than 50 years in the dynamics will help identify the risk factor for AD.

The problem is clear, but a number of questions arise in connection with the above-mentioned. If oxidative stress is more or less present in the erythrocytes of all elderly people and is a risk factor for dementia, why does this risk factor "work" for some people, while others, with the same risk factor, live to a very old age, maintaining "bright mind" and working capacity? The same question arises with regard to the concentration of 2,3-DPG reduction and the energy metabolism rate in the erythrocytes in general. It is obvious that the answers to these questions can only be obtained after identification of the reasons causing a global energy metabolism disorder, an increase of oxidative stress that are the basis of quick aging, affection of erythrocytes and that lead to a disruption of their functional capacity and early death. In other words, it is necessary to find out, under what influence factors (endogenous and exogenous) the reserve capacity of erythrocytes to withstand the stress that they are constantly exposed to, which circulate from the lungs to the tissues, decreases too soon.

Another problem is the lack of absolute knowledge of the hemopoiesis status in older people and especially in stressful situations that require intensification of the formation of blood cells. Numerous data indicate that the functions of basal hemopoiesis, which maintains the number of blood cells within the norm, changes insignificantly with age (Sansoni et al., 1993; Bagnara et al., 2000), whereas the reserve capacity of the bone marrow to resist stressful situations requiring its activation, even in healthy elderly people, reduces significantly with age (Williams et al., 1986; Globerson, 1999). For example, during bacterial infection or other periods of high hematopoietic demand, the formation of blood becomes "flaccid" and badly regulated, paradoxically (Rothstein, 1993), which makes it possible to

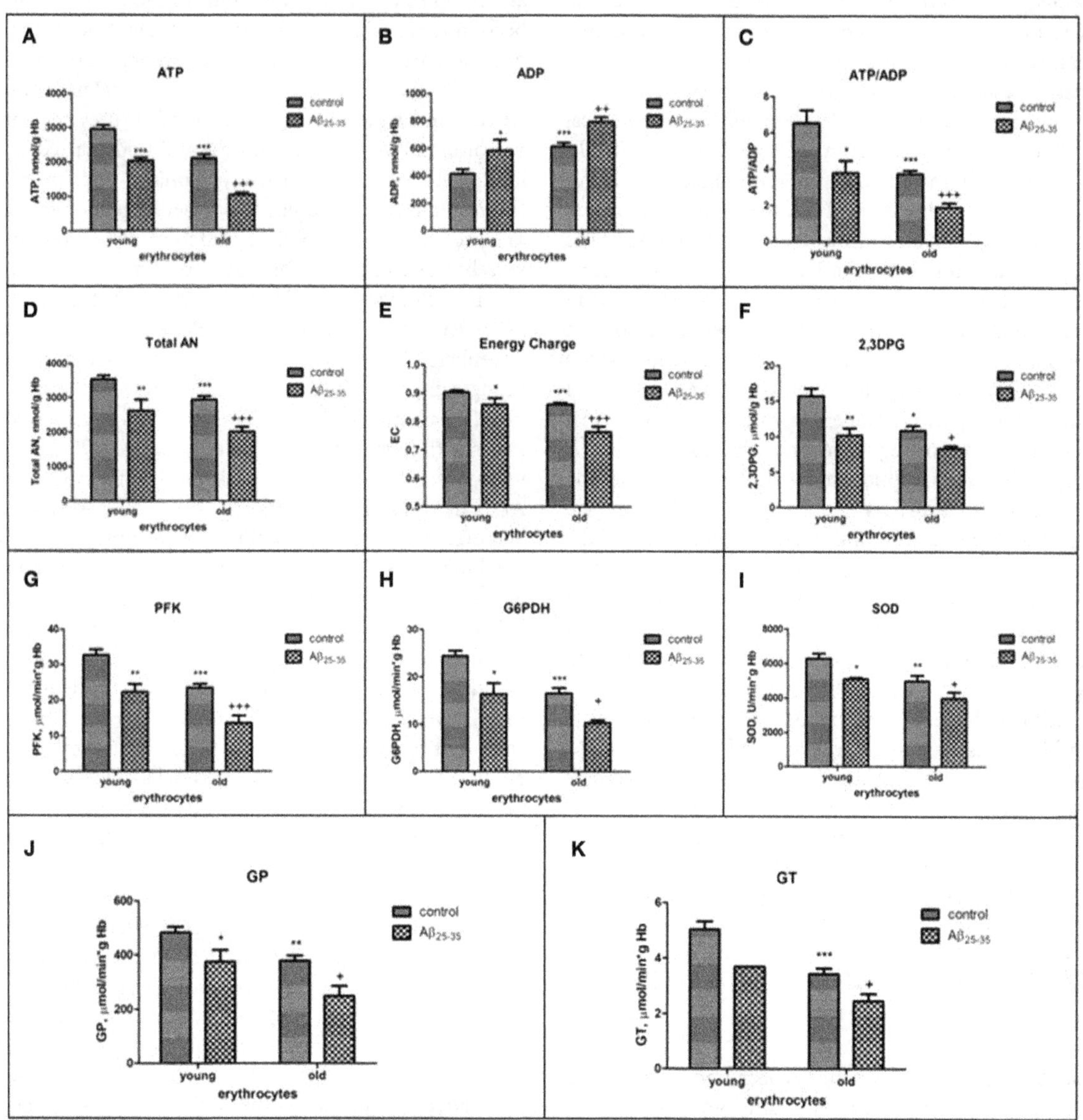

FIGURE 2 | The effects of Aβ25-35 on the parameters of the adenylate system, concentration of 2,3–DPG and activities of some glycolytic and antioxidant enzymes activities in young and old erythrocytes (RBCs). **(A)** ATP, **(B)** ADP, **(C)** ratio ATP/ADP, **(D)** total adenine nucleotide pool size, **(E)** energy charge, **(F)** 2,3DPG, **(G–K)** activities of phosphofructokinase, glucose-6-phosphate dehydrogenase, superoxide dismutase, glutathione peroxidase, glutathione transferase, respectively. ATP and AN are expressed as micromol/g Hb, ADP as nmol/g Hb. AN, total adenine nucleotide pool size; EC, adenylate energy charge [EC = (ATP + 1/2ADP)/AN]; phosphofructokinase (PFK), glucose-6-phosphate dehydrogenase (G-6PDH), glutathione peroxidase (GP), glutathione transferase (GT) activities are expressed as IU/g hemoglobin (Hb); superoxide dismutase (SOD) is expressed as units/min per g Hb. One unit of SOD activity is defined as the amount of enzyme required to produce a 50% inhibition of the rate of p-nitrotetrazolium blue reduction. The results are the mean±SEM of 16 rats. Cells were incubated at 25°C for 30 min in 10 mmol/L potassium phosphate buffer, pH 7.4, containing 0.9% NaCl, 5 mmol/L KCl, and 10 μmol/L $A\beta_{25-35}$. Control was incubated with nontoxic $A\beta_{35-25}$. Significant differences are indicated: $^{*}P < 0.05$, $^{**}P < 0.01$, and $^{***}P < 0.001$ as compared to young cells; $^{+}P < 0.05$, $^{++}P < 0.01$, and $^{+++}P < 0.001$ as compared to the old control (one-way analysis of variance [ANOVA] with Bonferroni's multiple comparison test). Aβ indicates amyloid β.

assume that there is a hidden defect in the achievement of hematopoietic equilibrium in older people. Hence, the main question arises. Is such a hidden bone marrow defect typical for people with dementia? And does this defect lead only to the disruption of cellular equilibrium, or does it also cause the appearance of defective cells in the circulation that have not received adequate "strength reserve" in the bone marrow, and therefore they quickly age and get damaged in the bloodstream? It is clear that without the answers to these questions, it is impossible to evaluate the contribution of the impaired functional capacity of erythrocytes to the clinical symptoms of AD and other types of dementia. However, when dementia is exclusively referred to brain diseases, the attention of scientists is concentrated only on neurological symptoms, whereas all possible "defects" of erythrocytes, which cause pathological consequences for the brain, remain unexplored. We found only a few literature sources discussing the role of morphological changes that characterize the violation of the architecture of the erythrocyte membranes in the development of neurological symptoms characteristic of dementia (Mohanty et al., 2008). In particular, it has been shown that the appearance of atypical cells with altered morphological features, that is giant elongated erythrocytes with a nonhomogeneous membrane (acanthocytes or erythrocytes with numerous random spur-like cytoplasmic outgrowths) (Brecher and Bessis, 1972; Lan et al., 2015), occurs in advance (for several years) before the onset of memory disorders (Goodall et al., 1994). The mechanism of the acanthocytes emergence in the bloodstream is unknown, but since atypical cells are only a small part of the general population of normal erythrocytes, it has been suggested that the cause of their formation is related to a disruption in the synthesis of membrane structural proteins that occurs in the stage of erythrocyte formation in the bone marrow, although the possibility of the cell damage under the influence of unknown factors immediately after they come out from the bone marrow into the blood is not ruled out. Soluble amyloid peptides that are found in various cerebral vessels of the patients with AD [cerebral amyloid angiopathy (CAA)] and which, on the one hand, are capable to contact the cellular elements of blood, on the other—to damage the walls of blood vessels and cause a hemorrhage in the brain (Thanvi and Robinson, 2006), have recently been recognized as one of these factors. However, it is possible that the appearance of erythrocytes of the atypical form is associated with amyloids that circulate in the bloodstream and bind to the cell membrane (Kuo et al., 2000; Kiko et al., 2012) leading to its damage.

THE ROLE OF AMYLOID ANGIOPATHY IN ERYTHROCYTE DAMAGE

The fact that AD is a systemic disease has been known for a long time, dating back to the last century, when amyloid peptides were first detected in small vessels of the brains of patients with AD (Scholz, 1938). For the sake of justice, it is worth mentioning that the existence of amyloid peptides was known back in 1878 when Atkins discovered amyloids in the brain and blood vessels of the brain in a young patient with dementia caused by a head injury (Atkins, 1878). At that time, it has been also identified that amyloids accumulate in the brain vessels in patients with syphilis (Atkins, 1875), and epilepsy (Blocq and Marinesco, 1892) indicating that cerebral amyloidosis and CAA are accompanying a number of diseases.

As it is now well known, in patients with DA, amyloids (mainly $A\beta_{1-40}$) are found in the capillaries (Attems and Jellinger, 2004), arteries, arterioles, veins, and venules (Thal et al., 2002), which penetrate the leptomeningeal, cortical and subcortical areas of the brain (Weller et al., 2009), as well as in blood vessels supplying the hippocampus (Masuda et al., 1988). Localized in various structures of blood vessels (Wisniewski and Wegiel, 1994) and in contact with numerous cells (myocytes, pericytes), amyloids cause their damage (Vonsattel et al., 1991; Dalkara et al., 2011), as a result of which the membrane of the vessels seems to loosen, becoming unstable, which can eventually lead to the formation of an aneurysms, its rupture and cerebral hemorrhage (Thanvi and Robinson, 2006), that is, a condition that usually occurs with strokes and which irrespective of AD causes the formation of hematoma, lysis of erythrocytes, brain edema (Xi et al., 2006), local cell death, and memory damage (Pfeifer et al., 2002). Interestingly, the multiple microvascular pathology, mediated by the presence of amyloids in different structures of the blood vessels, was confirmed not only at postmortem examination, but also in life in virtually all patients with AD (Kalaria and Hedera, 1995; Farkas and Luiten, 2001; Bailey et al., 2004; Smith and Greenberg, 2009) regardless of the presence of atherosclerotic changes in the vessels. It should be noted, however, that CAA in AD patients is observed in 90–100% of cases, while brain zones with hemorrhage are detected only in 20–25% of patients with AD (Urbach, 2011). This means that brain damage in AD can occur for reasons not associated with CAA-induced hemorrhage. Indeed, a significant accumulation of amyloids in the brain vessels can cause their occlusion, thereby blocking blood flow, supplying the brain with oxygen and glucose (de la Torre and Stefano, 2000), and causing neurodegeneration of neurons and memory impairment (Thal et al., 2008, 2009). In addition, localized in endothelial cells lining the lumen of blood vessels (Michaud et al., 2013), amyloids are constantly in contact with erythrocytes circulating in the bloodstream, causing, on the one hand, their adhesion to endothelial cells, thereby violating the blood flow (Ravi et al., 2004), on the other—interacting with the membrane of erythrocytes, cause its modification and damage (Nicolay et al., 2007).

It was true that some studies have demonstrated that AD patients have increased RBC membrane injury suggesting the increased capability for erythrocyte lysis *in vivo* (Bosman et al., 1991; Goodall et al., 1994; Mattson et al., 1997; Solerte et al., 2000; Kosenko et al., 2009), as evidenced by the accumulation of free hemoglobin and iron in the brain of AD patients (Wu et al., 2004; Perry et al., 2008). The consequences of RBC lysis for the brain are well known (Xi et al., 1998). It has been shown that the appearance of free hemoglobin in the brain leads to rapid destruction of the hemato-encephalic barrier, DNA fragmentation, increased lipid peroxidation and global oxidative stress, development of the inflammatory process, vasoconstriction, hypoperfusion, brain atrophy (Alexander and LoVerme, 1980), memory impairment and death (Hackett and Anderson, 2000).

The lytic effect of amyloids was confirmed on the general population of erythrocytes. *In vitro* $A\beta$ induces rapid lysis of human and rat erythrocytes that can be either attenuated by antioxidants (Mattson et al., 1997) or amplified in the presence of inhibitors of glycolytic and antioxidant enzymes or Na^{+}, K^{+}-ATPase (Kosenko et al., 2008a), and suggested the role of RBC glycolysis, ion pumping capacity and antioxidant status in the bioactivity and erythrotoxicity of amyloids. Given the above, we assumed that the constant contact of erythrocytes with amyloids can cause not only the change and damage on the membrane structures, but also the metabolic/energy metabolism in the erythrocytes underlying the aging, integrity, and functional ability of the cells. This assumption does not contradict the known pathological consequence of chronic brain hypoperfusion, leading to reducing oxygen delivery to the brain (de la Torre, 2017). On the contrary, it clearly points to the possible existence of additional unspecified mechanisms, restricting the oxygen supply to the brain and, therefore, participating in the development of hypoxia and neurodegenerative processes specific to AD (Thal et al., 2009). However, the population of erythrocytes is not homogeneous, and the facts that the least resistance of old erythrocytes to endogenous and exogenous pathological factors caused by a reduced rate of energy metabolism, antioxidant defense, and strengthening of catabolic processes (Bonsignore et al., 1964; Shinozuka et al., 1994) are well established.

Data on the effect of amyloid peptides on erythrocytes of different ages at present are currently not available and are of special interest, since patients with AD are characterized by accelerated aging of erythrocytes in the bloodstream (Bosman et al., 1991). We have recently showed that sensibility of RBC to βA-induced hemolysis was in proportion to both cell age and βA concentration (Tikhonova et al., 2014). The inhibition of glucose consumption and lactate production by βA was found to occur in both cells type. However, greater demand for ATP of the Na^+, K^+ -ATPase, in combination with a more reduced capacity of the glycolytic pathway and 2,3-DPG levels in old cells lead to more pronounced imbalance between ATP and 2,3-DPG formation, total nucleotide changes and ion pumping in aging erythrocytes exposed to the amyloid. Interestingly, the decline in the levels of antioxidative, glycolytic enzymes, 2,3DPG, ATP, adenine nucleotide pool and the adenylate energy charge in young cells treated with amyloid were similar to that we found as occurring during *in vivo* red cell aging (control old erythrocytes). Thus, our data obtained show that even a limited contact of amyloid with erythrocytes is sufficient to transform young erythrocytes into old ones and that similar biochemical mechanisms can underlie the accelerated aging of cells in the bloodstream of patients with AD (Bosman et al., 1991) (**Figure 2**), that may be one of the main reasons of both inadequate supply of oxygen to the brain, and lysis of cells in circulation.

NOVEL THERAPEUTIC STRATEGY: PROBLEMS AND POSSIBLE SOLUTIONS

At present there are no medical drugs which are able to increase and improve perfusion of the brain of AD patients, since due to the absence of early diagnostics the use of any drug therapy, when the brain tissue is irreparably damaged, is late and inefficient (Hachinski and Munoz, 1997). Thus, it is very problematic "to repair" chronically damaged blood vessels of the brain and to restore their functional state with the preparations available, as well as it is hard "to cure diseased erythrocytes." This is connected, first of all, with the fact that real causes of "chronic disease" of erythrocytes during natural aging of the organism are unknown. One of the important problems, as noted above, is the absence of total knowledge on the hematopoietic status of the elderly, especially during long bed rest, accompanied by undernourishment, leads to a decrease in metabolism rate.

It is interesting to note that the problems in relation to the "disease" of erythrocytes arise during transfusion of the whole donor blood or packed RBC to the patients with different diseases in order to restore oxygen transport to the tissues and release carbonic acid from them. The main challenge is that all intracellular indices of erythrocytes change very quickly during the storage period of the donated blood leading to rapid cell aging (Lang et al., 2016). And if these indices are not corrected before blood transfusion this may result in irreparable consequences (Beutler et al., 1969). It has been shown, for example, that if during red blood cell transfusion intracellular ATP concentration of erythrocytes was lower by 40% compared to the normal cells, these erythrocytes were lysed to an excessive degree in blood flow of the recipient (Hamasaki et al., 1981). Transfusion of erythrocytes with low intracellular content of 2,3-DPG did not allow for quick restoration of adequate delivery of oxygen to the tissues. Taken together, these observations require development of the ways to increase the concentrations of ATP and 2,3-DPG in erythrocytes immediately before RBC transfusion to the patient (Beutler et al., 1969). Further studies in this field are actively undertaken, and multiple developments directed toward restoration of energy exchange in the stored erythrocytes are successively utilized by the physicians to save the patients life (Valeri and Hirsch, 1969). The main components restoring energy exchange in erythrocytes are glucose, adenine, ascorbate-2-phosphate, phosphoenolpyruvat or the cations and activators of glycolysis, which can penetrate into erythrocytes (Moore et al., 1981). It has been shown that different activators of enzymes introduced into the medium, where erythrocytes are stored, maintain normal concentration of ATP and 2,3-DPG for 1,5 months (Vora, 1987). However, although the scientists have made a considerable progress in solving the problems with regard to restoration of energy exchange disturbed during storage of erythrocytes, all the developments use modulators and activators, which are able to quickly and easily pass through the cell membrane of erythrocytes. This is a limitation for the use of the wider class of active compounds that are unable to be transported into the cells. We tried to circumvent this problem and developed a technology of the encapsulation of substrates and high molecular enzymes in erythrocytes under hypotonic conditions leading to the formation of pores in the membranes of erythrocytes (Seeman et al., 1973), enabling the enzymes with great molecular mass (Baker, 1967; Kosenko et al., 2008b; Godfrin et al., 2012; Kaminsky and Kosenko, 2012; Alexandrovich et al., 2017) to pass through the cells. For instance, we developed an approach on how to introduce regulatory glycolytic enzymes into erythrocytes, where the activity of these enzymes in erythrocytes of old animals and in the elderly decreased by 30–50% (Kaminsky et al., 2013). The data obtained showed that the encapsulation of even one regulatory enzyme in erythrocytes stimulated glycolysis to considerable extent. The signs of it were the increased rate of glucose consumption and the formation of lactate. Moreover, the erythrocytes obtained circulated in the animal's blood flow within many days, sustaining the activity of encapsulated enzymes, the normal level of ATP, 2,3-DPG and other metabolites of energy exchange and antioxidant defense (data not shown). These results obtained are important by two reasons. First, such technology can be applied to restore ATP, 2,3-DPG and other metabolites of energy exchange, the concentration of which is decreased sharply in erythrocytes in aging of the organism. Transfusion of own erythrocytes, possessing encapsulated enzymes, should theoretically reduce the risk of the onset of inadequate oxygen supply to the brain both in the elderly and in patients with AD. Secondly, investigations make the basis for further development of innovative personalized therapeutic strategy.

CONCLUSIONS

Presently, non-genetic Alzheimer's disease is classified as a neurodegenerative disorder. However, there is an impressive body of evidence indicating that AD is a systemic metabolic disease (Perry et al., 2003), and it has originated as a vascular disorder with the resultant impairment of the delivery and transport of essential nutrients, particularly glucose and oxygen resulting in an energy metabolic breakdown with the plaques and tangles found in the brain secondary to the effects of the vascular pathology (de la Torre, 2002a). Since erythrocyte serve as the only oxygen carrier and their ability to the binding, transport, and delivery of oxygen to tissues depends, first of all, on the energy metabolism and antioxidant status there is therefore a strong possibility that the disturbance of energy metabolism and oxidative enhancement in these cells may have a dramatic impact on destabilization of aerobic glucose metabolism in the brain and AD development. With regard to RBC-controlled brain vital activity there is incontrovertible evidence that even just a few minutes of oxygen deprivation (together with glucose) initiate significant brain dysfunction and chronic effect can ultimately result in the irreversible brain damage and permanent impairment of cognition. This implies that the cerebrometabolic abnormalities are the most common form of dementia (Chibber et al., 2016; Gonzalez-Reyes et al., 2016). However, although major mechanisms involved in brain damage due to metabolic abnormalities resulting from the oxygen deprivation including alterations in neurotransmission, defect of mitochondrial oxidative phosphorylation, disturbance of Ca^{2+} homeostasis, oxidative stress and eventually apoptotic or necrotic cell death are profound and obvious (Barreto et al., 2011; Cabezas et al., 2012, 2015; Avila Rodriguez et al., 2014; Toro-Urrego et al., 2016; Baez et al., 2017; Baez-Jurado et al., 2017a,b; Martin-Jiménez et al., 2017a,b; Shevtsova et al., 2017), no systematic programs of research have examined the relationship between the breach of the energy metabolism of erythrocytes in the causing of leading to cerebrometabolic abnormalities and dementia. One of the reasons of this paradox is the large number of reports stating that brain atrophy and degeneration of nerve cells, observed with dementia, can occur without cerebrovascular pathology, but only through the amyloid fault, leading to the struggle with amyloids, and not with the causes that "gave birth to them," and made the AD a permanently incurable disease with unknown etiology. In our view, a careful examination and reversing age-related metabolic/energetic changes in erythrocytes is an achievable goal and will provide these cells as a marker of a risk of inadequate brain oxygen supply, resulting the irreversible brain damage and permanent impairment of cognition. We also strongly believe that biochemical erythrocyte indicators (ATP, 2,3DPG, glucose, lactate and others), as well as the enzymes of glycolysis, pentose phosphate and Rapoport-Luebering shunt, antioxidant pathways all of which are responsible for interrelated metabolism and functional capacity of RBC should be studied (especially in people over 50 years, and in the dynamics) not only in research laboratories, but also in clinical settings that may provide a basis for innovative personalized therapeutic strategies.

The development of technologies to assist in restoration of erythrocyte energy metabolism must form an integral part of new therapeutic strategies in the treatment of a great variety of disorders accompanied by inadequate oxygen delivery. Similar studies just are gathering pace but have already marked a turning-point in our knowledge regarding AD and amyloid peptides that cannot be the only pharmacological target in the struggle against this devastating illness of human beings.

AUTHOR CONTRIBUTIONS

All of authors (EK, LT, CM, GB, GA, and YK) write manuscript, created figures, and proof final version of this manuscript.

ACKNOWLEDGMENTS

The reported study was funded by RFBR and Moscow region according to the research project No 17-44-500561.

REFERENCES

Ackerman, W. J. (1974). Stupor, bradycardia, hypotension and hypothermia. A presentation of Wernicke's encephalopathy with rapid response to thiamine. *West. J. Med.* 121, 428–429.

Ahlgren, S., Li, G. L., and Olsson, Y. (1996). Accumulation of beta-amyloid precursor protein and ubiquitin in axons after spinal cord trauma in humans: immunohistochemical observations on autopsy material. *Acta Neuropathol.* 92, 49–55. doi: 10.1007/s004010050488

Ajmani, R. S., and Rifkind, J. M. (1998). Hemorheological changes during human aging. *Gerontology* 44, 111–120. doi: 10.1159/000021993

Ajmani, R. S., Fleg, J. L., Demehin, A. A., Wright, J. G., O'Connor, F., Heim, J. M., et al. (2003). Oxidative stress and hemorheological changes induced by acute treadmill exercise. *Clin. Hemorheol. Microcirc.* 28, 29–40.

Albin, R. L., and Greenamyre, J. T. (1992). Alternative excitotoxic hypotheses. *Neurology* 42, 733–738. doi: 10.1212/WNL.42.4.733

Alexander, M. P., and LoVerme, S. R. (1980). Aphasia after left hemispheric intracerebral hemorrhage. *Neurology* 30, 1193–1202. doi: 10.1212/WNL.30.11.1193

Alexandrovich, Y. G., Kosenko, E. A., Sinauridze, E. I., Obydennyi, S. I., Kireev, I. I., Ataullakhanov, F. I., et al. (2017). Rapid elimination of blood alcohol using erythrocytes: mathematical modeling and *in vitro* study. *BioMed Res. Int.* 2017:5849593. doi: 10.1155/2017/5849593

Aliev, G. (2011). Oxidative stress induced-metabolic imbalance, mitochondrial failure, and cellular hypoperfusion as primary pathogenetic factors for the development of Alzheimer disease which can be used as a alternate and successful drug treatment strategy: past, present and future. *CNS Neurol. Disord. Drug Targets* 10, 147–148. doi: 10.2174/187152711794480492

Aliev, G., Obrenovich, M. E., Smith, M. A., and Perry, G. (2003a). Hypoperfusion, mitochondria failure, oxidative stress, and Alzheimer disease. *J. Biomed. Biotechnol.* 2003, 162–163. doi: 10.1155/S1110724303305029

Aliev, G., Smith, M. A., de la Torre, J. C., and Perry, G. (2004). Mitochondria as a primary target for vascular hypoperfusion and oxidative stress in Alzheimer's disease. *Mitochondrion* 4, 649–663. doi: 10.1016/j.mito.2004.07.018

Aliev, G., Smith, M. A., Obrenovich, M. E., de la Torre, J. C., and Perry, G. (2003b). Role of vascular hypoperfusion-induced oxidative stress and mitochondria failure in the pathogenesis of Azheimer disease. *Neurotox. Res.* 5, 491–504. doi: 10.1007/BF03033159

Alkire, M. T., Haier, R. J., Barker, S. J., Shah, N. K., Wu, J. C., and Kao, Y. J. (1995). Cerebral metabolism during propofol anesthesia in humans studied with positron emission tomography. *Anesthesiology* 82, 393–403. discussion: 27A. doi: 10.1097/00000542-199502000-00010

Alkire, M. T., Haier, R. J., Shah, N. K., and Anderson, C. T. (1997). Positron emission tomography study of regional cerebral metabolism in humans during isoflurane anesthesia. *Anesthesiology* 86, 549–557. doi: 10.1097/00000542-199703000-00006

Arai, H., Lee, V. M., Hill, W. D., Greenberg, B. D., and Trojanowski, J. Q. (1992). Lewy bodies contain beta-amyloid precursor proteins of Alzheimer's disease. *Brain Res.* 585, 386–390. doi: 10.1016/0006-8993(92)91242-7

Arnsten, A. F., and Goldman-Rakic, P. S. (1998). Noise stress impairs prefrontal cortical cognitive function in monkeys: evidence for a hyperdopaminergic mechanism. *Arch. Gen. Psychiatry* 55, 362–368. doi: 10.1001/archpsyc.55.4.362

Atkins, R. (1875). Half-yearly report on mental disease. *Dublin J. Med. Sci.* 314–331. doi: 10.1007/BF02975691

Atkins, R. (1878). On the morbid histology of the spinal cord in five cases of insanity. *Br. Med. J.* 2, 96–99. doi: 10.1136/bmj.2.916.96

Attems, J., and Jellinger, K. A. (2004). Only cerebral capillary amyloid angiopathy correlates with Alzheimer pathology–a pilot study. *Acta Neuropathol.* 107, 83–90. doi: 10.1007/s00401-003-0796-9

Atwood, C. S., Obrenovich, M. E., Liu, T., Chan, H., Perry, G., Smith, M. A., et al. (2003). Amyloid-beta: a chameleon walking in two worlds: a review of the trophic and toxic properties of amyloid-beta. *Brain Res. Brain Res. Rev.* 43, 1–16. doi: 10.1016/S0165-0173(03)00174-7

Atwood, C. S., Robinson, S. R., and Smith, M. A. (2002). Amyloid-β: redox-metal chelator and antioxidant. *J. Alzheimers Dis.* 4, 203–214. doi: 10.3233/JAD-2002-4310

Auer, R. N., and Siesjö, B. K. (1993). Hypoglycaemia: brain neurochemistry and neuropathology. *Baillieres Clin. Endocrinol. Metab.* 7, 611–625. doi: 10.1016/S0950-351X(05)80210-1

Auer, R., Kalimo, H., Olsson, Y., and Wieloch, T. (1985). The dentate gyrus in hypoglycemia: pathology implicating excitotoxin-mediated neuronal necrosis. *Acta Neuropathol.* 67, 279–288. doi: 10.1007/BF00687813

Avila Rodriguez, M., Garcia-Segura, L. M., Cabezas, R., Torrente, D., Capani, F., Gonzalez, J., et al. (2014). Tibolone protects T98G cells from glucose deprivation. *J. Steroid Biochem. Mol. Biol.* 144(Pt B), 294–303. doi: 10.1016/j.jsbmb.2014.07.009

Baez, E., Guio-Vega, G. P., Echeverria, V., Sandoval-Rueda, D. A., and Barreto, G. E. (2017). 4'-Chlorodiazepam protects mitochondria in T98G astrocyte cell line from glucose deprivation. *Neurotox. Res.* 32, 163–171. doi: 10.1007/s12640-017-9733-x

Baez-Jurado, E., Hidalgo-Lanussa, O., Guio-Vega, G., Ashraf, G. M., Echeverria, V., Aliev, G., et al. (2017a). Conditioned medium of human adipose mesenchymal stem cells increases wound closure and protects human astrocytes following scratch assay *in vitro*. *Mol. Neurobiol.* doi: 10.1007/s12035-017-0771-4. [Epub ahead of print].

Baez-Jurado, E., Vega, G. G., Aliev, G., Tarasov, V. V., Esquinas, P., Echeverria, V., et al. (2017b). Blockade of neuroglobin reduces protection of conditioned medium from human mesenchymal stem cells in human astrocyte model (T98G) under a *scratch* assay. *Mol. Neurobiol.* doi: 10.1007/s12035-017-0481-y. [Epub ahead of print].

Bagnara, G. P., Bonsi, L., Strippoli, P., Bonifazi, F., Tonelli, R., D'Addato, S., et al. (2000). Hemopoiesis in healthy old people and centenarians: well-maintained responsiveness of $CD34^+$ cells to hemopoietic growth factors and remodeling of cytokine network. *J. Gerontol. A Biol. Sci. Med. Sci.* 55, B61–B66. discussion: B67–B70. doi: 10.1093/gerona/55.2.B61

Bailey, T. L., Rivara, C. B., Rocher, A. B., and Hof, P. R. (2004). The nature and effects of cortical microvascular pathology in aging and Alzheimer's disease. *Neurol. Res.* 26, 573–578. doi: 10.1179/016164104225016272

Baker, R. F. (1967). Entry of ferritin into human red cells during hypotonic haemolysis. *Nature* 215, 424–425. doi: 10.1038/215424a0

Balin, B. J., and Appelt, D. M. (2001). Role of infection in Alzheimer's disease. *J. Am. Osteopath. Assoc.* 101, S1–S6.

Bapat, R. D., Supe, A. N., and Sathe, M. J. (1983). Management of small bowel perforation with intra- and post-operative lavages with povidone iodine. (A prospective study). *J. Postgrad. Med.* 29, 29–33.

Barreto, G., White, R. E., Ouyang, Y., Xu, L., and Giffard, R. G. (2011). Astrocytes: targets for neuroprotection in stroke. *Cent. Nerv. Syst. Agents Med. Chem.* 11, 164–173. doi: 10.2174/187152411796011303

Beal, M. F. (1992). Does impairment of energy metabolism result in excitotoxic neuronal death in neurodegenerative illnesses? *Ann. Neurol.* 31, 119–130. doi: 10.1002/ana.410310202

Beal, M. F., Swartz, K. J., Hyman, B. T., Storey, E., Finn, S. F., and Koroshetz, W. (1991). Aminooxyacetic acid results in excitotoxin lesions by a novel indirect mechanism. *J. Neurochem.* 57, 1068–1073. doi: 10.1111/j.1471-4159.1991.tb08258.x

Beutler, E., Meul, A., and Wood, L. A. (1969). Depletion and regeneration of 2,3-diphosphoglyceric acid in stored red blood cells. *Transfusion* 9, 109–115. doi: 10.1111/j.1537-2995.1969.tb05527.x

Bird, T. D. (2005). Genetic factors in Alzheimer's disease. *N. Engl. J. Med.* 352, 862–864. doi: 10.1056/NEJMp058027

Blass, J. P. (2002). Glucose/mitochondria in neurological conditions. *Int. Rev. Neurobiol.* 51, 325–376. doi: 10.1016/S0074-7742(02)51010-2

Blass, J. P. (2003). Cerebrometabolic abnormalities in Alzheimer's disease. *Neurol. Res.* 25, 556–566. doi: 10.1179/016164103101201995

Blass, J. P., and Gibson, G. E. (1991). The role of oxidative abnormalities in the pathophysiology of Alzheimer's disease. *Rev. Neurol.* 147, 513–525.

Blocq, P., and Marinesco, G. (1892). Sur les le'sions et la pathoge'nie del 'epilepsie dite essentielle. *Sem. Me'dical* 12, 445–446.

Bonsignore, A., Fornaini, G., Fantoni, A., Leoncini, G., and Segni, P. (1964). Relationship between age and enzymatic activities in human erythrocytes from normal and fava bean-sensitive subjects. *J. Clin. Invest.* 43, 834–842. doi: 10.1172/JCI104969

Bosman, G. J., Bartholomeus, I. G., de Man, A. J., van Kalmthout, P. J., and de Grip, W. J. (1991). Erythrocyte membrane characteristics indicate abnormal cellular aging in patients with Alzheimer's disease. *Neurobiol. Aging* 12, 13–18. doi: 10.1016/0197-4580(91)90033-G

Braak, H., and Braak, E. (1991). Neuropathological stageing of Alzheimer-related changes. *Acta Neuropathol.* 82, 239–259. doi: 10.1007/BF00308809

Brecher, G., and Bessis, M. (1972). Present status of spiculed red cells and their relationship to the discocyte-echinocyte transformation: a critical review. *Blood* 40, 333–344.

Brewer, G. J., Oelshlegel, F. J., Moore, L. G., and Noble, N. A. (1974). *In vivo* red cell glycolytic control and DPG-ATP levels. *Ann. N. Y. Acad. Sci.* 241, 513–523. doi: 10.1111/j.1749-6632.1974.tb21907.x

Brito-Moreira, J., Paula-Lima, A. C., Bomfim, T. R., Oliveira, F. B., Sepúlveda, F. J., De Mello, F. G., et al. (2011). Aβ oligomers induce glutamate release from hippocampal neurons. *Curr. Alzheimer Res.* 8, 552–562. doi: 10.2174/156720511796391917

Brooks, W. M., Stidley, C. A., Petropoulos, H., Jung, R. E., Weers, D. C., Friedman, S. D., et al. (2000). Metabolic and cognitive response to human traumatic brain injury: a quantitative proton magnetic resonance study. *J. Neurotrauma* 17, 629–640. doi: 10.1089/089771500415382

Bruce, D. G., Davis, W. A., Casey, G. P., Clarnette, R. M., Brown, S. G. A., Jacobs, I. G., et al. (2009). Severe hypoglycaemia and cognitive impairment in older patients with diabetes: the Fremantle diabetes study. *Diabetologia* 52, 1808–1815. doi: 10.1007/s00125-009-1437-1

Bubber, P., Haroutunian, V., Fisch, G., Blass, J. P., and Gibson, G. E. (2005). Mitochondrial abnormalities in Alzheimer brain: mechanistic implications. *Ann. Neurol.* 57, 695–703. doi: 10.1002/ana.20474

Butterworth, R. F. (2003). Hepatic encephalopathy–a serious complication of alcoholic liver disease. *Alcohol Res. Health* 27, 143–145.

Cabezas, R., Avila, M. F., Gonzalez, J., El-Bacha, R. S., and Barreto, G. E. (2015). PDGF-BB protects mitochondria from rotenone in T98G cells. *Neurotox. Res.* 27, 355–367. doi: 10.1007/s12640-014-9509-5

Cabezas, R., El-Bacha, R. S., Gonzalez, J., and Barreto, G. E. (2012). Mitochondrial functions in astrocytes: neuroprotective implications from oxidative damage by rotenone. *Neurosci. Res.* 74, 80–90 doi: 10.1016/j.neures.2012.07.008

Calderón-Garcidueñas, L., Mora-Tiscare-o, A., Ontiveros, E., Gómez-Garza, G., Barragán-Mejía, G., Broadway, J., et al. (2008a). Air pollution, cognitive deficits and brain abnormalities: a pilot study with children and dogs. *Brain Cogn.* 68, 117–127. doi: 10.1016/j.bandc.2008.04.008

Calderón-Garcidueñas, L., Solt, A. C., Henríquez-Roldán, C., Torres-Jardón, R., Nuse, B., Herritt, L., et al. (2008b). Long-term air pollution exposure is associated with neuroinflammation, an altered innate immune response, disruption of the blood-brain barrier, ultrafine particulate deposition, and accumulation of amyloid beta-42 and alpha-synuclein in children and young adults. *Toxicol. Pathol.* 36, 289–310. doi: 10.1177/0192623307313011

Chang, C.-Y., Liang, H.-J., Chow, S.-Y., Chen, S.-M., and Liu, D.-Z. (2007). Hemorheological mechanisms in Alzheimer's disease. *Microcirculation* 14, 627–634. doi: 10.1080/10739680701411056

Chen, X.-H., Siman, R., Iwata, A., Meaney, D. F., Trojanowski, J. Q., and Smith, D. H. (2004). Long-term accumulation of amyloid-β, β-secretase, presenilin-1, and caspase-3 in damaged axons following brain trauma. *Am. J. Pathol.* 165, 357–371. doi: 10.1016/S0002-9440(10)63303-2

Chibber, S., Alexiou, A., Alama, M. N., Barreto, G. E., Aliev, G., and Ashraf, G. M. (2016). A synopsis on the linkage between age-related dementias and vascular disorders. *CNS Neurol. Disord. Drug Targets* 15, 250–258. doi: 10.2174/1871527315666160202121809

Cho, J., King, J. S., Qian, X., Harwood, A. J., and Shears, S. B. (2008). Dephosphorylation of 2,3-bisphosphoglycerate by MIPP expands the regulatory capacity of the Rapoport-Luebering glycolytic shunt. *Proc. Natl. Acad. Sci. U.S.A.* 105, 5998–6003. doi: 10.1073/pnas.0710980105

Cholevas, V., Challa, A., Lapatsanis, P. D., and Andronikou, S. (2008). Changes in red cell phosphate metabolism of preterm and fullterm infants with perinatal problems during their first month of life. *Eur. J. Pediatr.* 167, 211–218. doi: 10.1007/s00431-007-0464-5

Connolly, A. M., and Volpe, J. J. (1990). Clinical features of bilirubin encephalopathy. *Clin. Perinatol.* 17, 371–379.

Conrad, C. D. (2006). What is the functional significance of chronic stress-induced CA3 dendritic retraction within the hippocampus? *Behav. Cogn. Neurosci. Rev.* 5, 41–60. doi: 10.1177/1534582306289043

Conrad, C. D., Galea, L. A., Kuroda, Y., and McEwen, B. S. (1996). Chronic stress impairs rat spatial memory on the Y maze, and this effect is blocked by tianeptine pretreatment. *Behav. Neurosci.* 110, 1321–1334. doi: 10.1037/0735-7044.110.6.1321

Cornish, R., Blumbergs, P. C., Manavis, J., Scott, G., Jones, N. R., and Reilly, P. L. (2000). Topography and severity of axonal injury in human spinal cord trauma using amyloid precursor protein as a marker of axonal injury. *Spine* 25, 1227–1233. doi: 10.1097/00007632-200005150-00005

Dalkara, T., Gursoy-Ozdemir, Y., and Yemisci, M. (2011). Brain microvascular pericytes in health and disease. *Acta Neuropathol.* 122, 1–9. doi: 10.1007/s00401-011-0847-6

Danon, D., Bologna, N. B., and Gavendo, S. (1992). Memory performance of young and old subjects related to their erythrocyte characteristics. *Exp. Gerontol.* 27, 275–285. doi: 10.1016/0531-5565(92)90055-5

De Felice, F. G., Velasco, P. T., Lambert, M. P., Viola, K., Fernandez, S. J., Ferreira, S. T., et al. (2007). Aβ oligomers induce neuronal oxidative stress through an N-methyl-D-aspartate receptor-dependent mechanism that is blocked by the Alzheimer drug memantine. *J. Biol. Chem.* 282, 11590–11601. doi: 10.1074/jbc.M607483200

De Felice, F. G., Wu, D., Lambert, M. P., Fernandez, S. J., Velasco, P. T., Lacor, P. N., et al. (2008). Alzheimer's disease-type neuronal tau hyperphosphorylation induced by Aβ oligomers. *Neurobiol. Aging* 29, 1334–1347. doi: 10.1016/j.neurobiolaging.2007.02.029

De Jong, G. I., Farkas, E., Stienstra, C. M., Plass, J. R., Keijser, J. N., de la Torre, J. C., et al. (1999). Cerebral hypoperfusion yields capillary damage in the hippocampal CA1 area that correlates with spatial memory impairment. *Neuroscience* 91, 203–210. doi: 10.1016/S0306-4522(98)00659-9

de la Torre, J. C. (2000a). Cerebral hypoperfusion, capillary degeneration, and development of Alzheimer disease. *Alzheimer Dis. Assoc. Disord.* 14(Suppl. 1), S72–S81. doi: 10.1097/00002093-200000001-00012

de la Torre, J. C. (2000b). Impaired cerebromicrovascular perfusion. Summary of evidence in support of its causality in Alzheimer's disease. *Ann. N. Y. Acad. Sci.* 924, 136–152. doi: 10.1111/j.1749-6632.2000.tb05572.x

de la Torre, J. C. (2002a). Alzheimer disease as a vascular disorder: nosological evidence. *Stroke* 33, 1152–1162. doi: 10.1161/01.STR.0000014421.15948.67

de la Torre, J. C. (2002b). Alzheimer's disease: how does it start? *J. Alzheimers Dis.* 4, 497–512. doi: 10.3233/JAD-2002-4606

de la Torre, J. C. (2017). Are major dementias triggered by poor blood flow to the brain? Theoretical considerations. *J. Alzheimers Dis.* 57, 353–371. doi: 10.3233/JAD-161266

de la Torre, J. C., and Mussivand, T. (1993). Can disturbed brain microcirculation cause Alzheimer's disease? *Neurol. Res.* 15, 146–153. doi: 10.1080/01616412.1993.11740127

de la Torre, J. C., and Stefano, G. B. (2000). Evidence that Alzheimer's disease is a microvascular disorder: the role of constitutive nitric oxide. *Brain Res. Brain Res. Rev.* 34, 119–136. doi: 10.1016/S0165-0173(00)00043-6

Demuro, A., Mina, E., Kayed, R., Milton, S. C., Parker, I., and Glabe, C. G. (2005). Calcium dysregulation and membrane disruption as a ubiquitous neurotoxic mechanism of soluble amyloid oligomers. *J. Biol. Chem.* 280, 17294–17300. doi: 10.1074/jbc.M500997200

Dodds, C., and Allison, J. (1998). Postoperative cognitive deficit in the elderly surgical patient. *Br. J. Anaesth.* 81, 449–462.

Dong, Y., Zhang, G., Zhang, B., Moir, R. D., Xia, W., Marcantonio, E. R., et al. (2009). The common inhalational anesthetic sevoflurane induces apoptosis and increases beta-amyloid protein levels. *Arch. Neurol.* 66, 620–631. doi: 10.1001/archneurol.2009.48

Duhm, J. (1971). Effects of 2,3-diphosphoglycerate and other organic phosphate compounds on oxygen affinity and intracellular pH of human erythrocytes. *Pflugers Arch.* 326, 341–356. doi: 10.1007/BF00586998

Farkas, E., and Luiten, P. G. (2001). Cerebral microvascular pathology in aging and Alzheimer's disease. *Prog. Neurobiol.* 64, 575–611. doi: 10.1016/S0301-0082(00)00068-X

Fita, I. G., Enciu, A. M., and Stanoiu, B. P. (2011). New insights on Alzheimer's disease diagnostic. *Rom. J. Morphol. Embryol.* 52, 975–979.

Funato, H., Yoshimura, M., Kusui, K., Tamaoka, A., Ishikawa, K., Ohkoshi, N., et al. (1998). Quantitation of amyloid beta-protein (A beta) in the cortex during aging and in Alzheimer's disease. *Am. J. Pathol.* 152, 1633–1640.

Gabuzda, D., Busciglio, J., Chen, L. B., Matsudaira, P., and Yankner, B. A. (1994). Inhibition of energy metabolism alters the processing of amyloid precursor protein and induces a potentially amyloidogenic derivative. *J. Biol. Chem.* 269, 13623–13628.

Giannakopoulos, P., Herrmann, F. R., Bussière, T., Bouras, C., Kövari, E., Perl, D. P., et al. (2003). Tangle and neuron numbers, but not amyloid load, predict cognitive status in Alzheimer's disease. *Neurology* 60, 1495–1500. doi: 10.1212/01.WNL.0000063311.58879.01

Gibson, G. E., and Huang, H.-M. (2002). Oxidative processes in the brain and non-neuronal tissues as biomarkers of Alzheimer's disease. *Front. Biosci. J. Virtual Libr.* 7, d1007–d1015. doi: 10.2741/gibson

Gibson, G. E., Jope, R., and Blass, J. P. (1975). Decreased synthesis of acetylcholine accompanying impaired oxidation of pyruvic acid in rat brain minces. *Biochem. J.* 148, 17–23. doi: 10.1042/bj1480017

Gibson, G. E., Pulsinelli, W., Blass, J. P., and Duffy, T. E. (1981). Brain dysfunction in mild to moderate hypoxia. *Am. J. Med.* 70, 1247–1254. doi: 10.1016/0002-9343(81)90834-2

Glenner, G. G., and Wong, C. W. (1984). Alzheimer's disease and Down's syndrome: sharing of a unique cerebrovascular amyloid fibril protein. *Biochem. Biophys. Res. Commun.* 122, 1131–1135. doi: 10.1016/0006-291X(84)91209-9

Globerson, A. (1999). Hematopoietic stem cells and aging. *Exp. Gerontol.* 34, 137–146. doi: 10.1016/S0531-5565(98)00069-2

Godfrin, Y., Horand, F., Franco, R., Dufour, E., Kosenko, E., Bax, B. E., et al. (2012). International seminar on the red blood cells as vehicles for drugs. *Expert Opin. Biol. Ther.* 12, 127–133. doi: 10.1517/14712598.2012.631909

Gong, Y., Chang, L., Viola, K. L., Lacor, P. N., Lambert, M. P., Finch, C. E., et al. (2003). Alzheimer's disease-affected brain: presence of oligomeric Aβ ligands (ADDLs) suggests a molecular basis for reversible memory loss. *Proc. Natl. Acad. Sci. U.S.A.* 100, 10417–10422. doi: 10.1073/pnas.1834302100

Gonzalez, J., Jurado-Coronel, J. C., Avila, M. F., Sabogal, A., Capani, F., and Barreto, G. E. (2015). NMDARs in neurological diseases: a potential therapeutic target. *Int. J. Neurosci.* 125, 315–327. doi: 10.3109/00207454.2014.940941

Gonzalez-Reyes, R. E., Aliev, G., Avila-Rodrigues, M., and Barreto, G. E. (2016). Alterations in glucose metabolism on cognition: a possible link between diabetes and dementia. *Curr. Pharm. Des.* 22, 812–818. doi: 10.2174/1381612822666151209152013

Goodall, H. B., Reid, A. H., Findlay, D. J., Hind, C., Kay, J., and Coghill, G. (1994). Irregular distortion of the erythrocytes (acanthocytes, spur cells) in senile dementia. *Dis. Markers* 12, 23–41. doi: 10.1155/1994/493810

Gov, N. S., and Safran, S. A. (2005). Red blood cell membrane fluctuations and shape controlled by ATP-induced cytoskeletal defects. *Biophys. J.* 88, 1859–1874. doi: 10.1529/biophysj.104.045328

Grammas, P., Yamada, M., and Zlokovic, B. (2002). The cerebromicrovasculature: a key player in the pathogenesis of Alzheimer's disease. *J. Alzheimers Dis.* 4, 217–223. doi: 10.3233/JAD-2002-4311

Guillozet, A. L., Weintraub, S., Mash, D. C., and Mesulam, M. M. (2003). Neurofibrillary tangles, amyloid, and memory in aging and mild cognitive impairment. *Arch. Neurol.* 60, 729–736. doi: 10.1001/archneur.60.5.729

Gyure, K. A., Durham, R., Stewart, W. F., Smialek, J. E., and Troncoso, J. C. (2001). Intraneuronal abeta-amyloid precedes development of amyloid plaques in down syndrome. *Arch. Pathol. Lab. Med.* 125, 489–492. doi: 10.1043/0003-9985(2001)125<0489:IAAPDO>2.0.CO;2

Hachinski, V., and Munoz, D. G. (1997). Cerebrovascular pathology in Alzheimer's disease: cause, effect or epiphenomenon? *Ann. N. Y. Acad. Sci.* 826, 1–6. doi: 10.1111/j.1749-6632.1997.tb48456.x

Hackett, M. L., and Anderson, C. S. (2000). Health outcomes 1 year after subarachnoid hemorrhage: an international population-based study. The Australian cooperative research on subarachnoid hemorrhage study Group. *Neurology* 55, 658–662. doi: 10.1212/WNL.55.5.658

Hamasaki, N., Ideguchi, H., and Ikehara, Y. (1981). Regeneration of 2,3-bisphosphoglycerate and ATP in stored erythrocytes by phosphoenolpyruvate: a new preservative for blood storage. *Transfusion* 21, 391–396. doi: 10.1046/j.1537-2995.1981.21481275994.x

Hamberger, A. C., Chiang, G. H., Nylén, E. S., Scheff, S. W., and Cotman, C. W. (1979). Glutamate as a CNS transmitter. I. Evaluation of glucose and glutamine as precursors for the synthesis of preferentially released glutamate. *Brain Res.* 168, 513–530. doi: 10.1016/0006-8993(79)90306-8

Hamberger, A., Huang, Y.-L., Zhu, H., Bao, F., Ding, M., Blennow, K., et al. (2003). Redistribution of neurofilaments and accumulation of β-amyloid protein after brain injury by rotational acceleration of the head. *J. Neurotrauma* 20, 169–178. doi: 10.1089/08977150360547080

Hardy, J., and Selkoe, D. J. (2002). The amyloid hypothesis of Alzheimer's disease: progress and problems on the road to therapeutics. *Science* 297, 353–356. doi: 10.1126/science.1072994

Hardy, J. A., and Higgins, G. A. (1992). Alzheimer's disease: the amyloid cascade hypothesis. *Science* 256, 184–185. doi: 10.1126/science.1566067

Hodes, J. E., Soncrant, T. T., Larson, D. M., Carlson, S. G., and Rapoport, S. I. (1985). Selective changes in local cerebral glucose utilization induced by phenobarbital in the rat. *Anesthesiology* 63, 633–639. doi: 10.1097/00000542-198512000-00013

Hoyer, S. (1996). Oxidative metabolism deficiencies in brains of patients with Alzheimer's disease. *Acta Neurol. Scand. Suppl.* 165, 18–24. doi: 10.1111/j.1600-0404.1996.tb05868.x

Hoyer, S. (2000). Brain glucose and energy metabolism abnormalities in sporadic Alzheimer disease. Causes and consequences: an update. *Exp. Gerontol.* 35, 1363–1372. doi: 10.1016/S0531-5565(00)00156-X

Hoyer, S., Oesterreich, K., and Wagner, O. (1988). Glucose metabolism as the site of the primary abnormality in early-onset dementia of Alzheimer type? *J. Neurol.* 235, 143–148. doi: 10.1007/BF00314304

Hsia, A. Y., Masliah, E., McConlogue, L., Yu, G. Q., Tatsuno, G., Hu, K., et al. (1999). Plaque-independent disruption of neural circuits in Alzheimer's disease mouse models. *Proc. Natl. Acad. Sci. U.S.A.* 96, 3228–3233. doi: 10.1073/pnas.96.6.3228

Jack, C. R., Lowe, V. J., Weigand, S. D., Wiste, H. J., Senjem, M. L., Knopman, D. S., et al. (2009). Serial PIB and MRI in normal, mild cognitive impairment and Alzheimer's disease: implications for sequence of pathological events in Alzheimer's disease. *Brain J. Neurol.* 132, 1355–1365. doi: 10.1093/brain/awp062

Joachim, C. L., Mori, H., and Selkoe, D. J. (1989). Amyloid beta-protein deposition in tissues other than brain in Alzheimer's disease. *Nature* 341, 226–230. doi: 10.1038/341226a0

Jobst, K. A., Smith, A. D., Barker, C. S., Wear, A., King, E. M., Smith, A., et al. (1992). Association of atrophy of the medial temporal lobe with reduced blood flow in the posterior parietotemporal cortex in patients with a clinical and pathological diagnosis of Alzheimer's disease. *J. Neurol. Neurosurg. Psychiatry* 55, 190–194. doi: 10.1136/jnnp.55.3.190

Johnson, R. M., Goyette, G., Ravindranath, Y., and Ho, Y.-S. (2005). Hemoglobin autoxidation and regulation of endogenous H_2O_2 levels in erythrocytes. *Free Radic. Biol. Med.* 39, 1407–1417. doi: 10.1016/j.freeradbiomed.2005.07.002

Jordan, B. D. (2000). Chronic traumatic brain injury associated with boxing. *Semin. Neurol.* 20, 179–185. doi: 10.1055/s-2000-9826

Kalaria, R. N., and Harik, S. I. (1989). Reduced glucose transporter at the blood-brain barrier and in cerebral cortex in Alzheimer disease. *J. Neurochem.* 53, 1083–1088. doi: 10.1111/j.1471-4159.1989.tb07399.x

Kalaria, R. N., and Hedera, P. (1995). Differential degeneration of the cerebral microvasculature in Alzheimer's disease. *Neuroreport* 6, 477–480. doi: 10.1097/00001756-199502000-00018

Kamal, A., Almenar-Queralt, A., LeBlanc, J. F., Roberts, E. A., and Goldstein, L. S. (2001). Kinesin-mediated axonal transport of a membrane compartment containing beta-secretase and presenilin-1 requires APP. *Nature* 414, 643–648. doi: 10.1038/414643a

Kamenetz, F., Tomita, T., Hsieh, H., Seabrook, G., Borchelt, D., Iwatsubo, T., et al. (2003). APP processing and synaptic function. *Neuron* 37, 925–937. doi: 10.1016/S0896-6273(03)00124-7

Kaminsky, Y., Poghosyan, A., Tikhonova, L., Palacios, H. H., Kamal, M. A., Kosenko, E., et al. (2012). Glycolytic and proteolytic metabolism in erythrocytes from elderly and demented patients. *Am. J. Neuroprotect. Neuroregeneration* 4, 1–5. doi: 10.1166/ajnn.2012.1039

Kaminsky, Y. G., and Kosenko, E. A. (2012). Argocytes containing enzyme nanoparticles reduce toxic concentrations of arginine in the blood. *Bull. Exp. Biol. Med.* 153, 406–408. doi: 10.1007/s10517-012-1727-3

Kaminsky, Y. G., Marlatt, M. W., Smith, M. A., and Kosenko, E. A. (2010). Subcellular and metabolic examination of amyloid-β peptides in Alzheimer disease pathogenesis: evidence for Aβ (25-35). *Exp. Neurol.* 221, 26–37. doi: 10.1016/j.expneurol.2009.09.005

Kaminsky, Y. G., Reddy, V. P., Ashraf, G. M., Ahmad, A., Benberin, V. V., Kosenko, E. A., et al. (2013). Age-related defects in erythrocyte 2,3-diphosphoglycerate metabolism in dementia. *Aging Dis.* 4, 244–255. doi: 10.14336/AD.2013.0400244

Kang, J.-E., Lim, M. M., Bateman, R. J., Lee, J. J., Smyth, L. P., Cirrito, J. R., et al. (2009). Amyloid-β dynamics are regulated by orexin and the sleep-wake cycle. *Science* 326, 1005–1007. doi: 10.1126/science.1180962

Kasa, P., Papp, H., and Pakaski, M. (2001). Presenilin-1 and its N-terminal and C-terminal fragments are transported in the sciatic nerve of rat. *Brain Res.* 909, 159–169. doi: 10.1016/S0006-8993(01)02679-8

Kiefmann, R., Rifkind, J. M., Nagababu, E., and Bhattacharya, J. (2008). Red blood cells induce hypoxic lung inflammation. *Blood* 111, 5205–5214. doi: 10.1182/blood-2007-09-113902

Kiko, T., Nakagawa, K., Satoh, A., Tsuduki, T., Furukawa, K., Arai, H., et al. (2012). Amyloid β levels in human red blood cells. *PLoS ONE* 7:e49620. doi: 10.1371/journal.pone.0049620

Klein, W. L., Krafft, G. A., and Finch, C. E. (2001). Targeting small Abeta oligomers: the solution to an Alzheimer's disease conundrum? *Trends Neurosci.* 24, 219–224. doi: 10.1016/S0166-2236(00)01749-5

Klepper, J., and Voit, T. (2002). Facilitated glucose transporter protein type 1 (GLUT1) deficiency syndrome: impaired glucose transport into brain– a review. *Eur. J. Pediatr.* 161, 295–304. doi: 10.1007/s00431-002-0939-3

Kontush, A., Berndt, C., Weber, W., Akopyan, V., Arlt, S., Schippling, S., et al. (2001). Amyloid-β is an antioxidant for lipoproteins in cerebrospinal fluid and plasma. *Free Radic. Biol. Med.* 30, 119–128. doi: 10.1016/S0891-5849(00)00458-5

Koo, E. H., Park, L., and Selkoe, D. J. (1993). Amyloid beta-protein as a substrate interacts with extracellular matrix to promote neurite outgrowth. *Proc. Natl. Acad. Sci. U.S.A.* 90, 4748–4752. doi: 10.1073/pnas.90.10.4748

Korol, D. L., and Gold, P. E. (1998). Glucose, memory, and aging. *Am. J. Clin. Nutr.* 67, 764S−771S.

Kosenko, E., Kaminsky, Y., Grau, E., Miñana,, M. D., Marcaida, G., Grisolía, S., et al. (1994). Brain ATP depletion induced by acute ammonia intoxication in rats is mediated by activation of the NMDA receptor and Na^{+},K^{+}-ATPase. *J. Neurochem.* 63, 2172–2178. doi: 10.1046/j.1471-4159.1994.63062172.x

Kosenko, E. A., Aliev, G., and Kaminsky, Y. G. (2016). Relationship between chronic disturbance of 2,3-diphosphoglycerate metabolism in erythrocytes and Alzheimer disease. *CNS Neurol. Disord. Drug Targets* 15, 113–123. doi: 10.2174/1871527314666150821103444

Kosenko, E. A., Aliev, G., Tikhonova, L. A., Li, Y., Poghosyan, A. C., and Kaminsky, Y. G. (2012). Antioxidant status and energy state of erythrocytes in Alzheimer dementia: probing for markers. *CNS Neurol. Disord. Drug Targets* 11, 926–932. doi: 10.2174/1871527311201070926

Kosenko, E. A., Solomadin, I. N., and Kaminskii, I. G. (2009). Effect of the beta-amyloid peptide Abeta25-35 and fullerene C60 on the activity of enzymes in erythrocytes. *Bioorg. Khim.* 35, 172–177.

Kosenko, E. A., Solomadin, I. N., Marov, N. V., Venediktova, N. I., Pogosian, A. S., and Kaminskĭ, I. G. (2008a). [Role of glycolysis and antioxidant enzymes in the toxicity of amyloid beta peptide Aβ25-35 to erythrocytes]. *Bioorg. Khim.* 34, 654–660.

Kosenko, E. A., Venediktova, N. I., Kudryavtsev, A. A., Ataullakhanov, F. I., Kaminsky, Y. G., Felipo, V., et al. (2008b). Encapsulation of glutamine synthetase in mouse erythrocytes: a new procedure for ammonia detoxification. *Biochem. Cell Biol. Biochim. Biol. Cell.* 86, 469–476. doi: 10.1139/O08-134

Kowluru, R., Bitensky, M. W., Kowluru, A., Dembo, M., Keaton, P. A., and Buican, T. (1989). Reversible sodium pump defect and swelling in the diabetic rat erythrocyte: effects on filterability and implications for microangiopathy. *Proc. Natl. Acad. Sci. U.S.A.* 86, 3327–3331. doi: 10.1073/pnas.86.9.3327

Kucukatay, V., Erken, G., Bor-Kucukatay, M., and Kocamaz, E. (2009). Effect of sulfite treatment on erythrocyte deformability in young and aged rats. *Toxicol. Mech. Methods* 19, 19–23. doi: 10.1080/15376510802175788

Kuo, Y. M., Emmerling, M. R., Vigo-Pelfrey, C., Kasunic, T. C., Kirkpatrick, J. B., Murdoch, G. H., et al. (1996). Water-soluble Aβ (N-40, N-42) oligomers in normal and Alzheimer disease brains. *J. Biol. Chem.* 271, 4077–4081. doi: 10.1074/jbc.271.8.4077

Kuo, Y. M., Kokjohn, T. A., Kalback, W., Luehrs, D., Galasko, D. R., Chevallier, N., et al. (2000). Amyloid-β peptides interact with plasma proteins and erythrocytes: implications for their quantitation in plasma. *Biochem. Biophys. Res. Commun.* 268, 750–756. doi: 10.1006/bbrc.2000.2222

Kuypers, F. A., Scott, M. D., Schott, M. A., Lubin, B., and Chiu, D. T. (1990). Use of ektacytometry to determine red cell susceptibility to oxidative stress. *J. Lab. Clin. Med.* 116, 535–545.

Kyles, A. E., Waterman, A. E., Livingston, A., and Vetmed, B. (1993). Antinociceptive effects of combining low doses of neuroleptic drugs and fentanyl in sheep. *Am. J. Vet. Res.* 54, 1483–1488.

Lambert, M. P., Barlow, A. K., Chromy, B. A., Edwards, C., Freed, R., Liosatos, M., et al. (1998). Diffusible, nonfibrillar ligands derived from Aβ1-42 are potent central nervous system neurotoxins. *Proc. Natl. Acad. Sci. U.S.A.* 95, 6448–6453. doi: 10.1073/pnas.95.11.6448

Lan, J., Liu, J., Zhao, Z., Xue, R., Zhang, N., Zhang, P., et al. (2015). The peripheral blood of Aβ binding RBC as a biomarker for diagnosis of Alzheimer's disease. *Age Ageing* 44, 458–464. doi: 10.1093/ageing/afv009

Lang, E., Pozdeev, V. I., Xu, H. C., Shinde, P. V., Behnke, K., Hamdam, J. M., et al. (2016). Storage of erythrocytes induces suicidal erythrocyte death. *Cell. Physiol. Biochem.* 39, 668–676. doi: 10.1159/000445657

Lang, F., Jilani, K., and Lang, E. (2015). Therapeutic potential of manipulating suicidal erythrocyte death. *Expert Opin. Ther. Targets* 19, 1219–1227. doi: 10.1517/14728222.2015.1051306

Larsen, V. H., Waldau, T., Gravesen, H., and Siggaard-Andersen, O. (1996). Erythrocyte 2,3-diphosphoglycerate depletion associated with hypophosphatemia detected by routine arterial blood gas analysis. *Scand. J. Clin. Lab. Investig. Suppl.* 224, 83–87. doi: 10.3109/00365519609088626

Lee, H.-G., Casadesus, G., Zhu, X., Takeda, A., Perry, G., and Smith, M. A. (2004). Challenging the amyloid cascade hypothesis: senile plaques and amyloid-beta as protective adaptations to Alzheimer disease. *Ann. N.Y. Acad. Sci.* 1019, 1–4. doi: 10.1196/annals.1297.001

Li, G. L., Farooque, M., Holtz, A., and Olsson, Y. (1995). Changes of β-amyloid precursor protein after compression trauma to the spinal cord: an experimental study in the rat using immunohistochemistry. *J. Neurotrauma* 12, 269–277. doi: 10.1089/neu.1995.12.269

Liberski, P. P. (2004). Amyloid plaques in transmissible spongiform encephalopathies (prion diseases). *Folia Neuropathol.* 42(Suppl. B), 109–119.

Llansola, M., Rodrigo, R., Monfort, P., Montoliu, C., Kosenko, E., Cauli, O., et al. (2007). NMDA receptors in hyperammonemia and hepatic encephalopathy. *Metab. Brain Dis.* 22, 321–335. doi: 10.1007/s11011-007-9067-0

Lue, L. F., Kuo, Y. M., Roher, A. E., Brachova, L., Shen, Y., Sue, L., et al. (1999). Soluble amyloid β peptide concentration as a predictor of synaptic change in Alzheimer's disease. *Am. J. Pathol.* 155, 853–862. doi: 10.1016/S0002-9440(10)65184-X

Luo, Y., Sunderland, T., Roth, G. S., and Wolozin, B. (1996). Physiological levels of β-amyloid peptide promote PC12 cell proliferation. *Neurosci. Lett.* 217, 125–128. doi: 10.1016/0304-3940(96)13087-1

MacDonald, R. (1977). Red cell 2,3-diphosphoglycerate and oxygen affinity. *Anaesthesia* 32, 544–553. doi: 10.1111/j.1365-2044.1977.tb10002.x

Manikandan, S., Padma, M. K., Srikumar, R., Jeya Parthasarathy, N., Muthuvel, A., and Sheela Devi, R. (2006). Effects of chronic noise stress on spatial memory of rats in relation to neuronal dendritic alteration and free radical-imbalance in hippocampus and medial prefrontal cortex. *Neurosci. Lett.* 399, 17–22. doi: 10.1016/j.neulet.2006.01.037

Mann, D. M., Jones, D., South, P. W., Snowden, J. S., and Neary, D. (1992). Deposition of amyloid beta protein in non-Alzheimer dementias: evidence for a neuronal origin of parenchymal deposits of β protein in neurodegenerative disease. *Acta Neuropathol.* 83, 415–419. doi: 10.1007/BF00713534

Marcus, D. L., and Freedman, M. L. (1997). Decreased brain glucose metabolism in microvessels from patients with Alzheimer's disease. *Ann. N. Y. Acad. Sci.* 826, 248–253. doi: 10.1111/j.1749-6632.1997.tb48476.x

Marcus, D. L., de Leon, M. J., Goldman, J., Logan, J., Christman, D. R., Wolf, A. P., et al. (1989). Altered glucose metabolism in microvessels from patients with Alzheimer's disease. *Ann. Neurol.* 26, 91–94. doi: 10.1002/ana.410260114

Martindale, J. L., Senecal, E. L., Obermeyer, Z., Nadel, E. S., and Brown, D. F. M. (2010). Altered mental status and hypothermia. *J. Emerg. Med.* 39, 491–496. doi: 10.1016/j.jemermed.2010.03.021

Martin-Jiménez, C. A., Gáitan-Vaca, D. M., Echeverria, V., González, J., and Barreto, G. E. (2017a). Relationship between obesity, alzheimer's disease, and Parkinson's disease: an astrocentric view. *Mol. Neurobiol.* 54, 7096–7115. doi: 10.1007/s12035-016-0193-8

Martin-Jiménez, C. A., García-Vega, Á., Cabezas, R., Aliev, G., Echeverria, V., González, J., et al. (2017b). Astrocytes and endoplasmic reticulum stress: a bridge between obesity and neurodegenerative diseases. *Prog. Neurobiol.* 158, 45–68. doi: 10.1016/j.pneurobio.2017.08.001

Masuda, J., Tanaka, K., Ueda, K., and Omae, T. (1988). Autopsy study of incidence and distribution of cerebral amyloid angiopathy in Hisayama, Japan. *Stroke* 19, 205–210. doi: 10.1161/01.STR.19.2.205

Matsumoto, Y. (1995). [The function of red blood cells during experimental hemorrhagic and endotoxic shock]. *Masui* 44, 342–348.

Mattson, M. P., Begley, J. G., Mark, R. J., and Furukawa, K. (1997). Aβ25-35 induces rapid lysis of red blood cells: contrast with Abeta1-42 and examination of underlying mechanisms. *Brain Res.* 771, 147–153. doi: 10.1016/S0006-8993(97)00824-X

Mattson, M. P., Cheng, B., Davis, D., Bryant, K., Lieberburg, I., and Rydel, R. E. (1992). beta-Amyloid peptides destabilize calcium homeostasis and render human cortical neurons vulnerable to excitotoxicity. *J. Neurosci. Off. J. Soc. Neurosci.* 12, 376–389.

McCully, K., Chance, B., and Giger, U. (1999). *In vivo* determination of altered hemoglobin saturation in dogs with M-type phosphofructokinase deficiency. *Muscle Nerve* 22, 621–627. doi: 10.1002/(SICI)1097-4598(199905)22:5<621::AID-MUS11>3.0.CO;2-D

McGeer, E. G., McGeer, P. L., Harrop, R., Akiyama, H., and Kamo, H. (1990). Correlations of regional postmortem enzyme activities with premortem local glucose metabolic rates in Alzheimer's disease. *J. Neurosci. Res.* 27, 612–619. doi: 10.1002/jnr.490270422

McLean, C. A., Cherny, R. A., Fraser, F. W., Fuller, S. J., Smith, M. J., Vbeyreuther, K., et al. (1999). Soluble pool of Aβ amyloid as a determinant of severity of neurodegeneration in Alzheimer's disease. *Ann. Neurol.* 46, 860–866. doi: 10.1002/1531-8249(199912)46:6<860::AID-ANA8>3.0.CO;2-M

Meier-Ruge, W., and Bertoni-Freddari, C. (1996). The significance of glucose turnover in the brain in the pathogenetic mechanisms of Alzheimer's disease. *Rev. Neurosci.* 7, 1–19. doi: 10.1515/REVNEURO.1996.7.1.1

Meier-Ruge, W., Iwangoff, P., and Reichlmeier, K. (1984). Neurochemical enzyme changes in Alzheimer's and Pick's disease. *Arch. Gerontol. Geriatr.* 3, 161–165. doi: 10.1016/0167-4943(84)90007-4

Michaud, J.-P., Bellavance, M.-A., Préfontaine, P., and Rivest, S. (2013). Real-time *in vivo* imaging reveals the ability of monocytes to clear vascular amyloid β. *Cell Rep.* 5, 646–653. doi: 10.1016/j.celrep.2013.10.010

Miklossy, J., Kis, A., Radenovic, A., Miller, L., Forro, L., Martins, R., et al. (2006). Beta-amyloid deposition and Alzheimer's type changes induced by Borrelia spirochetes. *Neurobiol. Aging* 27, 228–236. doi: 10.1016/j.neurobiolaging.2005.01.018

Mohanty, J. G., Eckley, D. M., Williamson, J. D., Launer, L. J., and Rifkind, J. M. (2008). Do red blood cell-beta-amyloid interactions alter oxygen delivery in Alzheimer's disease? *Adv. Exp. Med. Biol.* 614, 29–35. doi: 10.1007/978-0-387-74911-2_4

Moore, G. L., Ledford, M. E., and Brummell, M. R. (1981). Improved red blood cell storage using optional additive systems (OAS) containing adenine, glucose and ascorbate-2-phosphate. *Transfusion* 21, 723–731. doi: 10.1046/j.1537-2995.1981.21682085764.x

Moreira, P. I., Zhu, X., Liu, Q., Honda, K., Siedlak, S. L., Harris, P. L., et al. (2006). Compensatory responses induced by oxidative stress in Alzheimer disease. *Biol. Res.* 39, 7–13. doi: 10.4067/S0716-97602006000100002

Morishima-Kawashima, M., Oshima, N., Ogata, H., Yamaguchi, H., Yoshimura, M., Sugihara, S., et al. (2000). Effect of apolipoprotein E allele epsilon4 on the initial phase of amyloid β-protein accumulation in the human brain. *Am. J. Pathol.* 157, 2093–2099. doi: 10.1016/S0002-9440(10)64847-X

Morris, C. R., Suh, J. H., Hagar, W., Larkin, S., Bland, D. A., Steinberg, M. H., et al. (2008). Erythrocyte glutamine depletion, altered redox environment, and pulmonary hypertension in sickle cell disease. *Blood* 111, 402–410. doi: 10.1182/blood-2007-04-081703

Murr, L. E., Soto, K. F., Garza, K. M., Guerrero, P. A., Martinez, F., Esquivel, E. V., et al. (2006). Combustion-generated nanoparticulates in the El Paso, TX, USA/Juarez, Mexico Metroplex: their comparative characterization and potential for adverse health effects. *Int. J. Environ. Res. Public. Health* 3, 48–66. doi: 10.3390/ijerph2006030007

Nakamura, J., Koh, N., Sakakibara, F., Hamada, Y., Wakao, T., Hara, T., et al. (1995). Polyol pathway, 2,3-diphosphoglycerate in erythrocytes and diabetic neuropathy in rats. *Eur. J. Pharmacol.* 294, 207–214. doi: 10.1016/0014-2999(95)00531-5

Ni, Y., Zhao, X., Bao, G., Zou, L., Teng, L., Wang, Z., et al. (2006). Activation of β2-adrenergic receptor stimulates gamma-secretase activity and accelerates amyloid plaque formation. *Nat. Med.* 12, 1390–1396. doi: 10.1038/nm1485

Nicolay, J. P., Gatz, S., Liebig, G., Gulbins, E., and Lang, F. (2007). Amyloid induced suicidal erythrocyte death. *Cell. Physiol. Biochem.* 19, 175–184. doi: 10.1159/000099205

Novelli, A., Reilly, J. A., Lysko, P. G., and Henneberry, R. C. (1988). Glutamate becomes neurotoxic via the N-methyl-D-aspartate receptor when intracellular energy levels are reduced. *Brain Res.* 451, 205–212. doi: 10.1016/0006-8993(88)90765-2

Nunomura, A., Perry, G., Pappolla, M. A., Friedland, R. P., Hirai, K., Chiba, S., et al. (2000). Neuronal oxidative stress precedes amyloid-β deposition in down syndrome. *J. Neuropathol. Exp. Neurol.* 59, 1011–1017. doi: 10.1093/jnen/59.11.1011

Omalu, B. I., DeKosky, S. T., Minster, R. L., Kamboh, M. I., Hamilton, R. L., and Wecht, C. H. (2005). Chronic traumatic encephalopathy in a National Football League player. *Neurosurgery* 57, 128–134. discussion: 128–134. doi: 10.1227/01.NEU.0000163407.92769.ED

Pankowska, E., Szypowska, A., Wysocka, M., and Lipka, M. (2005). [The role of 2,3-DPG in nerve conduction of children with type 1 diabetes]. *Endokrynol. Diabetol. Chor. Przemiany Materii Wieku Rozw.* 11, 207–210.

Papassotiriou, I., Kister, J., Griffon, N., Abraham, D. J., Kanavakis, E., Traeger-Synodinos, J., et al. (1998). Synthesized allosteric effectors of the hemoglobin molecule: a possible mechanism for improved erythrocyte oxygen release capability in hemoglobinopathy H disease. *Exp. Hematol.* 26, 922–926.

Papp, H., Pakaski, M., and Kasa, P. (2002). Presenilin-1 and the amyloid precursor protein are transported bidirectionally in the sciatic nerve of adult rat. *Neurochem. Int.* 41, 429–435. doi: 10.1016/S0197-0186(02)00014-1

Parikh, S. S., and Chung, F. (1995). Postoperative delirium in the elderly. *Anesth. Analg.* 80, 1223–1232.

Pascual, J. M., Wang, D., Lecumberri, B., Yang, H., Mao, X., Yang, R., et al. (2004). GLUT1 deficiency and other glucose transporter diseases. *Eur. J. Endocrinol.* 150, 627–633. doi: 10.1530/eje.0.1500627

Perry, G., Nunomura, A., Raina, A. K., Aliev, G., Siedlak, S. L., Harris, P. L. R., et al. (2003). A metabolic basis for Alzheimer disease. *Neurochem. Res.* 28, 1549–1552. doi: 10.1023/A:1025678510480

Perry, G., Smith, M. A., McCann, C. E., Siedlak, S. L., Jones, P. K., and Friedland, R. P. (1998). Cerebrovascular muscle atrophy is a feature of Alzheimer's disease. *Brain Res.* 791, 63–66. doi: 10.1016/S0006-8993(98)00006-7

Perry, R. T., Gearhart, D. A., Wiener, H. W., Harrell, L. E., Barton, J. C., Kutlar, A., et al. (2008). Hemoglobin binding to A β and HBG2 SNP association suggest a role in Alzheimer's disease. *Neurobiol. Aging* 29, 185–193. doi: 10.1016/j.neurobiolaging.2006.10.017

Pfeifer, L. A., White, L. R., Ross, G. W., Petrovitch, H., and Launer, L. J. (2002). Cerebral amyloid angiopathy and cognitive function: the HAAS autopsy study. *Neurology* 58, 1629–1634. doi: 10.1212/WNL.58.11.1629

Pike, K. E., Savage, G., Villemagne, V. L., Ng, S., Moss, S. A., Maruff, P., et al. (2007). β-amyloid imaging and memory in non-demented individuals: evidence for preclinical Alzheimer's disease. *Brain J. Neurol.* 130, 2837–2844. doi: 10.1093/brain/awm238

Plum, F., and Posner, J. B. (1972). The diagnosis of stupor and coma. *Contemp. Neurol. Ser.* 10, 1–286.

Ponizovsky, A. M., Barshtein, G., and Bergelson, L. D. (2003). Biochemical alterations of erythrocytes as an indicator of mental disorders: an overview. *Harv. Rev. Psychiatry* 11, 317–332. doi: 10.1080/10673220390264258

Pretorius, E., Olumuyiwa-Akeredolu, O.-O. O., Mbotwe, S., and Bester, J. (2016). Erythrocytes and their role as health indicator: using structure in a patient-orientated precision medicine approach. *Blood Rev.* 30, 263–274. doi: 10.1016/j.blre.2016.01.001

Quastel, J. H. (1932). Biochemistry and mental disorder. *Lancet* 220, 1417–1419. doi: 10.1016/S0140-6736(00)97278-7

Rabini, R. A., Petruzzi, E., Staffolani, R., Tesei, M., Fumelli, P., Pazzagli, M., et al. (1997). Diabetes mellitus and subjects' ageing: a study on the ATP content and ATP-related enzyme activities in human erythrocytes. *Eur. J. Clin. Invest.* 27, 327–332. doi: 10.1046/j.1365-2362.1997.1130652.x

Ravi, L. B., Mohanty, J. G., Chrest, F. J., Jayakumar, R., Nagababu, E., Usatyuk, P. V., et al. (2004). Influence of beta-amyloid fibrils on the interactions between red blood cells and endothelial cells. *Neurol. Res.* 26, 579–585. doi: 10.1179/016164104225016227

Reddy, P. H. (2006). Amyloid precursor protein-mediated free radicals and oxidative damage: implications for the development and progression of Alzheimer's disease. *J. Neurochem.* 96, 1–13. doi: 10.1111/j.1471-4159.2005.03530.x

Resnick, L. M., Gupta, R. K., Barbagallo, M., and Laragh, J. H. (1994). Is the higher incidence of ischemic disease in patients with hypertension and diabetes related to intracellular depletion of high energy metabolites? *Am. J. Med. Sci.* 307(Suppl. 1), S66–S69.

Richards, R. S., Wang, L., and Jelinek, H. (2007). Erythrocyte oxidative damage in chronic fatigue syndrome. *Arch. Med. Res.* 38, 94–98. doi: 10.1016/j.arcmed.2006.06.008

Richardson, J. T. (1990). Cognitive function in diabetes mellitus. *Neurosci. Biobehav. Rev.* 14, 385–388. doi: 10.1016/S0149-7634(05)80060-0

Riegel, B., Bennett, J. A., Davis, A., Carlson, B., Montague, J., Robin, H., et al. (2002). Cognitive impairment in heart failure: issues of measurement and etiology. *Am. J. Crit. Care Off. Publ. Am. Assoc. Crit. Care Nurses* 11, 520–528.

Rifkind, J. M., Abugo, O. O., Peddada, R. R., Patel, N., Speer, D., Balagopalakrishna, C., et al. (1999). Maze learning impairment is associated with stress hemopoiesis induced by chronic treatment of aged rats with human recombinant erythropoietin. *Life Sci.* 64, 237–247. doi: 10.1016/S0024-3205(98)00559-1

Roberts, G. W., Allsop, D., and Bruton, C. (1990). The occult aftermath of boxing. *J. Neurol. Neurosurg. Psychiatry* 53, 373–378. doi: 10.1136/jnnp.53.5.373

Rönnbäck, L., and Hansson, E. (2004). On the potential role of glutamate transport in mental fatigue. *J. Neuroinflammation* 1:22. doi: 10.1186/1742-2094-1-22

Ronquist, G., and Waldenström, A. (2003). Imbalance of plasma membrane ion leak and pump relationship as a new aetiological basis of certain disease states. *J. Intern. Med.* 254, 517–526. doi: 10.1111/j.1365-2796.2003.01235.x

Roselli, F., Tirard, M., Lu, J., Hutzler, P., Lamberti, P., Livrea, P., et al. (2005). Soluble β-amyloid1-40 induces NMDA-dependent degradation of postsynaptic density-95 at glutamatergic synapses. *J. Neurosci. Off. J. Soc. Neurosci.* 25, 11061–11070. doi: 10.1523/JNEUROSCI.3034-05.2005

Rothstein, G. (1993). Hematopoiesis in the aged: a model of hematopoietic dysregulation? *Blood* 82, 2601–2604.

Sakuta, S. (1981). Blood filtrability in cerebrovascular disorders, with special reference to erythrocyte deformability and ATP content. *Stroke* 12, 824–828. doi: 10.1161/01.STR.12.6.824

Samaja, M., Crespi, T., Guazzi, M., and Vandegriff, K. D. (2003). Oxygen transport in blood at high altitude: role of the hemoglobin-oxygen affinity and impact of the phenomena related to hemoglobin allosterism and red cell function. *Eur. J. Appl. Physiol.* 90, 351–359. doi: 10.1007/s00421-003-0954-8

Sansoni, P., Cossarizza, A., Brianti, V., Fagnoni, F., Snelli, G., Monti, D., et al. (1993). Lymphocyte subsets and natural killer cell activity in healthy old people and centenarians. *Blood* 82, 2767–2773.

Schmitt, F. A., Davis, D. G., Wekstein, D. R., Smith, C. D., Ashford, J. W., and Markesbery, W. R. (2000). "Preclinical" AD revisited: neuropathology of cognitively normal older adults. *Neurology* 55, 370–376. doi: 10.1212/WNL.55.3.370

Schneider, J. A., Arvanitakis, Z., Bang, W., and Bennett, D. A. (2007). Mixed brain pathologies account for most dementia cases in community-dwelling older persons. *Neurology* 69, 2197–2204. doi: 10.1212/01.wnl.0000271090.28148.24

Scholz, W. (1938). Studien zur Pathologie der Hirngefasse II. Die drusige Entartung der Hirnarterien und capillarien. *Z Ges Neurol. Psychiat.* 162, 694–715. doi: 10.1007/BF02890989

Seeman, P., Cheng, D., and Iles, G. H. (1973). Structure of membrane holes in osmotic and saponin hemolysis. *J. Cell Biol.* 56, 519–527. doi: 10.1083/jcb.56.2.519

Selkoe, D. J. (2007). Developing preventive therapies for chronic diseases: lessons learned from Alzheimer's disease. *Nutr. Rev.* 65, S239–S243. doi: 10.1301/nr.2007.dec.S239-S243

Selkoe, D. J. (2008). Soluble oligomers of the amyloid β-protein impair synaptic plasticity and behavior. *Behav. Brain Res.* 192, 106–113. doi: 10.1016/j.bbr.2008.02.016

Shevtsova, E. F., Vinogradova, D. V., Neganova, M. E., Avila-Rodriguez, M., Ashraf, G. M., Barreto, G. E., et al. (2017). Mitochondrial permeability transition pore as a suitable target for neuroprotective agents against Alzheimer's Disease. *CNS Neurol. Disord. Drug Targets* 16, 677–685. doi: 10.2174/1871527316666170424114444

Shi, J., Xiang, Y., and Simpkins, J. W. (1997). Hypoglycemia enhances the expression of mRNA encoding β-amyloid precursor protein in rat primary cortical astroglial cells. *Brain Res.* 772, 247–251. doi: 10.1016/S0006-8993(97)00827-5

Shinozuka, T., Miyamoto, T., Hirazono, K., Ebisawa, K., Murakami, M., Kuroshima, Y., et al. (1994). Follow-up laparoscopy in patients with ovarian cancer. *Tokai J. Exp. Clin. Med.* 19, 53–59.

Simpson, I. A., Chundu, K. R., Davies-Hill, T., Honer, W. G., and Davies, P. (1994). Decreased concentrations of GLUT1 and GLUT3 glucose transporters in the brains of patients with Alzheimer's disease. *Ann. Neurol.* 35, 546–551. doi: 10.1002/ana.410350507

Simpson, I. A., and Davies, P. (1994). Reduced glucose transporter concentrations in brains of patients with Alzheimer's disease. *Ann. Neurol.* 36, 800–801. doi: 10.1002/ana.410360522

Simpson, P. J., Mickelson, J., Fantone, J. C., Gallagher, K. P., and Lucchesi, B. R. (1988). Reduction of experimental canine myocardial infarct size with prostaglandin E1: inhibition of neutrophil migration and activation. *J. Pharmacol. Exp. Ther.* 244, 619–624.

Singh, V. K., Cheng, J. F., and Leu, S. J. (1994). Effect of substance P and protein kinase inhibitors on beta-amyloid peptide-induced proliferation of cultured brain cells. *Brain Res.* 660, 353–356. doi: 10.1016/0006-8993(94)91313-7

Smith, C. D., Carney, J. M., Starke-Reed, P. E., Oliver, C. N., Stadtman, E. R., Floyd, R. A., et al. (1991). Excess brain protein oxidation and enzyme dysfunction in normal aging and in Alzheimer disease. *Proc. Natl. Acad. Sci. U.S.A.* 88, 10540–10543. doi: 10.1073/pnas.88.23.10540

Smith, D. H., Chen, X.-H., Iwata, A., and Graham, D. I. (2003). Amyloid β accumulation in axons after traumatic brain injury in humans. *J. Neurosurg.* 98, 1072–1077. doi: 10.3171/jns.2003.98.5.1072

Smith, E. E., and Greenberg, S. M. (2009). β-amyloid, blood vessels, and brain function. *Stroke* 40, 2601–2606. doi: 10.1161/STROKEAHA.108.536839

Smith, M. A., Casadesus, G., Joseph, J. A., and Perry, G. (2002a). Amyloid-β and tau serve antioxidant functions in the aging and Alzheimer brain. *Free Radic. Biol. Med.* 33, 1194–1199. doi: 10.1016/S0891-5849(02)01021-3

Smith, M. A., Drew, K. L., Nunomura, A., Takeda, A., Hirai, K., Zhu, X., et al. (2002b). Amyloid-β, tau alterations and mitochondrial dysfunction in Alzheimer disease: the chickens or the eggs? *Neurochem. Int.* 40, 527–531. doi: 10.1016/S0197-0186(01)00123-1

Smith, M. A., Hirai, K., Hsiao, K., Pappolla, M. A., Harris, P. L., Siedlak, S. L., et al. (1998). Amyloid-β deposition in Alzheimer transgenic mice is associated with oxidative stress. *J. Neurochem.* 70, 2212–2215. doi: 10.1046/j.1471-4159.1998.70052212.x

Smith, M. A., Joseph, J. A., and Perry, G. (2000). Arson. Tracking the culprit in Alzheimer's disease. *Ann. N. Y. Acad. Sci.* 924, 35–38. doi: 10.1111/j.1749-6632.2000.tb05557.x

Solerte, S. B., Ceresini, G., Ferrari, E., and Fioravanti, M. (2000). Hemorheological changes and overproduction of cytokines from immune cells in mild to moderate dementia of the Alzheimer's type: adverse effects on cerebromicrovascular system. *Neurobiol. Aging* 21, 271–281. doi: 10.1016/S0197-4580(00)00105-6

Storey, E., Hyman, B. T., Jenkins, B., Brouillet, E., Miller, J. M., Rosen, B. R., et al. (1992). 1-Methyl-4-phenylpyridinium produces excitotoxic lesions in rat striatum as a result of impairment of oxidative metabolism. *J. Neurochem.* 58, 1975–1978. doi: 10.1111/j.1471-4159.1992.tb10080.x

Tabaton, M., and Gambetti, P. (2006). Soluble amyloid-β in the brain: the scarlet pimpernel. *J. Alzheimers Dis.* 9, 127–132. doi: 10.3233/JAD-2006-9S315

Tabaton, M., and Piccini, A. (2005). Role of water-soluble amyloid-β in the pathogenesis of Alzheimer's disease. *Int. J. Exp. Pathol.* 86, 139–145. doi: 10.1111/j.0959-9673.2005.00428.x

Teller, J. K., Russo, C., DeBusk, L. M., Angelini, G., Zaccheo, D., Dagna-Bricarelli, F., et al. (1996). Presence of soluble amyloid beta-peptide precedes amyloid plaque formation in Down's syndrome. *Nat. Med.* 2, 93–95. doi: 10.1038/nm0196-93

Terry, R. D., Masliah, E., Salmon, D. P., Butters, N., DeTeresa, R., Hill, R., et al. (1991). Physical basis of cognitive alterations in Alzheimer's disease: synapse loss is the major correlate of cognitive impairment. *Ann. Neurol.* 30, 572–580. doi: 10.1002/ana.410300410

Tesco, G., Koh, Y. H., Kang, E. L., Cameron, A. N., Das, S., Sena-Esteves, M., et al. (2007). Depletion of GGA3 stabilizes BACE and enhances beta-secretase activity. *Neuron* 54, 721–737. doi: 10.1016/j.neuron.2007.05.012

Thal, D. R., Capetillo-Zarate, E., Larionov, S., Staufenbiel, M., Zurbruegg, S., and Beckmann, N. (2009). Capillary cerebral amyloid angiopathy is associated with vessel occlusion and cerebral blood flow disturbances. *Neurobiol. Aging* 30, 1936–1948. doi: 10.1016/j.neurobiolaging.2008.01.017

Thal, D. R., Ghebremedhin, E., Rüb, U., Yamaguchi, H., Del Tredici, K., and Braak, H. (2002). Two types of sporadic cerebral amyloid angiopathy. *J. Neuropathol. Exp. Neurol.* 61, 282–293. doi: 10.1093/jnen/61.3.282

Thal, D. R., Griffin, W. S. T., and Braak, H. (2008). Parenchymal and vascular Aβ-deposition and its effects on the degeneration of neurons and cognition in Alzheimer's disease. *J. Cell. Mol. Med.* 12, 1848–1862. doi: 10.1111/j.1582-4934.2008.00411.x

Thanvi, B., and Robinson, T. (2006). Sporadic cerebral amyloid angiopathy–an important cause of cerebral haemorrhage in older people. *Age Ageing* 35, 565–571. doi: 10.1093/ageing/afl108

Tikhonova, L. A., Kaminsky, Y. G., Reddy, V. P., Li, Y., Solomadin, I. N., Kosenko, E. A., et al. (2014). Impact of amyloid β25-35 on membrane stability, energy metabolism, and antioxidant enzymes in erythrocytes. *Am. J. Alzheimers Dis. Other Demen.* 29, 685–695. doi: 10.1177/1533317514534757

Toro-Urrego, N., Garcia-Segura, L. M., Echeverria, V., and Barreto, G. E. (2016). Testosterone protects mitochondrial function and regulates neuroglobin expression in astrocytic cells exposed to glucose deprivation. *Front. Aging Neurosci.* 8:152. doi: 10.3389/fnagi.2016.00152

Tsirka, A., Challa, A., and Lapatsanis, P. D. (1990). Red cell phosphate metabolism in preterm infants with idiopathic respiratory distress syndrome. *Acta Paediatr. Scand.* 79, 763–768. doi: 10.1111/j.1651-2227.1990.tb11552.x

Urbach, H. (2011). Comment on: Brain Microbleeds and Alzheimer's disease: innocent observation or key player?: Cordonnier C, van der Flier WM. Brain. 2011;134:335-44. *Clin. Neuroradiol.* 21, 43–44. doi: 10.1007/s00062-011-0063-8

Uryu, K., Chen, X.-H., Martinez, D., Browne, K. D., Johnson, V. E., Graham, D. I., et al. (2007). Multiple proteins implicated in neurodegenerative diseases accumulate in axons after brain trauma in humans. *Exp. Neurol.* 208, 185–192. doi: 10.1016/j.expneurol.2007.06.018

Valeri, C. R., and Hirsch, N. M. (1969). Restoration *in vivo* of erythrocyte adenosine triphosphate, 2,3-diphosphoglycerate, potassium ion, and sodium ion concentrations following the transfusion of acid-citrate-dextrose-stored human red blood cells. *J. Lab. Clin. Med.* 73, 722–733.

van der Zwaluw, C. S., Valentijn, S. A. M., Nieuwenhuis-Mark, R., Rasquin, S. M. C., and van Heugten, C. M. (2011). Cognitive functioning in the acute phase poststroke: a predictor of discharge destination? *J. Stroke Cerebrovasc. Dis.* 20, 549–555. doi: 10.1016/j.jstrokecerebrovasdis.2010.03.009

van Groen, T., Puurunen, K., Mäki, H.-M., Sivenius, J., and Jolkkonen, J. (2005). Transformation of diffuse beta-amyloid precursor protein and beta-amyloid deposits to plaques in the thalamus after transient occlusion of the middle cerebral artery in rats. *Stroke* 36, 1551–1556. doi: 10.1161/01.STR.0000169933.88903.cf

Vanhanen, M., Koivisto, K., Karjalainen, L., Helkala, E. L., Laakso, M., Soininen, H., et al. (1997). Risk for non-insulin-dependent diabetes in the normoglycaemic elderly is associated with impaired cognitive function. *Neuroreport* 8, 1527–1530. doi: 10.1097/00001756-199704140-00041

van Wijk, R., and van Solinge, W. W. (2005). The energy-less red blood cell is lost: erythrocyte enzyme abnormalities of glycolysis. *Blood* 106, 4034–4042. doi: 10.1182/blood-2005-04-1622

Velliquette, R. A., O'Connor, T., and Vassar, R. (2005). Energy inhibition elevates β-secretase levels and activity and is potentially amyloidogenic in APP transgenic mice: possible early events in Alzheimer's disease pathogenesis. *J. Neurosci.* 25, 10874–10883. doi: 10.1523/JNEUROSCI.2350-05.2005

Villain, N., Desgranges, B., Viader, F., de la Sayette, V., Mézenge, F., Landeau, B., et al. (2008). Relationships between hippocampal atrophy, white matter disruption, and gray matter hypometabolism in Alzheimer's disease. *J. Neurosci.* 28, 6174–6181. doi: 10.1523/JNEUROSCI.1392-08.2008

Vonsattel, J. P., Myers, R. H., Hedley-Whyte, E. T., Ropper, A. H., Bird, E. D., and Richardson, E. P. (1991). Cerebral amyloid angiopathy without and with cerebral hemorrhages: a comparative histological study. *Ann. Neurol.* 30, 637–649. doi: 10.1002/ana.410300503

Vora, S. (1987). Metabolic manipulation of key glycolytic enzymes: a novel proposal for the maintenance of red cell 2,3-DPG and ATP levels during storage. *Biomed. Biochim. Acta* 46, S285–S289.

Walsh, D. M., Klyubin, I., Fadeeva, J. V., Cullen, W. K., Anwyl, R., Wolfe, M. S., et al. (2002). Naturally secreted oligomers of amyloid β protein potently inhibit hippocampal long-term potentiation *in vivo*. *Nature* 416, 535–539. doi: 10.1038/416535a

Walsh, D. M., and Selkoe, D. J. (2004). Deciphering the molecular basis of memory failure in Alzheimer's disease. *Neuron* 44, 181–193. doi: 10.1016/j.neuron.2004.09.010

Wang, J., Dickson, D. W., Trojanowski, J. Q., and Lee, V. M. (1999). The levels of soluble versus insoluble brain Aβ distinguish Alzheimer's disease from normal and pathologic aging. *Exp. Neurol.* 158, 328–337. doi: 10.1006/exnr.1999.7085

Webster, M. T., Pearce, B. R., Bowen, D. M., and Francis, P. T. (1998). The effects of perturbed energy metabolism on the processing of amyloid precursor protein in PC12 cells. *J. Neural Transm.* 105, 839–853. doi: 10.1007/s007020050098

Weller, R. O., Boche, D., and Nicoll, J. A. R. (2009). Microvasculature changes and cerebral amyloid angiopathy in Alzheimer's disease and their potential impact on therapy. *Acta Neuropathol.* 118, 87–102. doi: 10.1007/s00401-009-0498-z

Whitson, J. S., Selkoe, D. J., and Cotman, C. W. (1989). Amyloid β protein enhances the survival of hippocampal neurons *in vitro*. *Science* 243, 1488–1490. doi: 10.1126/science.2928783

Williams, L. H., Udupa, K. B., and Lipshitz, D. A. (1986). Evaluation of the effect of age on hematopoiesis in the C57BL/6 mouse. *Exp. Hematol.* 14, 827–832.

Wimo, A., and Prince, M. (2010). *World Alzheimer Report 2010: The Global Economic Impact of Dementia*. Alzheimer's Disease International, London.

Wirths, O., Multhaup, G., and Bayer, T. A. (2004). A modified β-amyloid hypothesis: intraneuronal accumulation of the β-amyloid peptide–the first step of a fatal cascade. *J. Neurochem.* 91, 513–520. doi: 10.1111/j.1471-4159.2004.02737.x

Wisniewski, H. M., and Wegiel, J. (1994). Beta-amyloid formation by myocytes of leptomeningeal vessels. *Acta Neuropathol.* 87, 233–241. doi: 10.1007/BF00296738

Wu, C.-W., Liao, P.-C., Yu, L., Wang, S.-T., Chen, S.-T., Wu, C.-M., et al. (2004). Hemoglobin promotes Aβ oligomer formation and localizes in neurons and amyloid deposits. *Neurobiol. Dis.* 17, 367–377. doi: 10.1016/j.nbd.2004.08.014

Xi, G., Keep, R. F., and Hoff, J. T. (1998). Erythrocytes and delayed brain edema formation following intracerebral hemorrhage in rats. *J. Neurosurg.* 89, 991–996. doi: 10.3171/jns.1998.89.6.0991

Xi, G., Keep, R. F., and Hoff, J. T. (2006). Mechanisms of brain injury after intracerebral haemorrhage. *Lancet Neurol.* 5, 53–63. doi: 10.1016/S1474-4422(05)70283-0

Xie, Z., Culley, D. J., Dong, Y., Zhang, G., Zhang, B., Moir, R. D., et al. (2008). The common inhalation anesthetic isoflurane induces caspase activation and increases amyloid β-protein level *in vivo*. *Ann. Neurol.* 64, 618–627. doi: 10.1002/ana.21548

Xie, Z., Dong, Y., Maeda, U., Alfille, P., Culley, D. J., Crosby, G., et al. (2006a). The common inhalation anesthetic isoflurane induces apoptosis and increases amyloid β protein levels. *Anesthesiology* 104, 988–994. doi: 10.1097/00000542-200605000-00015

Xie, Z., Dong, Y., Maeda, U., Moir, R., Inouye, S. K., Culley, D. J., et al. (2006b). Isoflurane-induced apoptosis: a potential pathogenic link between delirium and dementia. *J. Gerontol. A. Biol. Sci. Med. Sci.* 61, 1300–1306. doi: 10.1093/gerona/61.12.1300

Xie, Z., Moir, R. D., Romano, D. M., Tesco, G., Kovacs, D. M., and Tanzi, R. E. (2004). Hypocapnia induces caspase-3 activation and increases Aβ production. *Neurodegener. Dis.* 1, 29–37. doi: 10.1159/000076667

Yoshida, K., Furuse, M., Izawa, A., Iizima, N., Kuchiwaki, H., and Inao, S. (1996). Dynamics of cerebral blood flow and metabolism in patients with cranioplasty as evaluated by 133Xe CT and 31P magnetic resonance spectroscopy. *J. Neurol. Neurosurg. Psychiatry* 61, 166–171. doi: 10.1136/jnnp.61.2.166

Yu, N.-N., Wang, X.-X., Yu, J.-T., Wang, N.-D., Lu, R.-C., Miao, D., et al. (2010). Blocking β2-adrenergic receptor attenuates acute stress-induced amyloid β peptides production. *Brain Res.* 1317, 305–310. doi: 10.1016/j.brainres.2009.12.087

Zhang, B., Dong, Y., Zhang, G., Moir, R. D., Xia, W., Yue, Y., et al. (2008). The inhalation anesthetic desflurane induces caspase activation and increases amyloid β-protein levels under hypoxic conditions. *J. Biol. Chem.* 283, 11866–11875. doi: 10.1074/jbc.M800199200

Zhu, X., Smith, M. A., Honda, K., Aliev, G., Moreira, P. I., Nunomura, A., et al. (2007). Vascular oxidative stress in Alzheimer disease. *J. Neurol. Sci.* 257, 240–246. doi: 10.1016/j.jns.2007.01.039

17

Insulin Resistance as a Therapeutic Target in the Treatment of Alzheimer's Disease: A State-of-the-Art Review

Christian Benedict[1] *and Claudia A. Grillo*[2*]

[1] *Department of Neuroscience, Uppsala University, Uppsala, Sweden,* [2] *Department of Pharmacology, Physiology and Neuroscience, University of South Carolina-School of Medicine, Columbia, SC, United States*

***Correspondence:**
Claudia A. Grillo
cgrillo@uscmed.sc.edu

Research in animals and humans has shown that type 2 diabetes and its prodromal state, insulin resistance, promote major pathological hallmarks of Alzheimer's disease (AD), such as the formation of amyloid plaques and neurofibrillary tangles (NFT). Worrisomely, dysregulated amyloid beta (Aβ) metabolism has also been shown to promote central nervous system insulin resistance; although the role of tau metabolism remains controversial. Collectively, as proposed in this review, these findings suggest the existence of a mechanistic interplay between AD pathogenesis and disrupted insulin signaling. They also provide strong support for the hypothesis that pharmacologically restoring brain insulin signaling could represent a promising strategy to curb the development and progression of AD. In this context, great hopes have been attached to the use of intranasal insulin. This drug delivery method increases cerebrospinal fluid concentrations of insulin in the absence of peripheral side effects, such as hypoglycemia. With this in mind, the present review will also summarize current knowledge on the efficacy of intranasal insulin to mitigate major pathological symptoms of AD, i.e., cognitive impairment and deregulation of Aβ and tau metabolism.

Keywords: intranasal insulin, diabetes, mild cognitive impairment, amyloid beta, neurofibrillary tangles

BACKGROUND

Alzheimer's disease (AD) is a devastating disease characterized by a loss or decline in memory and other intellectual functions that can lead to impairments in everyday performance. AD affects 1 in 10 people ages 65 or older, and represents 60–70% of cases of dementia (Barker et al., 2002). At the macroscopic level, brain atrophy is the key neuropathological element of AD; at the microscopic level, the hallmarks of the disease are amyloid plaques, neurofibrillary tangles (NFT), and extensive neuronal loss. The principal proteinaceous component of amyloid plaques is the amyloid beta (Aβ) peptide, a 38–43 amino acid peptide produced from the cleavage of the transmembrane amyloid precursor protein (APP) by 2 enzymes: β-secretase and γ-secretase (Golde et al., 2000; Hardy and Selkoe, 2002). The active enzymatic component of the γ-secretase complex, presenilin, cleaves APP at several sites within the membrane to produce Aβ peptides of different lengths such as Aβ38, Aβ40, and Aβ42. The Aβ aggregation process is affected by the interaction of Aβ with the Aβ binding molecules such as apolipoprotein E (apoE) in the extracellular space (Kim et al., 2009). Human apoE has three common alleles (ε2, ε3, and ε4). The ε4 allele confers a genetic risk factor for AD; conversely, ε2 allele plays a protective role (Corder et al., 1993; Strittmatter et al., 1993). Aβ clearance from the interstitial fluid (ISF) depends on molecules such as neprilysin and insulin-degrading enzyme (IDE), as well as CSF and ISF bulk flow (Qiu et al., 1998; Jiang et al., 2017). The other hallmark of AD, the NFTs, are intracellular structures composed predominantly by hyperphosphorylated tau (Grundke-Iqbal et al., 1986; Goedert et al., 1988; Wischik et al., 1988). Tau is synthesized in all neurons and is also present in glial cells. Tau is a microtubule-associated protein that binds to tubulin and stabilizes microtubules. Under physiological conditions tau phosphorylation/dephosphorylation is a dynamic process essential for tau functionality. Phosphorylation of tau induces its release from microtubules and facilitates axonal vesicle transport, when tau is dephosphorylated it binds again to tubulin (Mandelkow et al., 2004). Hyperphosphorylation of tau can be a consequence of an imbalance of tau kinase and phosphatase activity. When tau suffers a hyperphosphorylation process, the protein dissociates from microtubules and self-aggregates forming NFTs observed in cell bodies and dystrophic neurites of the patients with AD. There is strong evidence that neurofibrillary pathology contributes to neuronal dysfunction and correlates with the clinical progression of AD. It has been suggested this is likely partly through pathways downstream of Aβ. However, Aβ is not the only factor that stimulates tau deposition. Other factors such as tau levels, its sequence and its phosphorylation state also contribute to tau aggregation and toxicity (Holtzman et al., 2012). Moreover, tau-related brain damage in AD might progress independently of Aβ (Small and Duff, 2008). Recent studies of Aβ plaques and tau-related neurodegeneration showed that they progress gradually in a sequential but temporally overlapping profile (Jack and Holtzman, 2013). The presence of Aβ plaques in the brain is the first detectable biomarker, followed by CSF tau proteins; whereas the cognitive deficit is the last event in the progression of AD (Jack et al., 2013). Taking into account these parameters, it is estimated that AD pathology probably begins 10–15 years prior to cognitive decline. In other words, it takes more than one decade of protein misfolding and aggregation until substantial neurodegeneration is developed and cognitive decline shows as the main symptom of this progressing disease (Perrin et al., 2009; Jack et al., 2010). Remarkably, this gradual evolvement of the AD provides a window for early intervention.

The brain utilizes ~20% of all glucose in a process that is mainly insulin independent. However, insulin receptors are widely distributed throughout the brain, with high concentrations in the olfactory bulb, hypothalamus and hippocampus (Fernandez and Torres-Alemán, 2012). The central function of insulin receptors ranges from regulation of whole-body energy metabolism in the hypothalamus (Woods et al., 1979; Brief and Davis, 1984; Hallschmid et al., 2004; Grillo et al., 2007; Benedict et al., 2011; Thienel et al., 2017) to modulation of memory at hippocampal level (Park et al., 2000; McNay et al., 2010; Grillo et al., 2015). Similarly to AD, reductions in insulin sensitivity (i.e., insulin resistance) occur years before the patients start to experience the symptoms and are diagnosed with diabetes (Dankner et al., 2009). Insulin resistance increases AD risk by at least two-fold (Sims-Robinson et al., 2010), and this deleterious effect can be due to the disruption of the function of the brain vasculature (Biessels and Reijmer, 2014; Frosch et al., 2017), and/or direct effects on Aβ aggregation or tau phosphorylation.

In recent years, type 2 diabetes and its prodromal state, insulin resistance (a pathological condition in which cells fail to respond normally to the hormone insulin), have been identified as risk factors for developing sporadic AD. For instance, a recent meta-analysis of longitudinal population-based studies (involving 1,746,777 individuals) has shown that the risk of AD is increased by about 50% in diabetic people compared to the general population (Zhang et al., 2017). The mechanistic pathways that might link impaired insulin signaling, particularly that of the brain and AD have been subject of intensive research in recent years, and will be comprehensively reviewed herein. These findings provide strong support for the hypothesis that pharmacologically restoring brain insulin signaling could be a promising novel strategy to curb the development and progression of AD. In this context, intranasal insulin administration has emerged as a very promising therapy for AD. With this in mind, one of the objectives of the current review is to summarize clinical trials and discuss the efficacy of intranasal insulin to improve major pathological symptoms of AD, i.e., cognitive dysfunction and deregulation of Aβ and tau metabolism. Additionally, we discuss some pre-clinical and clinical studies using drugs that enhance insulin sensitivity to ameliorate AD symptoms.

INSULIN RESISTANCE, BRAIN STRUCTURE, AND COGNITIVE FUNCTIONS

Clinical and pre-clinical studies consistently show an association between type 2 diabetes (and its prodromal state insulin resistance) and cognitive dysfunction. Additionally, the literature shows numerous examples of cognitive improvements due to insulin treatment.

Preclinical Studies

AD Models and Insulin Resistance

Insulin administration has been shown to ameliorate memory deficits and reverse diet-induced increases of Aβ levels in the brain of 3xTg-AD mice (Vandal et al., 2014). In the hippocampi of another AD mice model (APP/PS1 Tg), impairments in the insulin signaling were also reported (Bomfim et al., 2012). In addition, *in vivo* and *in vitro* experiments show that Aβ induces serine phosphorylation of insulin receptor substrate 1 (IRS-1) instead of tyrosine phosphorylation (Bomfim et al., 2012); this switch has been described as a major mechanism that triggers peripheral insulin resistance (Hirosumi et al., 2002). On the other hand, acute intrahippocampal administration of Aβ (1–42) impairs insulin signaling, decreasing phosphorylation of Akt and plasma membrane translocation of the insulin-sensitive glucose transporter 4, and these molecular effects were accompanied by deficits in spatial memory (Pearson-Leary and McNay, 2012).

Although it takes from 10 to 15 years after Aβ starts to aggregate to observe cognitive impairments in AD patients, an acute effect of Aβ upon cognition cannot be ruled out, especially taking into account the disruption in insulin signaling. Whether the same mechanism applies to human brains remains to be elucidated.

Diabetes Models and Cognitive Function

Experimental animal models of type 2 diabetes show impairments in hippocampal-based memory performance (Li et al., 2002; Winocur et al., 2005), deficits in hippocampal neuroplasticity including decreases in neuronal spine density and neurogenesis (Stranahan et al., 2008) and decreases in synaptic transmission (Kamal et al., 2013), whereas bolstering insulin signaling mitigates Aβ-induced synapse loss in mature cultures of hippocampal neurons (De Felice et al., 2009). Ultimately, the long-term consequences of diabetes-induced neuroplasticity deficits are reflected in cognitive impairments (Biessels and Reagan, 2015). Indeed, insulin resistance is a crucial contributor to the adverse effects on hippocampal cognitive function (de la Monte, 2012), and the literature consistently shows many examples that support the positive effects of insulin on cognitive function in rodent models. In this regard, central insulin administration improves spatial memory in a dose-dependent fashion in male rats (Haj-ali et al., 2009), whereas intrahippocampal insulin microinjections enhanced memory consolidation and retrieval (Moosavi et al., 2007). Acute delivery of insulin into the rat hippocampus also promotes spatial memory in the alternation test (McNay et al., 2010), and transiently enhances hippocampal-dependent memory in the inhibitory avoidance test (Stern et al., 2014). Nisticó et al. reported that mice with haploinsufficiency of insulin receptor β-subunit showed reduced hippocampal LTP and deficits in recognition memory (Nisticò et al., 2012). Concurrently, in a model of hippocampal-specific insulin resistance, rats showed deficits in LTP and spatial memory especially in long-term memory (Grillo et al., 2015).

Clinical Studies

AD and Insulin Resistance

Similar to preclinical studies, clinical studies show that disturbed insulin metabolism is a risk factor for cognitive dysfunction, brain atrophy, and dementia. There is evidence that insulin receptor density decreases in aging, and insulin signaling is impaired in AD (Frölich et al., 1998, 1999). In addition, post-mortem brain tissue from AD patients shows decreased insulin mRNA (Steen et al., 2005), suggesting a deficit in brain insulin signaling. Furthermore, brain tissue from AD patients without diabetes show insulin signaling impairments (Bruehl et al., 2010; De Felice and Ferreira, 2014; Yarchoan and Arnold, 2014).

Interestingly, a seminal work of Convit et al. describes memory deficits and hippocampal atrophy in individuals with impaired glucose metabolism (Convit et al., 2003). Conversion from mild cognitive impairment (MCI) to AD is higher in individuals with impaired glycemia compared to normoglycemic patients (Morris et al., 2014), suggesting that baseline glycemia and insulin resistance play key roles on cognitive decline and AD progression. Cognitive impairment is accompanied by whole-brain volume loss, although no difference was observed in hippocampal volume. In another study performed in healthy adults at risk for AD, the individuals that are strongly positive for Aβ (determined by Pittsburgh compound B tomography) show increased glucose metabolism in specific brain areas but not atrophy or cognitive loss compared to Aβ negative or Aβ indeterminate (Johnson et al., 2014). This potentially opens the opportunity to start an early intervention to prevent AD progression even in individuals that do not manifest abnormalities in peripheral glucose metabolism.

In a cross sectional study performed in cognitively healthy elderly individuals, it was shown that insulin resistance negatively correlates with verbal fluency performance and brain volume, especially in areas related to speech production (Benedict et al., 2012). However, there was no correlation when diabetic or cognitively impaired subjects were examined in an 11-year follow-up study carried out to examine a nationally representative adult population in Finland (Ekblad et al., 2017). Both studies concur that insulin resistance even in healthy individuals has a deleterious effect on verbal fluency performance. A recent cross-sectional study in late middle-aged participants at risk for AD showed that insulin resistance in normoglycemia has a positive correlation with Aβ deposition in frontal and temporal areas (Willette et al., 2015). It is important to note that these individuals are at risk for AD, whereas in previous studies in which type 2 diabetes was not associated with Aβ deposition or NFT, the brains were from patients without risk of AD (Nelson et al., 2009; Ahtiluoto et al., 2010). Furthermore, when cognitively asymptomatic middle-aged adults with a parental family history of AD were assessed, insulin resistance was associated with higher Aβ42 and long-term memory impairments (Hoscheidt et al., 2016).

When the other hallmark feature of AD, NFT, was considered, some studies suggest a link between insulin resistance and abnormal phosphorylation of tau protein (Liu et al., 2009). Insulin resistance is associated with higher P-Tau 181 and Total Tau in the CSF of asymptomatic late-middle-aged adults with risk factors for AD (APOEε4 carriers) and the association is negative for the APOEε4 non-carriers; whereas there is no effect on CSF Aβ42 levels (Starks et al., 2015). This suggests that insulin resistance may increase the susceptibility for tau pathology especially in the APOEε4 carriers.

Diabetic Patients and AD Hallmarks

Diabetes increases the odds of cognitive decline 1.2- to 1.5-fold compared to non-diabetic patients (Cukierman et al., 2005). Initial imaging studies in type 2 diabetic patients showed cortical and subcortical atrophy involving several brain regions accompanied by deficits in regional cerebral perfusion and vasoreactivity (Last et al., 2007) that ultimately may contribute to the cognitive dysfunction observed in elderly subjects with diabetes. In this regard, Crane et al. showed that higher glucose levels represent a risk factor for dementia in patients with or without diabetes. Unfortunately although hyperglycemia could result from decreases in insulin sensitivity, insulin levels were not reported (Crane et al., 2013). In a subsequent study, using glucose and hemoglobin A1c levels to characterize glucose exposure over 5 years before death, the same group did not find an association between glucose levels and NFT and dementia in people without diabetes treatment history (Crane et al., 2016). In spite of the effort to find the hallmark features of AD in the brain of type 2 diabetes patient, post-mortem studies were not able to show increased Aβ deposition or neurofibrillary tangles (Nelson et al., 2009; Ahtiluoto et al., 2010). More recent studies using Pittsburgh compound B to detect amyloid plaques mainly consisting of insoluble fibrils of Aβ—also failed to associate type 2 diabetes and Aβ aggregation (Thambisetty et al., 2013; Roberts et al., 2014). However, it must be noted that the load of insoluble Aβ does not correlate well with disease progression (Engler et al., 2006). Clinical evidence confirms that diabetes accelerates cognitive function decline, although, the mechanism still remains to be elucidated and it does not necessarily include the hallmark features of AD.

In a study performed in adults with prediabetes or early type 2 diabetes without cognitive impairment, insulin resistance was associated with reduced cerebral glucose metabolic rate (CMRglu) in frontal, parietotemporal and cingulate regions. During a memory task, individuals with diabetes showed a different pattern of CMRglu (more diffuse and extensive activation) and more difficulties in recalling items compared to healthy adults (Baker et al., 2011). This pattern is similar to that observed in prodromal or early AD as well as in non-symptomatic APOEε4 carriers; possibly these changes in CMRglu may try to compensate the disruption in the neuroarchitectural network that normally supports the cognitive task (Bookheimer et al., 2000; Sperling et al., 2010).

LINKING INSULIN RESISTANCE AND AD: POSSIBLE MOLECULAR MECHANISMS

Insulin Signaling Pathway

Although it is not clear how insulin resistance manifests in the central nervous system (CNS), many evidences suggest that different steps of the insulin signaling pathway might be altered (Biessels and Reagan, 2015). Importantly, changes in the insulin receptor expression cannot be ruled out especially in the brains of AD patients (Steen et al., 2005; Moloney et al., 2010). The first step in the insulin pathway activation, the receptor autophosphorylation, is followed by the Tyr phosphorylation of IRS1; however, in AD brains many groups reported increases in p(Ser)-IRS1, a marker of insulin resistance, instead of p(Tyr)-IRS1 (Steen et al., 2005; Moloney et al., 2010; Bomfim et al., 2012; Talbot et al., 2012; **Figure 1**). In addition, higher levels of p-JNK which can stimulate Ser-phosphorylation of IRS1 have been also reported in AD brains (Bomfim et al., 2012; Talbot et al., 2012; **Figure 1**). What leads to this switch in the insulin pathway observed in insulin resistance and AD remains to be elucidated. Recent studies from the Kapogiannis lab. show that plasma exosomes from AD patients exhibit higher pSer-IRS-1 levels and lower pTyr-IRS-1 compared to control subjects, suggesting that these biomarkers might be associated with the brain atrophy observed in AD. In fact, using neural-origin exosomes isolated by immunoprecipitation for L1 CAM, a positive correlation was observed between brain volume and pTyr-IRS-1; while the correlation was negative for pSer-IRS-1 (Mullins et al., 2017). This innovative methodology supports the hypothesis that central insulin resistance could be developed by changes in insulin signaling similarly to the changes described in the periphery and at the same time provides a potential brain-specific insulin resistance biomarker to study brain atrophy with a non-invasive and relatively simple procedure.

Clearance and Degradation of Aβ

Another possible mechanism that could explain why insulin resistance increases the risk of AD is through the clearance and degradation of Aβ. Insulin degrading enzyme (IDE) not only breaks down insulin but also degrades Aβ. In insulin resistance with high levels of insulin, IDE is saturated by insulin and it is less effective at Aβ degradation (Qiu et al., 1998; **Figure 1**). Clearance of Aβ is significantly decreased in rats treated with high doses of insulin (Shiiki et al., 2004). Conversely, inhibition of PI3K, a key step in the insulin pathway, suppresses APP cleavage and secretase activity, leading to decreases in Aβ production (Stöhr et al., 2013). In a mouse model of AD with neuron specific knockout of insulin receptor, Stöhr et al. (2013) observed reduction in Aβ levels and amyloid aggregation, suggesting that insulin signaling has an important effect upon Aβ deposition. In humans in a hyperinsulinemic-euglycemic clamp, insulin improved declarative memory, and increased CSF Aβ in older participants (Watson et al., 2003). In other studies using the same type of clamp, plasma and CSF Aβ was increased along with markers of inflammation (Fishel et al., 2005). These data suggest that hyperinsulinemia can regulate levels of Aβ. However, we have to take into account that these are acute effects observed after transient increases of insulin, whereas in type 2 diabetes hyperinsulinemia is chronic and therefore the long-term effect on Aβ degradation, cognitive function and AD progression could be different.

Glymphatic Clearance

An alternative mechanism by which insulin resistance exacerbates AD progression could include the clearance of the extracellular amyloid plaques. Decreases in the clearance of interstitial fluid in the hippocampus was observed in an experimental model of diabetes, and the cognitive deficits observed in the diabetic rats were inversely correlated to the retention of the contrast agent used to determine glymphatic clearance (Jiang et al., 2017). This is one of the first demonstrations that the system responsible for clearing brain extracellular solutes is affected by diabetes and might explain how insulin resistance may contribute to the initiation and progress of AD.

Fasting Insulin Levels

The two extremes of fasting insulin levels (lower and upper 15th percentiles) increase the risk of dementia in a longitudinal study performed in Japanese-American elderly men (Peila et al., 2004). In both cases, lack of insulin or excess of insulin due to insulin resistance lead to the convergent development of dementia. This finding is supported by studies in rodent models in which low levels of brain insulin and impaired insulin signaling preceded Aβ aggregation in a mouse model of AD (Chua et al., 2012). In other mouse model of AD, damaging the pancreatic cells that synthesize insulin leads to increases in Aβ levels (Wang et al., 2010). However, the lack of insulin resulting from the damage of the insulin-producing cells produces hyperglycemia that can also increase Aβ aggregation (MacAuley et al., 2015; Chao et al., 2016), making it difficult to elucidate if the increases in extracellular Aβ are due to the hypoinsulinemia and/or the glucotoxicity. Interestingly, lower levels of insulin produces decreases in IDE levels with the consequent increment in Aβ deposition.

Although the majority of the studies show that central insulin resistance in AD individuals has a deleterious effect, some studies in rodents have shown that deficiency in insulin receptor signaling in the brain can have a protective effect against Aβ deposition and even can extend lifespan (Freude et al., 2009; Stöhr et al., 2013). Deletion of insulin-like growth factor-1 receptor (IGF-1R) or insulin receptor in a mouse model of AD decreases APP processing delaying Aβ aggregation. However, only IGF-1R deficiency reduces premature mortality. According to cell based experiments inhibition of the PI3-kinase suppresses APP cleavage and decreases the secretases activity. This can explain the reduction in Aβ aggregation, but the differential effect on mortality remains still unknown.

Another question that remains unresolved is the time course of potential pre-diabetes relative to AD pathology and cognitive impairment. Recent studies from MacKlin et al. (2017) showed that APP/PS1 transgenic mice exhibit glucose intolerance at 2 months of age whereas Aβ accumulation and cognitive decline are not evident until 8–9 months of age. The metabolic deficit appears earlier and persists until the AD pathology and cognitive symptoms occur, indicating that at least in this model peripheral metabolic dysregulation precedes AD pathology (MacKlin et al., 2017).

Tau Hyperphosphorylation

The hypothesis that diabetes can facilitate tau pathology through induction of hyperphosphorylation of tau is supported

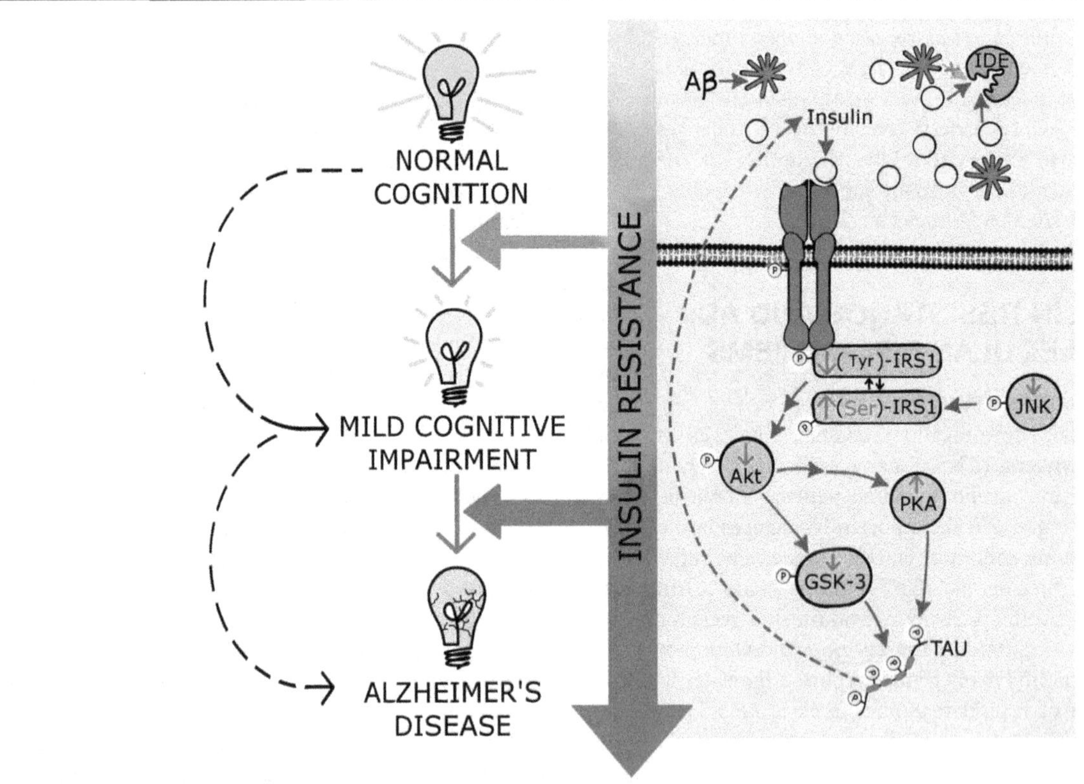

FIGURE 1 | Molecular mechanisms linking insulin resistance and Alzheimer's disease. Central insulin receptors are activated similarly to peripheral insulin receptors. This activation includes the autophosphorylation of the receptor followed by phosphorylation of other components of the cascade such as IRS1, Akt, and GSK-3. Insulin resistance results in stimulation of Ser-phosphorylation of IRS1 instead of normal Tyr-phosphorylation. Additionally, insulin resistance decreases p-JNK favoring the p(Ser)-IRS1. Insulin resistance also results in decreased phosphorylation of Akt affecting several downstream components of the insulin pathway, including GSK-3; this increment of the dephosphorylated form of GSK-3 (active state) stimulates tau hyperphosphorylation and NFT formation. Moreover, decreased activity of Akt induces PKA which also contributes to tau phosphorylation. Hyperphosphorylated tau further impairs insulin signaling. Additionally, the high levels of insulin, exhibited in insulin resistance states, compete with the Aβ for the insulin degrading enzyme (IDE) that is in charge of degrading both insulin and Aβ, affecting the clearance of Aβ. Through these multiple molecular mechanisms, insulin resistance might accelerate mild cognitive impairment as well as AD development and progression. See text for details.

by different molecular mechanisms. Under physiological conditions, insulin stimulates Akt phosphorylation that subsequently leads to Ser-phosphorylation of glycogen synthase kinase 3 (GSK3) and inactivates this enzyme. The active form of GSK3 stimulates tau phosphorylation and NFT formation (**Figure 1**). Hyperphosphorylation of tau may induce tau missorting which can lead to synaptic dysfunction and cognitive impairments (Wang and Mandelkow, 2016). Therefore, insulin resistance reduces p-Akt and p(Ser)-GSK3, and these decreases have also been described in postmortem brain tissue from patients with AD (Steen et al., 2005; Liu et al., 2011). Conversely, other groups reported the opposite: they observed increases in p-Akt and p(Ser)-GSK3 in AD brain samples (Pei et al., 2003; Griffin et al., 2005; Yarchoan et al., 2014). Therefore, there is no consensus about the participation of the phosphorylation/dephosphorylation processes of Akt and GSK3 upon the development of tau pathologies.

The impact of insulin resistance upon tau phosphorylation and cognition remains controversial. For instance, neuron-specific insulin receptor KO mice show higher levels of phosphorylated tau due to activation of GSK3 (Schubert et al., 2004). However, these mice have no memory impairments in spite of the higher levels of p-tau. Conversely, peripheral insulin administration increased abnormal phosphorylation of tau at Ser202 in a dose-dependent fashion in the CNS (Freude et al., 2005). On the other hand, in a model of obesity-associated hyperinsulinemia without changes in glucose homeostasis, no differences were observed in tau phosphorylation, the expression of the tau-kinases and tau-phosphatases (Becker et al., 2012). Although epidemiological studies show that diabetes is a risk factor for AD, there are still discrepancies about how insulin sensitivity modulates hyperphosphorylation of tau. A recent study in mice and monkeys demonstrates that chronic hyperinsulinemia leads to hyperphosphorylation of tau (Sajan et al., 2016; **Figure 1**). It is important to notice that in this last study the animal models exhibit hyperglycemia whereas in the Becker's study the animals were normoglycemic. Even though insulin sensitivity plays a crucial role on AD progress; the impact of glucotoxicity upon the neurodegenerative development cannot be ruled out.

Central insulin signaling dysregulation precedes the onset of peripheral insulin resistance in two mice models of AD, Tg2576 and 3xTg-AD. However, phosphorylation of several components of the insulin signaling cascade was differentially altered in both mouse models. Whereas phosphorylation of Akt and GSK3β showed the same trend in both models, p(Ser)-IRS1 and pPI3K were increased in Tg2576 and decreased in 3xTg-AD. These differences might be due to the tau pathology developed in 3xTg-AD mice (Velazquez et al., 2017).

Recently, a new contributor to the association between insulin signaling and tau pathology has been identified. In an animal model of insulin deficiency protein kinase A (PKA), a potent tau kinase, was activated. These effects on PKA and tau phosphorylation were confirmed by *in vitro* studies (van der Harg et al., 2017; **Figure 1**). Interestingly, insulin administration to diabetic rats was able to reverse both effects, emphasizing the potential of insulin treatment to ameliorate taupathies including AD.

Modulation of Insulin Signaling by Tau

Although the effects of insulin resistance upon tau pathogenesis has been studied (for review see El Khoury et al., 2014) the effects of tau pathology upon insulin signaling has been less explored. Marcianik et al. recently proposed a new function for tau by suggesting that tau might regulate brain insulin signaling (**Figure 1**). This concept was based on the observation that deletion of tau impairs insulin signaling in the hippocampus. In addition the anorexigenic effect of insulin acting on the hypothalamus is disrupted in these tau knockout mice. These new findings suggest a bidirectional effect between insulin resistance and tau loss-of-function, which ultimately might impair cognitive function in AD individuals (Marciniak et al., 2017). However, it would be interesting to discern between central and peripheral insulin sensitivity since tau is also expressed in pancreatic cells and its phosphorylation/dephosphorylation play an important role in insulin trafficking and release (Maj et al., 2016).

Figure 1 depicts some of the possible molecular mechanisms that link insulin resistance with MCI and AD, and shows how the progression of insulin resistance parallels the impairments in cognitive function.

INTRANASAL INSULIN AS A TREATMENT FOR ALZHEIMER'S DISEASE

Enhancing brain insulin function has recently emerged as a possible approach to mitigate AD symptoms and pathophysiology. An effective way to centrally administer insulin is via intranasal delivery. Using this route of administration insulin travels via convective bulk flow along perivascular pathways following the olfactory and trigeminal nerves and importantly bypassing the BBB. In this way, insulin can reach the hippocampus and the cortex in 15–30 mins (Chapman et al., 2013; Lochhead et al., 2015). Importantly, intranasal insulin does not reach the peripheral circulation (Born et al., 2002), thereby avoiding peripheral hypoglycemia (for advantages and disadvantages/possible side effects of intranasal insulin administration, see **Panel 1**). Clinical and preclinical studies have shown beneficial effects of intranasal insulin upon Aβ aggregation, NFT and cognitive function.

Intranasal Insulin in Diabetic and Healthy Individuals

In a recent study, acute intranasal insulin improved visuospatial memory in type 2 diabetic subjects as well as in the control individuals and this positive effect was due to regional vasoreactivity, especially vasodilatation in the anterior brain regions, such as insular cortex that regulates attention-related task performance (Novak et al., 2014). The same group of investigators demonstrated that intranasal insulin increases resting-state connectivity between the hippocampus and the medial frontal cortex compared to placebo and other default

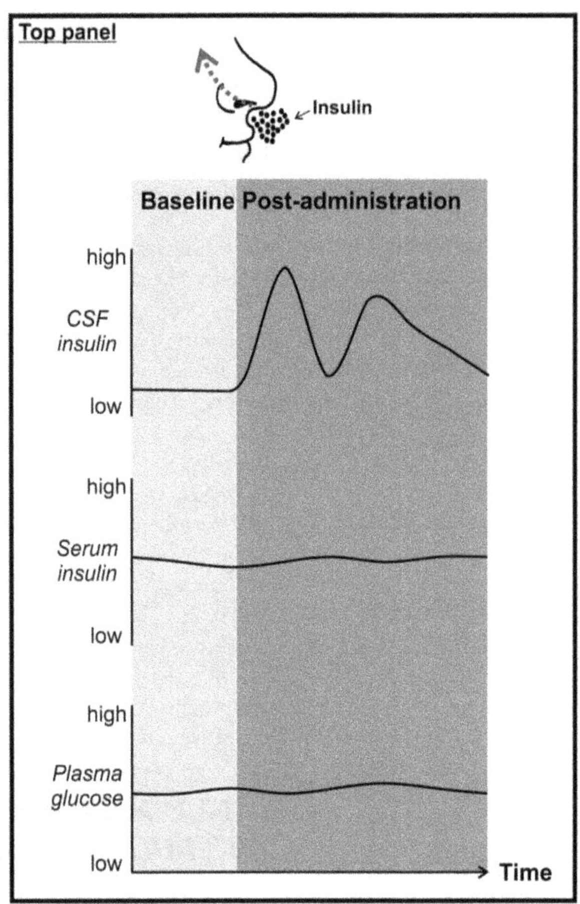

Bottom panel

Therapeutic benefits of intranasal insulin therapy: Non-invasive; can be self-administered; no risk of hypoglycemia; little or no effect on plasma insulin concentration.

Possible side effects/disadvantages of intranasal insulin therapy: Mild rhinitis; nosebleeds; the optimal treatment schedule has not yet been established and long-term safety data are scarce; preferential affinity of insulin-degrading enzyme (IDE) for insulin results in insulin-mediated inhibition of the degradation of beta-amyloid; possibility of brain insulin receptor desensitization as a result of chronic treatment with intranasal insulin; current evidence suggests that intranasal insulin is less effective in improving cognitive functions in APOE4-positive patients; there is no assessment of how effective intranasal insulin is, in comparison with current 'gold standard' treatment (e.g. Donepezil).

Panel 1 | Top: Proposed effects of intranasal insulin on cerebrospinal fluid (CSF) insulin, serum insulin, and plasma glucose concentrations. **Bottom**: Therapeutic benefits and possible side effects of intranasal insulin.

mode network (DMN) regions in type 2 diabetic patients. Moreover, the lower connectivity between the hippocampus and the medial frontal cortex observed in diabetic subjects was increased by intranasal insulin to a level comparable to control individuals (Zhang et al., 2015). Intranasal insulin administration was also tested in healthy individuals showing beneficial effects on cognitive function. Chronic intranasal insulin improved declarative memory (word recall) and enhanced mood (less anger and more self-confidence) in healthy male and female subjects (Benedict et al., 2004). Interestingly, these positive effects can be enhanced by using a rapid—acting insulin analog (Benedict et al., 2007). In addition to these chronic effects, transient increase of brain insulin levels improved delayed (10 min) but not immediate odor-cued recall of spatial memory in young men (Brünner et al., 2015). Interestingly, single dose intranasal insulin reduces food intake in healthy normal-weight males but not in females; conversely, hippocampus-dependent memory and working memory were improved in females, but not in males (Benedict et al., 2008). These findings could be seen as support for the hypothesis that women are more sensitive to the enhancement of hippocampus-dependent memory, whereas men are more susceptible to the anorexigenic effect of insulin. However, when obese men were long-term treated (8 weeks) with intranasal insulin although no changes were observed in body weight and adiposity, declarative memory and mood were improved similarly to normal-weight men (Hallschmid et al., 2008). It has moreover been demonstrated that intranasal insulin may normalize stress axis activity in humans by reducing cortisol levels (Benedict et al., 2004; Bohringer et al., 2008; Thienel et al., 2017). This inhibitory effect may also contribute to the positive impact on cognitive function. Finally, intranasal insulin administration has been shown to increase electroencephalogram delta power during non-rapid-eye-movement sleep in young adults (Feld et al., 2016). Sleep is a time period during which newly acquired memories are consolidated (Diekelmann and Born, 2010; Cedernaes et al., 2016) and cellular waste products accumulating in the ISF of the brain during wakefulness (such as soluble Aβ) are removed (Xie et al., 2013; Cedernaes et al., 2017). With these beneficial effects of sleep in mind, it could be speculated that intranasal insulin administration timed before sleep onset may have the strongest memory-improving and brain health-promoting therapeutic potential in humans.

Intranasal Insulin in Individuals With MCI or AD

Chronic intranasal insulin administration (4 months) in patients with MCI or mild to moderate AD improved delayed memory, preserved general cognition and functional abilities and these changes were associated with changes in Aβ42 level and tau/Aβ42 ratio in CSF. In addition, insulin impaired progression avoiding decreases in cerebral glucose metabolic rate in the parietotemporal, frontal, precuneus, and cuneus regions (Craft et al., 2012). Since no deleterious side effects were observed with this prolonged treatment, intranasal insulin emerges as an effective therapeutic approach for patients with MCI or AD. In a recent study aimed to compare regular insulin with long acting insulin (detemir) in adults with MCI or AD, the regular insulin showed improvements in memory after 2 and 4 months compared with placebo, whereas no significant effects were observed for the detemir-assigned group compared with the placebo group. Moreover, regular insulin treatment was associated with preserved volume on MRI and with reduction in the tau-P181/Aβ42 ratio (Craft et al., 2017).

APOE Status and Intranasal Insulin in Individuals With MCI or AD

Acute intranasal insulin improved verbal memory in ApoE ε4 negative subjects with MCI compared to ApoE ε4 positive or normal individuals (Reger et al., 2006). Interestingly and unexpectedly ApoE ε4 positive patients worsen their memory performance after insulin administration, suggesting differences in insulin metabolism due to the expression of ApoE ε4. Although both sexes were tested, gender differences were not analyzed. In a different study the same group found that repeated intranasal insulin improved verbal memory, attention and functional status compared to placebo-treated group in patients with MCI or early AD that was accompanied by increases in the short form of the beta-amyloid peptide (Reger et al., 2008b). This investigative group also found differential dose-response curves for intranasal insulin administration depending on ApoE ε4 allele: ApoE ε4 negative had a peak in verbal memory performance at 20 IU whereas ApoE ε4 positive patients showed memory decline after insulin treatment (Reger et al., 2008a). Interestingly, higher dose (60 IU) had a detrimental effect on memory in both groups (ApoE ε4 positive and negative).

A chronic study of 4 months of daily administration of intranasal insulin showed that men and women improved their cognitive function with 20 IU insulin, but just men benefited with higher dose (40 IU). When ApoE ε4 carriage was evaluated, the results showed that whereas ApoE ε4 negative men improved ApoE ε4 negative women worsened and the ApoE ε4 positive counterparts remained cognitively stable (Claxton et al., 2013). Conversely, using a long-lasting insulin analog (detemir), the results were also influenced by ApoE status; in ApoE ε4 carriers memory improvements were observed whereas non-carriers showed impairments (Claxton et al., 2015). The mechanistic basis of APOE-related treatment differences remains unknown. Collectively, these data highlight the importance of the APOE status upon the changes observed in cognition after intranasal insulin treatment. Since the treatment status can lead to beneficial or detrimental effects, it is crucial to take into account the APOE status when assessing the eligibility of the patients to participate in theses therapeutic approaches.

Insulin Sensitizer Agents and AD

Since insulin has beneficial effects upon memory in individuals with or without MCI or AD, it is logical to hypothesize that drugs that increase insulin sensitivity might also have a positive effect. In this regard, members of the incretin family were considered as prime candidates to ameliorate the MCI and AD symptoms. Within the incretin family, Glucagon-like peptide-1 (GLP-1) was one of the first to be tested. GLP-1 and its receptors (GLP-1Rs) are not just expressed in the pancreas and in the vascular endothelium, they are also found in the CNS, especially in the hypothalamus, hippocampus, cerebral cortex, and olfactory bulb (Lockie, 2013). Several studies have shown the importance of GLP-1 signaling on cognitive function, and many preclinical studies have been performed to evaluate the potential protective role of GLP-1 on the brain (Calsolaro and Edison, 2015). *In vitro* Aβ oligomers impaired axonal transport and this effect was prevented by treatment with a GLP-1R agonist that is used to treat diabetes; moreover this anti-diabetes agent decreases the serine phosphorylation of IRS-1 in hippocampus improving the cognitive function in a mice model of AD (Bomfim et al., 2012). This preclinical study establishes the molecular basis to investigate the potential therapeutic effect of GLP-1 agonists to prevent or treat AD in the clinical setting.

GLP-1 analogs have a dual role: in the periphery they modulate insulin release and centrally they enhance synaptic plasticity and even are able to reverse impairments induced by Aβ oligomers (McClean et al., 2010). In addition to facilitate insulin signaling, GLP-1 analogs have neuroprotective effects *per se*. Chronic treatment with liraglutide, a long-acting GLP-1R agonist, prevented memory decline, synapse loss, synaptic plasticity impairments, decreased the Aβ aggregation, and neuroinflammation, and increased the expression of young neurons in APP/PS1 mice, suggesting that liraglutide has preventive effects at the early stage of AD (McClean et al., 2011). Interestingly, liraglutide also showed restorative effects in the later stages of the disease in 14 months-old APP/PS1 mice (McClean and Hölscher, 2014). Since liraglutide has preventive and restorative effects upon pathological hallmarks of AD, this incretin hormone has been tested in clinical trials in AD patients. Six months of liraglutide treatment did not have any effect on Aβ deposition in the temporal and occipital lobes compared to placebo-treated patients; glucose metabolism (CMRglu) decreased in placebo patients, whereas liraglutide-treated patients exhibited a trend to increase it; and cognitive function was not improved (Gejl et al., 2016). Although preclinical data were very promising in the clinical setting liraglutide failed to reverse the hallmarks of AD.

The insulin-sensitizing drug metformin, used to treat insulin resistance, was thought as a possible alternative to ameliorate the AD symptomatology. In a placebo-controlled crossover study conducted in non-diabetic patients with MCI or early AD, metformin was able to improve executive function without changes in cerebral blood flow (Koenig et al., 2017). The beneficial effects of metformin are also supported by other study that showed that 1 year of treatment improved total recall compare to baseline in overweight/obese patients with MCI (Luchsinger et al., 2016).

It is important to note that so far these insulin sensitizer agents have not been administered via intranasal route. Therefore, the efficacy of these drugs depends on the peripheral effects and the ability to cross the BBB; and these could explain the differences when compared to the intranasal insulin.

CONCLUDING REMARKS

Available evidence, as reviewed herein, suggests that central nervous system insulin resistance is frequently found in patients with AD (Freiherr et al., 2013). Worrisomely, central insulin resistance promotes major pathological hallmarks of AD that can be found in the brain long before the clinical onset of this devastating disease, such as the formation of Aβ plaques and neurofibrillary tangles (Jack and Holtzman, 2013). On the other hand, deregulated Aβ and tau metabolism has also been shown to promote central insulin resistance (Bruehl et al., 2010; De Felice and Ferreira, 2014; Yarchoan and Arnold, 2014). This suggests the existence of a mechanistic interplay between AD pathogenesis and insulin resistance. In an attempt to interrupt this vicious cycle, in recent years particular attention has been devoted to clinical trials testing effects of intranasal insulin on cognition, daily function, and AD biomarkers. This drug delivery method increases CSF concentrations of insulin in the absence of peripheral side effects such as hypoglycemia (Born et al., 2002). Collectively, results deriving from these clinical trials so far are promising in that they demonstrated beneficial effects on cognition, mood, and metabolic integrity of the brain in patients with MCI or early AD (Reger et al., 2008a,b; Craft et al., 2012, 2017; Claxton et al., 2015). However, many unanswered questions remain, such as which dose of intranasal insulin is optimal to improve cognition, preserve brain metabolism, and reduce possible side effects in AD patients? Are effects of intranasal insulin on cognition and brain health augmented when combined with insulin sensitivity-increasing interventions, such as GLP-1 infusions or exercise programs? Does the time of the day modulate central nervous system effects of intranasal insulin (e.g., morning vs. evening)? Does a chronic treatment with intranasal insulin lead to desensitization of brain insulin signaling, as seen in peripheral tissues (Kupila et al., 2003)? Notwithstanding these questions, the currently available scientific evidence provides a sufficiently strong basis for the hypothesis that counteracting insulin resistance represents a promising therapeutic target in the treatment of AD. Whether intranasal insulin represents such candidate therapy remains to be elucidated in future trials.

AUTHOR CONTRIBUTIONS

All authors listed have made a substantial, direct, and intellectual contribution to the work, and approved it for publication.

ACKNOWLEDGMENTS

The authors would like to thank Victoria Macht for design and preparation of **Figure 1**. The work of CB is supported by the Novo Nordisk Foundation (NNF14OC0009349), the Swedish Brain Foundation, and the Swedish Research Council (2015-03100). The work of CG is supported by the National Science Foundation, NSF IOS-1656626 (USA), and the National Institutes of Health CTT COBRE, P20 GM109091-03 (USA). The funders did not have any role in design of the review, interpretation of the discussed literature, or in the writing process. We apologize to the many researchers who have contributed to the field and who because of space constraints have not been cited herein.

REFERENCES

Ahtiluoto, S., Polvikoski, T., Peltonen, M., Solomon, A., Tuomilehto, J., Winblad, B., et al. (2010). Diabetes, Alzheimer disease, and vascular dementia: a population-based neuropathologic study. *Neurology* 75, 1195–1202. doi: 10.1212/WNL.0b013e3181f4d7f8

Baker, L. D., Cross, D. J., Minoshima, S., Belongia, D., Watson, G. S., and Craft, S. (2011). Insulin resistance and Alzheimer-like reductions in regional cerebral glucose metabolism for cognitively normal adults with prediabetes or early type 2 diabetes. *Arch. Neurol.* 68, 51–57. doi: 10.1001/archneurol.2010.225

Barker, W. W., Luis, C. A., Kashuba, A., Luis, M., Harwood, D. G., Loewenstein, D., et al. (2002). Relative frequencies of Alzheimer disease, Lewy body, vascular and frontotemporal dementia, and hippocampal sclerosis in the State of Florida Brain Bank. *Alzheimer Dis. Assoc. Disord.* 16, 203–212. doi: 10.1097/00002093-200210000-00001

Becker, K., Freude, S., Zemva, J., Stöhr, O., Krone, W., and Schubert, M. (2012). Chronic peripheral hyperinsulinemia has no substantial influence on tau phosphorylation *in vivo*. *Neurosci. Lett.* 516, 306–310. doi: 10.1016/j.neulet.2012.04.022

Benedict, C., Brede, S., Schiöth, H. B., Lehnert, H., Schultes, B., Born, J., et al. (2011). Intranasal insulin enhances postprandial thermogenesis and lowers postprandial serum insulin levels in healthy men. *Diabetes* 60, 114–118. doi: 10.2337/db10-0329

Benedict, C., Brooks, S. J., Kullberg, J., Burgos, J., Kempton, M. J., Nordenskjöld, R., et al. (2012). Impaired insulin sensitivity as indexed by the HOMA score is associated with deficits in verbal fluency and temporal lobe gray matter volume in the elderly. *Diabetes Care* 35, 488–494. doi: 10.2337/dc11-2075

Benedict, C., Hallschmid, M., Hatke, A., Schultes, B., Fehm, H. L., Born, J., et al. (2004). Intranasal insulin improves memory in humans. *Psychoneuroendocrinology* 29, 1326–1334. doi: 10.1016/j.psyneuen.2004.04.003

Benedict, C., Hallschmid, M., Schmitz, K., Schultes, B., Ratter, F., Fehm, H. L., et al. (2007). Intranasal insulin improves memory in humans: superiority of insulin aspart. *Neuropsychopharmacology* 32, 239–243. doi: 10.1038/sj.npp.1301193

Benedict, C., Kern, W., Schultes, B., Born, J., and Hallschmid, M. (2008). Differential sensitivity of men and women to anorexigenic and memory-improving effects of intranasal insulin. *J. Clin. Endocrinol. Metab.* 93, 1339–1344. doi: 10.1210/jc.2007-2606

Biessels, G. J., and Reagan, L. P. (2015). Hippocampal insulin resistance and cognitive dysfunction. *Nat. Rev. Neurosci.* 16, 660–671. doi: 10.1038/nrn4019

Biessels, G. J., and Reijmer, Y. D. (2014). Brain changes underlying cognitive dysfunction in diabetes: what can we learn from MRI? *Diabetes* 63, 2244–2252. doi: 10.2337/db14-0348

Bohringer, A., Schwabe, L., Richter, S., and Schachinger, H. (2008). Intranasal insulin attenuates the hypothalamic–pituitary–adrenal axis response to psychosocial stress. *Psychoneuroendocrinology* 33, 1394–1400. doi: 10.1016/j.psyneuen.2008.08.002

Bomfim, T. R., Forny-Germano, L., Sathler, L. B., Brito-Moreira, J., Houzel, J.-C., Decker, H., et al. (2012). An anti-diabetes agent protects the mouse brain from defective insulin signaling caused by Alzheimer's disease–associated Aβ oligomers. *J. Clin. Invest.* 122, 1339–1353. doi: 10.1172/JCI57256

Bookheimer, S. Y., Strojwas, M. H., Cohen, M. S., Saunders, A. M., Pericak-Vance, M. A., Mazziotta, J. C., et al. (2000). Patterns of brain activation in people at risk for Alzheimer's disease. *N. Engl. J. Med.* 343, 450–456. doi: 10.1056/NEJM200008173430701

Born, J., Lange, T., Kern, W., McGregor, G. P., Bickel, U., and Fehm, H. L. (2002). Sniffing neuropeptides: a transnasal approach to the human brain. *Nat. Neurosci.* 5, 514–516. doi: 10.1038/nn849

Brief, D. J., and Davis, J. D. (1984). Reduction of food intake and body weight by chronic intraventricular insulin infusion. *Brain Res. Bull.* 12, 571–575.

Bruehl, H., Sweat, V., Hassenstab, J., Polyakov, V., and Convit, A. (2010). Cognitive impairment in nondiabetic middle-aged and older adults is associated with insulin resistance. *J. Clin. Exp. Neuropsychol.* 32, 487–493. doi: 10.1080/13803390903224928

Brünner, Y. F., Kofoet, A., Benedict, C., and Freiherr, J. (2015). Central insulin administration improves odor-cued reactivation of spatial memory in young men. *J. Clin. Endocrinol. Metab.* 100, 212–219. doi: 10.1210/jc.2014-3018

Calsolaro, V., and Edison, P. (2015). Novel GLP-1 (glucagon-like peptide-1) analogues and insulin in the treatment for Alzheimer's disease and other neurodegenerative diseases. *CNS Drugs* 29, 1023–1039. doi: 10.1007/s40263-015-0301-8

Cedernaes, J., Osorio, R. S., Varga, A. W., Kam, K., Schiöth, H. B., and Benedict, C. (2017). Candidate mechanisms underlying the association between sleep-wake disruptions and Alzheimer's disease. *Sleep Med. Rev.* 31, 102–111. doi: 10.1016/j.smrv.2016.02.002

Cedernaes, J., Sand, F., Liethof, L., Lampola, L., Hassanzadeh, S., Axelsson, E. K., et al. (2016). Learning and sleep-dependent consolidation of spatial and procedural memories are unaltered in young men under a fixed short sleep schedule. *Neurobiol. Learn. Mem.* 131, 87–94. doi: 10.1016/j.nlm.2016.03.012

Chao, A.-C., Lee, T.-C., Juo, S.-H. H., and Yang, D.-I. (2016). Hyperglycemia increases the production of amyloid beta-peptide leading to decreased endothelial tight junction. *CNS Neurosci. Ther.* 22, 291–297. doi: 10.1111/cns.12503

Chapman, C. D., Frey, W. H., Craft, S., Danielyan, L., Hallschmid, M., Schiöth, H. B., et al. (2013). Intranasal treatment of central nervous system dysfunction in humans. *Pharm. Res.* 30, 2475–2484. doi: 10.1007/s11095-012-0915-1

Chua, L.-M., Lim, M.-L., Chong, P.-R., Hu, Z. P., Cheung, N. S., and Wong, B.-S. (2012). Impaired neuronal insulin signaling precedes Aβ42 accumulation in female AβPPsw/PS1ΔE9 mice. *J. Alzheimers Dis.* 29, 783–791. doi: 10.3233/JAD-2012-111880

Claxton, A., Baker, L. D., Hanson, A., Trittschuh, E. H., Cholerton, B., Morgan, A., et al. (2015). Long-acting intranasal insulin detemir improves cognition for adults with mild cognitive impairment or early-stage Alzheimer's disease dementia. *J. Alzheimers Dis.* 44, 897–906. doi: 10.3233/JAD-141791

Claxton, A., Baker, L. D., Wilkinson, C. W., Trittschuh, E. H., Chapman, D., Watson, G. S., et al. (2013). Sex and ApoE genotype differences in treatment response to two doses of intranasal insulin in adults with mild cognitive impairment or Alzheimer's disease. *J. Alzheimers. Dis.* 35, 789–797. doi: 10.3233/JAD-122308

Convit, A., Wolf, O. T., Tarshish, C., and de Leon, M. J. (2003). Reduced glucose tolerance is associated with poor memory performance and hippocampal atrophy among normal elderly. *Proc. Natl. Acad. Sci. U.S.A.* 100, 2019–2022. doi: 10.1073/pnas.0336073100

Corder, E. H., Saunders, A. M., Strittmatter, W. J., Schmechel, D. E., Gaskell, P. C., Small, G. W., et al. (1993). Gene dose of apolipoprotein E type 4 allele and the risk of Alzheimer's disease in late onset families. *Science* 261, 921–923.

Craft, S., Baker, L. D., Montine, T. J., Minoshima, S., Watson, G. S., Claxton, A., et al. (2012). Intranasal insulin therapy for Alzheimer disease and amnestic mild cognitive impairment. *Arch. Neurol.* 69:29. doi: 10.1001/archneurol.2011.233

Craft, S., Claxton, A., Baker, L. D., Hanson, A. J., Cholerton, B., Trittschuh, E. H., et al. (2017). Effects of regular and long-acting insulin on cognition and Alzheimer's disease biomarkers: a pilot clinical trial. *J. Alzheimers Dis.* 57, 1325–1334. doi: 10.3233/JAD-161256

Crane, P. K., Walker, R. L., Sonnen, J., Gibbons, L. E., Melrose, R., Hassenstab, J., et al. (2016). Glucose levels during life and neuropathologic findings at autopsy among people never treated for diabetes. *Neurobiol. Aging* 48, 72–82. doi: 10.1016/j.neurobiolaging.2016.07.021

Crane, P. K., Walker, R., Hubbard, R. A., Li, G., Nathan, D. M., Zheng, H., et al. (2013). Glucose levels and risk of dementia. *N. Engl. J. Med.* 369, 540–548. doi: 10.1056/NEJMoa1215740

Cukierman, T., Gerstein, H. C., and Williamson, J. D. (2005). Cognitive decline and dementia in diabetes–systematic overview of prospective observational studies. *Diabetologia* 48, 2460–2469. doi: 10.1007/s00125-005-0023-4

Dankner, R., Chetrit, A., Shanik, M. H., Raz, I., and Roth, J. (2009). Basal-state hyperinsulinemia in healthy normoglycemic adults is predictive of type 2 diabetes over a 24-year follow-up: a preliminary report. *Diabetes Care* 32, 1464–1466. doi: 10.2337/dc09-0153

De Felice, F. G., and Ferreira, S. T. (2014). Inflammation, defective insulin signaling, and mitochondrial dysfunction as common molecular denominators connecting type 2 diabetes to Alzheimer disease. *Diabetes* 63, 2262–2272. doi: 10.2337/db13-1954

De Felice, F. G., Vieira, M. N. N., Bomfim, T. R., Decker, H., Velasco, P. T., Lambert, M. P., et al. (2009). Protection of synapses against Alzheimer's-linked toxins: insulin signaling prevents the pathogenic binding of Abeta oligomers. *Proc. Natl. Acad. Sci. U.S.A.* 106, 1971–1976. doi: 10.1073/pnas.0809158106

de la Monte, S. M. (2012). Brain insulin resistance and deficiency as therapeutic targets in Alzheimer's disease. *Curr. Alzheimer Res.* 9, 35–66. doi: 10.2174/156720512799015037

Diekelmann, S., and Born, J. (2010). The memory function of sleep. *Nat. Rev. Neurosci.* 11, 114–126. doi: 10.1038/nrn2762

Ekblad, L. L., Rinne, J. O., Puukka, P., Laine, H., Ahtiluoto, S., Sulkava, R., et al. (2017). Insulin resistance predicts cognitive decline: an 11-year follow-up of a nationally representative adult population sample. *Diabetes Care* 40, 751–758. doi: 10.2337/dc16-2001

El Khoury, N. B., Gratuze, M., Papon, M.-A., Bretteville, A., and Planel, E. (2014). Insulin dysfunction and Tau pathology. *Front. Cell. Neurosci.* 8:22. doi: 10.3389/fncel.2014.00022

Engler, H., Forsberg, A., Almkvist, O., Blomquist, G., Larsson, E., Savitcheva, I., et al. (2006). Two-year follow-up of amyloid deposition in patients with Alzheimer's disease. *Brain* 129, 2856–2866. doi: 10.1093/brain/awl178

Feld, G. B., Wilhem, I., Benedict, C., Rüdel, B., Klameth, C., Born, J., et al. (2016). Central nervous insulin signaling in sleep-associated memory formation and neuroendocrine regulation. *Neuropsychopharmacology* 41, 1540–1550. doi: 10.1038/npp.2015.312

Fernandez, A. M., and Torres-Alemán, I. (2012). The many faces of insulin-like peptide signalling in the brain. *Nat. Rev. Neurosci.* 13, 225–239. doi: 10.1038/nrn3209

Fishel, M. A., Watson, G. S., Montine, T. J., Wang, Q., Green, P. S., Kulstad, J. J., et al. (2005). Hyperinsulinemia provokes synchronous increases in central inflammation and β-amyloid in normal adults. *Arch. Neurol.* 62, 1539–1544. doi: 10.1001/archneur.62.10.noc50112

Freiherr, J., Hallschmid, M., Frey, W. H., Brünner, Y. F., Chapman, C. D., Hölscher, C., et al. (2013). Intranasal insulin as a treatment for Alzheimer's disease: a review of basic research and clinical evidence. *CNS Drugs* 27, 505–514. doi: 10.1007/s40263-013-0076-8

Freude, S., Hettich, M. M., Schumann, C., Stohr, O., Koch, L., Kohler, C., et al. (2009). Neuronal IGF-1 resistance reduces A accumulation and protects against premature death in a model of Alzheimer's disease. *FASEB J.* 23, 3315–3324. doi: 10.1096/fj.09-132043

Freude, S., Plum, L., Schnitker, J., Leeser, U., Udelhoven, M., Krone, W., et al. (2005). Peripheral hyperinsulinemia promotes tau phosphorylation *in vivo*. *Diabetes* 54, 3343–3348. doi: 10.2337/diabetes.54.12.3343

Frölich, L., Blum-Degen, D., Bernstein, H.-G., Engelsberger, S., Humrich, J., Laufer, S., et al. (1998). Brain insulin and insulin receptors in aging and sporadic Alzheimer's disease. *J Neural Transm.* 105:423. doi: 10.1007/s007020050068

Frölich, L., Blum-Degen, D., Riederer, P., and Hoyer, S. (1999). A disturbance in the neuronal insulin receptor signal transduction in sporadic Alzheimer's disease. *Ann. N. Y. Acad. Sci.* 893, 290–293.

Frosch, O. H., Yau, P. L., Osorio, R. S., Rusinek, H., Storey, P., and Convit, A. (2017). Insulin resistance among obese middle-aged is associated with decreased cerebrovascular reactivity. *Neurology* 89, 249–255. doi: 10.1212/WNL.0000000000004110

Gejl, M., Gjedde, A., Egefjord, L., Møller, A., Hansen, S. B., Vang, K., et al. (2016). In Alzheimer's disease, 6-month treatment with GLP-1 analog prevents decline of brain glucose metabolism: randomized, placebo-controlled, double-blind clinical trial. *Front. Aging Neurosci.* 8:108. doi: 10.3389/fnagi.2016.00108

Goedert, M., Wischik, C. M., Crowther, R. A., Walker, J. E., and Klug, A. (1988). Cloning and sequencing of the cDNA encoding a core protein of the paired helical filament of Alzheimer disease: identification as the microtubule-associated protein tau. *Proc. Natl. Acad. Sci. U.S.A.* 85, 4051–4055.

Golde, T. E., Eckman, C. B., and Younkin, S. G. (2000). Biochemical detection of Aβ isoforms: implications for pathogenesis, diagnosis, and treatment of Alzheimer's disease. *Biochim. Biophys. Acta* 1502, 172–187. doi: 10.1016/S0925-4439(00)00043-0

Griffin, R. J., Moloney, A., Kelliher, M., Johnston, J. A., Ravid, R., Dockery, P., et al. (2005). Activation of Akt/PKB, increased phosphorylation of Akt substrates and loss and altered distribution of Akt and PTEN are features of Alzheimer's disease pathology. *J. Neurochem.* 93, 105–117. doi: 10.1111/j.1471-4159.2004.02949.x

Grillo, C. A., Piroli, G. G., Lawrence, R. C., Wrighten, S. A., Green, A. J., Wilson, S. P., et al. (2015). Hippocampal insulin resistance impairs spatial learning and synaptic plasticity. *Diabetes* 64, 3927–3936. doi: 10.2337/db15-0596

Grillo, C. A., Tamashiro, K. L., Piroli, G. G., Melhorn, S., Gass, J. T., Newsom, R. J., et al. (2007). Lentivirus-mediated downregulation of hypothalamic insulin receptor expression. *Physiol. Behav.* 92, 691–701. doi: 10.1016/j.physbeh.2007.05.043

Grundke-Iqbal, I., Iqbal, K., Tung, Y. C., Quinlan, M., Wisniewski, H. M., and Binder, L. I. (1986). Abnormal phosphorylation of the microtubule-associated protein tau (tau) in Alzheimer cytoskeletal pathology. *Proc. Natl. Acad. Sci. U.S.A.* 83, 4913–4917.

Haj-ali, V., Mohaddes, G., and Babri, S. H. (2009). Intracerebroventricular insulin improves spatial learning and memory in male Wistar rats. *Behav. Neurosci.* 123, 1309–1314. doi: 10.1037/a0017722

Hallschmid, M., Benedict, C., Schultes, B., Born, J., and Kern, W. (2008). Obese men respond to cognitive but not to catabolic brain insulin signaling. *Int. J. Obes.* 32, 275–282. doi: 10.1038/sj.ijo.0803722

Hallschmid, M., Benedict, C., Schultes, B., Fehm, H.-L., Born, J., and Kern, W. (2004). Intranasal insulin reduces body fat in men but not in women. *Diabetes* 53, 3024–3029. doi: 10.2337/diabetes.53.11.3024

Hardy, J., and Selkoe, D. J. (2002). The amyloid hypothesis of Alzheimer's disease: progress and problems on the road to therapeutics. *Science* 297, 353–356. doi: 10.1126/science.1072994

Hirosumi, J., Tuncman, G., Chang, L., Görgün, C. Z., Uysal, K. T., Maeda, K., et al. (2002). A central role for JNK in obesity and insulin resistance. *Nature* 420, 333–336. doi: 10.1038/nature01137

Holtzman, D. M., Mandelkow, E., and Selkoe, D. J. (2012). Alzheimer Disease in 2020. *Cold Spring Harb. Perspect. Med.* 2:a011585. doi: 10.1101/cshperspect.a011585

Hoscheidt, S. M., Starks, E. J., Oh, J. M., Zetterberg, H., Blennow, K., Krause, R. A., et al. (2016). Insulin resistance is associated with increased levels of cerebrospinal fluid biomarkers of Alzheimer's disease and reduced memory function in at-risk healthy middle-aged adults. *J. Alzheimers Dis.* 52, 1373–1383. doi: 10.3233/JAD-160110

Jack, C. R., and Holtzman, D. M. (2013). Biomarker modeling of Alzheimer's disease. *Neuron* 80, 1347–1358. doi: 10.1016/j.neuron.2013.12.003

Jack, C. R., Knopman, D. S., Jagust, W. J., Petersen, R. C., Weiner, M. W., Aisen, P. S., et al. (2013). Tracking pathophysiological processes in Alzheimer's disease: an updated hypothetical model of dynamic biomarkers. *Lancet Neurol.* 12, 207–216. doi: 10.1016/S1474-4422(12)70291-0

Jack, C. R., Knopman, D. S., Jagust, W. J., Shaw, L. M., Aisen, P. S., Weiner, M. W., et al. (2010). Hypothetical model of dynamic biomarkers of the Alzheimer's pathological cascade. *Lancet Neurol.* 9, 119–128. doi: 10.1016/S1474-4422(09)70299-6

Jiang, Q., Zhang, L., Ding, G., Davoodi-Bojd, E., Li, Q., Li, L., et al. (2017). Impairment of the glymphatic system after diabetes. *J. Cereb. Blood Flow Metab.* 37, 1326–1337. doi: 10.1177/0271678X16654702

Johnson, S. C., Christian, B. T., Okonkwo, O. C., Oh, J. M., Harding, S., Xu, G., et al. (2014). Amyloid burden and neural function in people at risk for Alzheimer's disease. *Neurobiol. Aging* 35, 576–584. doi: 10.1016/j.neurobiolaging.2013.09.028

Kamal, A., Ramakers, G. M. J., Gispen, W. H., Biessels, G. J., and Al Ansari, A. (2013). Hyperinsulinemia in rats causes impairment of spatial memory and learning with defects in hippocampal synaptic plasticity by involvement of postsynaptic mechanisms. *Exp. Brain Res.* 226, 45–51. doi: 10.1007/s00221-013-3409-4

Kim, J., Basak, J. M., and Holtzman, D. M. (2009). The role of apolipoprotein E in Alzheimer's disease. *Neuron* 63, 287–303. doi: 10.1016/j.neuron.2009.06.026

Koenig, A. M., Mechanic-Hamilton, D., Xie, S. X., Combs, M. F., Cappola, A. R., Xie, L., et al. (2017). Effects of the insulin sensitizer metformin in alzheimer disease: pilot data from a randomized placebo-controlled crossover study. *Alzheimer Dis. Assoc. Disord.* 31, 107–113. doi: 10.1097/WAD.0000000000000202

Kupila, A., Sipilä, J., Keskinen, P., Simell, T., Knip, M., Pulkki, K., et al. (2003). Intranasally administered insulin intended for prevention of type 1 diabetes-a safety study in healthy adults. *Diabetes. Metab. Res. Rev.* 19, 415–420. doi: 10.1002/dmrr.397

Last, D., Alsop, D. C., Abduljalil, A. M., Marquis, R. P., de Bazelaire, C., Hu, K., et al. (2007). Global and regional effects of type 2 diabetes on brain tissue volumes and cerebral vasoreactivity. *Diabetes Care* 30, 1193–1199. doi: 10.2337/dc06-2052

Li, X. L., Aou, S., Hori, T., and Oomura, Y. (2002). Spatial memory deficit and emotional abnormality in OLETF rats. *Physiol. Behav.* 75, 15–23. doi: 10.1016/S0031-9384(01)00627-8

Liu, Y., Liu, F., Grundke-Iqbal, I., Iqbal, K., and Gong, C.-X. (2011). Deficient brain insulin signalling pathway in Alzheimer's disease and diabetes. *J. Pathol.* 225, 54–62. doi: 10.1002/path.2912

Liu, Y., Liu, F., Grundke-Iqbal, I., Iqbal, K., and Gong, C.-X. (2009). Brain glucose transporters, O -GlcNAcylation and phosphorylation of tau in diabetes and Alzheimer's disease. *J. Neurochem.* 111, 242–249. doi: 10.1111/j.1471-4159.2009.06320.x

Lochhead, J. J., Wolak, D. J., Pizzo, M. E., and Thorne, R. G. (2015). Rapid transport within cerebral perivascular spaces underlies widespread tracer distribution in the brain after intranasal administration. *J. Cereb. Blood Flow Metab.* 35, 371–381. doi: 10.1038/jcbfm.2014.215

Lockie, S. H. (2013). Glucagon-like peptide-1 receptor in the brain: role in neuroendocrine control of energy metabolism and treatment target for obesity. *J. Neuroendocrinol.* 25, 597–604. doi: 10.1111/jne.12039

Luchsinger, J. A., Perez, T., Chang, H., Mehta, P., Steffener, J., Pradabhan, G., et al. (2016). Metformin in amnestic mild cognitive impairment: results of a pilot randomized placebo controlled clinical trial. *J. Alzheimers. Dis.* 51, 501–514. doi: 10.3233/JAD-150493

MacAuley, S. L., Stanley, M., Caesar, E. E., Yamada, S. A., Raichle, M. E., Perez, R., et al. (2015). Hyperglycemia modulates extracellular amyloid-β concentrations and neuronal activity *in vivo*. *J. Clin. Invest.* 125, 2463–2467. doi: 10.1172/JCI79742

MacKlin, L., Griffith, C. M., Cai, Y., Rose, G. M., Yan, X.-X., and Patrylo, P. R. (2017). Glucose tolerance and insulin sensitivity are impaired in APP/PS1 transgenic mice prior to amyloid plaque pathogenesis and cognitive decline. *Exp. Gerontol.* 88, 9–18. doi: 10.1016/j.exger.2016.12.019

Maj, M., Hoermann, G., Rasul, S., Base, W., Wagner, L., and Attems, J. (2016). The microtubule-associated protein tau and its relevance for pancreatic beta cells. *J. Diabetes Res.* 2016:1964634. doi: 10.1155/2016/1964634

Mandelkow, E.-M., Thies, E., Trinczek, B., Biernat, J., and Mandelkow, E. (2004). MARK/PAR1 kinase is a regulator of microtubule-dependent transport in axons. *J. Cell Biol.* 167, 99–110. doi: 10.1083/jcb.200401085

Marciniak, E., Leboucher, A., Caron, E., Ahmed, T., Tailleux, A., Dumont, J., et al. (2017). Tau deletion promotes brain insulin resistance. *J. Exp. Med.* 214, 2257–2269. doi: 10.1084/jem.20161731

McClean, P. L., and Hölscher, C. (2014). Liraglutide can reverse memory impairment, synaptic loss and reduce plaque load in aged APP/PS1 mice, a model of Alzheimer's disease. *Neuropharmacology* 76, 57–67. doi: 10.1016/j.neuropharm.2013.08.005

McClean, P. L., Gault, V. A., Harriott, P., and Hölscher, C. (2010). Glucagon-like peptide-1 analogues enhance synaptic plasticity in the brain: a link between diabetes and Alzheimer's disease. *Eur. J. Pharmacol.* 630, 158–162. doi: 10.1016/j.ejphar.2009.12.023

McClean, P. L., Parthsarathy, V., Faivre, E., and Holscher, C. (2011). The diabetes drug liraglutide prevents degenerative processes in a mouse model of Alzheimer's disease. *J. Neurosci.* 31, 6587–6594. doi: 10.1523/JNEUROSCI.0529-11.2011

McNay, E. C., Ong, C. T., McCrimmon, R. J., Cresswell, J., Bogan, J. S., and Sherwin, R. S. (2010). Hippocampal memory processes are modulated by insulin and high-fat-induced insulin resistance. *Neurobiol. Learn. Mem.* 93, 546–553. doi: 10.1016/j.nlm.2010.02.002

Moloney, A. M., Griffin, R. J., Timmons, S., O'Connor, R., Ravid, R., and O'Neill, C. (2010). Defects in IGF-1 receptor, insulin receptor and IRS-1/2 in Alzheimer's disease indicate possible resistance to IGF-1 and insulin signalling. *Neurobiol. Aging* 31, 224–243. doi: 10.1016/j.neurobiolaging.2008.04.002

Moosavi, M., Naghdi, N., and Choopani, S. (2007). Intra CA1 insulin microinjection improves memory consolidation and retrieval. *Peptides* 28, 1029–1034. doi: 10.1016/j.peptides.2007.02.010

Morris, J. K., Vidoni, E. D., Honea, R. A., Burns, J. M., and Alzheimer's Disease Neuroimaging Initiative (2014). Impaired glycemia increases disease progression in mild cognitive impairment. *Neurobiol. Aging* 35, 585–589. doi: 10.1016/j.neurobiolaging.2013.09.033

Mullins, R. J., Mustapic, M., Goetzl, E. J., and Kapogiannis, D. (2017). Exosomal biomarkers of brain insulin resistance associated with regional atrophy in Alzheimer's disease. *Hum. Brain Mapp.* 38, 1933–1940. doi: 10.1002/hbm.23494

Nelson, P. T., Smith, C. D., Abner, E. A., Schmitt, F. A., Scheff, S. W., Davis, G. J., et al. (2009). Human cerebral neuropathology of Type 2 diabetes mellitus. *Biochim. Biophys. Acta* 1792, 454–469. doi: 10.1016/j.bbadis.2008.08.005

Nisticò, R., Cavallucci, V., Piccinin, S., Macrì, S., Pignatelli, M., Mehdawy, B., et al. (2012). Insulin receptor β-subunit haploinsufficiency impairs hippocampal late-phase, LTP, and recognition memory. *Neuromol. Med.* 14, 262–269. doi: 10.1007/s12017-012-8184-z

Novak, V., Milberg, W., Hao, Y., Munshi, M., Novak, P., Galica, A., et al. (2014). Enhancement of vasoreactivity and cognition by intranasal insulin in type 2 diabetes. *Diabetes Care* 37, 751–759. doi: 10.2337/dc13-1672

Park, C. R., Seeley, R. J., Craft, S., and Woods, S. C. (2000). Intracerebroventricular insulin enhances memory in a passive-avoidance task. *Physiol. Behav.* 68, 509–514. doi: 10.1016/S0031-9384(99)00220-6

Pearson-Leary, J., and McNay, E. C. (2012). Intrahippocampal administration of amyloid-β(1-42) oligomers acutely impairs spatial working memory, insulin signaling, and hippocampal metabolism. *J. Alzheimers Dis.* 30, 413–422. doi: 10.3233/JAD-2012-112192

Pei, J.-J., Khatoon, S., An, W.-L., Nordlinder, M., Tanaka, T., Braak, H., et al. (2003). Role of protein kinase B in Alzheimer's neurofibrillary pathology. *Acta Neuropathol.* 105, 381–392. doi: 10.1007/s00401-002-0657-y

Peila, R., Rodriguez, B. L., White, L. R., and Launer, L. J. (2004). Fasting insulin and incident dementia in an elderly population of Japanese-American men. *Neurology* 63, 228–233. doi: 10.1212/01.WNL.0000129989.28404.9B

Perrin, R. J., Fagan, A. M., and Holtzman, D. M. (2009). Multimodal techniques for diagnosis and prognosis of Alzheimer's disease. *Nature* 461, 916–922. doi: 10.1038/nature08538

Qiu, W. Q., Walsh, D. M., Ye, Z., Vekrellis, K., Zhang, J., Podlisny, M. B., et al. (1998). Insulin-degrading enzyme regulates extracellular levels of amyloid beta-protein by degradation. *J. Biol. Chem.* 273, 32730–32738.

Reger, M. A., Watson, G. S., Frey, W. H., Baker, L. D., Cholerton, B., Keeling, M. L., et al. (2006). Effects of intranasal insulin on cognition in memory-impaired older adults: modulation by APOE genotype. *Neurobiol. Aging* 27, 451–458. doi: 10.1016/j.neurobiolaging.2005.03.016

Reger, M. A., Watson, G. S., Green, P. S., Baker, L. D., Cholerton, B., Fishel, M. A., et al. (2008a). Intranasal insulin administration dose-dependently modulates verbal memory and plasma amyloid-beta in memory-impaired older adults. *J. Alzheimers Dis.* 13, 323–331. doi: 10.3233/JAD-2008-13309

Reger, M. A., Watson, G. S., Green, P. S., Wilkinson, C. W., Baker, L. D., Cholerton, B., et al. (2008b). Intranasal insulin improves cognition and modulates -amyloid in early AD. *Neurology* 70, 440–448. doi: 10.1212/01.WNL.0000265401.62434.36

Roberts, R. O., Knopman, D. S., Cha, R. H., Mielke, M. M., Pankratz, V. S., Boeve, B. F., et al. (2014). Diabetes and elevated hemoglobin A1c levels are associated with brain hypometabolism but not amyloid accumulation. *J. Nucl. Med.* 55, 759–764. doi: 10.2967/jnumed.113.132647

Sajan, M., Hansen, B., Ivey, R., Sajan, J., Ari, C., Song, S., et al. (2016). Brain insulin signaling is increased in insulin-resistant states and decreases in FOXOs and PGC-1α and increases in Aβ1-40/42 and phospho-tau may Abet Alzheimer development. *Diabetes* 65, 1892–1903. doi: 10.2337/db15-1428

Schubert, M., Gautam, D., Surjo, D., Ueki, K., Baudler, S., Schubert, D., et al. (2004). Role for neuronal insulin resistance in neurodegenerative diseases. *Proc. Natl. Acad. Sci. U.S.A.* 101, 3100–3105. doi: 10.1073/pnas.0308724101

Shiiki, T., Ohtsuki, S., Kurihara, A., Naganuma, H., Nishimura, K., Tachikawa, M., et al. (2004). Brain insulin impairs amyloid- (1-40) clearance from the brain. *J. Neurosci.* 24, 9632–9637. doi: 10.1523/JNEUROSCI.2236-04.2004

Sims-Robinson, C., Kim, B., Rosko, A., and Feldman, E. L. (2010). How does diabetes accelerate Alzheimer disease pathology? *Nat. Rev. Neurol.* 6, 551–559. doi: 10.1038/nrneurol.2010.130

Small, S. A., and Duff, K. (2008). Linking Aβ and tau in late-onset Alzheimer's disease: a dual pathway hypothesis. *Neuron* 60, 534–542. doi: 10.1016/j.neuron.2008.11.007

Sperling, R. A., Dickerson, B. C., Pihlajamaki, M., Vannini, P., LaViolette, P. S., Vitolo, O. V., et al. (2010). Functional alterations in memory networks in early Alzheimer's disease. *Neuromol. Med.* 12, 27–43. doi: 10.1007/s12017-009-8109-7

Starks, E. J., Patrick O'Grady, J., Hoscheidt, S. M., Racine, A. M., Carlsson, C. M., Zetterberg, H., et al. (2015). Insulin resistance is associated with higher cerebrospinal fluid tau levels in asymptomatic APOEε4 carriers. *J. Alzheimers. Dis.* 46, 525–533. doi: 10.3233/JAD-150072

Steen, E., Terry, B. M., Rivera, E. J., Cannon, J. L., Neely, T. R., Tavares, R., et al. (2005). Impaired insulin and insulin-like growth factor expression and signaling mechanisms in Alzheimer's disease–is this type 3 diabetes? *J. Alzheimers Dis.* 7, 63–80. doi: 10.3233/JAD-2005-7107

Stern, S. A., Chen, D. Y., and Alberini, C. M. (2014). The effect of insulin and insulin-like growth factors on hippocampus- and amygdala-dependent long-term memory formation. *Learn. Mem.* 21, 556–563. doi: 10.1101/lm.0293 48.112

Stöhr, O., Schilbach, K., Moll, L., Hettich, M. M., Freude, S., Wunderlich, F. T., et al. (2013). Insulin receptor signaling mediates APP processing and β-amyloid accumulation without altering survival in a transgenic mouse model of Alzheimer's disease. *Age* 35, 83–101. doi: 10.1007/s11357-011-9333-2

Stranahan, A. M., Arumugam, T. V., Cutler, R. G., Lee, K., Egan, J. M., and Mattson, M. P. (2008). Diabetes impairs hippocampal function through glucocorticoid-mediated effects on new and mature neurons. *Nat. Neurosci.* 11, 309–317. doi: 10.1038/nn2055

Strittmatter, W. J., Saunders, A. M., Schmechel, D., Pericak-Vance, M., Enghild, J., Salvesen, G. S., et al. (1993). Apolipoprotein E: high-avidity binding to beta-amyloid and increased frequency of type 4 allele in late-onset familial Alzheimer disease. *Proc. Natl. Acad. Sci. U.S.A.* 90, 1977–1981.

Talbot, K., Wang, H.-Y., Kazi, H., Han, L.-Y., Bakshi, K. P., Stucky, A., et al. (2012). Demonstrated brain insulin resistance in Alzheimer's disease patients is associated with IGF-1 resistance, IRS-1 dysregulation, and cognitive decline. *J. Clin. Invest.* 122, 1316–1338. doi: 10.1172/JCI59903

Thambisetty, M., Metter, E. J., Yang, A., Dolan, H., Marano, C., Zonderman, A. B., et al. (2013). Glucose intolerance, insulin resistance, and pathological features of alzheimer disease in the baltimore longitudinal study of aging. *JAMA Neurol.* 70 1167–1172. doi: 10.1001/jamaneurol.2013.284

Thienel, M., Wilhelm, I., Benedict, C., Born, J., and Hallschmid, M. (2017). Intranasal insulin decreases circulating cortisol concentrations during early sleep in elderly humans. *Neurobiol. Aging* 54, 170–174. doi: 10.1016/j.neurobiolaging.2017.03.006

van der Harg, J. M., Eggels, L., Bangel, F. N., Ruigrok, S. R., Zwart, R., Hoozemans, J. J. M., et al. (2017). Insulin deficiency results in reversible protein kinase A activation and tau phosphorylation. *Neurobiol. Dis.* 103, 163–173. doi: 10.1016/j.nbd.2017.04.005

Vandal, M., White, P. J., Tremblay, C., St-Amour, I., Chevrier, G., Emond, V., et al. (2014). Insulin reverses the high-fat diet-induced increase in brain a and improves memory in an animal model of Alzheimer disease. *Diabetes* 63, 4291–4301. doi: 10.2337/db14-0375

Velazquez, R., Tran, A., Ishimwe, E., Denner, L., Dave, N., Oddo, S., et al. (2017). Central insulin dysregulation and energy dyshomeostasis in two mouse models of Alzheimer's disease. *Neurobiol. Aging* 58, 1–13. doi: 10.1016/j.neurobiolaging.2017.06.003

Wang, X., Zheng, W., Xie, J.-W., Wang, T., Wang, S.-L., Teng, W.-P., et al. (2010). Insulin deficiency exacerbates cerebral amyloidosis and behavioral deficits in an Alzheimer transgenic mouse model. *Mol. Neurodegener.* 5:46. doi: 10.1186/1750-1326-5-46

Wang, Y., and Mandelkow, E. (2016). Tau in physiology and pathology. *Nat. Rev. Neurosci.* 17, 5–21. doi: 10.1038/nrn.2015.1

Watson, J. M., Sherwin, R. S., Deary, I. J., Scott, L., and Kerr, D. (2003). Dissociation of augmented physiological, hormonal and cognitive responses to hypoglycaemia with sustained caffeine use. *Clin. Sci.* 104, 447–454. doi: 10.1042/cs1040447

Willette, A. A., Johnson, S. C., Birdsill, A. C., Sager, M. A., Christian, B., Baker, L. D., et al. (2015). Insulin resistance predicts brain amyloid deposition in late middle-aged adults. *Alzheimers Dement.* 11, 504.e1–510.e1. doi: 10.1016/j.jalz.2014.03.011

Winocur, G., Greenwood, C. E., Piroli, G. G., Grillo, C., a, Reznikov, L. R., Reagan, L. P., et al. (2005). Memory impairment in obese Zucker rats: an investigation of cognitive function in an animal model of insulin resistance and obesity. *Behav. Neurosci.* 119, 1389–1395. doi: 10.1037/0735-7044.119.5.1389

Wischik, C. M., Novak, M., Thøgersen, H. C., Edwards, P. C., Runswick, M. J., Jakes, R., et al. (1988). Isolation of a fragment of tau derived from the core of the paired helical filament of Alzheimer disease. *Proc. Natl. Acad. Sci. U.S.A.* 85, 4506–4510.

Woods, S. C., Lotter, E. C., McKay, L. D., and Porte, D. (1979). Chronic intracerebroventricular infusion of insulin reduces food intake and body weight of baboons. *Nature* 282, 503–505.

Xie, L., Kang, H., Xu, Q., Chen, M. J., Liao, Y., Thiyagarajan, M., et al. (2013). Sleep drives metabolite clearance from the adult brain. *Science* 342, 373–377. doi: 10.1126/science.1241224

Yarchoan, M., and Arnold, S. E. (2014). Repurposing diabetes drugs for brain insulin resistance in Alzheimer disease. *Diabetes* 63, 2253–2261. doi: 10.2337/db14-0287

Yarchoan, M., Toledo, J. B., Lee, E. B., Arvanitakis, Z., Kazi, H., Han, L.-Y., et al. (2014). Abnormal serine phosphorylation of insulin receptor substrate 1 is associated with tau pathology in Alzheimer's disease and tauopathies. *Acta Neuropathol.* 128, 679–689. doi: 10.1007/s00401-014-1328-5

Zhang, H., Hao, Y., Manor, B., Novak, P., Milberg, W., Zhang, J., et al. (2015). Intranasal insulin enhanced resting-state functional connectivity of hippocampal regions in type 2 diabetes. *Diabetes* 64, 1025–1034. doi: 10.2337/db14-1000

Zhang, J., Chen, C., Hua, S., Liao, H., Wang, M., Xiong, Y., et al. (2017). An updated meta-analysis of cohort studies: diabetes and risk of Alzheimer's disease. *Diabetes Res. Clin. Pract.* 124, 41–47. doi: 10.1016/j.diabres.2016.10.024

Permissions

All chapters in this book were first published by Frontiers; hereby published with permission under the Creative Commons Attribution License or equivalent. Every chapter published in this book has been scrutinized by our experts. Their significance has been extensively debated. The topics covered herein carry significant findings which will fuel the growth of the discipline. They may even be implemented as practical applications or may be referred to as a beginning point for another development.

The contributors of this book come from diverse backgrounds, making this book a truly international effort. This book will bring forth new frontiers with its revolutionizing research information and detailed analysis of the nascent developments around the world.

We would like to thank all the contributing authors for lending their expertise to make the book truly unique. They have played a crucial role in the development of this book. Without their invaluable contributions this book wouldn't have been possible. They have made vital efforts to compile up to date information on the varied aspects of this subject to make this book a valuable addition to the collection of many professionals and students.

This book was conceptualized with the vision of imparting up-to-date information and advanced data in this field. To ensure the same, a matchless editorial board was set up. Every individual on the board went through rigorous rounds of assessment to prove their worth. After which they invested a large part of their time researching and compiling the most relevant data for our readers.

The editorial board has been involved in producing this book since its inception. They have spent rigorous hours researching and exploring the diverse topics which have resulted in the successful publishing of this book. They have passed on their knowledge of decades through this book. To expedite this challenging task, the publisher supported the team at every step. A small team of assistant editors was also appointed to further simplify the editing procedure and attain best results for the readers.

Apart from the editorial board, the designing team has also invested a significant amount of their time in understanding the subject and creating the most relevant covers. They scrutinized every image to scout for the most suitable representation of the subject and create an appropriate cover for the book.

The publishing team has been an ardent support to the editorial, designing and production team. Their endless efforts to recruit the best for this project, has resulted in the accomplishment of this book. They are a veteran in the field of academics and their pool of knowledge is as vast as their experience in printing. Their expertise and guidance has proved useful at every step. Their uncompromising quality standards have made this book an exceptional effort. Their encouragement from time to time has been an inspiration for everyone.

The publisher and the editorial board hope that this book will prove to be a valuable piece of knowledge for researchers, students, practitioners and scholars across the globe.

List of Contributors

Daria Laptinskaya and Iris-Tatjana Kolassa
Clinical and Biological Psychology, Institute of Psychology and Education, Ulm, University, Ulm, Germany
Department of Psychology, University of Konstanz, Konstanz, Germany

Franka Thurm
Department of Psychology, University of Konstanz, Konstanz, Germany
Faculty of Psychology, TU Dresden, Dresden, Germany

Christine A. F. von Arnim
Department of Neurology, Ulm University, Ulm, Germany

Olivia C. Küster and Patrick Fissler
Clinical and Biological Psychology, Institute of Psychology and Education, Ulm University, Ulm, Germany
Department of Neurology, Ulm University, Ulm, Germany

Winfried Schlee
Department for Psychiatry and Psychotherapy, University Hospital Regensburg, Regensburg, Germany

Stephan Kolassa
SAP (Switzerland) AG, Tägerwilen, Switzerland

Shreyasi Chatterjee and Amritpal Mudher
Centre of Biological Sciences, University of Southampton, Southampton, United Kingdom

Mudsser Azam and Qazi Mohd Rizwanul Haq
Department of Biosciences, Jamia Millia Islamia, New Delhi, India

Arif Tasleem Jan, Safikur Rahman, Angham M. S. Almigeiti, Duk Hwan Choi, Eun Ju Lee and Inho Choi
Department of Medical Biotechnology, Yeungnam University, Gyeongsan, South Korea

Mudsser Azam and Qazi Mohd Rizwanul Haq
Department of Biosciences, Jamia Millia Islamia, New Delhi, India

Md. Sahab Uddin and Abdullah Al Mamun
Department of Pharmacy, Southeast University, Dhaka, Bangladesh

Anna Stachowiak
Department of Experimental Embryology, Institute of Genetics and Animal Breeding, Polish Academy of Sciences, Magdalenka, Poland

Nikolay T. Tzvetkov
Department of Molecular Biology and Biochemical Pharmacology, Institute of Molecular Biology "Roumen Tsanev", Bulgarian Academy of Sciences, Sofia, Bulgaria

Shinya Takeda
Department of Clinical Psychology, Tottori University Graduate School of Medical Sciences, Tottori, Japan

Adrian M. Stankiewicz
Department of Molecular Biology, Institute of Genetics and Animal Breeding, Polish Academy of Sciences, Magdalenka, Poland
Institute of Genetics and Animal Breeding of the Polish Academy of Sciences, Jastrzebiec, Poland

Atanas G. Atanasov
Department of Molecular Biology, Institute of Genetics and Animal Breeding, Polish Academy of Sciences, Magdalenka, Poland
Department of Pharmacognosy, University of Vienna, Vienna, Austria

Leandro B. Bergantin
Department of Pharmacology, Federal University of São Paulo, São Paulo, Brazil

Mohamed M. Abdel-Daim
Department of Pharmacology, Suez Canal University, Ismailia, Egypt
Department of Ophthalmology and Micro-technology, Yokohama City University, Yokohama, Japan

Shreedarshanee Devi, Rashmi Yadav, Pratibha Chanana and Ranjana Arya
School of Biotechnology, Jawaharlal Nehru University, New Delhi, India

Jian Bao, Yacoubou A. R. Mahaman and Rong Liu
Key Laboratory of Ministry of Education of China for Neurological Disorders,
Department of Pathophysiology, School of Basic Medicine and the Collaborative Innovation Center for Brain Science, Tongji Medical College, Huazhong University of Science and Technology, Wuhan, China

Jian-Zhi Wang and Xiaochuan Wang
Key Laboratory of Ministry of Education of China for Neurological Disorders, Department of Pathophysiology, School of Basic Medicine and the Collaborative Innovation Center for Brain Science, Tongji Medical College, Huazhong University of Science and Technology, Wuhan, China
Co-innovation Center of Neuroregeneration, Nantong University, Nantong, China

Zhiguo Zhang
School of Medicine and Health Management, Tongji Medical College, Huazhong University of Science and Technology, Wuhan, China

Bin Zhang
Department of Genetics and Genomic Sciences, Icahn School of Medicine at Mount Sinai, New York, NY, United States

Anna Brzecka
Department of Pulmonology and Lung Cancer, Wroclaw Medical University, Wroclaw, Poland

Jerzy Leszek
Department of Psychiatry, Wroclaw Medical University, Wroclaw, Poland

Ghulam Md Ashraf
King Fahd Medical Research Center, King Abdulaziz University, Jeddah, Saudi Arabia

Maria Ejma
Department of Neurology, Wroclaw Medical University, Wroclaw, Poland

Marco F. Ávila-Rodriguez
Facultad de Ciencias de la Salud, Universidad del Tolima, Ibagué, Colombia

Anna N. Samsonova
Institute of Physiologically Active Compounds of the Russian Academy of Sciences, Chernogolovka, Russia

Nagendra S. Yarla
Department of Biochemistry and Bioinformatics, School of Life Sciences, Institute of Science, Gandhi Institute of Technology and Management University, Visakhapatnam, India

Vadim V. Tarasov and Vladimir N. Chubarev
Institute for Pharmaceutical Science and Translational Medicine, Sechenov First Moscow State Medical University, Moscow, Russia

George E. Barreto
Departamento de Nutrición y Bioquímica, Facultad de Ciencias, Pontificia Universidad Javeriana, Bogotá, Colombia
Instituto de Ciencias Biomédicas, Universidad Autónoma de Chile, Santiago, Chile

Gjumrakch Aliev
Institute of Physiologically Active Compounds of the Russian Academy of Sciences, Chernogolovka, Russia
GALLY International Biomedical Research and Consulting LLC, San Antonio, TX, United States
School of Health Science and Healthcare Administration, University of Atlanta, Johns Creek, GA, United States

Manuel Menendez-Gonzalez
Servicio de Neurologia, Hospital Universitario Central de Asturias, Oviedo, Spain Department of Cellular Morphology and Biology, University of Oviedo, Oviedo, Spain Instituto de Investigacion Sanitaria del Principado de Asturias, Oviedo, Spain

Huber S. Padilla-Zambrano
Centro de Investigaciones Biomedicas (CIB), University of Cartagena, Cartagena, Colombia

Gabriel Alvarez
HealthSens, S.L., Oviedo, Spain

Estibaliz Capetillo-Zarate
Departamento de Neurociencias, Universidad del Pais Vasco (UPV/EHU), Leioa, Spain El Centro de Investigación Biomédica en Red sobre Enfermedades Neurodegenerativas, Madrid, Spain
Achucarro Basque Center for Neuroscience, Leioa, Spain
Ikerbasque, Basque Foundation for Science, Bilbao, Spain

Cristina Tomas-Zapico
Instituto de Investigacion Sanitaria del Principado de Asturias, Oviedo, Spain
Department of Functional Biology, University of Oviedo, Oviedo, Spain

Agustin Costa
Department of Physical and Analytical Chemistry, University of Oviedo, Oviedo, Spain

Yang Xin
Department of Pharmacy, The Fifth Affiliated Hospital of Guangzhou Medical University, Guangzhou, China
Fifth Clinical School of Guangzhou Medical University, Guangzhou, China

Liu Ting and Hu Guoyan
Fifth Clinical School of Guangzhou Medical University, Guangzhou, China

Chen Diling, Yang Jian, Tang Xiaocu, Shuai Ou, Zheng Chaoqun and Xie Yizhen
State Key Laboratory of Applied Microbiology Southern China, Guangdong Provincial Key Laboratory of Microbial Culture Collection and Application, Guangdong Open Laboratory of Applied Microbiology, Guangdong Institute of Microbiology, Guangzhou, China

Liang Hualun
Department of Pharmacy, The Second Clinical Medical College of Guangzhou University of Chinese Medicine, Guangzhou, China

Lai Guoxiao
State Key Laboratory of Applied Microbiology Southern China, Guangdong Provincial Key Laboratory of Microbial Culture Collection and Application, Guangdong Open Laboratory of Applied Microbiology, Guangdong Institute of Microbiology, Guangzhou, China
College of Pharmacy, Guangxi University of Traditional Chinese Medicine, Nanning, China

Zhao Jun
Department of Obstetrics, Guangdong Women and Children Hospital, Guangzhou, China

Devesh Tewari and Archana N. Sah
Department of Pharmaceutical Sciences, Faculty of Technology, Kumaun University, Nainital, India

Lukasz Huminiecki and Jarosław O. Horbańczuk
Institute of Genetics and Animal Breeding of the Polish Academy of Sciences, Jastrzebiec, Poland

Andrei Mocan
Department of Pharmaceutical Botany, Iuliu Hat,ieganu University of Medicine and Pharmacy, Cluj Napoca, Romania
ICHAT and Institute for Life Sciences, University of Agricultural Sciences and Veterinary Medicine, Cluj-Napoca, Romania

Atanas G. Atanasov
Institute of Genetics and Animal Breeding of the Polish Academy of Sciences, Jastrzebiec, Poland
Department of Pharmacognosy, University of Vienna, Vienna, Austria

Guilin Meng
Shanghai Tenth People's Hospital, Tongji University School of Medicine, Shanghai, China
School of Computer Science and Informatics, Indiana University, Bloomington, IN, United States

Aiping Jin, Yanxin Zhao and Xueyuan Liu
Shanghai Tenth People's Hospital, Tongji University School of Medicine, Shanghai, China

Xiaoye Ma
Shanghai Tenth People's Hospital, Tongji University School of Medicine, Shanghai, China

Xiulin Meng
Houma People's Hospital, Linfen, China

Gengping Zhang
Library of Tongji University, Shanghai, China

Xiaolin Hu
School of Life Sciences, Tsinghua University, Beijing, China

Weicong Ren
Department of Psychology, Hebei Normal University, Shijiazhuang, China
Key Laboratory of Brain Aging and Cognitive Neuroscience of Hebei Province, Hebei Medical University, Shijiazhuang, China
Center on Aging Psychology, Key Laboratory of Mental Health, Institute of Psychology, Chinese Academy of Sciences, Beijing, China

Zhijie Zhang
Department of Psychology, Hebei Normal University, Shijiazhuang, China
Key Laboratory of Brain Aging and Cognitive Neuroscience of Hebei Province, Hebei Medical University, Shijiazhuang, China

Juan Li
Center on Aging Psychology, Key Laboratory of Mental Health, Institute of Psychology, Chinese Academy of Sciences, Beijing, China

Jiang Ma
Department of Rehabilitation, First Hospital of Shijiazhuang, Shijiazhuang, China

Mingwei Wang
Key Laboratory of Brain Aging and Cognitive Neuroscience of Hebei Province, Hebei Medical University, Shijiazhuang, China
Department of Neurology, First Hospital of Hebei Medical University, Shijiazhuang, China

Safikur Rahman
Department of Medical Biotechnology, Yeungnam University, Gyeongsan, South Korea

Ayyagari Archana
Department of Microbiology, Swami Shraddhanand College, University of Delhi, New Delhi, India

Arif Tasleem Jan
School of Biosciences and Biotechnology, Baba Ghulam Shah Badshah University, Rajouri, India

Rinki Minakshi
Institute of Home Economics, University of Delhi, New Delhi, India

Jiao Liu, Guohua Zheng, Jinsong Wu and Kun Hu
College of Rehabilitation Medicine, Fujian University of Traditional Chinese Medicine, Fuzhou, China

Lidian Chen and Weilin Liu
College of Rehabilitation Medicine, Fujian University of Traditional Chinese Medicine, Fuzhou, China
Fujian Key Laboratory of Rehabilitation Technology, Fujian University of Traditional Chinese Medicine, Fuzhou, China

Jing Tao
College of Rehabilitation Medicine, Fujian University of Traditional Chinese Medicine, Fuzhou, China
Fujian Key Laboratory of Rehabilitation Technology, Fujian University of Traditional Chinese Medicine, Fuzhou, China
Department of Psychiatry, Massachusetts General Hospital and Harvard Medical School, Charlestown, MA, United States

Jian Kong and Natalia Egorova
Department of Psychiatry, Massachusetts General Hospital and Harvard Medical School, Charlestown, MA, United States

Zengjian Wang
Department of Psychiatry, Massachusetts General Hospital and Harvard Medical School, Charlestown, MA, United State
Developmental and Educational Psychology, South China Normal University, Guangzhou, China

Xiangli Chen
Department of Rehabilitation Psychology and Special Education, University of Wisconsin-Madison, Madison, WI, United States

Xiehua Xue and Ming Li
Affiliated Rehabilitation Hospital, Fujian University of Traditional Chinese Medicine, Fuzhou, China

Xiuling Nie and Suiren Wan
State Key laboratory of Bioelectronics, School of Biological Sciences and Medical Engineering, Southeast University, Nanjing, China

Yu Sun
State Key laboratory of Bioelectronics, School of Biological Sciences and Medical Engineering, Southeast University, Nanjing, China
Institute of Cancer and Genetic Science, University of Birmingham, Birmingham, United Kingdom

Hui Zhao and Yun Xu
Department of Neurology, Affiliated Drum Tower Hospital of Nanjing University Medical School, Nanjing, China

Renyuan Liu, Xueping Li, Sichu Wu, Zhao Qing and Bing Zhang
Department of Radiology, Affiliated Drum Tower Hospital of Nanjing University Medical School, Nanjing, China

Zuzana Nedels and Jakub Hort
Department of Neurology, Memory Clinic, 2nd Faculty of Medicine, Charles University in Prague, Motol University Hospital, Prague, Czechia
International Clinical Research Center, St. Anne's University Hospital Brno, Brno, Czech Republic

Elena A. Kosenko, Lyudmila A. Tikhonova and Yury G. Kaminsky
Institute of Theoretical and Experimental Biophysics, Russian Academy of Sciences, Pushchino, Russia

Carmina Montoliu
Fundación Investigación Hospital Clínico, INCLIVA Instituto Investigación Sanitaria, Valencia, Spain

George E. Barreto
Departamento de Nutrición y Bioquímica, Facultad de Ciencias, Pontificia Universidad Javeriana, Bogotá, Colombia
Instituto de Ciencias Biomédicas, Universidad Autónoma de Chile, Santiago, Chile

Gjumrakch Aliev
GALLY International Biomedical Research Institute Inc., San Antonio, TX, United States

Christian Benedict
Department of Neuroscience, Uppsala University, Uppsala, Sweden

Claudia A. Grillo
Department of Pharmacology, Physiology and Neuroscience, University of South Carolina-School of Medicine, Columbia, SC, United States

Index

Printed in the USA
CPSIA information can be obtained
at www.ICGtesting.com
JSHW051626061123
51533JS00005B/124